DEVELOPMENT OF VERTEBRATE ANATOMY

DEVELOPMENT OF VERTEBRATE ANATOMY

JOY B. PHILLIPS

Department of Zoology
Drew University
Madison, New Jersey

WITH 470 ILLUSTRATIONS

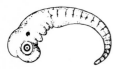
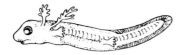
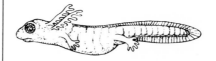

Saint Louis
THE C. V. MOSBY COMPANY
1975

Library of Congress Cataloging in Publication Data

Phillips, Joy B   1917-
    Development of vertebrate anatomy.

    1. Morphogenesis. 2. Morphology (Animals).
3. Vertebrates—Anatomy. I. Title. [DNLM:
1. Vertebrates—Embryology. QL959 P561d]
QL799.P47   596'.04   74-14876
ISBN 0-8016-3927-1

CB/CB/B 9 8 7 6 5 4 3 2 1

PREFACE

Biological knowledge has undergone a spectacular growth during the twentieth century. However, undergraduate students have only a limited amount of time in which to assimilate basic biological principles from this vast array of information. The pressures of contemporary science and society demand that their courses contain an introduction to molecular biology, to environmental science, and to life at the organismic level. Therefore those responsible for guiding undergraduates through their early training and exposing them to up-to-date biological knowledge are forced to reevaluate their curriculum and to condense, combine, or eliminate certain aspects of biological information traditionally included.

Anatomy and embryology are merely facets of the general topic of morphology. Each adds to the understanding of the other, since the adult is only one stage in the development of the individual. It is logical, therefore, to combine the two approaches in a study of the processes involved in the development of adult vertebrates. The formation of this body structure is known as morphogenesis and is the subject of this text.

The book examines those developmental processes that lead to the establishment of the primitive embryonic form of vertebrates. It focuses on the similar, but not identical, patterns of development that give rise to the gametes, zygote, blastula, gastrula, neurula, and generalized body organization. During later stages of development the unique characteristics of the specific animal are established and the definitive body form of the adult makes its appearance. This basic plan of adult structure evident in vertebrates, although sometimes obscured by adaptive modifications, is presented in detail.

The book is divided into three main sections. The last section is arranged according to germ layer derivation of the various systems and emphasizes the similarity of developmental patterns among vertebrate classes. Despite the great diversity of animal form, *Development of Vertebrate Anatomy* tries to make the student aware of common morphological themes. It is these themes that strengthen the probability of a common ancestry for all vertebrates.

A special word of acknowledgment should go to Michael Carpenter for his patience and skill in producing the fine illustrations for this book.

JOY B. PHILLIPS

CONTENTS

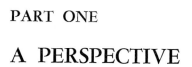

PART ONE

A PERSPECTIVE

CHAPTER 1

INTRODUCTION

The aim of this book is to acquaint the student with the structural composition, the *morphology*, of the chordates. Although all chordates are considered, we are specifically interested in the architecture of those animals classified as belonging to the subphylum *Vertebrata*. Common morphologic themes run throughout vertebrate history despite the great diversity of animal form, function, development and habitat. A blue whale is over 100 feet long and a mouse only a few inches, yet they share many characteristics. The streamlined cyclostomes at one end of the vertebrate scale and the mammalian tetrapods at the other have a common body plan. The bones composing the foreleg of the frog are similar to those of the cat. All vertebrate embryos have gill slits at some stage of their development. These common characteristics, held by the many diverse forms of vertebrate life, occur not by chance but, it is believed, because they all descended from a common ancestor. The concept of *evolution* explains this relatedness.

Vertebrate structure can be studied by several methods and at various levels of organization. Two comparative approaches (comparative anatomy and comparative embryology) focus at the levels of cells, organs, and systems. The comparative anatomist examines adult structure. He tries to draw relationships based on fossil evidence (paleontology), similarity of origin and structure of two organs in different species of animals (homologies), and the resemblances that exist in present-day vertebrates. The comparative embryologist is interested in studying the embryonic origin of vertebrate structure. He seeks basic developmental plans and compares the deviations from this plan that occur in the various classes. Embryonic patterns tend to be conservative. That is, once a successful pathway for organ formation is established in the embryo, those developmental processes are apparently selected and maintained even as animals evolve into higher forms. It is not surprising, then, that this basic uniformity of developmental processes in vertebrates should lead to a uniformity of adult structure.

Comparative anatomy and comparative embryology are different facets of the general topic of morphology. Each adds to the understanding of

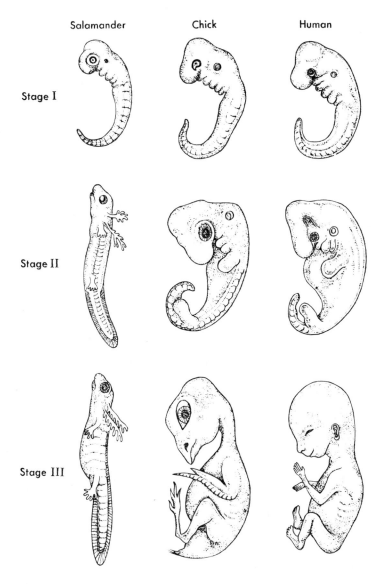

Fig. 1-1
Comparable stages in the development of three vertebrates. Similar basic processes during formative stages bring about embryonic forms resembling one another (stage I). By stage III, unique characteristics of the specific vertebrates are established. (From Turney, T.: Introduction to biology, St. Louis, 1973, The C. V. Mosby Co.)

the other, since the adult is only one stage in the development of the individual. It is logical, therefore, to combine the two approaches in a study of the processes involved in the development of adult vertebrate body form. The development of this body form is known as *morphogenesis* and is the subject of this text.

The structures of every embryo and every adult animal living today reflect a history of hundreds of millions of years. The evolution of these organs plays an important role in both anatomy and embryology. It is not the object of this book to trace these lines of descent; this is a part of the subject matter of evolution. However, in examining the basic forms of vertebrates, we have not been blind to the matter of descent as we accumulate evidence that points to close relationships between groups of animals. This relationship is also expressed in the similarity of developmental patterns. We shall find in vertebrates a common, basic pattern in the sequence of developmental steps leading to the construction of the adult body. This basic design of both embryo and adult strengthens the probability of a common ancestry for all vertebrates.

The organ system of an embryonic vertebrate resembles in its formative stages the same organ system in a different vertebrate embryo. Fig. 1-1 shows some common embryonic forms. In some cases they are difficult to distinguish. During later stages of development, the animal establishes its unique characteristics and the definitive body form of the adult makes its appearance. During the early part of the nineteenth century, Karl Ernst von Baer recognized the tendency of vertebrates to follow common developmental procedures and described his observations of the unfolding of vertebrate structure in a series of steps that have become known as von Baer's laws. We shall refer to von Baer again later in the text.

The object of this book is to examine those developmental processes that lead to the establishment of the primitive embryonic form of vertebrates. We will concentrate on the similar, but not identical, plans of development that give rise to the blastula, gastrula, neurula, and generalized body organization. The basic plan of adult structure evident in vertebrates, although sometimes obscured by adaptive modifications, is presented in detail.

By the very nature of their approach comparative anatomists and comparative embryologists emphasize the differences among animals. However, this book is an attempt to combine the two approaches, to present a unifying picture of vertebrate structure. We shall stress the *similarities* that exist among vertebrates and mention differences when groups of animals deviate from this common plan.

MORPHOGENESIS
Preformation and epigenesis

Long before there was such a thing as the modern sciences of embryology, or genetics, or a theory of evolution, biologists tried to explain how an egg can give rise to a complex, highly organized adult and why offspring resemble their parents. Hippocrates studied the development of the hen's egg and Aristotle was interested in the embryology of many animals. As long ago as 1651, Harvey, who did not possess a microscope and had not seen a mammalian egg, theorized about the developmental process. He said, "All animals, even those that produce their young alive, including man himself, are evolved out of an egg." He described the organs of the higher animals as successively forming out of the materials of the egg, each part forming anew. This process of progressive unfolding, *epigenesis*, is the oldest theory attempting to explain development, and was supported and promoted by Aristotle. Some form of this concept can be traced back to at least the twelfth century B.C. It was the beginning of an attempt to explain biological phenomena previously assumed to arise spontaneously and by divine direction.

Jan Swammerdam (1637) is credited with popularizing the *preformation theory*, although it too had been suggested by Aristotle. Swammerdam believed that the embryo developed from previously created parts, rather than from a series of new formations. According to him, all the characteristics of the adult were present in miniature and needed only the proper environment to develop. The preformation theory appealed to biologists of the day, and they soon became divided into two rival schools, the ovists and the animalculists (spermatists). Each believed the egg or sperm to contain the actual embryo. With the aid of the newly invented microscope, and their imaginations, entire figures complete with arms and legs, were seen coiled within the sperm or egg. Fig. 1-2 illustrates one artist's conception of the "homunculus," or little man.

The sperm seemed superfluous to the ovists and was often considered to be a parasite swimming in the semen. The animalculists, on the other hand, considered the egg merely a source of nutritional material for the embryo within the sperm. The ovists finally won the argument when it was realized that certain insects developed parthenogenetically (from unfertilized eggs). Since each adult generation contained the eggs of the next, and that one, the eggs of

the next, etc., there soon evolved the ridiculous picture of an infinite number of individuals contained within the egg. The *encasement theory* was a logical extension of the preformist position.

The belief that all organs were ready-formed in the egg or sperm at first stifled the curiosity of the eighteenth-century anatomists. There were no new ideas until 1759 when C. F. Wolff began his careful and systematic study of developing chick embryos and their eggs. The ova contained no adult, only a homogeneous, unstructured mass. Wolff demonstrated that the organs of the chick embryo were not present in the egg in the beginning, but gradually formed out of the unorganized egg as development continued. The epigenetic theory again gained prominence.

The preformists and epigenesists laid the foundation for our present interpretation of development, and the rise of molecular biology added another dimension. Since those early days, we have gained a concept of the gene and an insight into its role in developmental and evolutionary processes. The improved light microscope and the electron microscope reveal much about the structure of cells, and refined chemical techniques permit the analysis of physiological processes. However, as with so many historical concepts, when expressed in modern terminology, one is surprised at some of the lasting insights offered by these eighteenth-century anatomists.

Both these concepts (epigenesis and preformation) have something to offer our modern interpretation of development. However, they appear to function in a complementary rather than a mutually exclusive way. We now know that the genes are handed down from generation to generation and that they have directive influences. These *preformed elements* guide the maturation of the egg and sperm as well as the development of the future organism. The genes, with their coded information, interact during development with a *progressively changing* (epigenetic) *microenvironment*. Many of the characteristics of the adult are not represented at all in the zygote, but they unfold at various times during development according to the instructions packaged in the genes. Normal development results from a

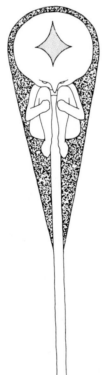

Fig. 1-2
The early animalculist (spermatist) believed that each sperm contained a curled figure of the little man or "homunculus." Complete in body form, including arms and legs, he waited for the opportunity to be released and to grow.

succession of organized, sequential steps that transform the fertilized egg into a new adult state. It is the *interaction between preformed and epigenetic influences that is responsible for the development of the new individual.* These processes are collectively called "morphogenesis."

Morphogenetic processes

Common developmental processes lead to the formation of adult vertebrate organs. Although they are discussed in detail later in the text, we now summarize these formative procedures to give a perspective of the events to follow. Similar mechanisms occur in both the shark embryo and in the embryo of man, as well as in all organisms in between. They are programmed from the beginning (preformed) and follow a set of instructions encoded in the nucleus of the fertilized egg. Fig. 1-3 presents in diagrammatic form a summary of these events, further expanded as follows:

1. All vertebrates reproduce sexually and form when special generative cells, the gametes (eggs and sperm), fuse and give rise to a zygote *(fertilization).* The gametes represent a physical link with the previous generation and manifest a continuity between successive generations. "Development" actually begins before fertilization, since the initiation of both cytoplasmic and nuclear maturation of these generative cells occurs before they are released from the gonads. These cells differ from other body cells in that they undergo a special type of mitosis (meiosis) that reduces the chromosome number to half (haploid number). As a result of fertilization, the chromosomes of the zygote are returned to the normal diploid number for the particular species.

2. The fertilized egg divides (cleaves) into many smaller cells (blastomeres) until it reaches a *blastula stage.* During cleavage various areas of the cytoplasm become bound by new cell membranes isolating them from one another. At each division, there is genetic replication and each blastomere contains the same genetic information as its parent. However, since the cytoplasm in the egg is not homogeneous, each cleavage plane may divide the cytoplasm into two unlike cells. The cytoplasmic environment in which a particular set of genes finds itself may not be identical to the environment of the parent genes.

3. The materials composing the egg are sorted out and rearranged as the cytoplasm is packaged in the many dozens of blastomeres. The cells (or groups of cells) composing the blastula move by various types of *morphogenetic movements* into new spatial relationships with one another, giving rise to the gastrula stage. The cells establish themselves in layers. Embryologists distinguish three *germ layers: ectoderm, endoderm,* and *mesoderm.*

4. The cells of these layers interact and influence one another *(induction)* in a manner controlled by their genetic makeup. As development continues, there is a progressive increase in the interrelationship and interdependence among cells. Some are destined to form certain structures as far back as the egg, when their protoplasm lay unbound by cell membranes and continuous with the contents of the general egg "pool." Other cells usually become *determined,* that is, their destiny becomes set, when they interact in their new environment during the gastrula stage.

5. There is an increase in mass of the organism or its parts because of the increase in protoplasm. *Growth* includes synthesis as well as catabolism; energy consumption and storage; and excretion. In the formation of the blastomeres, cell divisions result in smaller cells; there is no increase in total protoplasm. However, in the later stages, newly formed cells return to the size of the parent cell through growth processes.

6. The gastrula elongates, and its layers arrange themselves according to a fundamental plan common to all vertebrates and inherent in all vertebrate genes. This basic design consists of six tubes of potentially active cells. There is a solid rod, the noto-

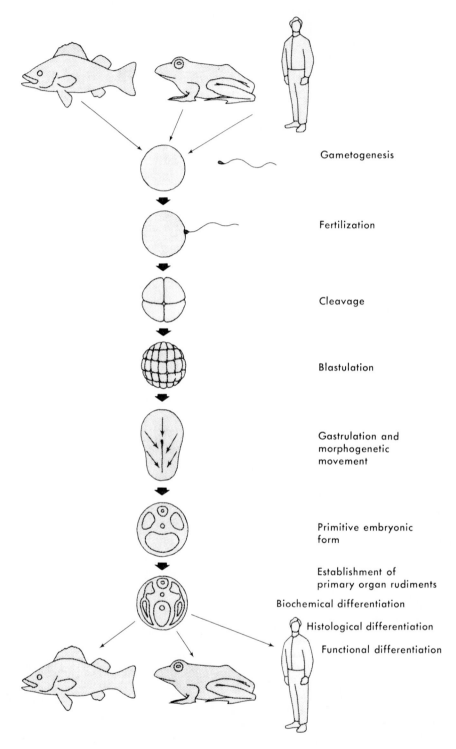

Gametogenesis

Fertilization

Cleavage

Blastulation

Gastrulation and
morphogenetic
movement

Primitive embryonic
form

Establishment of
primary organ rudiments

Biochemical differentiation

Histological differentiation

Functional differentiation

Fig. 1-3
Summary of the common developmental processes that lead to the formation of adult vertebrate organs. See text for discussion.

chord, running down the length of the body, a dorsally located neural tube, a ventrally placed gut tube, and a mesodermal tube on both sides. All of this is enclosed by a body tube. We refer to this stage as the *primitive embryonic form* of vertebrates. Refer to Fig. 1-3.

7. The various layers of the gastrula give rise to *primary organ rudiments*, sometimes referred to as *primordia*, or *anlagen*, (pronounced on'log'n), the forerunners of the future organs. The cells that compose these embryonic structures begin to diverge metabolically along different lines of development, initiating organogenesis. New unique systems of proteins appear that *differentiate* them chemically from their neighbors and from the cells of the past. Gene-cytoplasmic interaction brings about this process of differentiation.

8. *Histologic differentiation* follows biochemical differentiation, and groups of similar cells aggregate to form tissues. The tissues, in turn, join other tissues to form organs, and the organs combine with others to give rise to the various organ systems.

9. Organs, and the systems they compose, develop at different rates and at different times. The circulatory system is one of the first systems to arise. The nervous system also forms early, although a part of its development is completed after birth (postnatal development). When the numbers, and kinds of organs, their positions in the embryo, and their specific features are established, the *morphological plan* of the specific animal is revealed, and differences between the classes become apparent. For example, vascular gill slits, but no lungs, develop in shark embryos; gill slits develop in the mammalian embryo as well, but they are never vascular and are transitory structures.

10. Certain common functions are necessary for the continued existence of all animals. The organ systems interact to carry out these vital physiological needs. All vertebrates have a shape maintained by an endoskeleton, within which these processes occur. Food must be obtained from outside sources, broken down, and made available for growth, repair, and maintenance of the organism. A source of energy is one of the primary needs of the animal. It allows the animal to move about and the machinery of the body to operate. Energy conversions are basically chemical processes, and both food and oxygen must be conveyed to the cells where chemical reactions can take place. Some of the products of metabolism are toxic and must be removed. Finally, the animal must be able to reproduce.

Vertebrates evolved nine major organ systems that handle these physiologic needs. These systems can be categorized according to the germ layers from which they primarily originate. The *nervous* and *integumentary* systems arise from ectoderm; the *digestive* and *respiratory* systems develop from endoderm; and all other systems, *skeletal, muscular, circulatory,* and *urogenital systems,* develop from mesoderm. An exception is the coordinating *endocrine system* composed of glands derived from all three germ layers. Of course, most adult organs are composite structures, and contain cells derived from more than one germ layer.

Genetic control of development

When fertilization occurs, the two gametes bring to the zygote its genetic endowment, the genome. A zygote is a diploid cell (double set of chromosomes) from which the multicellular adult develops. Through thousands of successive cell divisions (mitosis) the nuclear contents of the one-celled zygote are faithfully replicated (duplicated) and transferred to daughter cells. In the vertebrates, this can result ultimately in an adult with a billion or more cells. Since the hereditary material of each cell is an exact copy of the original set of genetic information held in the nucleus of the zygote, all daughter cells are genetically identical to one another and to the parent cell from which they arose.

An analysis of this genetic material, carried by chromosomes, shows that three different chemical substances compose it: proteins, deoxyribonucleic acid (DNA), and ribonucleic acid (RNA). In higher organisms it is the DNA of the chromosomes that contains the genetic code and determines the phenotype (appearance) of the organism. *Genes,* specific areas or units of the DNA molecule, control these traits. The genes exist in alternative forms, known as *alleles,* and give rise to different versions of the same trait. Some genes have as many as 100 different alleles. The genes are distinct from one another and are arranged in a specific pattern along the chromosomes.

The genetic material in the nucleus contains a set of instructions that dictates what is to be synthesized during development. We are speaking primarily of proteins that have several functions. A large group of these proteins are enzymes that catalyze the chemical reactions occurring in the cells of the organism. Another type includes the structural proteins that are involved in setting up the basic structure of the cells and tissues (such as membranes); they influence the external and internal forms of the individual. A third type of protein is responsible for movement (such as muscle).

The coding of the DNA molecule determines the kind and linkage sequence of the available 20 amino acids (the building blocks of the protein molecule) and therefore the synthesis of the specific protein. A special kind of RNA, called messenger RNA, carries the genetic instructions from the nucleus to the cytoplasmic ribosomes where it is used as a template for protein synthesis.

The first proteins to form in the egg are probably the enzymes that will enable the egg to begin its synthetic activities. For example, in most animals, oocytes synthesize food reserves (yolk) and store them in the cytoplasm. This occurs while the egg is still in the ovary. Since enzymes are proteins, the DNA code in the oocyte nucleus describes the specific structures, and therefore properties, of these catalysts. It is the enzymes that determine the types of protein formed and where and how they will be formed. The appearance (phenotype) of the individual depends on the synthesis and ultimate distribution of proteins during morphogenesis.

MORPHOGENETIC PROBLEMS

Two large problems confront the student of morphology. One concerns *ontogeny,* the development of the individual, and the other, *phylogeny,* the evolution of groups of animals. The embryologist, concerned with ontogeny, considers the fundamental question to be: How do cells that are genetically identical to one another, give rise to cells that differ morphologically, physiologically, and biochemically? More specifically, how does one cell "know" how to become a liver cell and another, a muscle fiber?

This question is the topic of much embryologic research. It involves *differentiation,* a rather ambiguous term with several levels of interpretation. Incorporated into the definition of the word is the concept that some kind of progressive, orderly change is going on. It can refer to development as a whole; how an egg becomes a new individual. It can refer to how cells or parts of an organism differ from one another and from their parent cells. Or it can relate to the development of specific cell types. For example, in a muscle cell differentiation occurs at the biochemical level first, then histologic level, and finally functional level. The contractile element of a muscle cell differs from the synthetic machinery of the gland cell. These differences allow each cell to do a specific kind of work.

Differentiation obviously plays an important role in morphogenesis although other processes such as growth, morphogenetic movements, and metabolic activities are also involved. Presumably all the cells have identical genetic composition, resulting from the uniformity of mitotic divisions. However, each cell's inheritance, in some way, directs it along a specific developmental pathway that may differ from that of an adjacent cell. Since the coding sequence of DNA determines all the proteins that can be made, the cells contain the codes for all proteins. Therefore, if there is a need for a particular type of protein (type A, for example), the cell must have some mechanism by which it restricts or "turns off" the synthesizing processes it does not need and "turns on" those that it does need. For example, the cell does not synthesize messenger RNA specific for type B proteins (transcription). Since the ribosomes never receive the instructions for producing B protein, there is no synthesis of the specific B enzyme out in the cytoplasm. A developmental process, therefore, can proceed only along those pathways for which synthetic activities are available.

Differentiation cannot be explained on the basis of the sorting out of genetic material (since each cell contains the same genome). Rather, we shall have to turn to the microenvironment in which the genetic material finds itself. As noted earlier, the introduction of variety occurs among the cytoplasms of the daughter cells when the cleavage planes divide the heterogeneous eggplasm into small membrane-contained packages. These differences in the microenvironments in some way activate or inhibit the expression of the various genes. The distribution of identical nuclear compositions in A and B microenvironments causes the cell with A to start down one pathway and the cell with B cytoplasm to begin another. These A and B environments do not necessarily mean the presence of different kinds of molecules; they may differ merely in concentration (number of molecules) of some particular substance.

At the danger of oversimplification, perhaps at this time we can summarize the available data and briefly suggest a modern interpretation of differentiation. Cell differentiation results when the cell's inheritance interacts with its environment. Ontogeny is the sum total of the activities that go on between the time the egg is first formed and the final stages of development of the individual.

Anatomists are concerned with the problem of phylogeny and the diversity expressed among the different vertebrates that overlays their common characteristics. If all vertebrates are related to one another through common ancestry, how did modifications occur to the genetic makeup of these ancestral cells to give rise to the various classes of animals within the subphylum? How was diversity of structure imposed upon the unity that was provided by the chromosomes of the first hypothetical ancestor?

Phylogenetic changes require enormous expanses of time, as suggested by Fig. 1-4. When we discussed differentiation of the embryo, we talked about sequential changes that occurred in hours, days, or years. Now we refer

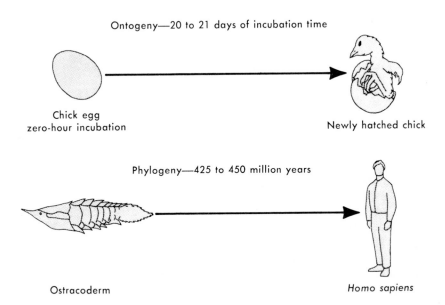

Ontogeny—20 to 21 days of incubation time

Chick egg
zero-hour incubation

Newly hatched chick

Phylogeny—425 to 450 million years

Ostracoderm

Homo sapiens

Fig. 1-4
Comparison of developmental and evolutionary times. Development of an embryo occurs in hours, days, or a year or two; evolutionary time involves millions of years. The fossils of the first vertebrates (ostracoderms) date back 500 million years. The oldest fossils of *Homo sapiens* are 100,000 years old.

to a concept of *evolutionary time*, a concept difficult to grasp. When we speak of the ancestral vertebrates, we refer to those animals that first appeared 500 million years ago! There is evidence that modern genera are at least a million years old. On the other hand the archiac mammals are relatively young, since their fossil record dates back only 150 million years. Paleontologists consider those changes rapid that occur in only 1 or 2 million years. Like our definition of embryonic development, the definition of organic evolution implies the development of specific characteristics by a sequence of changes from a simple to a more complex state. Since these alterations appear during the course of evolutionary time, they are, indeed, gradual.

The fossil record preserves some of the modifications that occurred. Scientists determine the age of these records by a process of dating based on the fact that radioactive elements decay at a constant rate. All living things contain a carbon isotope, carbon 14, that starts to decay when the individual is buried. For fossil records of 40,000 years old or less, carbon-14 decay determines the age of the fossil deposit. For older records, the decay of uranium 238 to form lead 206 acts as a radioactive clock.

Through these records of past forms of life, we have some idea as to when major groups of organisms appeared. However, the numerous fossils represent only a small portion of the organisms that existed in the past, and the information they offer is often biased. The formation of a fossil occurs when the animal is buried in some way. In general, it represents the aquatic vertebrates or those living near streams or ponds and not those existing in the mountains and highlands. The soft remains of most animals were quickly consumed by other organisms. Thus, a fossil consists mostly of preserved hard parts, such as bones and teeth. So we probably know more about *vertebrates* from these fossil records than about animals of other phyla. From these data, paleontologists deduce something about the shape of the animal, its posture, what it ate, and how it moved. The size of the skull relates to its intelligence. The bone scars tell us something about the attachment and size of muscles.

The changes that gradually occurred from ancestral to modern times culminated in the structure of the animals we see on earth today. During this time many forms became extinct, leaving gaps in what must have been a continuous line of successive stages. As a result, isolated groups of animals were established. A good fossil record, however, demonstrates the existence of many transitional forms in some of these groups. For example, the dog and bear families are considered related, but one has no difficulty in differentiating between them. However, 20 million years ago animals intermediate between the bear and dog existed with characteristics so common to both that they were difficult to categorize. It is because of the loss of these generalized intermediate forms that the dog and bear appear so distinctively different to us today and we are able to classify them as two separate families.

Because of the extinction of various intermediate forms, it is not always possible to see relationships between animals. In tracing *homologies* we seek to establish the basic pattern of an anatomical plan. The concept of homologies gained great importance in the latter part of the nineteenth century when the principles of evolution became the accepted mode of thought. Scientists presumed that the structure of any living group of animals had descended from a similar structure in a common ancestor.

The study of homologies usually applies to structural rather than physiological identities. Homologous structures need not resemble one another in shape, size, color, or function. Rather, the term "homologous" refers to structures that have been produced by similar developmental processes. The swim bladder of the fish and the lungs of the tetrapods are homologous structures, since both arose from a posterior pharyngeal pouch. Another often quoted example is that of the anterior pharyngeal pouch of the primitive fish that evolved into the spiracle of the shark and the eustachian tube and middle ear of man. Although each organ is adapted for a different function, their apparent evolution from a common ancestral gill pouch is a strong argument for a common evolutionary origin.

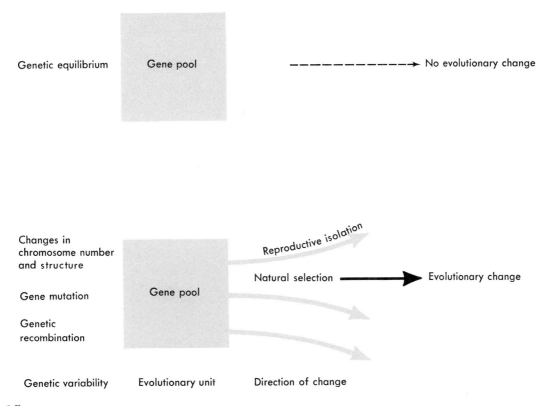

Fig. 1-5
Diagram to illustrate how interaction between genetic variability and the changing environment produces adaptive changes.

MODERN CONCEPT OF EVOLUTION

The raw materials of evolution are the genes and chromosomes. From an evolutionary standpoint, it is the population of pooled genes of all individuals within the population that is important. A population of individuals is an *evolutionary unit*. Each individual is, of course, genetically unique and rarely are two individuals within a population identical, since each member may possess a different allele for the same characteristic. It is possible to calculate the number of different alleles present in a population and to determine their percentage among the total number of alleles present in the pool. If isolated spatially from a similar group of animals, the genetic composition of any one group of organisms tends to be stable from one generation to another. When such *genetic equilibrium* occurs, there is no evolutionary change.

The status quo is upset, as suggested in Fig. 1-5, when variability appears in the gene pool or when environmental changes occur.

Although many facts are not available to us, there is general agreement that certain forces acting over the millions of years are responsible for the course of evolution, or *phylogeny*, as it is often called. These forces operate by changing the composition of the gene pool. Certain basic processes contribute to evolution: gene mutation, changes in chromosome number and structure, genetic recombinations, natural selection, and reproductive isolation. The first three, all equally important, occur within the gametes of the individual and provide variability. Without variability there could be no change; without natural selection and reproductive isolation there could be no direction to the change. Some authorities believe that genetic drift plays at least a minor role in evolution. Genetic drift, the random fluctuations of genes, occurs in many small populations and affects the genetic composition. It changes the equilibrium of the gene pool by chance rather than by natural selection.

As indicated previously, genes of present-day species exist in several forms, or alleles. Mutations must have arisen in the population of our hypothetical ancestors and brought about these changes in gene form. Mutations affect the genetic pool by increasing the number of alleles available at any one point (locus) on the chromosomes. This, in turn, increases variability. In modern times the use of x rays and other ionizing radiations, heat, ultraviolet light, and certain chemicals experimentally produce mutations in the laboratory. These are referred to as mutagenic substances. However, mutations also occur spontaneously in nature. A mutation results in a permanent change at the gene locus because of alterations in the nucleotide sequence of the gene. This might be caused by part of a chromosome breaking off and becoming physically lost (deletions), or parts of a chromosome translocating or inverting. Changes in the sequence of nucleotides that make up the genetic code alter the set of instructions available for protein synthesis. The new code carried by the messenger RNA reflects itself in the type of protein synthesized. Alterations in the properties and functions of the protein express themselves in the cell of which they are a part. Most mutations are lethal since any mutation that interferes with the basic processes that go on in the cell will be deleterious to the organism. Smaller changes can often be tolerated better than larger ones can be.

In higher organisms further variability is obtained by the very nature of the reproductive process. Meiosis reduces the chromosome number in the egg and sperm to the haploid state and the new individual begins when these two nonidentical gametes fuse. New gene combinations occur because of crossing over, and the phenotype reflects the expression of this duplicate set of genes.

The importance of natural selection was first presented by Darwin before a meeting of the Linnaean Society in London in 1858. He perceived that most populations had an enormous reproductive ability, yet this potentiality was seldom realized. The constant struggle for existence allowed only some of the population to survive. Darwin also noted that variations constantly appeared in nature. He realized that any organism possessing a characteristic that gave it a greater advantage over its neighbor in coping with the problems of existence was ensured a greater chance of survival. Those animals that possessed the advantage not only survived but also reproduced and therefore became the dominant forms in the population. The selection of those heritable variations that occur and prove advantageous to the organism as it struggles for existence is referred to as *natural selection*. Darwin's hypothesis, somewhat refined, remains acceptable today. Continued selection, generation after generation, apparently produces sufficient accumulative changes that eventually new forms appear.

Since natural selection preserves those organisms with advantageous variations, their underlying genetic factors are thus preserved. Such a set of genetic factors has adaptive value. Adaptation refers to the ability of the organism to fit to its environment, survive, and produce young. As an example, the amniotic egg, with its protective membranes, made it possible for aquatic animals to adapt to severe seasonal changes. Those animals with genes that directed the formation of these fetal membranes survived their environmental stress and continued to reproduce. Eventually, this led to land animals that became the dominant organisms of the time.

The ability of the animal to control its body temperature through internal mechanisms is another example of a change that freed the organism (birds and mammals) from dependence on environmental conditions. A constant internal temperature allowed physiological processes to continue at all times. Also, the increased metabolism that goes on at a higher temperature allowed greater levels of activity, resulting in the evolution of flight.

SUGGESTED READINGS

1. Aristotle: On the generation of animals (translated by Arthur Platt). Reprinted in Hutchins, R. M., editor: Great books of the Western world, Chicago, 1952, Encyclopaedia Britannica, Inc.
2. Dillon, L. S.: Evolution: Concepts and consequences, St. Louis, 1973, The C. V. Mosby Co.
3. Harvey, W.: On the generation of animals (translated by Robert Willis). Reprinted in Hutchins, R. M., editor: Great books of the Western world, Chicago, 1952, Encyclopaedia Britannica, Inc.
4. Saunders, J. W., Jr.: Animal morphogenesis, Current concepts in biology series, New York, 1968, The MacMillan Co.
5. Savage, J. M.: Evolution, Modern biology series, New York, 1963, Holt, Rinehart, & Winston.
6. Stebbins, G. L.: Processes of organic evolution, Concepts of modern biology series, New York, 1971, Prentice-Hall, Inc.
7. Weiss, P.: Principles of development, New York, 1939, Holt & Co.

CHAPTER 2

CHORDATES

PHYLUM CHORDATA

The fossil record reveals that 100 million years of invertebrate development passed before the first animal with a backbone made its appearance. During this period the ancestors of the vertebrates also evolved. These ancestral forms were probably soft bodied and therefore left no fossil remains; we know them only through their modern representatives. Small marine animals living today are believed to resemble those early primitive forms. They constitute a closely allied group of animals collectively known as the *protochordates*. Together with the vertebrates, they compose the phylum Chordata. They are of importance to us because they are the simplest animals with structures similar to the vertebrates; at the same time, some of their characteristics link them with the invertebrates, specifically, the echinoderms.

The phylum Chordata is usually divided into three or four subphyla, depending upon the classification system used. All the members of the Hemichordata do not consistently demonstrate all of the chordate characteristics, and for this reason, some taxonomists place them in a separate but related phylum. Others find them closer to the chordates than any group of animals besides the echinoderms and consider them to be the lowest and simplest form of chordate life. This lack of taxonomic agreement is sometimes confusing to the student, but one should remember that classifications are made by experts in the fields and that all experts do not always agree on all points. Usually the disagreements are of a minor nature. We shall consider the hemichordates to be a separate phylum, but since they may offer a clue to the link between chordates and invertebrates, we shall consider them briefly.

Examples of the phylum Hemichordata are the simply constructed Enteropneusta (acorn worm) and the flowerlike Pterobranchia. The acorn worm *(Dolichoglossus)*, shown in Fig. 2-1, is a small, wormlike creature with a body consisting of an anterior proboscis, a collar, and an elongated trunk. The trunk region possesses gill slits that allow the water to pass from the inside of the animal to the outside. An extension of the gut into the proboscis forms a stiff rodlike structure referred to as a stomo-chord, not considered homologous to the noto-chord of higher forms. A dorsal solid nerve strand may be found in the collar region. Even more interesting, the larva of the acorn worm, the tornaria, is almost identical to the larva of some echinoderms (Fig. 2-2). In fact, for a long time the two were not distinguished. They vary only in the pattern of the cilia.

Another example of a hemichordate is the pterobranch. It is a tiny animal that lives in colonial fashion in the deep ocean. Each animal contains feathery arms that are attached to a body that, in turn, is anchored by an extensible stalk to the gelatinous tube in which it lives.

A proboscis and collar are located at the base of the arms, as shown in Fig. 2-3. Of the characteristics associated with chordates, the ptero-branchs have only gill slits. There are no signs of the notochord and hollow dorsal nerve cord.

Protochordates

Most biologists agree that the Urochordata should be a subphylum of the Chordata. Generally referred to as tunicates, the sea squirts and ascidians belong to this group. They are marine and many are sessile, usually attaching themselves to rocks or some other stationary object. They are filter feeders. The water, with all of its food material and debris, passes into

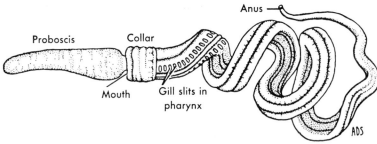

Fig. 2-1
Dolichoglossus is a marine enteropneust. It possesses two of the chordate characteristics, since it has a dorsal hollow nerve cord, and the pharyngeal wall exhibits a series of gill slits leading to the exterior. Most investigators do not consider the stiff rodlike structure in the proboscis (the stomochord) to be homologous with the notochord of the chordates. (From Kent, G. C.: Comparative anatomy of the vertebrates, ed. 3, St. Louis, 1973, The C. V. Mosby Co.)

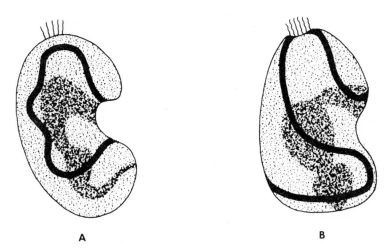

Fig. 2-2
Comparison of larval forms of, **A**, acorn worm (Hemichordata) and, **B**, sea cucumber (Echinodermata). For a long time these two ciliated larvae were both considered to belong to the echinoderms.

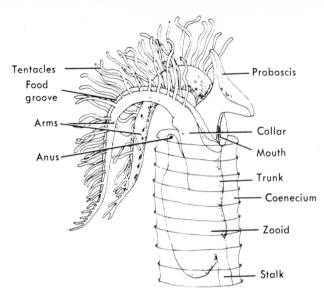

Tentacles
Food groove
Arms
Anus
Proboscis
Collar
Mouth
Trunk
Coenecium
Zooid
Stalk

Fig. 2-3
Basic body plan of the pterobranch is similar to that of the Enteropneusta. Some forms of these hemichordates live together in anastomosing gelatinous tubes, extending their tentacles through terminal openings as shown in this example of an individual pterobranch. They attach to the walls of the tube by an extensible stalk (peduncle) that can pull them inside the tube if necessary. (From Hickman, C. P., Biology of the invertebrates, ed. 2, St. Louis, 1973, The C. V. Mosby Co.)

the barrel-shaped pharynx through an incurrent siphon. The many gill slits located in the pharynx allow the water to pass out of the pharynx into a specialized atrial cavity and then on to the outside by way of the excurrent siphon. Any food particles present in the water sink to the bottom of the pharynx and are conveyed through the short gut. The adult tunicate, as exemplified by *Molgula manhattensis* (Fig. 2-4), does not resemble any chordate. A rough tunic covers its barrel-shaped body. It possesses only gill slits, but its free-swimming larval stage shows the other chordate characteristics. The larva is often shaped like a tadpole and, in fact, is referred to as a tunicate tadpole (Fig. 2-5). It has a notochord in the tail region and also possesses a dorsal hollow nerve cord and gill slits, all three chordate characteristics. After swimming about for a short period, the tadpole undergoes metamorphosis. It loses its tail and attaches itself to some object. The nerve cord is reduced to a single ganglion and only the gill slits remain.

The second subphylum of the phylum Chordata is the Cephalochordata, composed of two genera. A group of marine species collectively known as amphioxus belongs to the *Branchiostoma*, the most numerous genus. A diagram of a specimen is shown in Fig. 2-6. Amphioxus is especially interesting to us for two reasons. Its egg demonstrates in simplest form the developmental stages followed by the embryos of higher forms. In the following pages we shall refer many times to these embryonic stages and to some of the processes that bring about their development. Amphioxus also demonstrates the typical body plan of the vertebrate. It resembles the ammocoetes larva of those jawless fish belonging to the most primitive vertebrate class, Petromyzontes.

We shall only describe the general characteristics of amphioxus at this time, since some of its systems are discussed in detail later. Amphioxus is a slender animal, about 2 inches long, that usually lies partly buried in the sand.

It is also a filter feeder. The beating of the buccal cirri that encircle the oral hood at the anterior end of the animal causes the water with its food particles to enter the vestibule, or oral cavity. A membrane, the velum, containing an opening, the mouth, separates the oral cavity from the pharynx. Velar tentacles act as a sieve,

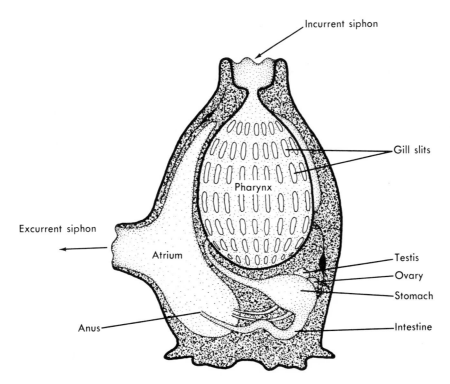

Fig. 2-4
Mature tunicate. Water and food are taken into the large barrel-shaped pharynx by way of the incurrent siphon. The food is mixed with mucus and enters the stomach; the water moves through the gill slits into the atrial cavity, eventually passing to the outside by way of the excurrent siphon.

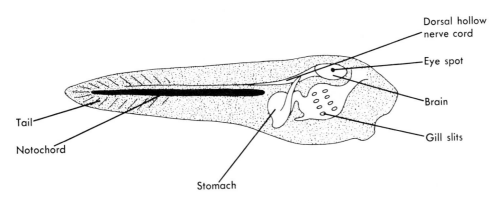

Fig. 2-5
"Tadpole" larva of some tunicates has a tiny brain and a dorsal hollow nerve cord. A notochord is present in the well-developed tail and gill slits in the pharynx. After swimming about, the larva attaches itself to a suitable substratum, undergoes metamorphosis, and develops into the sessile adult.

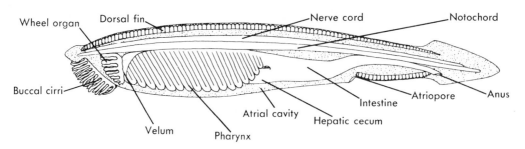

Fig. 2-6
Schematic drawing of amphioxus, a primitive chordate.

preventing any large pieces of debris from passing through the mouth into the gut. Water sweeps through the mouth into the pharynx. It then passes by way of the numerous gill slits, into a specialized atrial cavity and on to the outside through the atriopore. The food, mixed with the mucus secreted by the wheel organ, falls to the floor of the pharynx into a groove, the endostyle. The beating cilia convey the food around the sides of the pharynx to the dorsally located epibranchial groove. The food moves down the groove to the intestine.

A cross section of amphioxus (Fig. 2-7) demonstrates the systems of vertebrates in their simplest form. Familiarity with this body plan will aid in understanding the more complex architecture of higher organisms. Although amphioxus lacks a heart, the circulatory system consists of paired anterior and posterior cardinal veins that bring blood from the two regions of the body. These veins join one another at the ducts of Cuvier and merge at the ventral region to form a large pulsating vessel under the pharynx. This vessel drives the blood dorsally through many aortic arches located between the gill slits. These arches open into the dorsal aorta which carries the blood into the head region and down the length of the body.

The muscular system of amphioxus is similar to that of the lowest vertebrate. Its body wall consists of muscles, segmentally arranged. Each segment extends from the dorsal to the ventral body wall and is angled in the middle to form a V. A notochord runs the length of the body, projecting into the head region to a point anterior to the nerve cord. This characteristic is responsible for the name Cephalochordata

(*kephalē*, 'head'; *chordata*, 'cords'). The nervous system is not much more than a dorsal hollow cord; there is only a slight enlargment, the cerebral vesicle, in the brain region. Amphioxus is either male or female, with fertilization occurring in the surrounding water. Only the excretory system is unlike the higher vertebrates. It resembles that of the invertebrates and consists of segmentally arranged nephridia.

Common vertebrate characteristics

The majority of the chordates belong to the subphylum Vertebrata. These animals not only possess the three common chordate structures, but also share other similar characteristics. The basic vertebrate body plan may be described as follows:

All vertebrates demonstrate *bilateral symmetry*, that is, their body can be divided into two mirror images. This symmetry is imposed as early as the first cleavage in some animals. Each animal also has anterior and posterior regions as well as dorsal, ventral, and lateral surfaces. The possession of this type of body plan (as opposed to radial symmetry) allows the animal a greater degree of activity.

The embryo of vertebrates displays limited *segmentation*. Unlike some of the invertebrates, the external body is never divided into a repetitious series of body parts. The arrangement of myotomes, the primordia of the muscles, demonstrates this segmentation. They are first laid down in the embryo in a series of blocklike somites, which are concentrations of mesoderm. The adults of lower vertebrates retain these divisions, but they are lost in the higher forms. The formation of the vertebrae, the arrangement of spinal nerves, and the early development of some kidney tubules also reflect the segmentation concept seen in all vertebrates.

Vertebrates have a large body cavity, the *coelom,* established during the gastrula stage of development and retained in the adult. Many of the organs of the body are arranged around the coelom or suspended in it by mesenteries. The coelom divides into an anterior pericardial cavity, containing the heart, and a more posterior abdominal, or peritoneal, cavity. This latter cavity becomes the pleuroperitoneal cavity of lower lung-bearing vertebrates, but is further divided into pleural and peritoneal cavities in higher forms.

All vertebrates possess an *endoskeleton,* which includes among other structures, the segmented vertebrae of the backbone. Of course, the name of the subphylum is derived from this particular characteristic. It first appears in the embryo as a cartilaginous replica of the adult structure, but is usually replaced with bone in the adult. The members of the classes Myxini, Petromyzontes, and Chondrichthyes are three exceptions. In these animals, the embryonic cartilaginous skeletal material is retained in the adult. Bone is a very hard, uniquely vertebrate tissue, composed of a matrix impregnated with calcium phosphate. Since the earliest vertebrates possessed bone, we assume that these groups of vertebrates lost the

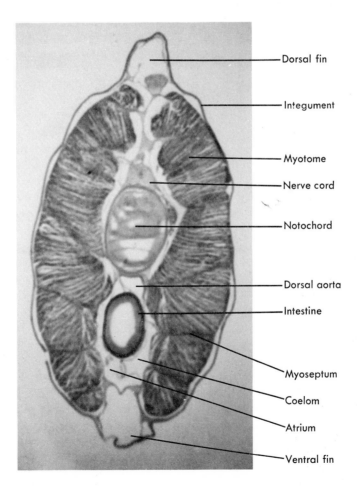

Fig. 2-7
Transverse section through intestinal region of amphioxus demonstrating the simple chordate body plan.

ability to form bone; such a loss is considered a *degenerate characteristic* rather than a primitive one.

Vertebrates have *muscles* that enable them to move parts of their body or the body as a whole. Some of them are voluntary, under the control of the individual's will, especially the large skeletal muscles; others are involuntary and, with the exception of cardiac muscle, form an integral part of most organs. All vertebrate muscles have basically the same biochemical and physiological properties, but based on the assembly of their ultrastructure, they are usually referred to as skeletal, cardiac, and smooth muscle.

The nervous system of all vertebrates shows *cephalization*. There is a growth and increase in complexity of the dorsal hollow nerve cord at the anterior end of the animal to give rise to a brain. Special senses also appear, and eyes, olfactory organs, and one to three semicircular canals are usually present. In the embryo, the anterior region of the cord divides, first into three and then five basic brain vesicles. The remaining part of the nerve cord is the spinal cord. Both somatic and autonomic spinal nerves are given off on each side of the body in each segment. They consist of a sensory root and a motor root capable of carrying out reflex action.

Unlike the protochordates, all vertebrates have a muscular pump, the heart, that sends blood throughout the body. The *circulatory system* is one of the first systems to be established in the embryo. Blood leaves the heart by way of arteries and returns in the veins. Tiny capillaries connect the two vessels, making the vertebrate circulatory system a closed system. An accessory lymphatic system returns tissue fluid to the heart. The blood of vertebrates consists of plasma (the liquid part) and the formed elements— erythrocytes (red blood cells) and leukocytes (white blood cells). The erythrocytes contain hemoglobin, the oxygen-carrying compound of vertebrates.

The gut, or *digestive system*, is a continuous tube within the body tube. The anterior opening is the mouth and the posterior opening, the anus. The gill slits develop in the walls of the pharynx. In the embryo, outpocketings (diverticula) from the gut tube give rise to other common structures. The lung buds (in those vertebrates that have lungs), liver, gallbladder, pancreas, and, in some cases, the urinary bladder all develop from the embryonic gut and are retained as adult structures.

The *excretory system* of vertebrates consists primarily of a filtering system composed of kidney tubules, or nephrons. Liquid filters from the blood vessels of the kidney's glomerulus through two thin layers of cells into a cuplike structure, Bowman's capsule. The urine may or may not be concentrated as it moves through the tubules. Kidney ducts collect the urine and convey it either to the cloaca, to a urinary bladder, or directly to the outside.

Normally, vertebrates are either male or female, although sex reversals do occur and hermaphrodites exist, especially among lower animals. All vertebrates *reproduce sexually* and their reproductive system consists of gonads, either ovaries or testes, and a series of ducts. The gonads release the eggs or sperm into reproductive ducts that carry the generative cells to the outside. Cyclostomes are an exception since they lack ducts, instead shedding the gametes directly into the body cavity from which they escape to the outside via special pores. Fertilization occurs either externally or internally; in the latter case, intromittent organs usually develop in association with the reproductive tract.

The *interaction of the nervous and endocrine systems* integrates the life processes of vertebrates. The nervous system detects changes in the internal and external environments. A quick response to such changes is brought about by way of the nervous system acting through the effector organs, usually muscles or glands. The endocrine system utilizes the circulatory system to carry its chemical messengers (hormones), and thus its response is slower. Unlike the invertebrates whose life processes are controlled by neurosecretions, in vertebrates the endocrine cells exist as discrete organs. Although the structures of the endocrine organs resemble one another throughout the various classes of vertebrates, the chemistry and action of many of the hormones have changed phylogenetically.

Vertebrate classes

Students often have a difficult time remembering names when they are first introduced to taxonomic and anatomic terms. Most terms are descriptive and represent combinations of certain roots usually derived from Latin or Greek. For example, *ichthyes* refers to 'fishes,' *chondro-* means 'cartilage,' and *osteo-*, 'bone.' When the above are combined, they describe the two basic classes of fish. You will meet these words throughout the book in various other combinations. For example, we shall refer to osteoblasts, which are embryonic bone-forming cells, or refer to Teleostei, fishes with skeletons entirely of bone (*teleios*, 'complete').

Animals belonging to 11 different classes are usually grouped together under the subphylum Vertebrata. These animals all possess the general chordate and vertebrate characteristics, as well as characteristics unique for their particular group (class). We have no difficulty in telling the members apart, for example, a fish from a frog, a lizard from a cat, etc. However, it should again be emphasized that fossil records of vertebrates show many forms between fish and amphibian, amphibian and reptiles, and reptiles and mammals. Thus vertebrate life is a continuum. Although the modern classes of vertebrates have distinguishing characteristics that set them apart from one another, it is likely that in past ages their genetic relationships were no further apart than present-day genera or families. They are apparent to us today because of the extinction in between of large groups of animals.

The vertebrates can be divided into two general categories: those lower aquatic vertebrates with fishlike forms and those with four limbs, the tetrapods. In some of the latter forms the limbs may have been lost or modified.

Two superclasses compose the fishlike forms: the Cyclostomata and the Gnathostomata. Under the superclass Cyclostomata, animals without jaws, the lowest three classes are grouped together. The members of the class *Ostracodermi* (see Fig. 2-10) are all extinct. Usually these animals lacked paired appendages; some had only one dorsal nostril between the eyes, and all were covered with an armor of heavy bony plates. Their head region was greatly expanded and occupied by a large gill chamber. They are of significance because their fossils are the oldest and most primitive of all the vertebrates. The *Petromyzontes*, represented by the modern lamprey, and the *Myxini*, the hagfish, make up the other classes of jawless fish. Their eel-like bodies are soft and scaleless. They lack fins and jaws and their round mouths are often used as suckers. They have cartilaginous skeletons and a single nostril. They are predaceous.

The rest of the vertebrates have jaws and are grouped as *Gnathostomata* ('jaw mouths'). The members of the class Placodermi (Fig. 2-11) apparently evolved from ostracoderm-like ancestors but are now all extinct. Many of them retained their bony armor and added bony spines and spires. They had both pectoral and pelvic paired fins.

When the placoderms became extinct, three classes of fish took their place, the *Chondrichthyes,* the *Holocephali*, and the *Osteichthyes*. The sharks and skates belong to the first class. They all have cartilaginous skeletons as the name Chondrichthyes implies. The chimaeras compose the Holocephali. Their nostrils are double; they have well-formed jaws with teeth, a spiracle, and an exoskeleton of placoid scales, representing all that is left of the placoderm armor. They lack air bladders. The bony fish belong to the *Osteichthyes,* a class considered older than that of the sharks. The modern food fish of economic value belong to this class. The body is covered with bony scales and the gills by a bony operculum. Their nostrils are double, and they have swim bladders, or in a few cases, lungs.

Four classes represent the animals usually referred to as tetrapods. The vertebrates belonging to the class *Amphibia* usually live near water; they represent transitional stages between aquatic and terrestrial animals. They are cold-blooded (cannot maintain constant body temperature). Their bodies are usually naked, but a few have bony scales. Although the larvae use gills as a breathing organ, most adults have lungs. A few adults have both structures. The larva undergoes metamorphosis and changes into the adult stage. The ventricle of the heart is undivided. The embryo develops without benefit of membranes, this characteristic being the main difference between the amphibian and the truly terrestrial animal.

The *Reptilia* are the first wholly terrestrial forms (although some are aquatic), because they have evolved the amniote egg. This egg contains membranes that protect the embryo from desiccation and allows it to be laid on land. The reptilian body is covered with keratinized scales and its skin has few glands. Reptiles are poikilothermic (cold-blooded). They have a three-chambered heart, but the ventricle is partially divided. They breathe exclusively by lungs. The young resemble the parent, and thus there is no metamorphosis.

The class *Aves* consists of vertebrates whose forelimbs are modified to form wings and whose skin is covered with feathers. They are homeothermic (warm-blooded), possess a four-chambered heart, and lay eggs. Only extinct birds had teeth. Birds demonstrate complex behavior patterns indicating an increase in the development of the brain.

The class *Mammalia* contains the archaic egg-laying mammals, the pouched forms, and the placental animals. They all have hair, an internal temperature control, circulatory improvements, and use their diaphragm to breathe. With the exception of the Prototheria, the females have mammary glands with nipples and suckle their young. When compared with the reptiles, mammals demonstrate a greater capacity for intelligent activity. Association centers develop, offering the potential for learning, memory, and consciousness.

As shown in Table 2-1, there are many general ways of categorizing vertebrates other than into fishlike forms and tetrapods. All such schemes reveal general characteristics about the animals. They may be divided into those animals without jaws (Cyclostomata) and those with jaws (Gnathostomata), those with eggs spawned into the water (anamniote), and those that protect their developing embryos from the desiccation of a land environment by membranes such as an amnion (amniotes). There are those vertebrates that reflect the temperature of their environment (poikilothermic) and those that have developed a homeostatic temperature control (homoiothermic). Usually, each of these advanced general characteristics has progressively allowed the vertebrate to probe his environment further than did the lower forms.

TABLE 2-1. Classification of vertebrates

Superclass	Class	Examples	Presence of jaws	Egg type	Temperature control	Habitat of majority
Cyclostomata	Ostracodermi	Extinct ostracoderms	No			
	Petromyzontes	Lampreys		Anamniote	Poikilothermic	Aquatic
	Myxini	Hagfishes				
Gnathostomata	Placodermi	Acanthodians, arthrodires, antiarchs—all extinct	Yes			
	Chondrichthyes	Sharks, rays, skates				
	Holocephali	Chimaeras				
	Osteichthyes	Higher bony fish				
	Amphibia	Frogs, toads, newts, salamanders				Intermediate
	Reptilia	Lizards, snakes, turtles, crocodiles, alligators		Amniote		Terrestrial
	Aves	All birds			Homoiothermic	
	Mammalia	Egg-laying forms: anteater and duckbill platypus				
		Pouched forms: kangaroo, opossum, etc.				
		Placental forms: mouse, cow, man, etc.				

PHYLOGENETIC ORIGINS

Amphioxus is important not only because it has a simple body plan similar to the vertebrates, but also because it may point forward to the evolution of the vertebrates and backward toward their origins. Modern amphioxus is a specialized chordate that has had as much time to undergo an independent evolution as the vertebrates. It is not surprising that over this period of time it should develop many characteristics not found in modern vertebrates. Amphioxus, itself, is not considered the ancestor of vertebrates but, rather, may share a similar type of ancestor, with the two forms separating from one another as far back as the Precambrian times. There are no fossil remains of these early animals and any relationships must be deduced from the modern examples.

Amphioxus has many characteristics similar to the larva of the lamprey, a member of the lowest group of living vertebrates, the cyclostomes. In fact, the larva is so different from the adult lamprey that for many years its relationship was not recognized and it was given the separate generic name of *Ammocoetes*. Both amphioxus and ammocoetes spend their time burrowed in the mud, and if one accepts the neotenic origin of amphioxus (see below), they both are larval forms. A cross section through the two animals shows a similar anatomical plan (Figs. 2-7 and 2-8) although the ammocoetes is more advanced; it has a brain, major sense organs, a

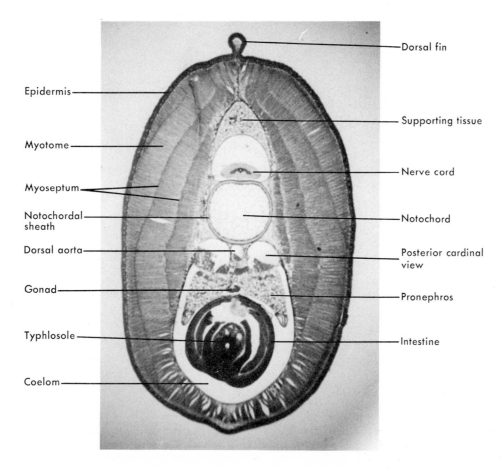

Fig. 2-8
Transverse section through intestinal region of ammocoetes larva. A comparison with Fig. 2-7 shows a similar anatomical plan with that of amphioxus.

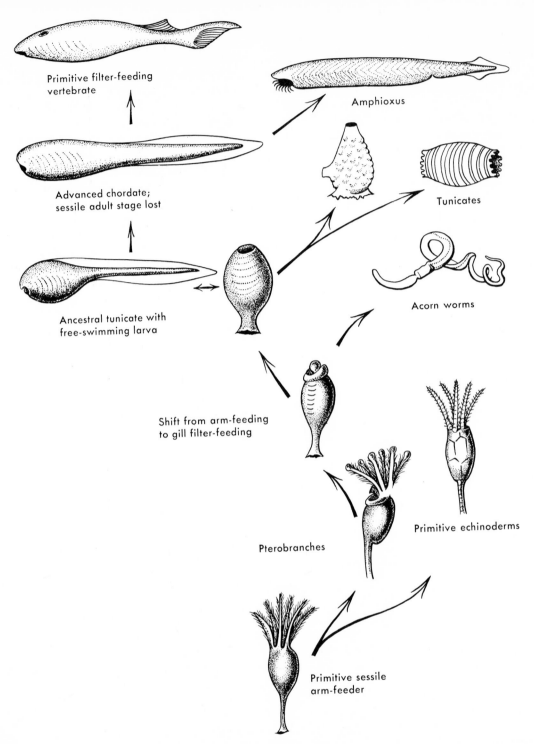

Primitive filter-feeding
vertebrate

Amphioxus

Advanced chordate;
sessile adult stage lost

Tunicates

Ancestral tunicate with
free-swimming larva

Acorn worms

Shift from arm-feeding
to gill filter-feeding

Primitive echinoderms

Pterobranches

Primitive sessile
arm-feeder

Fig. 2-9
Family tree suggesting the evolution of amphioxus and the early vertebrates from primitive arm-feeding, sessile ancestors. Such simple forms may have been ancestral to both pterobranchs and primitive echinoderms. A shift from arm
feeding to a gill filter-feeding system produced sessile tunicate-like forms. If the free swimming stages of such an
adult became capable of reproduction, a line of animals could be established in which the adult stages were lost. Such
a line would lead to amphioxus and to the primitive filter-feeding vertebrates. (From Romer, A. S.: The vertebrate
story, Chicago, 1959, University of Chicago Press.)

pulsating heart, and other structures that amphioxus lacks. Some biologists suggest that both amphioxus and the ammocoetes larva arose from a common ancestral stock and that the lamprey larva later evolved its adult stage.

There are those who regard amphioxus as the larval stage of a vertebrate, a larva that developed reproductive capabilities. Such a condition is known as *neoteny*. Once the larva was able to reproduce, the adult stage was superfluous and became extinct. The other theory suggests that amphioxus evolved from a free-swimming larva of some sessile ancestor. This evolutionary pathway is diagrammed in Fig. 2-9. If this latter pathway is assumed, the hypothetical adult ancestor may have been a sessile filter feeder reminiscent of today's tunicate. If we push back further along this evolutionary line, we see that such an animal could have given rise to modern tunicates as well as to animals leading to vertebrates. If the free-swimming stage of such a sessile adult became capable of reproduction, a line of animals could have been established in which the adult sessile stage was eventually lost. It would be this line that led to amphioxus and to the vertebrates.

Romer (1967) suggests that the tunicate-like form evolved from a sessile animal with gill slits and a noselike proboscis. Such an ancestor, no doubt, gave rise to the acorn worm, those specialized creatures of today classified as the boundary between chordates and invertebrates. The numerous gill slits have only to be reduced and arms added to shift from a filter feeder to an arm-feeding organism. This assumes that the ocean was the ancestral home since these tiny arm feeders were all marine. Their ciliated arms helped to push food into their mouths as they remained attached to the floor of the ocean. They consisted primarily of a digestive system and were passive in their feeding habits. Such a primitive, sessile, arm feeder could have been ancestral to both the modern pterobranchs (Hemichordata) and the crinoids, primitive echinoderms that grow on stalks. Romer summarizes this line of vertebrate evolution in Fig. 2-9 and suggests the pterobranch-tunicate-amphioxus-ammocoetes pathway of development.

Although almost every phylum in the animal kingdom has been suggested as leading to vertebrates, best evidence links the chordates with the echinoderms. The similarity of developmental patterns offers one indication of this relationship. We mentioned earlier the bilaterally symmetrical larvae of the Hemichordata and Echinodermata. In chordates, hemichordates, and echinoderms, cleavage is radial and gastrulation is similar. In many of these embryos mesoderm forms from pouches that evaginate from the gut. The blastopore is located at the posterior end of the body and the skeleton is mesodermal in origin. Other invertebrates follow different developmental processes. There are also biochemical similarities among the groups. The energy source for muscle contraction in vertebrates is creatine phosphate, but in most invertebrates, arginine is present in place of creatine. Analysis reveals that both amino acids, creatine and arginine, are present in echinoderms, tunicates, and some hemichordates. The study of blood proteins offers additional information. Serological tests show that the proteins in the sera of the lower chordates and echinoderms are similar to one another but not to those of the other invertebrates. All these remarkable similarities tend to link the chordates to the echinoderms and lead to the inescapable conclusion that the two groups of animals had a common ancestor.

STAGES IN VERTEBRATE EVOLUTION

Some of the changes that occurred to vertebrates in the evolutionary past led to their extinction, some led to their success within a particular environment, and a few led to their further evolutionary development. Looking back over evolutionary growth, one can discern a pattern. Out of evolutionary experimentation, one divergent line crosses through the ecological barrier into a new ecological zone. The movement from water to land is an example. Since there is no immediate competition in this new zone, the divergent line (reptiles, for example) adapts to the new environment and flourishes. Once established, the new line undergoes divergent growth and through special adaptations invades all aspects of the environment (adaptive radiation). For example, the reptiles invaded not only the land and the air, but they even returned to the water. The evolutionary pattern is repeated when a new divergent line is able to cross into a new ecological zone.

Although changes were going on continually, many of which were of great adaptive value to the individual, we shall consider only those that contributed to the evolution of the mammal. This will limit the scope of our discussion and relate more directly to the animals we shall study. Reference to the classification of the phylum Chordata listed at the end of this chapter can reveal what forms are omitted from our discussion.

Although most changes modified previously established structures, a few evolved into innovations that allowed the organism to adapt itself to a completely new way of life. The ability to control body temperature is one of the important changes that enabled Aves and Mammalia to evolve. Some authorities list seven sequential steps leading to the evolution of placental animals. Understand that we cannot actually speak of single "steps" in the evolution of any one class of vertebrates. The term should be considered in a broad, collective sense. One of our seven steps actually involves a number of individual genetic changes that took place over a period of evolutionary time. For example, fossil evidence reveals that the shift in the quadrate and articular bones from the lower jaw of reptiles to the ear of mammals was a gradual process, but we speak of the shift as if it were one step. Using the migration of these bones as a guide (through the fossil record), one has difficulty telling where the reptiles leave off and the mammals begin.

The earliest vertebrates were the ostracoderms, which date back to the early Paleozoic times (Figs. 2-10 and 2-11). They were filter feeders, but had a distinct advantage over the ancestral tunicate type in that they were motile. The development of a *strong swimming tail* allowed them to move from place to place and seek out more advantageous feeding grounds. They had a small round opening for a mouth and lacked jaws. The ostracoderms resembled the tunicate larva since they had an expanded head region and tail, but differed in that they were encased in bony armor. Bone, considered to be a unique vertebrate characteristic, appears suddenly on the scene. In some cases it was present only as bony armor; an endoskeleton was lacking. In other examples an internal skeleton also developed. The large eurypterids, invertebrates that dominated the freshwaters of this period, preyed upon these early vertebrates. Their bony

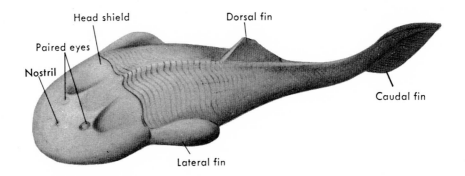

Fig. 2-10
Earliest fossil vertebrates are represented by the ostracoderms, filter feeders that date back to early Paleozoic times. They developed a strong swimming tail, were covered by bony armor, and may have had an internal skeleton. Since they were motile, they had an advantage over tunicate type of ancestors and could move about seeking more advantageous feeding grounds. They had a small round mouth and lacked jaws. They became extinct during Devonian times. (From Hickman, C. P., Sr., Hickman, C. P., Jr., and Hickman, F. M.: Integrated principles of zoology, ed. 5, St. Louis, 1974, The C. V. Mosby Co.)

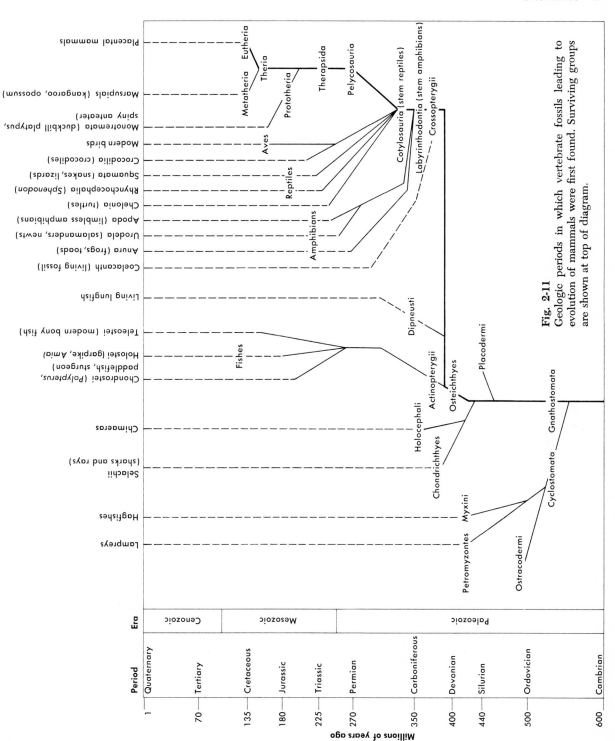

Fig. 2-11
Geologic periods in which vertebrate fossils leading to evolution of mammals were first found. Surviving groups are shown at top of diagram.

armor as well as their increased ability to swim probably helped in the defense of these early vertebrates.

There are no ostracoderms living at the present time; by the end of the Devonian period they had vanished, leaving in their place the eel-like lampreys and hagfishes. These modern forms have retained certain primitive characteristics (lack of jaws and fins), but they also show degenerative characteristics (lack of bone). They have developed certain specialized characteristics unique to them, including the adhesive disklike mouth and rasping tongue that allow them to attach to and live parasitically on other fishes. The modern cyclostome represents a branch off the main line of evolution. An ancestral form more like the ostracoderm gave rise to the placoderms.

The appearance of *jaws with teeth* was the second major change in structure. The jaws of the gnathostomes evolved from the anterior skeletal bars used to support the gill slits of round-mouthed forms. Teeth are bony scales that once covered the surface of the animal (such as the ostracoderm) and migrated inward over the jaws. The biting jaw allowed the animal to change from a filter feeder to one that was more predaceous, from a passive, defensive animal to one that was actively aggressive.

The first jawed animals to appear in the fossil records of the Silurian period were the *placoderms* (see Fig. 2-12). Since they were also armored at first, they resembled the ostracoderms, but as time passed, the armor decreased. Freed of a cumbersome, heavy, bony encasement and possessing a biting mouth, the animal darted about hunting food and escaping from its predators. The appearance of paired fins aided in this freedom. The placoderms became extinct before the close of the Paleozoic, but from them evolved three classes of more advanced fish, the Chondrichthyes, Holocephali, and Osteichthyes.

The Chondrichthyes are the cartilaginous fish of which the shark is an example. Since bone is considered to be a vertebrate characteristic, one can assume that they have lost their bony condition and retained the embryonic form of skeletal material. A cartilaginous skeleton is considered a degenerate characteristic in the shark and is an example of an evolutionary change considered regressive. The evolution of all structures does not always proceed from the simple to the complex, but, as indicated above, may show degenerative characteristics. Although the shark is widely used for dissection in the anatomy laboratory as an illustration of simple vertebrate form, it is not in the evolutionary line of higher vertebrates and is not discussed in detail at this time.

The fish that belong to the class Osteichthyes all have a bony skeleton. They can be divided

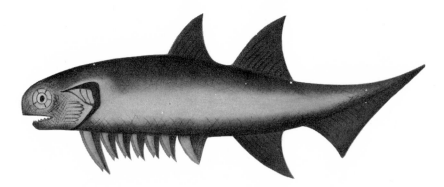

Fig. 2-12
Appearance of jaws and teeth was the second major evolutionary change found in the early vertebrates. They were present in the armored placoderms that arose in the late Silurian period. They later became free of their cumbersome armor and, possessing a biting mouth and fins, darted about hunting food and escaping from predators. (From Hickman, C. P., Sr., Hickman, C. P., Jr., and Hickman, F. M.: Integrated principles of zoology, ed. 4, St. Louis, 1970, The C. V. Mosby Co.)

into the ray-finned fishes, subclass *Actinopterygii;* the lobe-finned fishes, the *Crossopterygii;* and the lungfish, the *Dipneusti.* The ray-finned fish compose the majority of fishes and gave rise to the successful fishes of modern times. They are the fish of great economic value.

It is from the Crossopterygii that land animals evolved. These fish had *fleshy-lobed* fins, as shown in Fig. 2-13, and their skeleton was not unlike those of the primitive amphibians. The skeletons in both the fins and girdles were strengthened, a step representing a major advance over the previous fishes. Unlike the horny ray-supported fins of the Actinopterygii, the fleshy-lobed fins contained bony skeletal supports. They could now use the fins to push themselves over the bottom of the ponds when the water became shallow. As the ponds and streams dried up, those fish with fleshy-lobed fins used them to find another pond. Many of them had developed a skull similar to that of amphibians and higher vertebrates and also *internal nares,* or *choanae.* The crossopterygian fish flourished during the Devonian time and then declined. They left the coelacanths, a side branch that survives today in the Indian Ocean and possibly elsewhere.

A third subclass, the Dipneusti, contains the modern lungfish. Although these fish have many characteristics similar to land animals, they are probably a related group rather than in the direct evolutionary line. They are significant, however, since their relationship suggests that the crossopterygian fish may also have had *lungs* that functioned when their water became fouled. Lungs, as they first evolved, were not for land use. Rather, when environmental conditions became unfavorable, they tided the animal over until the rains came. Once the water became filled with oxygen, the gills could again function. Some geologists interpret the continental sediments to indicate the presence of severe seasonal droughts during the Devonian period. Fish that lacked lungs and had to depend only on gills, obviously, could not survive. The presence of lungs in fish is very old, dating back 400 million years ago.

The Crossopterygii gave rise to the Labyrinthodontia, a superorder, sometimes referred to as the "stem amphibians" (Fig. 2-14). These amphibians, now extinct, dominated the late Paleozoic era and Triassic period. It was the labyrinthodonts that first invaded land, not to explore it, but to find new pools as each pool dried up during the periods of seasonal droughts. The earliest amphibian probably resembled a fish, except that it lacked median fins and used short sturdy legs that had developed from the fleshy-lobed fins of the crossopterygian fish. The *presence of legs and lungs* initiated the development of tetrapods. The living orders of amphibians, the frogs and toads (Anura), the

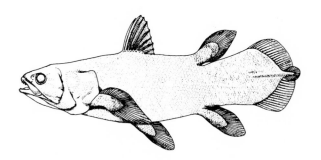

Fig. 2-13
It is from the Crossopterygii that land animals are believed to have evolved. Many of these fish developed internal nares, were lung breathers, and had a skeleton that resembled the primitive amphibians. Unlike the horny supported fins of the Actinopterygii, the fleshy-lobed fins contained jointed bony skeletal supports. The fins could be used to push the fish over the bottom of the ponds when the water became shallow or to find another home when the streams and ponds disappeared. (From Hickman, C. P., Sr., Hickman, C. P., Jr., and Hickman, F. M.: Integrated principles of zoology, ed. 4, St. Louis, 1970, The C. V. Mosby Co.)

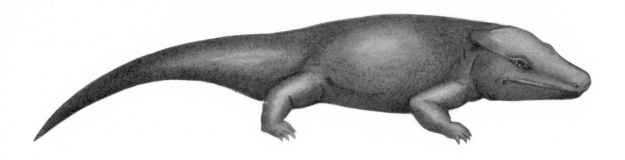

Fig. 2-14
The labyrinthodonts, primitive amphibians, demonstrate both crossopterygian and amphibian features. Their head was covered with bony scales and their limbs, extending at right angles from the body, resembled the fleshy-lobed fins of their fish ancestors. They were the first animals to invade land. Some of them suggest transitional forms leading to the first reptiles. (From Hickman, C. P., Sr., Hickman, C. P., Jr., and Hickman, F. M.: Integrated principles of zoology, ed. 4, St. Louis, 1970, The C. V. Mosby Co.

newts and salamanders (Urodela), and some wormlike forms (Apoda) evolved from a later type of amphibian, one different from the branch that gave rise to the reptiles. As these modern amphibians evolved, the labyrinthodonts gave rise to the stem reptiles and then passed into extinction. The amphibians represented an intermediate form, occupying a borderline niche, part terrestrial and part aquatic. Most of them never became completely terrestrial. Although the adults wander far from the ancestral ponds, they are tied to water by the larval stages, which remain aquatic. The eggs of amphibians cannot develop completely devoid of moisture.

It was the reptiles that took advantage of the next evolutionary advancement, the formation of the *amniote egg*. The *cotylosaurs*, the first reptiles, probably resembled the amphibians structurally as depicted in Fig. 2-15. These stem reptiles, however, differed in their mode of reproduction.

The reptilian embryo during its development became wrapped in three egg membranes: amnion, chorion, and allantois. A protective shell was deposited around the egg. A yolk sac supplied food to the embryo as it developed within its confined space. The amnion, filled with fluid, surrounded the embryo and represented essentially a bit of the ancestral pond carried onto land. Since both the amphibians and stem reptiles were, no doubt, amphibious at this time, it appears that the adaptation of the egg to a land environment occurred before the animals themselves invaded the land. The development of amniote eggs, like the evolution of limbs, allowed the animals possessing these characteristics to survive a fluctuating environment. At first, the membrane-covered egg ensured development of aquatic forms during seasons of drought. Later, its adaptation to a land environment opened the possibility of a terrestrial existence to vertebrates. The amniote egg permitted reptiles to leave their aquatic environment and to explore land habitats. They were even able to live in deserts, an environment incompatible with other forms.

From the cotylosaurs (stem reptiles) evolved all other reptiles—turtles, lizards, snakes, crocodiles, and dinosaurs. Reptiles became the dominant group during the Mesozoic era.

One of the principles of evolution is that new species do not arise from the most advanced or complex animals, but from simple unspecialized forms. Before the reptiles underwent their great radiation that led to the experimentation of many forms, two other groups evolved. One gave rise to the birds. A different and earlier stock, the *pelycosaurs*, evolved from

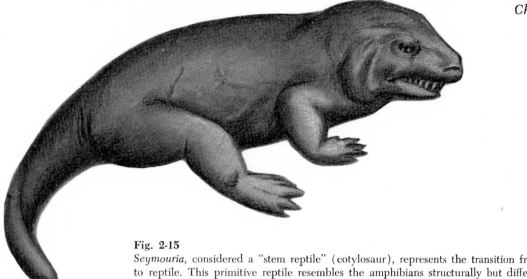

Fig. 2-15
Seymouria, considered a "stem reptile" (cotylosaur), represents the transition from amphibian to reptile. This primitive reptile resembles the amphibians structurally but differs in its mode of reproduction. The development of the amniote egg enabled the cotylosaurs to establish a land existence. (From Hickman, C. P., Sr., Hickman, C. P., Jr., and Hickman, F. M.: Integrated principles of zoology, ed. 4, St. Louis, 1970, The C. V. Mosby Co.)

the stem reptile and ultimately gave rise to mammals. At first these reptiles walked with the sprawled-out pose of the amphibians. Later, the legs were drawn under the body as shown in Fig. 2-16. The small, mammal-like reptiles, the therapsids, with more efficient locomotion became the dominant forms of the late Permian and Triassic periods. Their skulls and teeth placed them halfway between typical reptiles and primitive mammals. These forms continued to exist in small groups during the dominance of the carnivorous dinosaurs, but they disappeared in the Jurassic, leaving in their place mammalian descendants that differed little from themselves. The transition from reptiles to mammals took approximately 100 million years. When the dinosaurs became extinct, the mammals were able to take over as the ruling forms.

The earliest mammals were four footed and active. Their *cerebral hemispheres had increased in size* and there was potential for more coordinated action than had been present in their reptilian ancestors. They were able to *maintain their body temperature* and were therefore less limited in habitat. The presence of hair represents another of their adaptations. Mammals, in general, showed *improved reproductive patterns.* For example, a placental connection developed between the mother and the embryo allowing the mother to nourish and maintain the young inside her body for a longer period of time. In addition, the presence of *mammary glands* provided further protection for the young by extending their period of dependence on the parent.

Mammals can be divided into two main groups (subclasses): the Prototheria and the Theria. The Prototheria are represented by the archaic egg-laying mammals, which include the duckbill platypus and spiny anteater of Australia. Their skeletal characteristics and chromosomes are so different from other mammals that some suggest they may have descended from the therapsids independently of other mammals. The subclass Theria consists of mammals that bear their young alive. Two different methods evolved. The metatherian animals bore their young alive in an immature stage and continued their development within a pouch. The eutherian animals developed an efficient placenta and retained the young within the uterus for a longer period of time. Man evolved from the Eutheria.

There has been a succession of progressively more modified and highly complex vertebrates during the past half billion years. The influence of adaptation and competition resulted in the sequence leading to the mammals. This sequence, summarized in Fig. 2-11, is as follows:

Ostracodermi, Placodermi, Crossopterygii, Labyrinthodontia, Cotylosauria, Pelycosauria, Therapsida, and Eutheria. The habitat from which
the vertebrates arose (marine or freshwater)

is still disputed, as are the habitats in which
the various classes evolved (cold, semiarid,
tropical). Perhaps we shall never know all the
facts leading to the descent of man.

CLASSIFICATION OF CHORDATES

Phylum Hemichordata
    Class Pterobranchia—colonial forms
    Class Enteropneusta—acorn worms
Phylum Chordata
  Subphylum Urochordata—tunicates
  Subphylum Cephalochordata—amphioxus
  Subphylum Vertebrata—animals with backbones
    Superclass Cyclostomata—jawless vertebrates
      Class Ostracodermi—extinct heavy-armored fish
      Class Myxini—hagfishes
      Class Petromyzontes—lampreys
    Superclass Gnathostomata—jawed vertebrates
      Class Placodermi—extinct jawed vertebrates
      Class Chondrichthyes (Elasmobranchii)—fish with cartilaginous skeletons
        Subclass Selachii—sharks, dogfishes
          Order Squaliformes—sharks and rays
          Order Rajiformes—skates
      Class Holocephali—chimaeras
      Class Osteichthyes—fish with bony skeletons
        Subclass Actinopterygii—ray-finned fish, gills covered with operculum
          Order Chondrostei—primitive fish with cartilage in skeleton, largely extinct
          Order Holostei—dominant during Mesozoic, now represented by garpike and *Amia*
          Order Teleostei—dominant fishes of modern times
        Subclass Dipneusti—lungfish
        Subclass Crossopterygii—fish with fleshy-lobed fins and choanae; ancestral to land vertebrates
      Class Amphibia—first land-living vertebrates without amniote egg
        Order Labyrinthodontia—gave rise to reptiles, now extinct
        Order Anura—frogs, toads
        Order Urodela—salamanders, newts
        Order Apoda—wormlike amphibians of the tropics
        Three extinct orders, in addition
      Class Reptilia—first amniotes
        Subclass Anapsida
          Order Cotylosauria—stem reptile from which other forms are derived, all extinct
          Order Chelonia—turtles
        Subclass Synapsida—extinct forms
          Order Pelycosauria—primitive mammal-like reptiles
          Order Therapsida—advanced mammal-like reptiles
        Subclass Synaptosauria—extinct forms
        Subclass Ichthyopterygia—extinct forms specialized for life in the seas
        Subclass Lepidosauria—one extinct form
          Order Rhynchocephalia—living *Sphenodon* of New Zealand
          Order Squamata—lizards, snakes
        Subclass Archosauria
          Order Thecodontia—extinct ancestors of birds, dinosaurs, etc.
          Order Crocodilia—crocodiles, alligators
      Class Aves—vertebrates with feathers
      Subclass Archeornithes—primitive toothed birds
      Subclass Neornithes—modern birds

Class Mammalia—vertebrates with hair
    Subclass Prototheria—egg-laying mammals
        Order Monotremata—duckbill platypus, spiny anteater
    Subclass Theria—young born alive
      Infraclass Metatheria
        Order Marsupialia—young born in immature state; represented by kangaroo,
          opossum
      Infraclass Eutheria—young retained in body of mother until development com-
        pleted; nourishment, excretion, respiration carried out by efficient placenta
        Order Insectivora—moles, shrews
        Order Dermoptera—flying lemur
        Order Chiroptera—bats
        Order Primates—monkey, apes, man
        Order Edentata—sloths
        Order Pholidota—scaly anteater
        Order Rodentia—rats, mice, squirrels
        Order Lagomorpha—rabbits
        Order Carnivora—dogs, cats, seals
        Order Cetacea—whales, porpoises
        Order Tubulidentata—aardvark
        Order Proboscidea—elephants
        Order Hyracoidea—cony
        Order Sirenia—manatee
        Order Perissodactyla—horse, zebra
        Order Artiodactyla—cattle, deer, sheep

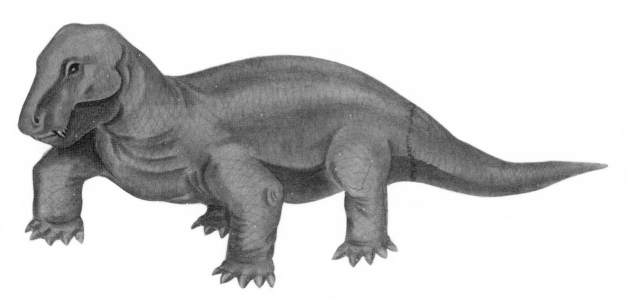

Fig. 2-16
Cynognathus is an example of the Therapsida, one of the mammal-like reptiles of the Triassic period. Many were small and insignificant in size but some were as big as a large dog. Their legs were drawn under their body, enabling more efficient locomotion. They are usually considered the group from which mammals stemmed. (From Hickman, C. P., Sr., Hickman, C. P., Jr., and Hickman, F. M.: Integrated principles of zoology, ed. 4, St. Louis, 1970, The C. V. Mosby Co.)

SUGGESTED READINGS

1. Barrington, E. J. W.: The biology of Hemichordata and Protochordata, San Francisco, 1965, W. H. Freeman & Co., Publishers.
2. Berrill, N. J.: The origin of the vertebrates, New Jersey, 1955, Oxford University Press.
3. Griffin, D. R.: Animal structure and function, Modern Biology Series, New York, 1962, Holt, Rinehart & Winston.
4. Romer, A. S.: The vertebrate body, Philadelphia, 1962, W. B. Saunders Co.
5. Romer, A. S.: Major steps in vertebrate evolution, Science **158:**1629-1637, 1967.
6. Young, J. Z.: The life of vertebrates, Oxford, 1950, Clarendon Press.

CHAPTER 3

REPRODUCTIVE SYSTEM

VERTEBRATE REPRODUCTIVE SYSTEM

The perpetuation of the species is ensured either sexually by union of sperm and egg or asexually by fission or budding. Although asexual reproduction occurs in some chordates (the Urochordata), vertebrate animals have evolved a reproductive system consisting of ovaries or testes, which produce and nurture the gametes, and ducts that transport the eggs or sperm.

Fertilization may take place either internally or externally. If fertilization is external, the female deposits her eggs in the water (spawns) and the male fertilizes them during the process. Although the sperm remain viable for several hours, the egg soon loses its ability to become fertilized, perhaps because of the absorption of water by its jelly coats, which then act as a barrier to sperm penetration. Intromittent organs develop in those animals (mainly terrestrial) with internal fertilization and aid in guiding the sperm to the female reproductive tract. Accessory sexual structures present in the male compensate for the lack of an aquatic environment by secreting a fluid medium for the sperm. Since the sperm are hardly more than sacks of chromosomes, this material, the semen, also provides nourishment for them and induces their motility. The type of fertilization practiced by a few vertebrates, such as newts and salamanders, does not fall into either of the above categories. The male of these animals deposits immobile sperm in small gelatinous packets called spermatophores, on twigs and debris near the female, and she picks them up with her cloacal lips and stores them. Fertilization occurs internally as the eggs leave the oviducts.

The number of eggs released by the vertebrate animal during a breeding period shows a definite relationship to the type of fertilization practiced. Fishes and amphibians ovulate large numbers of eggs. Since the adults abandon the eggs after they are spawned and show no further interest in their fate, the prodigious numbers ensure species survival. For example, it is estimated that a population of Pacific herring releases from 8 to 75 billion eggs each year. Most of them hatch (95%), but only 0.1% survive long enough to reach maturity.

On the other hand, in those species in which the young are nurtured within the body of the mother until the time of birth, only a few eggs are usually released during a reproductive cycle. Normally, a human female ovulates only one.

The vertebrate reproductive system, like all systems in the body, is under the control of chemical agents or *hormones*. Ductless or *endocrine* glands of the body generally produce the hormones, which basically function by modifying cellular metabolism. As a result, they coordinate and integrate the adjustments made by the body to living conditions. Changes in structure, function, or development of the individual organs reflect hormonal control and result in the maintenance of a stable state. The vertebrate reproductive system is an excellent example of a system operating under endocrine control. The cyclic changes in structure, function, and behavior associated with the female reproductive cycle can be correlated with fluctuations in hormone secretion.

Hormones of the hypothalamus and pituitary glands regulate these cycles and the steroid sex hormones produced by the testis or ovary (androgen, estrogen, and progesterone) maintain them. In general, these substances are masculinizing, feminizing, and pregnancy-maintaining, respectively. Integration of the complex factors involved in controlling the sexual cycles is critical. A specific developmental period is essential for each species, and this must be correlated to coincide with that period of the year in which the environmental factors are best suited for development and postnatal care.

Although structural changes in the reproductive system no doubt occurred over the ages, the reproductive organs in present-day vertebrates are essentially similar to one another, despite the fact that they may vary in size, shape, or position within the body. In view of this basic similarity the study of the reproductive system of any vertebrate serves as an illustrative example of the group as a whole.

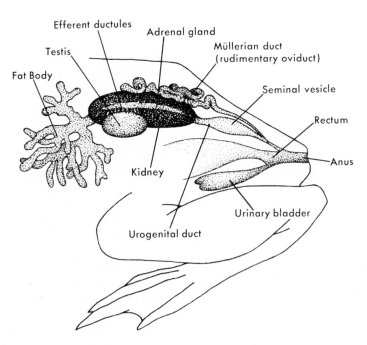

Fig. 3-1
Urogenital system of adult male frog.

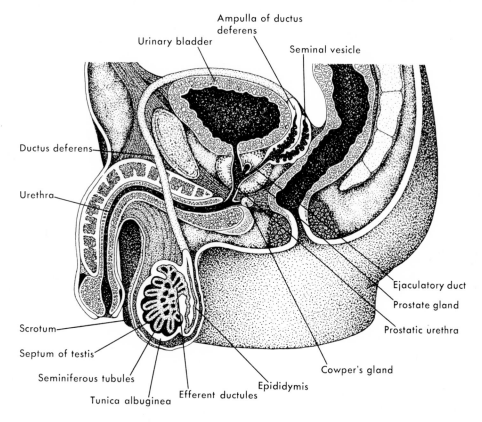

Ampulla of ductus deferens

Urinary bladder

Seminal vesicle

Ductus deferens

Urethra

Ejaculatory duct

Prostate gland

Prostatic urethra

Scrotum

Septum of testis

Seminiferous tubules

Cowper's gland

Tunica albuginea

Efferent ductules

Epididymis

Fig. 3-2
Diagram of adult human male reproductive system.

MALE SYSTEM
Structure of vertebrate testes

The reproductive system of most males consists of a pair of testes, sperm-conducting ducts, and certain accessory tissues. In all vertebrates the testes perform two essential functions necessary for reproduction. They act both as an *exocrine* organ and an endocrine gland, since they produce sperm and also secrete the male hormone. The testes of most vertebrates are located in the upper part of the abdominal cavity lateral to or just anterior to the kidneys as shown for the frog in Fig. 3-1. A double fold of the peritoneal mesentery, the *mesorchium,* usually suspends them from the dorsal wall. In the majority of mammals, however, the testes do not remain in this position within the abdominal cavity, but descend posteriorly into the scrotal sacs as illustrated for man in Fig. 3-2.

Each testis is covered by a thin layer of peritoneal epithelium under which lies a tough connective tissue capsule, the *tunica albuginea.* In some animals septa extend radially to the capsule, thus partitioning the gland into smaller areas; in other cases the testis is lobular or segmented. *Seminiferous tubules,* which produce the sex cells, and *interstitial tissue,* which secretes androgen (the general term for the male hormone), compose the testis regardless of its shape, size, or location.

The tubules may be short (ampulla) or long and tortuous, but in either case their walls usually consist of an outer connective tissue capsule, a thin basement membrane, and a lining of stratified epithelium. Spermatogenesis occurs in these seminiferous tubules. By a series of rapid cell divisions the *spermatogonia,* undifferentiated sex cells located beneath the basement membrane, transform into mature *spermatozoa* and pass into the lumen of the tubules. A cross section through the tubules (Fig. 3-3) reveals many stages of differentiating sperm, usually in more or less distinct layers, located between the basement membrane and the cavity of the tubule. It is possible by repeated cell division of a small number of spermatogonial cells to produce several million sperm each reproductive cycle. It is estimated in man that any single ejaculation releases about 300 million sperm.

Interspersed among the spermatogonia of the seminiferous tubule is a second type of cell, the sustentacular or *Sertoli cell* shown in Fig. 4-9. These cells, wedged between the many layers of cells undergoing division, extend from the basement membrane to the lumen. They help provide structure to the tubule and function as nurse cells for the sperm. The mature sperm has no way of manufacturing its food and must depend upon some external source for its nutritive materials. The heads of several mature sperm embed in membrane folds of the Sertoli cells, where they apparently receive nourishment and remain until released into the genital tract of the male.

In general, most male vertebrates have mature sperm only during breeding periods, whereas during periods of sexual quiescence the tubules undergo changes in which large amounts of lipid material accumulate. There are exceptions to this general statement, however, since some vertebrates have mature sperm the year round. Amphibia and certain male mammals, such as man, remain spermatogenically active. Not all spermatogonia within a tubule mature at one time, since some must remain as reserve cells for future sperm. In some anuran testes, for example, one lobe of the testis may contain active sperm, whereas in an adjacent lobe, all

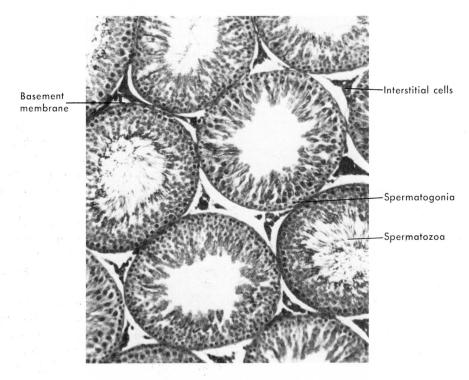

Basement membrane

Interstitial cells

Spermatogonia

Spermatozoa

Fig. 3-3
Transverse section through seminiferous tubules showing stages of differentiating sperm located in layers between basement membrane and the cavity of the tubule. Mature sperm are present in some of the cavities. (× 100.)

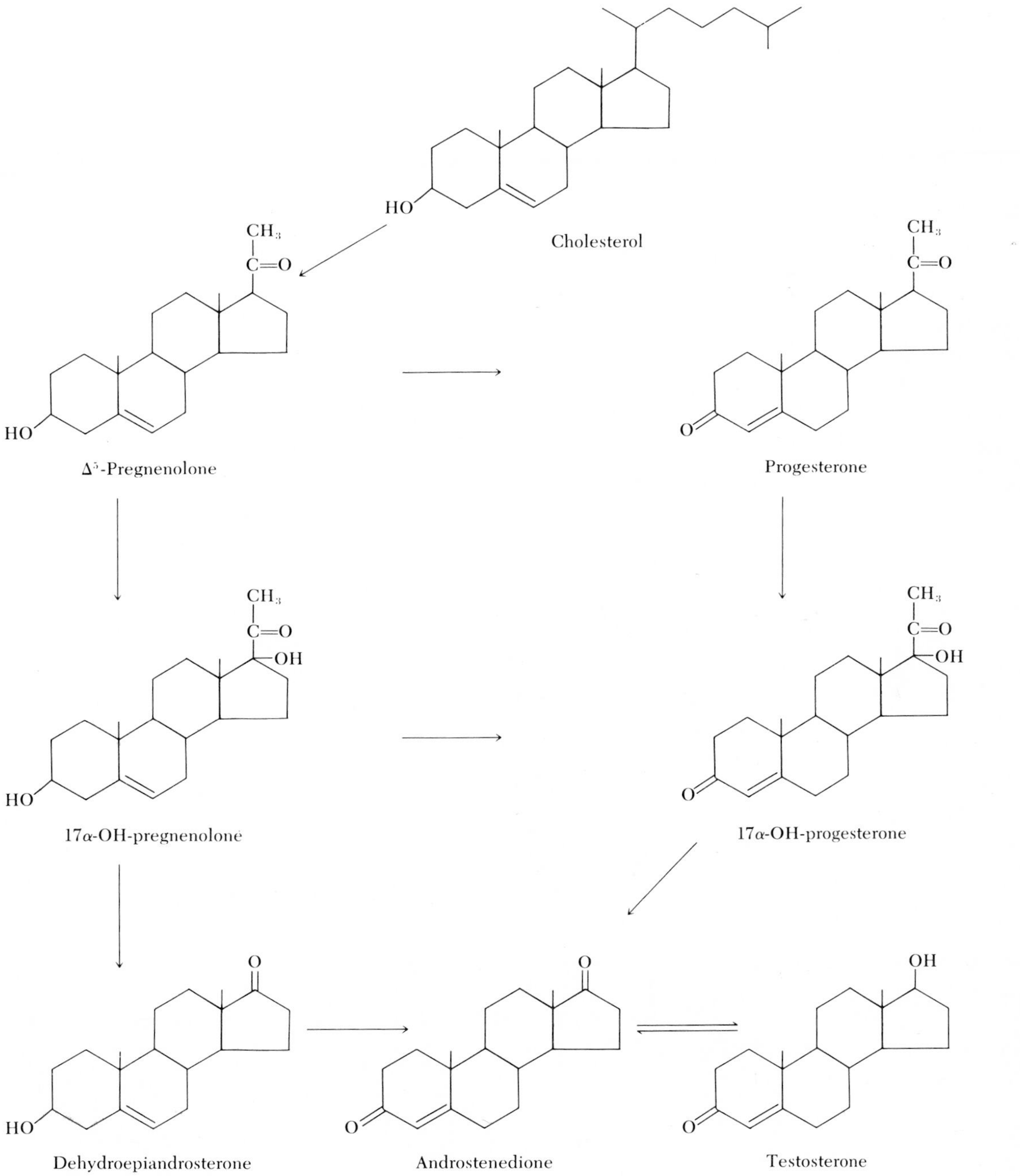

Fig. 3-4
Possible pathway of gonadal synthesis of testosterone and androstenedione, the two main androgens secreted by the testis.

the spermatogonia remain in a quiescent state. In man, one area of seminiferous tubules may be actively producing mature sperm whereas another area may be inactive.

The seminiferous tubules usually anastomose (join together) at their distal ends and empty into straight tubules. These tubules empty into a network of sinuses or channels known as the *rete tubules.* In man, the rete tubules converge to form 12 to 14 *efferent ductules,* which transport the sperm from the testis to the sperm duct. The efferent ductules are located in the mesorchium of lower animals. The ductules appear as thin threads leading from the testis to the anterior end of the sperm duct and may be seen even in a preserved animal if the mesentery is held up to the light.

The *interstitial cells,* or *Leydig cells,* of the testes produce androgen, the masculinizing hormone. These cells, located between the seminiferous tubules, are obvious in the mammal but may exist in less typical forms in other vertebrates. Although the testes are the main androgen-secreting organs, other structures contain the necessary enzymatic machinery for producing the hormone. For example, the ovary, adrenal cortex, and probably the placenta also are capable of synthesizing the male steroid androgen. Testosterone and androstenedione are the main androgens secreted by the testes. These compounds contain 19 carbon atoms and possess methyl groups at C-10 and C-13. Their possible pathway of synthesis in the gonads is given in Fig. 3-4.

The male hormone primarily facilitates spermatogenesis in vertebrates. It also stimulates protein synthesis and growth and maintains the development of those structures associated with

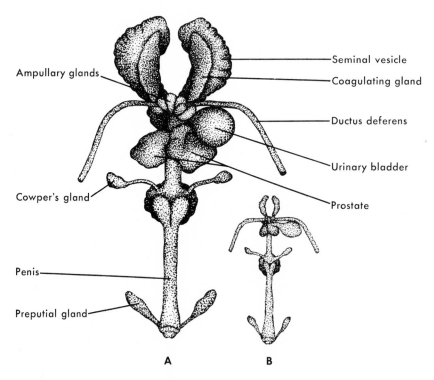

Fig. 3-5

Effect of castration on the genital tract of rats. Both animals were castrated at 30 days of age and autopsied 6 months later. The tracts are drawn to scale. Daily injections of testosterone proprionate for 20 days before autopsy were able to bring the accessory reproductive organs of castrated littermate **A** to approximate normal state. Castrated littermate **B** received no replacement therapy and shows atrophied accessory organs. (Redrawn from Turner, C. D., and Bagnara, J. T.: General endocrinology, ed. 5, Philadelphia, Philadelphia, 1971, W. B. Saunders Co.)

"maleness." The reproductive ducts and the accessory structures are small and undeveloped in those animals that have not reached puberty and in those adult males that are in between breeding cycles. The secretion of the gonadal hormones induces them to become functional. Castration of the male demonstrates the dependence of the ducts and accessory organs on the hormones for maintaining a structurally functional state. Removal of the mammalian testes causes the *ductus deferens, epididymis, prostate,* and *seminal vesicles* to atrophy and soon to resemble the prepubertal state. The effect of castration is shown in Fig. 3-5. Replacement therapy, that is, injection of the proper hormone in correct dosages, restores the male ducts and accessory glands to their normal state.

The secondary sex characteristics in the male are also under the control of androgens. These are characteristics that differentiate one sex from another but have nothing to do with the production of ova and sperm or their transport. They may, however, enhance the attractiveness of one sex for another or aid in the care of the young after hatching or birth. The horns of sheep, plumage of birds, claws of turtle, anal fin of fish, and hair patterns and voice timber of human beings are all examples of secondary sex characteristics; castration suppresses their expression. The comb of birds is so sensitive to androgenic hormones that its reaction consti-

tutes an assay method (capon test) as may be seen in Fig. 3-6. The comb and wattles of the capon resemble those of the hen rather than the cock. In the capon test the castrated cocks are injected with the test material. The degree of growth of comb and wattles from the castrated condition indicates the presence or absence of the male hormone in the test material.

Descent of mammalian testes

In most vertebrates the male gonads retain their position in the upper part of the peritoneal cavity. In the mammal, however, the testes change position during development and migrate posteriorly and ventrally, with the extent depending on the species. This process is depicted in Fig. 3-7. In the eutherian and marsupial mammals the testes descend into the scrotal sacs where they may remain temporarily during the breeding season (bats, moles, and rodents) or permanently, as in man. The descent of the testes of the human male normally occurs about the seventh or ninth month of gestation. If the testes remain within the abdominal cavity and do not descend into the sacs, the condition is called *cryptorchidism.* When it happens to both testes, the individual is sterile, since no sperm will develop. Fig. 3-8 demonstrates the effects of experimentally induced unilateral cryptorchidism in the adult rat. The shrunken left testis was confined to the abdominal cavity

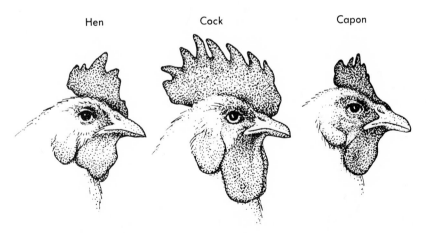

Hen	Cock	Capon

Fig. 3-6
Effect of castration on the secondary sex characteristics of birds. The comb and wattles of the capon resemble those of the hen more than those of the cock.

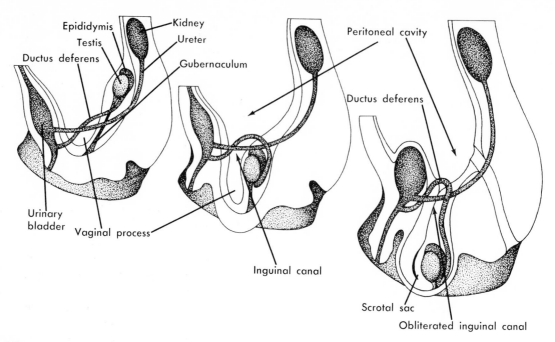

Fig. 3-7
Descent of human testis. The testis is technically never actually in the cavity of the scrotal sac but is covered by the peritoneal epithelium. See text for description.

for a period of time; the right testis occupied its normal position in the scrotal sac. The cryptorchid testis was sterile but sperm was present in the right. Mature sperm are sensitive to the high temperatures of the abdomen but the lower scrotal temperature, 1 to 8 centigrade degrees cooler, promotes spermatogenesis. Spermatogonia, on the other hand, are more resistant to temperature and die only after prolonged exposure to heat. The scrotal sacs, therefore, apparently have a temperature-regulating function, and knowledge of this fact led some Orientals to take hot baths as a form of birth control.

Although the cryptorchid individual is sterile, he retains all of his secondary sex characteristics, since the interstitial cells secrete the male hormone at either temperature. Cryptorchidism emphasizes the dual role of the testis; its endocrine activities remain normal under conditions that inhibit its exocrine functions. Birds lack scrotal sacs. Although they have a higher body temperature than mammals, they are able to function spermatogenically. Possibly, in these animals the air sacs wrap around the testes in

the abdominal cavity and keep them cooler than the other visceral organs.

The scrotal sacs form as evaginated coelomic pouches in the floor of the abdominal cavity, and in early development are continuous with the body cavity by way of the *inguinal canal.* This canal remains in those animals in which there is temporary testicular displacement, but is obliterated in those in which there is permanent testicular descent. The skin, muscle, and connective tissue of the body wall form the wall of the scrotal pouches, and the peritoneal epithelium furnishes their lining. They may remain as two separate cavities but usually fuse and form a single scrotum with a partition between them. The testis is never actually in the cavity of the scrotal sac, since it is always *retroperitoneal,* that is, technically outside the peritoneal cavity, and covered by the peritoneal epithelium (see Fig. 3-7). The *gubernaculum,* which represents the posterior differentiation of the mesorchium, anchors the testis to the floor of the scrotum. As the testis descends into the scrotal sac, it carries with it the blood and lymph vessels, the nerves, and the sperm duct. These structures constitute the *spermatic cord.*

Male ducts and accessory structures

The cyclostomes, such as the lamprey, release their sperm cells into their body cavity, from which they escape to the outside through germinal pores. There are no sperm-conducting ducts in these animals. All other male vertebrates have both reproductive ducts that transport the sperm to the outside and accessory structures that contribute to the nutrition, maturation, and motility of the sperm. In most vertebrates the sperm is unable to fertilize an egg until it has come into contact with the secretions of these accessory glands.

The sperm released into the lumina of the seminiferous tubules are immobile, and the pressure of accumulated fluid is believed to move them along to the rete tubules. There is some evidence that in the frog the fluid accumulates because of the conversion of an acid mucopolysaccharide, hyaluronic acid, into its component parts. Van Oordt et al., 1958, showed that when this occurred, water is taken up in the seminiferous tubule from the surrounding capillaries. The force of the current is great enough to loosen the sperm bundles from the Sertoli cells and move them toward the efferent ducts. Spermatozoa collect in the tubules of the rete testes and then pass to the efferent ductules where the beating of the ciliated epithelium aid in further movement of the sperm toward the epididymis. The epididymis in man is a highly coiled elongated tube, 15 to 20 feet long, which adheres closely to the surface of the testes. Because of its great length, it can store countless spermatozoa. In the lower animals the seminal vesicle also takes over this function.

The sperm duct is a confusing structure to many students, since it is assigned a variety of names in anatomy textbooks. Its specific name depends on the animal in which it is described or the functions it performs, that is, whether it conducts only sperm, or both sperm and

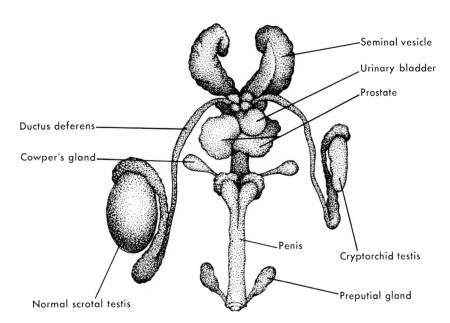

Fig. 3-8

Effect of unilateral cryptorchidism in the rat. The left testis was confined to the abdominal cavity for 6 months where it underwent regressive changes. Sperm were absent in the cryptorchid testis but were present in the testis allowed to remain in its normal position within the scrotal sac. Drawn to scale. (Redrawn from Turner, C. D., and Bagnara, J. T.: General endocrinology, ed. 5, Philadelphia, 1971, W. B. Saunders Co.)

urine. In reptiles, birds, and mammals the paired sperm ducts are composed of the anterior *epididymis,* which receives the sperm from the testes, and the *ductus deferens,* which carries it to the cloaca or urethra. As shown in Fig. 3-9, the duct has a thick muscular wall, adapted to fast transport of the sperm and functions only in sperm conduction in the amniote. The reproductive ducts of lower animals apparently evolved from the primitive urinary ducts and carry both sperm and urine to the outside. In these animals the epididymis and the anterior part of the duct serve to transport sperm, but renal tubules open into the more posterior regions of the duct and empty their contents also into the lumen. In the fishes and amphibians this duct is usually referred to as the wolffian, opisthonephric, or mesonephric duct, although the amniote term "ductus deferens" is also used.

It is the sperm duct, or ductus deferens, that opens into the cloaca of most vertebrates or the urethra of higher mammals. In such animals as the frog and salamander a dilation or lateral pocket forms from the sperm duct near the cloaca. These pockets are known as the *seminal vesicles.* Sperm collect here until released, and the organs therefore have a different structure as well as function from the seminal vesicles of mammals.

In these days of overpopulation a simple operation known as vasectomy is gaining popularity as a method of birth control. According to some reports 275,000 American males underwent surgery in 1970. Vasectomy is a surgical operation, usually performed in the surgeon's office in about 20 minutes, in which the ductus deferens is cut or tied off from the epididymis. Sperm thus no longer pass from the testes to the outside, but the "maleness" of the individual, which is under the control of androgens se-

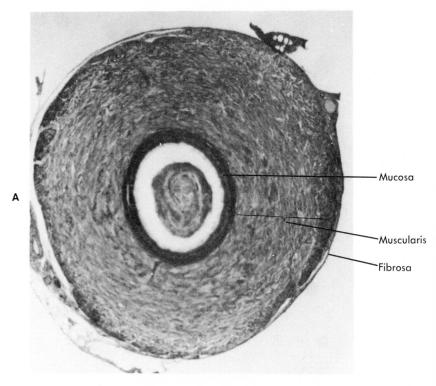

Mucosa

Muscularis

Fibrosa

Fig. 3-9
A, Wall of the ductus deferens consists of three layers: an inner mucosa, a middle muscularis, and an outer fibrosa. Transverse sections reveal the muscularis to be the thickest coat. (× 40.) **B,** A portion of the mucosa showing the ciliated epithelial cells lining the lumen. (× 450.)

creted by the interstitial cells, is not diminished. Perhaps the main advantages of this procedure are the lack of side effects (such as may be caused in the female by the Pill) and its great success as a form of contraception. Its main disadvantage is that it is not easily reversible in case there is a change of plans, divorce, or death of children.

In mammals the paired spermatic cords originate at the scrotal sac and pass through the muscles of the abdominal wall and into the peritoneal cavity. The ductus deferens separates from the spermatic cord, loops over the urinary ducts (the ureters), and turns posteriorly toward the median line (see Fig. 3-7). It passes along the dorsal surface of the bladder and enters the structure distal to the entrance of the urinary ducts from the kidneys. Posterior to the entrance of the ductus deferens the tube or duct that opens to the outside is called the *urethra*. The

relationship of these structures is shown in Fig. 3-2. Since the urethra originates in the bladder, it carries both urine and sperm.

Just before each ductus deferens terminates in the prostatic portion of the urethra it enlarges to form the *ampulla* and then gradually narrows to give rise to the *ejaculatory duct*. A prostate gland surrounds the urethra at this point, and the ejaculatory duct penetrates the gland as it joins the urethra. In most mammals, convoluted sacs known as the *seminal vesicles* open into the ejaculatory duct. The *bulbourethral glands*, or *Cowper's glands*, are located on the urethra posterior to the prostate. The penis encloses the terminal portion of the urethra.

The ampullary gland, prostate gland, seminal vesicle, and bulbourethral glands all have a typical glandular structure and secrete their substances into the lumen of the reproductive duct. Fig. 3-10 shows a section through the

B

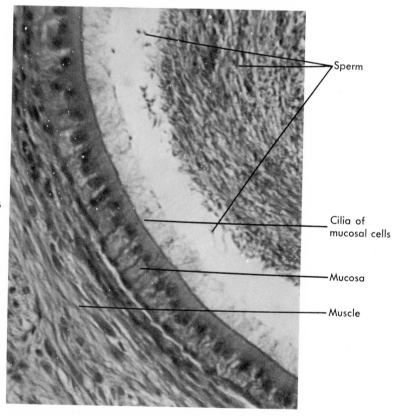

Sperm

Cilia of mucosal cells

Mucosa

Muscle

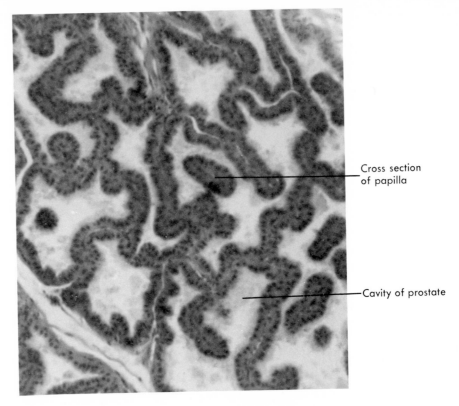

Cross section
of papilla

Cavity of prostate

Fig. 3-10
Section of cat prostate. This accessory male gland surrounds the urethra at its origin from the urinary bladder and empties its secretions into its lumen by way of several independent ducts. A cross section shows folds of epithelium projecting into the cavity of the gland. Some of the branching papillae appear as isolated islands. (× 100.)

prostate gland, demonstrating its glandular composition. Castration of the male animal demonstrates the dependence of these glands on hormonal control. The seminal vesicle is especially sensitive to androgen and undergoes cytological degeneration within 2 days after removal of the testes. The secretions of these glands, along with the spermatozoa and cellular debris from the reproductive tract, make up the *semen*. The volume of the semen from a single ejaculation varies from time to time and from individual to individual, but is around 2 to 6 ml. It is especially rich in fructose, an energy source for the motile sperm, secreted by the seminal vesicle. It is also rich in prostaglandins. These parahormones affect the circulation, smooth muscle, and nervous system, and are the subjects of much recent investigation.

The testes of vertebrates do not contain motile sperm. Contact with water or chemicals liberated by the egg induces motility in some animals. The secretions of the male reproductive tract and accessory glands are necessary to stimulate activity in the mammalian sperm. Secretions of the prostate appear especially important.

FEMALE SYSTEM
Structure of vertebrate ovary

The vertebrate ovary also functions both as an exocrine and as an endocrine organ. It produces ova and the steroid sex hormones estrogen and progesterone, which regulate the reproductive tract, secondary sex characteristics, and mating behavior of the female. The ovary is suspended from the dorsal body wall just behind the kidneys by a section of the peritoneum called the *mesovarium* and may be classified morphologically into either a solid or saccular type. Most vertebrates have a pair of ovaries, but a single structure is found in many fish, probably representing a fusing of the two original ovaries since it has a typical vertebrate structure. In some animals, birds for example, only one side of the reproductive tract develops and the ovary on the other side remains inactive or degenerates.

The external shape of the ovary varies according to the species and to the reproductive state of the individual. In the frog, during the breeding months the multilobed organ fills the body cavity, actually stretching the body wall. After ovulation, the ovary involutes and looks like a ruffled piece of mesentery. The ovary of birds is an enormous structure because of both the accumulation of yolk in individual eggs and of the fact that the female bird ovulates one egg per day for several months. The human ovary is a relatively small, walnut-shaped body measuring $4 \times 2 \times 1$ cm.

The *saccular* type of ovary, represented by the frog in Fig. 3-11, consists primarily of an outer area where the eggs are located and a lymph-filled central space, connecting with the cavities of other lobes. The *solid* ovary (Figs. 3-12 and 3-13) can be divided into two areas: an outer region, the *cortex*, containing many ova in various stages of development, and an inner *medulla*, consisting of irregularly arranged connective tissue, blood, and lymph vessels. *Interstitial cells*, similar to those found in the male, are embedded in the framework or *stroma* of the ovary, and are prominent in some species. A dense connective tissue layer, the *tunica albuginea*, covers the cortex. External to the tunic, the peritoneal epithelium surrounds the ovary. This epithelium was unfortunately named the *germinal epithelium* by the early biologists who believed that these cells were the source of the primordial germ cells, the future eggs and sperm. However, studies involving histochemical staining techniques demonstrate that the primordial germ cells originate in other areas of the body, outside the gonad, and migrate into it during development.

Regardless of the morphology of the ovary (saccular or solid) possessed by the vertebrate, the germ cells take up their position within the cortical region where clusters of epithelial cells surround each ovum and form a *follicle*. The follicular cells are believed to arise from the germinal epithelium. In electron micrographs protoplasmic connections extend from the follicle cells to the surface of the egg and evidently aid in providing nutrition for the growing oocyte (Fig. 4-12). For this reason, they are often referred to as "nurse cells." These follicular cells (along possibly with the *theca interna* cells) synthesize the hormone *estrogen*.

A young follicle, one whose wall is only one cell thick, is initially located in the cortex of the ovary embedded in the connective tissue stroma. The stroma contributes additional connective tissue cells to the follicle in the form of sheaths around the follicular epithelium. These sheaths differentiate into an external fibrous layer, the *theca externa*, and an inner vascular layer, the *theca interna*. As the number of connective tissue sheaths increase, the follicles move away from the periphery of the ovary into the deeper areas of the cortex.

When the oocyte matures in the *viviparous* mammal, the number of follicular cells increases because of cellular proliferation. Consequently, several layers of cells, known as the *membrana granulosa*, surround the mature ovum. Small cavities appear in spaces between the follicle cells and coalesce to form a large crescent-shaped, fluid-filled space, the *antrum*. At this stage the egg, eccentrically located within the follicle and surrounded by a small mass of granulosa cells, projects from one wall of the follicle into the antrum like a small peninsula. This condition is clearly shown in Fig. 3-12. The mature mammalian follicle with large antrum, ovum, membrana granulosa, theca interna, and theca externa is known as the *graafian follicle*. It may extend the width of the cortex, actually forming a bulge on the surface of the ovary. With the exception of the mammal, most vertebrate eggs are relatively large, because of the accumulation of yolk material. They fill their follicular cavities, leaving no room for the development of an antrum; only a small fluid-filled space remains between egg and

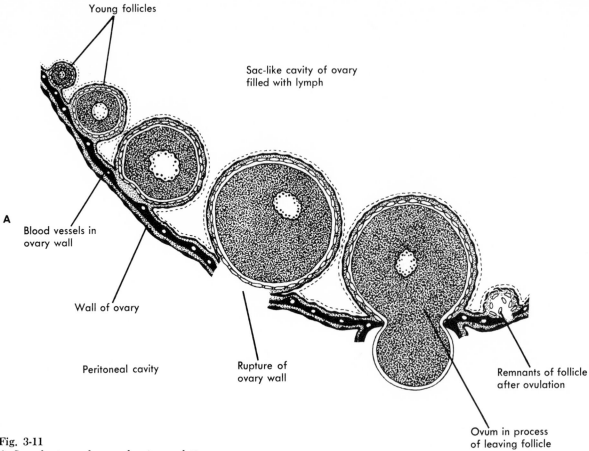

Young follicles

Sac-like cavity of ovary
filled with lymph

A

Blood vessels in
ovary wall

Wall of ovary

Peritoneal cavity

Rupture of
ovary wall

Remnants of follicle
after ovulation

Ovum in process
of leaving follicle

Fig. 3-11
A, Saccular type of ovary showing ovulation.

follicle wall. Consequently, in these animals the follicular cells are thin and not as conspicuous as those seen in the mammal.

In a newborn human infant as many as 400,000 follicles have been counted in serial sections of both ovaries. Whether this represents all the oogonia that the female will have during her lifetime is not clear, since there is no agreement about the formation of new oogonia after birth. In general, there is little evidence to demonstrate that new germ cells form postnatally. Many believe that the female possesses all the eggs in her ovary at birth that she will ever have. If this concept is correct, anything that destroys her oogonia leaves her sterile, since she will be unable to replace them. Of the 400,000 follicles present at birth only a few reach maturity. The human female is capable of reproducing for about 30 to 35 years,

that is, from puberty to the menopause. If the maturation and release of one egg occurs each month, only about 400 eggs will be ovulated. The rest will degenerate.

When the egg and follicle mature, the surface of the ovary thins because of the increased internal pressure. The wall becomes necrotic, ruptures, and releases the egg into the body cavity. This process of freeing the ovum from the ovary is called *ovulation* and is under the control of pituitary, hypothalamic, and ovarian hormones.

The number of eggs released from the ovary at any one time is determined genetically for each species. In those vertebrates that lay their eggs and then desert them, species survival depends on the production of large numbers of eggs, since the mortality is high. Certain fishes spawn several million eggs each season.

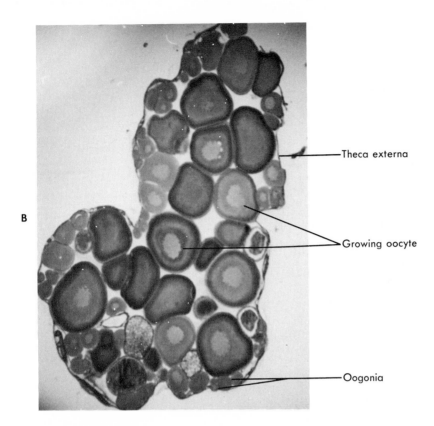

B

Theca externa

Growing oocyte

Oogonia

Fig. 3-11, cont'd
B, A section through a growing frog ovary. (× 40.)

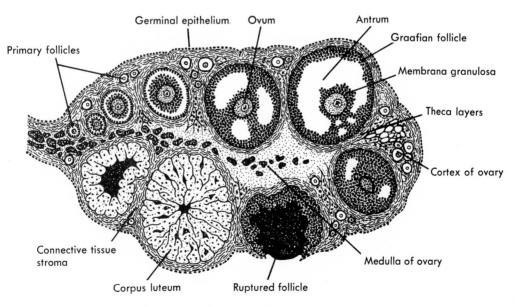

Germinal epithelium

Ovum

Antrum

Primary follicles

Graafian follicle

Membrana granulosa

Theca layers

Cortex of ovary

Connective tissue stroma

Corpus luteum

Ruptured follicle

Medulla of ovary

Fig. 3-12
Mammalian ovary showing successive stages of follicular growth.

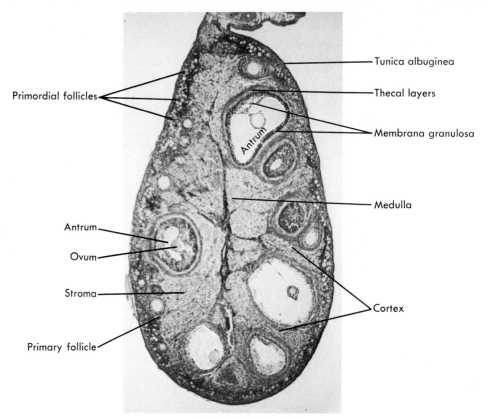

Primordial follicles

Antrum

Antrum

Ovum

Stroma

Primary follicle

Tunica albuginea

Thecal layers

Membrana granulosa

Medulla

Cortex

Fig. 3-13
Section through a maturing ovary. Many primordial follicles and several primary follicles are located in cortex. Note ovum, antrum, membrana granulosa, and theca layers of mature follicle. ($\times$ 4.)

Frogs shed as many as 2000 to 3000 eggs at one time. On the other hand, normally only one graafian follicle matures at any one cycle in the human female, but in those mammals that usually have multiple births, several follicles may mature and rupture, releasing eggs. The female dog may ripen seven or more follicles as compared to the sow that releases four to ten eggs each cycle.

In the human species fraternal, or *dizygotic twins* result when two separate eggs are ovulated and fertilized. These embryos have separate implantation sites and are assumed to be comparable to any other sibling (that is children born of the same parents but at different times). The tendency to bear two-egg twins appears inherited, although statistics are not complete and the mechanism is not understood. Hormone production, which is under control of the genes, may be the responsible factor in inducing multiple ovulations.

The development and maturation of ovarian follicles and the release of their eggs appear to be similar processes in all vertebrates. The granulosa cells of the ruptured mammalian follicle become filled with a yellow pigment. They transform into luteal cells, giving rise to the yellow body, or *corpus luteum*. This structure is capable of secreting estrogen but is considered the primary source of progesterone, the pregnancy hormone. The corpus luteum grows and functions for a certain period of time. If fertilization does not take place, it degenerates and transforms into a *corpus albicans,* which remains as a small scar on the ovary at the site of the former corpus luteum. If fertilization occurs, the corpus luteum remains for part or all of the duration of pregnancy. Luteal bodies form in representatives of every vertebrate class, and progesterone is present in some animals that lack corpora lutea. Endocrinologists are investigating the significance of these bodies in vertebrates other than mammals. There is evidence that they do not function as endocrine glands associated with pregnancy. Instead, they may have some kind of phagocytic activity in which they remove degenerating eggs or follicular debris (Hisaw, 1958). The corpus luteum may be an example of a structure whose function changed as animals evolved from the oviparous to the viviparous condition.

Female ducts

Most vertebrates are *oviparous;* that is, they lay eggs which range in size from almost microscopic to large heavy-shelled ones, and development occurs externally to the mother. Obviously, since no arrangement is made for the sperm to enter the shelled egg, fertilization must occur before the shell is secreted about the egg. In some cases the reproductive tract of the mother retains the fertilized eggs. The mother does not nourish the young directly, but they live off the food stored within the eggs. They hatch from the eggs within the confines of the mother's uterus and are brought forth alive. Such animals are *ovoviviparous;* certain sharks are examples. The marsupial and placental animals are *viviparous.* The eggs of these animals are small and almost devoid of yolk. The young remain within the uterus of the mother during developmental stages and are born as living replicas of the adult.

The period of development within the body of the mother varies with the species and is referred to as the *gestation* time. It may be anywhere from 20 to 21 days for the rat to 607 to 641 days for the elephant. See Table 3-1. The human embryo takes 270 to 295 days to complete its development. Viviparity requires structural modification of the reproductive tract. The establishment of an intimate association between mother and the embryo allows the young to receive food and excrete wastes. The formation of this intimate relationship is referred to as placentation. The structure formed, the placenta, develops partly from the maternal tis-

TABLE 3-1. Duration of gestation

Animal	Days[*]
Dogfish (*Mustelus canis*)	300
Opossum (marsupial)	12-13
Mouse	19-20
Rat	20-22
Red-necked wallaby (marsupial)	30
Rabbit	28-32
Squirrel	30-40
Giant kangaroo (marsupial)	39
Fox	52-63
Guinea pig	62-70
Dog	60-65
Cat	52-65
Lion	105-115
Pig	112-120
Sheep	145-155
Rhesus monkey	150-170
Chimpanzee	250
Man	270-295
Cow	275-290
Horse	330-345
Whale	334-365
Giraffe	400-480
Elephant	500-730

[*]Statistics obtained from various sources.

sues derived from the female reproductive tract (the uterine wall) and partly from extraembryonic tissues associated with the embryo.

Most vertebrates release their ova into the body cavity. The eggs of the cyclostomes (the lampreys and hagfish) leave the coelomic cavity by way of a pair of posteriorly placed abdominal pores. In all other vertebrates, a pair of *müllerian tubes,* or *oviducts,* conduct the ova to the outside. The anterior ends of these ducts are located near the ovary; the posterior ends empty into the cloaca of all chordates except mammals.

In general, the ovary is not attached to the oviduct. The anterior end of the duct is a fringed, ciliated funnel, the *infundibulum,* located near the ovary as shown for the human female in Fig. 3-14. When the follicle ruptures and releases ripe eggs, they are caught in the funnel-shaped *ostium* (opening). They begin their journey down the duct aided by the beating of the cilia. In animals such as the frog (see Fig. 3-15), the ovary is located some distance from the ostium. Cilia located on the

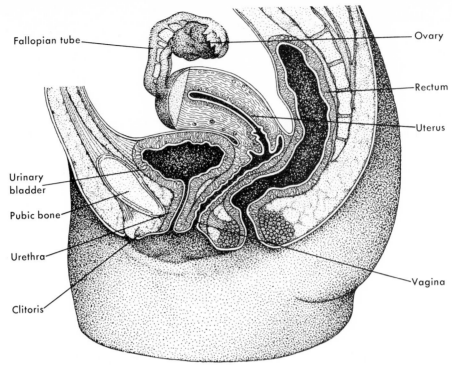

Fig. 3-14
Diagram of adult human female reproductive system.

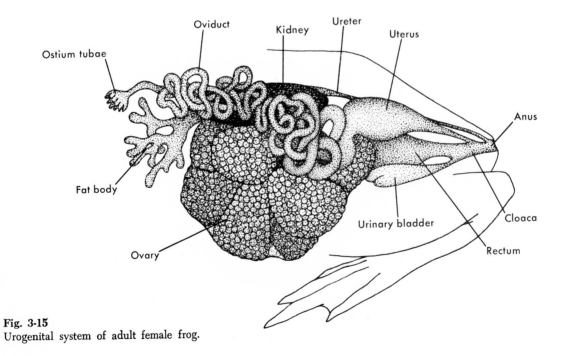

Fig. 3-15
Urogenital system of adult female frog.

viscera (liver, peritoneum, etc.) beat in the direction of the openings and help move the eggs toward the mouth of the oviduct. It takes about 2 hours for a newly ovulated frog's egg to reach one of these openings.

The oviduct, like the male reproductive duct, is more than a transport system. It changes the chemical makeup of the egg in some way so that it can be fertilized. Eggs obtained from the frog's ovary or coelomic cavity are not fertilizable. However, if they are removed from the oviduct a short distance posterior to the ostium, they can be induced to cleave by normal sperm suspension (Rugh, 1951).

Although these ducts are essentially similar in all vertebrates, various areas are modified and serve the needs of the particular animal. The walls of the frog's oviduct secrete three jelly coats about the ovum in the 2 to 4 hours it takes the egg to travel down the duct. The eggs are temporarily stored in the enlarged distal end, the highly elastic *uterus*. In birds and reptiles, on the other hand, a shell must also be deposited about the egg. In these animals the oviduct is divided into three regions; the *magnum*, in which albumen coats the ovum, the *isthmus*, where the secretion of soft shell membranes occur, and the *uterus*, in which the shell is deposited around the egg.

In the majority of vertebrates the two oviducts remain separated and terminate at the cloaca. However, in the mammals, as may be seen in Fig. 3-16, the anterior portion of the oviduct differentiates into a *fallopian tube*, which contains the ostium, and the muscular *uterus*, which is the site of embryonic implantation. In the egg-laying mammals (the monotremes) the uteri empty into the cloaca, but in the higher mammals the cloaca is modified and the uteri terminate in the *vagina*. In these mammals the uteri and vagina usually are fused to different degrees, although the fallopian tubes remain separated. Fusion of oviducts is shown diagrammatically in Fig. 3-16. For example, in the marsupials there is only fusion of the vaginas *(duplex type)*. On the other hand, in man and apes, both uteri and vaginas are fused along their entire length, and only the Fallopian tubes are separate *(simplex type)*. Carnivores and un-

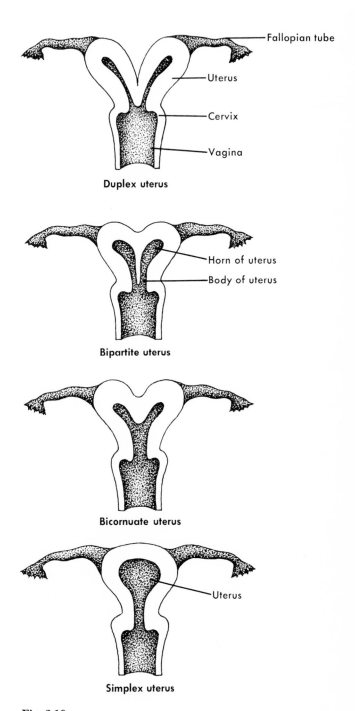

Fig. 3-16
Fusion of oviducts to form various types of mammalian uteri. See text for description.

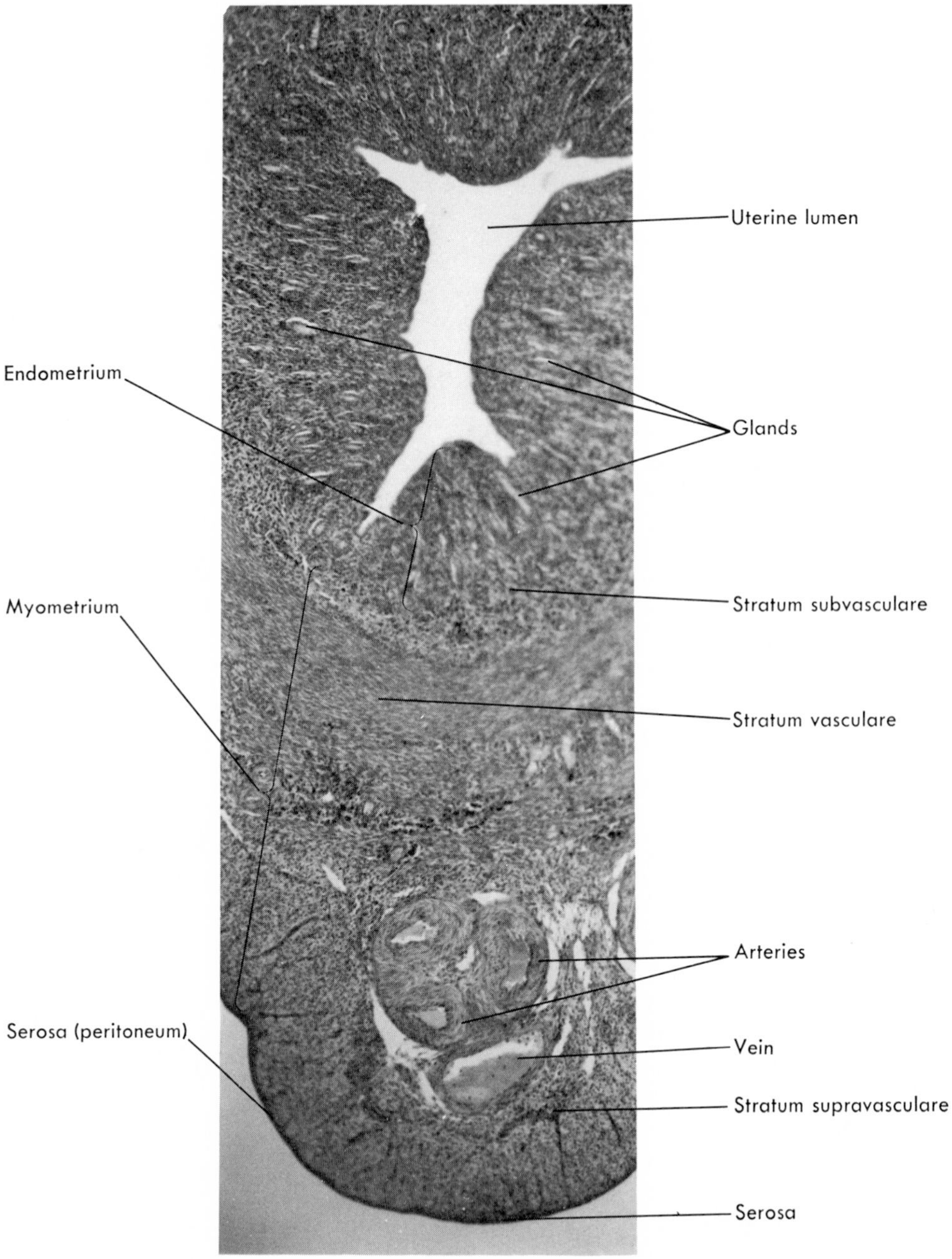

Uterine lumen

Endometrium

Glands

Myometrium

Stratum subvasculare

Stratum vasculare

Arteries

Serosa (peritoneum)

Vein

Stratum supravasculare

Serosa

Fig. 3-17
Part of wall of uterus showing three basic layers: endometrium, myometrium, and serosa. Many tubular glands present in the endometrium open directly into the lumen of the uterus. Large arteries and veins located in the stratum vasculare give the wall a spongy appearance. (× 10.)

gulates represent stages in between. The vaginas and lower parts of the uteri fuse to a single *body*, while the anterior parts of the uteri remain separate and make up the *horns* of the uterus. In the pregnant cat, the uterine horns become greatly enlarged, exhibiting a series of bulges containing the embryos. Some rodents have a *bipartite* type of oviduct in which a partition, representing the fused walls of the uteri, remain, but in the carnivores this partition is absent and only the horns remain separate (*bicornuate*).

The nonpregnant human uterus is a pear-shaped structure averaging about 7 cm. in length, the lumen of which conforms to the general shape of the structure. Anatomically the uterus is divided into an upper *body* with a dome-shaped top, the *fundus*, and a terminal *cervix*, which opens into the vagina. The fallopian tubes, which are about 15 cm. long, terminate in the lateral part of the uterine cavity. The lumen of the uterus is lined with a glandular membrane, the *endometrium*, and is especially adapted for implantation and maintenance of the embryo. The specific details of this process and the contribution of the endometrium toward the formation of the placenta are discussed in Chapter 9. The epithelial surface of the endometrium penetrates the deeper layers of the uterus to form tubular uterine glands, the growth of which are under the control of hormones. These glands may be seen in Fig. 3-17, showing a section through a mature uterus. The uterus walls consist of a large mass of smooth muscle, the *muscularis* or *myometrium*, with individual muscle cells varying in length according to the stage of the menstrual cycle. During pregnancy the mass of uterine tissue increases about 24 times because of an increase in both the number of muscle cells and fiber length. Some muscle cells in the pregnant uterus grow as much as 10 times their nonpregnant length.

The mesenteries, the *mesotubaria*, anchor the oviducts in place in the body. However, these structures have some independent movement. For example, there must be allowance for the growth of the uterus in the pregnant mammal. In these animals the mesotubarium develops into the *broad ligament* that supports the horns and body of the uterus and the blood vessels, lymphatics, and nerves that pass to it. A *round ligament*, believed to be comparable to the gubernaculum of the male, anchors the uterus to the posterior wall of the pelvis and is located at right angles to the broad ligament.

EXTERNAL GENITALIA

Most aquatic animals spawn their eggs or sperm directly into the water where fertilization occurs. Eggs accumulate in the uteri of the females and sperm in the seminal vesicles of males until deposited into the cloaca. Males and females merely come in proximity with one another and release their eggs or sperm. Most birds copulate by cloacal contact. Sperm is deposited in the female cloaca. Cilia, beating toward the ovarian end of the reproductive tract, aid the sperm in its passage up the oviduct to the infundibulum. Fertilization occurs in the anterior regions of the duct well before any membrane deposition begins about the egg.

In those lower animals that practice internal fertilization some structure such as the pelvic fins of the male shark or anal fin ray of fish are modified as accessory genital apparatuses to guide the sperm along the proper path. Erectile structures located either outside the cloaca (hemipenis of snakes and lizards) or inside the cloaca (introcloacal penis of turtles, crocodiles, and some birds) when inserted in the cloaca of the female, aid in the transfer and guidance of sperm to the female tract.

In both male and female embryos of placental mammals there is division of the cloaca during the later stages of organ formation. As a result, the openings of the urogenital ducts shift and the urinary bladder forms from the base of the allantois. The development of the external genitalia reflects the modification of the cloacal chamber. The details of this architectural change are best described in the chapter on urogenital development. It is sufficient to state here that the external genitalia of the male and of the female have a common embryonic origin. Development in the male includes the penis, an erectile copulatory organ, and a scrotum, which has already been described. In the female the labia minora border the opening of the vagina and the labia majora surround the clitoris (considered a homolog of the male penis).

REPRODUCTIVE CYCLES

The gonads of vertebrates are not independent structures and do not function continuously, but rather they fluctuate cyclically during the reproductive period of the individual's life. In most vertebrates the cycle is a yearly one and, in the temperate zone, many breed in the spring (when conditions are best for hatching or birth). This reproductive season alternates with a sexually quiescent one in which the ovaries and testes regress. The individual during this time is anatomically and physiologically incapable of reproducing. Domestication and selection modifies this basic pattern and some domestic birds and mammals carry on reproductive activity throughout the year. Higher primates, including man, can breed at any time.

During their reproductive season most poikilothermic (cold-blooded) vertebrates enter into a period of courtship that terminates in mating and spawning. The fertilized eggs are then abandoned by the adults who become reproductively inactive. The reproductive cycles of birds and mammals are more complex, involving periods of incubation or gestation that call for corresponding changes in adult behavior.

Control of reproductive cycles

The production of sperm or ova and the synthesis and release of the sex hormones do not occur randomly in vertebrates. *Gonadotrophic* (gonad-stimulating) *hormones*, produced by the anterior lobe of the pituitary gland (hypophysis) control the function of the gonads. These hypophyseal hormones are released into the bloodstream and carried to the ovary or testis where they produce their effect. The gonadotrophic hormones are believed to be the same in both male and female, differing quantitatively rather than qualitatively. The target organ itself (ovary or testis) determines the effect of their stimulation. The names given to these hormones refer to their functions in the female.

The pituitary gland releases two hormones that affect both the ovaries and testes—the *follicle stimulating hormone* (FSH) and the *luteinizing hormone* (LH). They control seasonal reproductive cycles as shown in Fig. 3-18. Two different cell types in the pituitary apparently produce these two hormones. Each hormone has a specific function although they also act synergistically; that is, they produce greater effects when administered together than when given separately at the same dose levels. The follicle stimulating hormone (FSH) acts on the seminiferous tubules in the male, where it stimulates spermatogenesis. In the female, it affects the growth of the follicular cells and the secretion of estrogen. The luteinizing hormone (LH), sometimes referred to as the *interstitial cell stimulating hormone* (ICSH), causes the interstitial cells of the testis (and perhaps the ovary) to secrete the male hormone. It also stimulates the luteal cells of the ovary to release progesterone. A third gonadotrophic hormone, *prolactin* or the *lactogenic hormone* (LTH), appears to affect only the ovary; no definite function has been ascribed to it in the testis. The ovaries and testes have little autonomous control over themselves, but are regulated by a feedback mechanism sensitive to fluctuating levels of gonadotrophic hormones circulating in the blood.

Concept of feedback regulation

Although the pituitary gland stimulates the gonads to secrete their hormones, a reciprocal interaction exists between the two organs. The activity of the pituitary is also inhibited by certain circulating levels of the sex steroids. This relationship has been termed *negative feedback*. At first, researchers believed that androgen, estrogen, or progesterone acted directly on the cells of the pituitary. If their circulating levels were high, they inhibited gonadotrophic secretion. On the other hand, if the circulating sex steroids fell below a certain level, the pituitary was stimulated to release more FSH and LH. A simple feedback mechanism (see Fig. 3-19) was hypothesized to explain the relationship that existed between the pituitary and its target organs, ovaries and testes. Investigations over the past two decades, however, indicate that the explanation is not so simple. Pituitary function can be modified by environmental and emotional factors that affect higher brain cen-

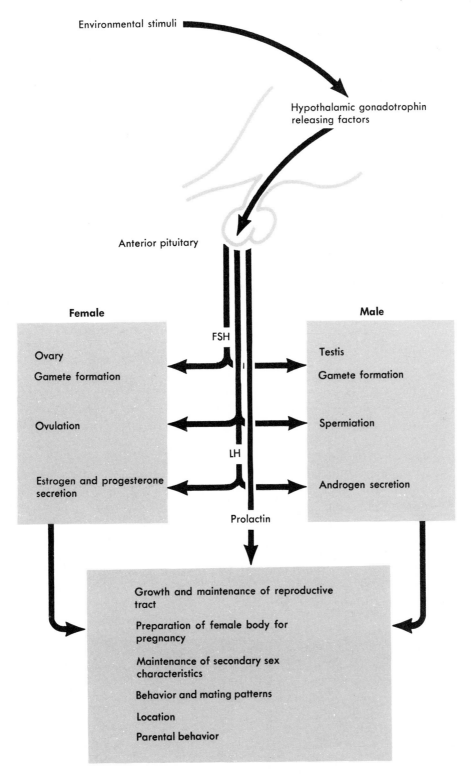

Fig. 3-18
Control of seasonal reproductive cycles by the pituitary hormones and hypothalamic factors.

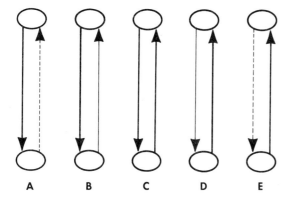

Fig. 3-19
Diagram of simple negative-feedback mechanism operating in endocrine control. At first the pituitary stimulates the gonads (target organ) to secrete their hormones, **A** and **B**. As the secretion of gonadal hormones increase, they in turn inhibit the secretion of trophic hormones by the pituitary, **C** to **E**. Eventually, the concentration of gonadal hormones falls, **A**, and the pituitary, released from its inhibition, once more secretes its trophic hormones.

ters; thus the original explanation of a simple feedback regulation must be expanded to include these nervous centers.

Apparently, the circulating steroid hormones act not only directly on the cells of the pituitary but also stimulate the chemoreceptors of certain brain centers sensitive to the steroid level. The amygdala, cerebellum, and median eminence contain centers sensitive to progesterone (Piva, Kalra, and Martini, 1973). These centers, in turn, induce the hypothalamus to release factors to the pituitary that travel to it by way of the hypophyseal portal system. These factors accelerate the release of gonadotrophins by the pituitary. It is the *hypothalamus,* therefore, that controls the reproductive cycles by regulating and maintaining pituitary function. It also reacts to sensory information received by way of the nervous system by adjusting the amount of gonadotrophins released into the bloodstream by the pituitary gland.

Data substantiate the hypothesis that the secretion of the sex hormones and ovulation are under the control of the "expanded" feedback mechanism described above. All information available at the present time, however, indicates that spermatogenesis is not regulated by such a mechanism. One can demonstrate that FSH, LH, and androgen affect spermatogenesis, but there is no known secretion by the seminiferous tubules that influences the pituitary gland. Removal of the pituitary (hypophysectomy) from an experimental animal causes the male reproductive tract to degenerate. Androgen restores the epithelium to a limited degree and allows spermatogenesis to continue, but a combination of androgen and pituitary hormones is needed to bring the animal back to a more normal functional state. Recent investigations with lower animals indicate that seasonal environmental factors, such as light and temperature, affect the hypothalamus, which, in turn, regulates gonadotrophic secretion. The response to these stimuli and rhythmic changes in sensitivity to the hormones by the germinal epithelium in the seminiferous tubules are factors that enter into the control of the seasonal production of the sperm.

Mammalian reproductive cycles

In general, the vertebrate breeding cycle of the male parallels that of the female, although exceptions certainly exist. Maturation and storage of the sperm occur, with the result that the sperm is prepared for insemination of the egg. The female vertebrate's seasonal cycle involves the interaction of the pituitary gonadotrophins and estrogen. These hormones stimulate her eggs to mature and be ovulated at the most propitious breeding period for her young.

Female mammals that follow an annual reproductive season pass through several shorter sexual cycles during the breeding period when she is more receptive of the male and when ovulation occurs spontaneously. See Table 3-2. During these short cycles, referred to as *estrous cycles,* many changes occur. The dominant event of the cycle is the maturation and release of the ova, which usually occurs at the time the female is most receptive to the male (periods of heat, or estrus). In animals other than the primates the length of the estrous cycle varies with the species (Table 3-2). It ranges from 4 to 5 days in the rat, 21 days in the cow, and 3 to 4 months in the dog. Animals who have two or

TABLE 3-2. Duration of estrous cycle

Animal	Days
Rat	4-5
Mouse	5
Guinea pig	16
Sheep	16
Asian elephant	21
Sow	21
Cow	21
Mare	21
Rhesus monkey	24-26
Woman	28
Opossum	28
Chimpanzee	35-37
Dog	90-120

more cycles within a breeding season are said to be *polyestrous,* as opposed to those with only one estrous cycle, *monestrous.*

The reproductive cycle of female primates is fundamentally comparable to the estrous cycle but is usually referred to as the *menstrual cycle.* Two main differences exist between the estrous cycle of most mammals and the menstrual cycle of primates. There is no peak of heightened sexual activity in the female primate, since she will accept the male throughout the cycle except during menstruation. The second difference is that the endometrium of the uterus is eroded at the end of the cycle and bleeding occurs. The primate cycle is approximately 28 days long, with ovulation occurring ordinarily midway between the two menstrual periods, or 12 to 15 days after the onset of menstruation. However, there is individual variation and some cycles are longer or shorter. Four basic hormones, interacting with one another, coordinate the sequence of events in the menstrual cycle. They are easily affected by any adjustment the body makes to changes or stress (by the hypothalamus). An understanding of this hormonal control explains the variability of the cycles within each individual female.

On the basis of events happening in the ovary, the menstrual cycle is divided into a *follicular stage,* in which estrogen is secreted, and a *luteal phase,* in which progesterone is produced. During the follicular phase FSH from the pituitary stimulates the follicles with their ova to mature

and to develop into graafian follicles. Estrogen, secreted by the follicle cells, increases in amount as the time of ovulation approaches, as shown in Fig. 3-20. The high levels of estrogen stimulate the development of the reproductive tract. The uterus thickens in preparation for possible implantation of a fertilized egg. The rising proportion of estrogen eventually blocks the release of FSH in the pituitary (negative-feedback regulation). When the level of circulating FSH falls, the secretion of LH by the pituitary increases.

At the end of the follicular phase there is an abrupt increase in the ovulation-inducing hormone (OIH). This hormone, released into the circulatory system, initiates a series of events in the ovary leading to the rupture of the follicular wall. LH is considered the principal component of OIH. Most investigators who have studied ovulation in mammals believe that a neuroendocrine mechanism is involved with its release. As a result of the neurogenic stimulus, neurohumoral agents travel from the hypothalamus to the pituitary causing it to release OIH. Hypothalamic centers are also sensitive to the levels of circulating estrogen and progesterone, and these ovarian steroids also play a role in stimulating or inhibiting hypothalamic activity.

After ovulation, the follicle cells transform into the glandular corpus luteum, and the second phase of the menstrual cycle begins. LH, the predominant gonadotrophin at this time, stimulates the corpus luteum to produce progesterone. In some animals, rats for example, lactogenic hormone is also necessary for the formation of the corpus luteum. Progesterone is sometimes referred to as the pregnancy hormone, since it induces the uterus to prepare for pregnancy in a more elaborate manner than did estrogen. The high circulating levels of both estrogen and progesterone inhibit the release of FSH from the pituitary. No new follicles can mature and be ovulated as long as the corpus luteum remains.

The human egg, barely visible to the naked eye, takes about 4 days to travel the 4½ inches down the fallopian tubes to the cavity of the uterus. If fertilized, it floats for 2 or 3 days living off the secretions of the uterus. About the sixth day after ovulation, the developing embryo

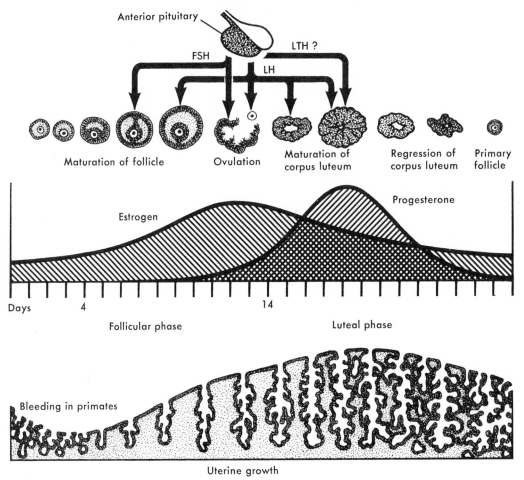

Fig. 3-20

Diagram of essential components of the estrous cycle. When estrogen and progesterone decrease at the end of the cycle, bleeding occurs in primates. See text for discussion of the cycle.

induces a *decidual reaction* in the endometrium, a reaction that is essential if implantation is to occur.

In the mouse and probably other animals, the pregnant uterine mucosa or decidua (so called because it will be shed at parturition) participates with the blastocyst (the early stages of mammalian development) to bring about this reaction. The estrogen-sensitized uterus releases substances that activate the blastocyst. One such substance has been identified as responsible for dissolving the zona pellucida. Others are believed to increase the metabolic rate of the blastocyst or to remove some inhibitor. Once the blastocyst is activated, the cells on the outer

wall of the blastocyst (trophoblast cells) increase in number and enlarge. In turn, the uterine endometrium is stimulated, possibly by some embryonic metabolic by-product, to undergo the decidual reaction. There is an increase in capillary permeability near the vicinity of the blastocyst; the stroma of the uterus fills with fluid; and the endometrium is eroded away at the site of implantation. The trophoblast of the developing embryo (blastocyst) invades the wall through this gap in the epithelium and soon is covered over by the endometrial cells. If pregnancy occurred, the pituitary continues to release LH; the corpus luteum remains active and secretes progesterone. Both ovulation and menstruation are suspended for the duration of pregnancy.

Once implantation is established, the uterine and embryonic tissues contribute to the formation of the placenta. This organ permits the diffusion of food and waste materials between the bloodstreams of the mother and the fetus. The placenta is also an endocrine organ and secretes estrogen and progesterone as well as gonadotrophins. These gonadotrophins are referred to as *chorionic gonadotrophins* to distinguish them from the hypophyseal gonadotrophins discussed above. For the first 3 months the state of pregnancy is maintained by progesterone from the corpus luteum; after 3 months, the progesterone secreted by the placenta dominates the situation. The third month of pregnancy, therefore, is a critical one, since the responsibility for the secretion of progesterone shifts from the corpus luteum to the placenta, and the control of this secretion from the gonadotrophin of the pituitary to the gonadotrophin of the placenta. Natural abortions occur most often at this time because of some kind of imbalance in hormonal control. Either the corpus luteum regresses too soon or the placenta is unprepared to take over the major secretory role at the time it is needed. In either case, the uterus is not maintained properly and the embryo loses its attachment to the uterine wall.

As a result of the secretion by the placenta, the chorionic gonadotrophin levels rise in the circulating fluids about the third month of pregnancy and some is excreted in the urine. The presence at this time of excess gonadotrophin in the urine is the basis of several definitive pregnancy tests. If pregnant urine is injected into immature mice or rats, the gonadotrophin, which is present and is mainly LH, induces corpora lutea or blood points to form in the ovaries (Aschheim-Zondek test). The South African toad is used also as a test animal. Injections of pregnancy urine into the dorsal lymph sacs of *Xenopus laevis* will cause the eggs to escape from the oviduct. Both of these tests are said to be sensitive enough to determine a rising level of gonadotrophins before the third month.

The presence of human chorionic gonadotrophin (HCG) in the urine and serum of preg-

nant women is the basis also for serologic tests for pregnancy. Antibodies against HCG (anti-HCG) are obtained by injecting a rabbit with HCG. Some of this anti-HCG is incubated with the patient's urine. If the individual is pregnant, the HCG present in her urine neutralizes the antibodies. Latex particles covered with HCG are added. If the antibodies are neutralized, the latex particles will not agglutinate and will remain in suspension. On the other hand, if the patient was not pregnant, no HCG will be present in her urine, and no reaction with the anti-HCG can occur. The antibodies present react with the latex particles that then agglutinate and fall to the bottom of the container. A turbid supernatant is interpreted as a positive test and a clear supernatant, a negative test for pregnancy.

If fertilization does not occur, the pituitary is signaled to stop releasing LH and, as a result, in about 10 days the corpus luteum degenerates. The low levels of estrogen and progesterone circulating in the blood are unable to maintain the uterus in its prepregnant state. A constriction of blood vessels and a shrinkage of mucosa occur, and blood and disintegrating endometrial cells are released into the lumen of the uterus. In the absence of pregnancy the release of FSH is no longer blocked, and it is again secreted into the system. This new FSH again acts on the follicles, stimulating one to grow and mature. Thus another cycle is begun.

Once the factors involved in maintaining the female menstrual cycle were understood, one could manipulate the hormones to induce ovulation and thereby increase fertility, or to inhibit ovulation and prevent pregnancy. As a result, fertility and birth control pills soon made their appearance on the market. Although these concoctions of hormones appear to the general public almost as miracle drugs, they are not without their hazards. Although they prevent conception, they also affect other cells and systems in the body as well. For example, they appear to increase risks of blood clots.

In treating sterility, one has difficulty knowing the exact amount of hormone to administer, since the sensitivity of each woman to the hormones varies. Her treatment becomes complicated if she is taking more than one drug, that is, if she is receiving medication for some unrelated ailment. We have already mentioned the synergistic effect of hormones (or drugs or chemicals). Usually the physician administers FSH to the patient in an attempt to stimulate her ovaries to produce a mature graafian follicle. He then induces her ovaries with LH to release the egg. Administration of an excess amount of hormone may cause multiple eggs to ripen and be ovulated. Recent multiple births by New Jersey, Australian, and South African women, all of whom were on fertility pills, attest to this fact.

The birth control pill acts in the opposite manner; it inhibits ovulation. As was mentioned earlier during the discussion of the menstrual cycle, ovulation is controlled by LH. If estrogen, progesterone, or synthetic steroids related to them are administered to the female, the release of LH will be blocked and no egg will be ovulated. When the tablets are discontinued, pituitary blockage is removed and LH is secreted. As a result, ovulation occurs, followed by normal menstruation.

SUGGESTED READINGS

1. Berrill, N. J.: The person in the womb, New York, 1968, Dodd, Mead, & Co.
2. Bloom, W., and Fawcett, D. W.: A textbook of histology, Philadelphia, 1968, W. B. Saunders Co.
3. Frye, B. E.: Hormonal control in vertebrates, New York, 1967, The Macmillan Co.
4. Frye, B. E.: Reproduction. In Watterman, A. J. (editor): Chordate structure and function, New York, 1971, The Macmillan Co.
5. Goodrich, E. S.: Studies on the structure and development of vertebrates, New York, 1958, Dover Publications, Inc.
6. Patt, D. I., and Patt, G. R.: Comparative vertebrate histology, New York, 1969, Harper & Row, Publishers.
7. Piva, F., Kalma, P. S., and Martini, L.: Participation of the amygdala and the cerebellum in the feedback effects of progesterone, Neuroendocrinology 11:229-239, 1973.
8. Hormones in reproduction, Book 3. In Austin, C. R., and Short, R. V. (editors): Reproduction in Mammals, Cambridge, 1972, University Press.
9. Reproductive patterns, Book 4. In Austin, C. R., and Short, R. V. (editors): Reproduction in Mammals, Cambridge, 1972, University Press.
10. Artificial Control of Reproduction, Book 5. In Austin, C. R., and Short, R. V. (editors): Reproduction in Mammals, Cambridge, 1972, University Press.
11. Turner, C. D., and Bagnara, J. T.: General endocrinology, Philadelphia, 1971, W. B. Saunders Co.

PART TWO

EARLY DEVELOPMENTAL PROCESSES

CHAPTER 4

MATURATION OF GAMETES

GAMETES

The *germ cells* give rise to the gametes of the individual. They provide the continuity between generations and are segregated early in development from *somatic cells,* which contribute to the formation of the body. The germ cells can be distinguished cytologically from the somatic cells in the differentiating gonad before it is possible to tell whether the embryo is female or male.

Certain cells located outside the gonad and even outside the body of the embryo (at earlier stages of development) are believed to be the precursors of the germ cells. These cells are the *primordial germ cells.* Many embryologists consider them to be the only cells destined to form the future gametes of the individual. They can be identified about 24 days after fertilization in the human embryo and after about 19 hours of incubation in the chick.

The fact that they are very early separated in the gonads, especially in the ovary, protects the germ cells from the diseases and injuries that somatic cells suffer, although they, too, can be affected by the poor environment of an unhealthy body. In the gonads, the germ cells develop into the oogonia or spermatogonia and proliferate. Eventually they transform into oocytes or spermatocytes and undergo nuclear and cytoplasmic maturation. As a result of nuclear maturation, a reduction occurs in the chromosome number in each gamete through the process of meiosis. When the egg cytoplasm matures, there is synthesis of RNA and some proteins—all the essentials for development. The egg stores these materials in its cytoplasm for future use by the embryo. The spermatozoon, on the other hand, discards its cytoplasm in favor of specializing in motility and consequently depends on its surroundings for its nourishment.

At the end of the maturation process the egg is ready for *ovulation* and the sperm for *spermiation* (release from the Sertoli cells). Passage through the respective gonadal ducts completes their structural and biochemical changes. The ova or sperm are prepared for a successful union at fertilization, a necessity for species survival in vertebrate animals where sexual reproduction is the rule.

COMPARISON OF SOMATIC AND GERM CELLS

When a cell divides mitotically, the chromosomes in the nucleus are distributed equally, qualitatively and quantitatively, between the two daughter cells. As a result each daughter cell is identical to the parent cell as far as genetic composition is concerned. All sexually derived individuals start out as one cell, the fertilized egg, which then divides repeatedly to give rise to a new individual. As a result, all cells of an embryo contain the same number and kind of chromosomes despite the fact that some cells will eventually differentiate into germ cells (ova and sperm), some into muscle cells, and some into skin or nerve cells in the adult body. Each cell carries the same code in the DNA of its chromosomes for all the morphogenetic or physiological activities that go on in the body of a particular species. The genes and the chromosomes of both the somatic and the germ cells are identical. It is not, then, their hereditary material that distinguishes between these two types of cells.

Actually, the capacity of the adult somatic cell to follow the coded instructions contained in the DNA of its genes appears to be limited. A skin cell may carry the code for all cellular activities, but it differentiates and functions only as a skin cell, and not as a germ cell or a muscle cell. Somewhere along the developmental pathway the destiny of the cell became fixed, its possibilities for differentiation were restricted. Embryologists say that it becomes *determined.* Its potentiality is limited or, at least, its ability to express all its potentiality is *partially repressed.* Despite the fact that the cell contains the code for all activities that go on in the organism's cells, most of these potentialities are somehow blocked and only particular functions are expressed by particular types of cell.

In some instances, the somatic cells can reproduce their own kind. A skin cell from the germinativum layer of the epidermis can undergo mitosis and form a new skin cell. A liver cell can give rise to another liver cell. But many cells cannot form new cells, for example, the highly differentiated nerve cell. However, none of the somatic cells can become whole individuals. Only certain cells in the body have the ability to develop into new organisms under normal conditions. These are the cells that carry the germ plasm and are segregated from the somatic cells early in development. They divide repeatedly by mitosis, undergo meiosis at their maturity, and differentiate into ova or sperm. The ova, as opposed to the somatic cells, are said to be harmoniously *totipotent,* since they possess the ability not only of forming the various types of tissues associated with the specific animal's body, but they also are capable of organizing it so that a total, fully formed individual is produced. These cells contain sufficient substrate, the proper mechanisms, and some kind of organizational center that allow them to express their total potentially and to give rise to a complete embryo.

The germ cells are considered to be highly specialized cells. They not only carry the genetic code, which is passed on to the next generation, but the ova also contain the "ingredients," the cytoplasm of the egg, out of which a new individual begins its development. The cytoplasm of most oocytes is highly basophilic; that is, it stains readily with basic dyes, indicating the presence of deoxyribonucleic and ribonucleic acids. This reaction is primarily from the presence of ribosomal RNA supplied by the nucleolus. However, messenger and transfer RNA is also present in the cytoplasm as well as DNA associated with the mitochondria. Generally, somatic cells do not have this high RNA content. During oogenesis the egg organizes itself, synthesizes messenger and ribosomal RNA, produces some proteins, and, in general, prepares itself for operating the cell during the early developmental stages. The sperm cannot form a new individual out of its own cytoplasm, since most of it is discarded as spermiogenesis takes place. However, the sperm have their own unique function, which is to add half of the genes (the paternal characteristics) to the individual and to trigger the egg in such a way that physiological mechanisms of the cell are set into operation and development is initiated.

Perhaps the most striking difference between the two cell types is the fact that somatic cells divide mitotically but are incapable of under-

TABLE 4-1. Comparison of mitotic and meiotic cell division

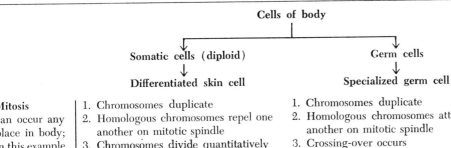

	Differentiated skin cell	Specialized germ cell	
Mitosis can occur any place in body; in this example, the skin	1. Chromosomes duplicate 2. Homologous chromosomes repel one another on mitotic spindle 3. Chromosomes divide quantitatively and are passed to daughter cells 4. Daughter cells all diploid	1. Chromosomes duplicate 2. Homologous chromosomes attract one another on mitotic spindle 3. Crossing-over occurs 4. Chromosome number is reduced to half and passed on to daughter cells 5. Daughter cells haploid	**Meiosis** occurs in testis in male; starts in ovary of female but may be completed in ducts or outside body after fertilization
	1. Gives rise to two new cells 2. Each daughter cell is genetically identical to parent cell 3. Each cell is diploid 4. Skin cell gives rise to skin cell; it is determined	1. Gives rise to ovum and three polar bodies or four sperm 2. Because of segregation, independent assortment and crossing over, gamete is not identical to parent cell 3. Each cell is haploid 4. Ovum contains potential to form complete individual; it is totipotent	

going *meiosis* and forming gametes, an essential process if normal development is to occur. These two types of cell divisions are compared in Table 4-1. The ability to divide *meiotically* is delegated only to a few cells of the embryo, those that become the germ cells. We do not understand the basic mechanisms causing the members of chromosomal pairs to repel each other as they line up on the spindle during mitosis, but to attract one another during meiosis. The ability to undergo meiosis is a unique characteristic of germ cells. No one has yet been able experimentally to induce this type of division in an animal somatic cell.

It is obvious that under normal circumstances the ability to give rise to a new organism is restricted to the egg. The fact that the egg can be activated artificially (without the aid of the sperm) and induced to develop into a total organism (parthenogenetically) indicates that the egg contains all the essential materials necessary for development.

If experimental evidence is considered, the distinction between germ cells and somatic cells is not as sharp and well defined as it appears to be in the normal developing organism. In fact, under laboratory conditions the somatic cell is revealed to retain many of its potentialities assumed lost when it differentiated.

The work of F. C. Steward and his colleagues (1964) with carrot plants raises some interesting speculations. Normally a carrot grows from a seed, but these investigators have been able to stimulate fully differentiated tissue of a mature carrot into active growth. When a cell of one of these mature plants was freed from its normal cellular (or tissue) environment, both the differentiated nucleus and the cytoplasm were capable of interacting in such a way that a new embryo developed. Small plugs from nongrowing areas of carrot root grown in coconut milk rapidly increased their weight. If individual cells were taken from the plugs and placed in separate fresh flasks of coconut milk, a few of these cells underwent mitosis and organized themselves into carrot embryos. In other words, each somatic cell behaved as if it were a fertilized egg. It passed through various embryonic stages and developed into a plantlet, which became a mature carrot plant when transplanted to soil. There obviously had been no irreversible changes in the nucleus or cytoplasm of the fully differentiated carrot cell. According to Steward's experimental results, the interrelationship of somatic cells maintains their specialized state. When separated from the environment of other cells, the differentiated somatic cell is capable of producing a new plant, a function under normal circumstances delegated only to the germ cells.

ORIGIN OF PRIMORDIAL GERM CELLS

Two types of cells are identified when the developing gonad is sectioned and stained. First there are small, somatic cells that will give rise to follicles, Sertoli cells, interstitial cells, and surface epithelium; and then there are large, round cells with vesicular nuclei considered *primordial germ cells.* It is these latter cells that many embryologists believe are destined to give rise to the eggs or sperm of the adult animal. They generally agree that the mesoderm of the germinal ridge is the source of somatic cells of the gonad. This ridge is a thickened longitudinal strip of tissue located lateral to the dorsal mesentery. However, the primordial cells appear to originate from a different source. One approach to their study has been to trace methodically their presence in the embryo backward in developmental time until they first appear. When this is done, various areas of the embryo outside the gonad reveal the presence of these primordial cells. They migrate from these areas into the germinal ridge either through ameboid movement or by way of the blood vessels.

Weisman's concept of biological immortality

The origin of the primordial cells has intrigued biologists for many years. The fact that these cells are set aside from the somatic cells early in development led August Weisman (1834-1914) to hypothesize that the body was composed of two distinct plasms: the somatoplasm, which gives rise to the body proper, and the germ plasm, which is transmitted from one generation to the next. He believed that the germ plasm was located in the nucleus of the cells and was distributed unequally during cell division, with the cells making up the organs receiving specific *determiners.* That is, cells destined to form the heart received heart determiners as opposed to brain or kidney determiners. This qualitative parceling out of nuclear determiners was an orderly process that occurred during divisions of the fertilized egg. Weisman believed that the determiners in the germ cells were not dispersed as in the soma. He speculated that the germ cells were set aside early in cleavage and were given a full complement of the material, and therefore these cells contained the hereditary determiners for all the cells of the body.

As a result of his hypothesis a kind of "biological immortality" was suggested in which molecules of germ plasm were passed unchanged from one generation to another. Weisman believed that the primordial germ cells were not derived from the embryo itself but from substance that could be traced directly to the parent germ cell, the germ plasm. This germ plasm did not contribute directly to the formation of the body of the new individual in each generation, but was set aside for the formation of the germ cells of the next generation. He suggested that the germ plasm grew by absorbing new materials, but its constituents remained unchanged from generation to generation.

Weisman's ideas about the physical continuity of the germ plasm and the unequal distribution of determiners during cleavage were postulated before the rediscovery of Mendel's work and, therefore, before genetics had reached its present state of knowledge. He knew nothing about chromosomes and genes but tried to work out some concept by which he could explain the passing of inherited characteristics from parent to embryo. Much of Weisman's work has *not* been supported by experimental evidence, but it was of value in posing the problems inherent in development. There is no experimental evidence that demonstrates the passage of specific molecules from one generation to another for all vertebrate animals. We do not believe that a stockpile of molecules was set up in the primeval sludge. What is inherited, it is agreed, is the pattern of development followed by the particular individual. This pattern is under the control of the genes, and it is the genes that replicate and are passed on to the next generation.

Modern concepts of germ plasm origin

Weisman's theories about the immortality of the germ plasm stimulated extensive investigation as biologists sought to verify or disprove his ideas by experimentation. The origin of the germ plasm is a difficult problem to solve, since a permanent, nontoxic method of marking the plasm is needed before it can be followed through successive generations. This labeling not only must be stable but also must be specific for the germ plasm, differentiating between it and the plasm of the somatic cells. No such technique is available at the present time.

There is evidence (Blackler, 1958) that a specific area of cytoplasm within the frog's egg is set aside early for the formation of the gametes. This cytoplasm located near the vegetal pole in the newly fertilized but uncleaved eggs of *Rana temporaria* and *Rana pipiens* stains with Azure A, a dye that selectively stains nucleic acids. The dye remains in those cells formed from this region during cleavage, labeling them as they take up their position in different locations in the embryo. The RNA-rich cytoplasm, first located in the vegetal region, segregates into cells that move to the middle of the endoderm below the gut cavity as indicated in Fig. 4-1. These cells contain the "germinal plasm" since they may be traced from the floor of the gut cavity to its roof, from here to the dorsal mesentery, and then into the germinal ridges. It is difficult to say whether the Azure A–stained cytoplasm is responsible for the specific qualities that differentiate germ plasm from somatoplasm, but it does indicate that a specific area in the fertilized egg is segregated early for gamete formation in the frog.

Another experimental procedure used to study the origin of the primordial germ cells involves the surgical removal of some of the cell layers of the embryo. The embryo of frogs in their early stages consists of an outer ectodermal layer or "tube" and an inner gut "tube" of endoderm; this is the "tube within a tube" body-plan arrangement associated with triploblastic (three germ layered) animals. The mesoderm is sandwiched between these two tubes. Embryologists are able to remove surgically the endodermal layers of cells and leave a shell of ectoderm and mesoderm. If this endodermal tube is removed from the frog embryo about the time the neural tube closes (the neurual stage), gonads develop but they are sterile. These results agree with the concept of primordial germ origin suggested

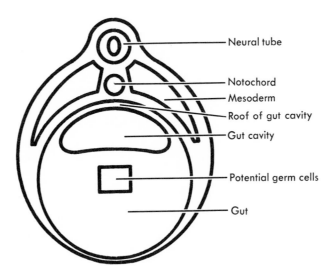

Neural tube

Notochord

Mesoderm

Roof of gut cavity

Gut cavity

Potential germ cells

Gut

Fig. 4-1
Drawing of transverse section through frog embryo. Primordial germ cells with RNA-rich cytoplasm move to middle of endoderm below gut cavity.

by Blackler for the frog—that gonadal somatic tissue develops from the mesoderm. On the other hand, the cells that give rise to the future gametes are derived from the endodermal cells and migrate into the gonadal primordium. Surgical removal of this endodermal layer excised the primordial germ cells with it; none were left to find their way to the rudimentary ovary or testes.

However, the gametes of all amphibians do not originate from this same endodermal source. If the endoderm from another embryo, one that differs in pigmentation, is inserted back into the shell, the host cells can be distinguished from the donor cells. The exchange of endodermal types in salamander embryos showed that the germ cells do not develop from the "marked" (pigmented) endoderm but rather from the host's tissue. These experiments and others suggest that the primordial germ cells in amphibians originate from at least two sources. In the frogs, evidence supports the endoderm as the source of the future germ cells, but in the salamanders they originate from the mesoderm. Regardless of the germ source in the amphibian embryo, authorities agree that the germ cells reach the site of the rudimentary gonad by ameboid movement.

In the chick, after about 30 hours of incubation, certain large cells identified as the primordial germ cells appear in a *crescentic* area in front of the head in the extraembryonic endoderm, that is, in tissues located outside the embryo proper. This is shown in Fig. 4-2. This area may be surgically removed, or destroyed by cauterizing with a hot needle or by irradiation, without disturbing the chick's development. Four days after their first appearance in this crescentic area of a normal chick embryo, the primordial germ cells are found in the rudimentary ovary when it is sectioned and stained (Fig. 4-3). On the other hand, no primordial cells appear in the developing gonad of the experimental animal (an embryo with this cres-

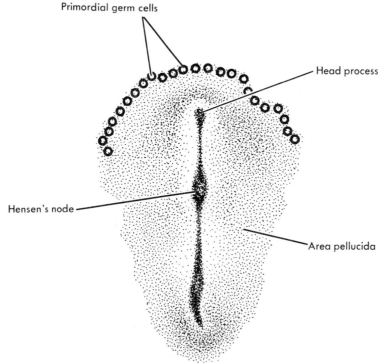

Fig. 4-2

Surface view of chick embryo after about 30 hours of incubation. Large primordial germ cells appear in the extraembryonic endoderm anterior to the head process.

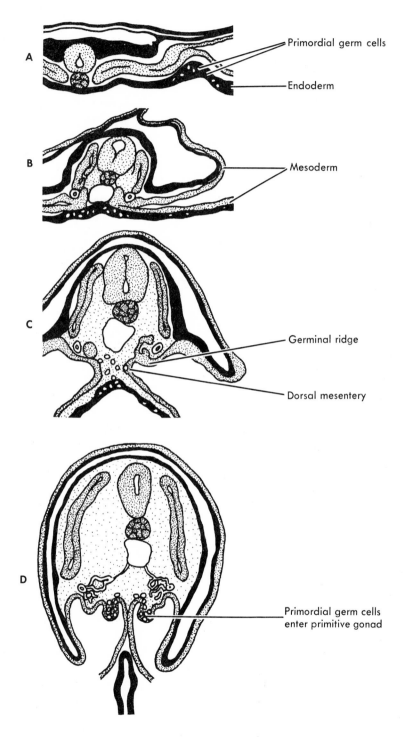

Fig. 4-3
Schematic sections through midregion of young chick embryos illustrating the migratory pathway of primordial germ cells. **A** and **B,** Germ cells originate in extraembryonic endoderm and migrate by way of blood vessels to region of gonadal primordia. **C,** Cells travel through dorsal mesentery to site of primitive gonad, **D.**

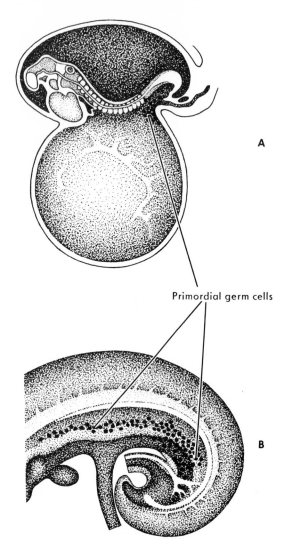

A

Primordial germ cells

B

Fig. 4-4
In human embryo, primordial germ cells first appear in
the posterior region of yolk sac, **A.** They undergo
mitosis and migrate by way of the dorsal mesentery into
the germinal ridge, **B.**

centic area removed) despite the fact that the
germinal ridge was not disturbed.

Unlike the amphibian the primordial germ
cells of the chick do not make their way through
the tissues by ameboid movement, but instead
they have been observed to penetrate the blood
vessels where they travel to the rudimentary
gonad by way of the vascular system. The cells
have been identified in the vascular system, and
although some are lost and degenerate, many

find their way to the proper site (Fig. 4-3, *C*).
The intriguing question of why or how these
cells selectively take up their position in the
rudimentary gonad belongs to the realm of experimental embryology.

In mammalian embryos, including man, the
primordial germ cells apparently arise from the
endodermal layer near the yolk sac. In the human embryos they have been identified at the
posterior end of the primitive streak, the area
posterior to the embryo. Later, they appear in
the endoderm of the hindgut when the embryo
is only a few millimeters in length, as shown
in Fig. 4-4. Although no experimental investigations have been carried out on human embryos,
in the mouse certain large cells, rich in alkaline
phosphatase and believed to be primordial germ
cells, can be selectively stained and their migratory path followed. In these animals cinemato-
graphic recordings reveal that the primary germ
cells migrate through the tissues as in the amphibian, by ameboid movements, possibly aided
by their ability to bring about lysis of cells and
membranes that block their path. They move
from the gut into the dorsal mesentery and then
into the germinal ridge. As they migrate, they
undergo repeated mitoses and multiply from
less than a hundred cells to a few thousand.

The fact that in the early stages of development these cells can be traced from some area
outside the rudimentary gonad into the developing gonad, does not necessarily indicate that
they are the precursors to the egg and the sperm.
There is a reciprocal relationship between a
gonad rudiment and gametes. The gametes need
the environment of the gonad in order to mature, and in some animals the rudimentary
gonad will not develop properly without the
gametes. Some authorities reason therefore, that
the primordial germ cells function only to induce the ovary or testes to form the gametes. In
many cases the primordial germ cells die without progressing further. There are some biologists who believe that all primordial germ
cells die once they make their way to the
gonadal primordium and induce it to differentiate. These investigators look to the gonadal
epithelium as the source of future gametes. They

are responsible for the term "germinal epithelium," which refers to the coelomic lining covering the ovary and testis.

As the gonad develops, there is a great proliferation of cells. The primordial cells become embedded in the mesoderm of the genital ridge and lose some of their differentiating characteristics (special staining affinities, for example). It is difficult, if not impossible, to tell one cell from another or to determine the origin of any one cell. The proliferating cells may be derived from the primordial germ cells, or from the germinal epithelium (surface epithelium) or from certain mesodermal cells composing the rudimentary gonad, or from a combination of these sources. At this time we cannot probe the question further and should now consider the development of the germ cells within the gonad.

FATE OF GERM CELLS IN GONAD

If the gonad develops into a testis, primitive germ cells proliferate, become surrounded by the cells of the future seminiferous tubules, and give rise to the *spermatogonia*. If the gonad becomes an ovary, cells cluster around each germ cell or *oogonium* and a *primary follicle* develops. Both gonads remain in this state of development until puberty.

The primordial germ cells divide mitotically. Although it is probably unnecessary to review mitosis at this time, a brief summary might be helpful before we consider meiosis. The number of chromosomes present in each cell is species specific: 46 for human cells, 8 for the fruitfly, and 4 for ascaris. This number is referred to as the *diploid* number. With the exception of the sex chromosomes, certain of the chromosomes resemble one another in size and shape and can be matched up in pairs, with the chromosomes of each pair, in fact, contributing to the same characteristics of an individual. These pairs of similar chromosomes are referred to as *homologous pairs*. Each chromosome is the homolog, or mate, of the other and contains similar, but not identical, sequences of genes. During mitosis each chromosome acts independently of its mate, apparently repelled rather than attracted to it.

In mitosis each chromosome replicates to form two chromatids (two potential chromosomes),

and during anaphase these chromatids separate and move to the poles of the spindle. The cell then divides. The chromosome number does not change as a result of this division, nor do the kinds of chromosomes vary, but each new cell retains the chromosomal content identical to the parent cell.

By now nearly every freshman biology student has been introduced to molecular biology, by the contributions of Watson and Crick, among others, who proposed a structure for DNA after examining the x-ray diffraction studies of Wilkins. Therefore, we shall summarize only the organization of the DNA molecule.

Based on available data, investigators deduced that DNA consists of two helically coiled polynucleotide chains. Three components make up this double helix. Phosphates and pentose sugars compose the ribbon or backbone of each chain. Nucleotide bases project as connecting bars between the two ribbons and hold together these two adjacent strands. Two nucleotide bases compose each connecting bar. The entire double-stranded structure is coiled, making a complete turn every 34 Å.

The DNA molecule uses only four nucleotide bases: adenine, thymine, cytosine, and guanine. These weakly organic bases vary in molecular size and join one another, forming specific combinations. Watson and Crick suggested a complementary nature for the two chains. Where adenine appears on one chain, the base pair opposite it is always thymine. Where guanine appears, cytosine must be opposite it. If one chain contains a particular sequence of bases, such as ACTTG, the sequence on the other chain must be the complement of the first, that is, it must be TGAAC. The double helix is of uniform diameter and these particular combinations of base pairs make connecting bars of the same length. Other combinations would be too long or too short to fit between the two ribbons.

With this brief review let us return to the process of mitosis where we are primarily concerned with the replication of the DNA molecule. Replication occurs during the interphase and is well separated from the four stages of mitosis that follow.

During this nondividing phase of a mitotic

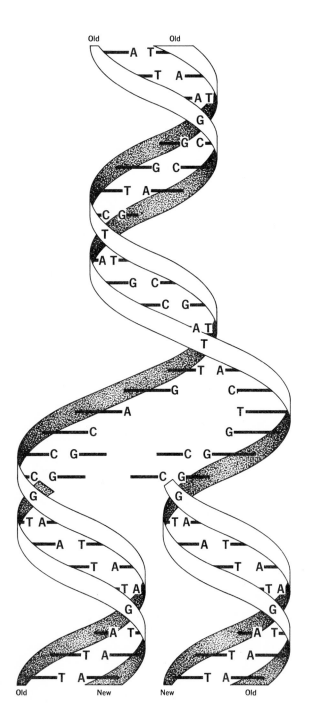

cycle, hydrogen bonds holding the base pairs together break, and the two component chains of the DNA molecule unwind and separate. Each chain then acts as a template for a new polynucleated chain. Each half of the original DNA chain attracts complementary nucleotides from the nuclear pool and forms a new chain identical to the one from which it separated (Fig. 4-5). As a result, two pairs of chains exist where before there was only one. Each newly formed double helix of DNA contains one "old" polynucleotide chain and one "new" one.

As the cells enter the prophase of the mitotic division, each chromosome is made up of two chromatids. Each chromatid consists of a double-stranded DNA molecule. The two chromatids are held together at one region by the centromere. At anaphase the centromeres divide and the two sister chromatids separate, each passing to the opposite pole. As a result of the DNA replication at interphase, each of the two new daughter cells receive identical complements of hereditary material.

J. Herbert Taylor demonstrated the replication of DNA during the mitotic cycle. He added radioactive thymidine to the medium in which he was growing some root tips. When the root-tip DNA replicated, it incorporated the labeled thymidine into its molecule. He then removed the tissue to fresh medium containing no labeled thymidine. After a further incubation period, he withdrew the cells at different intervals of time and fixed them at various mitotic stages. He followed the behavior of the chromatids by utilizing a technique called "autoradiography." A black dot appears in the photographic emulsion above the cell if radioactive thymidine is

Fig. 4-5
Diagram of a double-stranded DNA molecule. The ribbons symbolize the two phosphate-sugar chains and the horizontal lines the pairs of bases. Thymine always pairs with adenine, and cytosine pairs with guanine. During the interphase of a mitotic division the two component chains of the DNA molecules unwind, separate, and act as templates for new polynucleotide chains. From the nuclear pool each half of the original DNA chain attracts a complementary nucleotide, which will be identical to the alternate half of the original DNA molecule. (From Nagle, J. J.: Heredity and human affairs, St. Louis, 1974, The C. V. Mosby Co.)

incorporated into the chromosome. An absence of dots indicates that no radioactive thymidine is present. This technique enabled him to tell when the cell synthesized DNA. The results of his experiment are summarized in Fig. 4-6. Taylor found that both chromatids of each chromosome during the first mitosis were labeled; that is, they incorporated some of the radioactive material into a strand of DNA during the first replication. When the original double strand of DNA unwound and separated at interphase, each half of the chain attracted complementary nucleotides labeled with radioactive thymidine. Two chromatids were formed. Each chromatid contained one "old" unlabeled nucleotide chain and one "new" labeled nucleotide chain, identified by the presence of black dots in the photographic emulsion. At the next division, however, only one chromatid of each chromosome was

marked. This is as it should be if synthesis of DNA occurred again. During the interphase of the second mitotic division the double strand of DNA (one marked and one unmarked) unwind and separate. Again, each strand forms its complement from the nuclear pool—this time unmarked. Since only one strand of the DNA contains radioactive thymidine, only half of the chromatids formed are labeled. Taylor's experiment along with those of other investigators point to the fundamental feature of somatic and gonial mitosis, the replication of the chromosome and its equal distribution to the new cells.

NUCLEAR MATURATION
Meiosis

Meiosis is an universal process in sexual reproduction and occurs in both invertebrate and vertebrate animals, as well as higher plants.

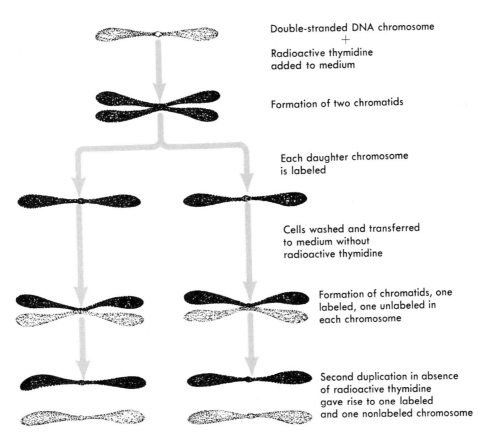

Double-stranded DNA chromosome
+
Radioactive thymidine added to medium

Formation of two chromatids

Each daughter chromosome is labeled

Cells washed and transferred to medium without radioactive thymidine

Formation of chromatids, one labeled, one unlabeled in each chromosome

Second duplication in absence of radioactive thymidine gave rise to one labeled and one nonlabeled chromosome

Fig. 4-6
Demonstration of duplication of chromosomes during mitosis.

Meiosis is a general term applied to the *nuclear maturation* of the gamete, either sperm or egg. It results in halving the chromosome number of these gametes. If some kind of mechanism did not exist by which the number of sperm and egg chromosomes were reduced by half, they would double each generation and soon fill the cell. The elimination of chromosomes during meiosis does not occur in an arbitrary manner. As a result of this type of cell division, the ovum or spermatozoon receives a single set of chromosomes, one from each pair of chromosomes, thus representing all the characteristics of the body. Since the chromosomes assort independently of one another, they give rise to a random combination of chromosomes to compose a new set. When a cell contains only one set of chromosomes, it is said to be *haploid*. The mechanics of meiosis are the same in either the egg or the sperm and may be considered as consisting of two cellular divisions but of only one chromosomal division. When it occurs in the egg, the process is known as *oogenesis* and when in the sperm, it is *spermatogenesis*.

Meiosis is a biological process taught in some form in almost every course in the biology curriculum. Yet it is one of the most confusing subjects to the student. Only an outline of the process is presented here and the student is urged to refer to a genetics book for details.

Three periods or stages are associated with meiosis: proliferation, growth, and nuclear maturation. The *proliferation stage* involves the germ cells in the gonads of the fetal animal. They undergo cell division, and by the time of birth, in the male mammal for example, the spermatogonia are lined up inside the basement membrane of the seminiferous tubules. In the female, the oogonia, surrounded by their follicle cells, are located in the cortex of the ovary where they are known as primary follicles. The speramatogonia and oogonial cells are diploid. There is no further growth or development of these cells until puberty, at which time FSH and LH, released by the pituitary, initiate and control their maturation.

Some of the spermatogonia and oogonia destined to become mature gametes start to enlarge and enter into the second stage of meiosis, the *growth stage*. They become the primary germ cells and are known as primary *spermatocytes* or *oocytes*. Other spermatogonia or oogonia remain as reserve cells and give rise to another wave or cycle of developing primary germ cells. In the male it takes about 3 weeks for a spermatogenic cycle to be completed; that is, for a primary spermatocyte to form and develop into a mature spermatozoon. This growth stage is more complex and plays a greater role in the maturation of the egg than in the sperm.

The third stage of meiosis involves a period of *nuclear maturation* by a special type of meiosis. At the beginning of prophase the diploid chromosomes (consisting of homologous pairs of chromosomes, a single set from each parent) find their mates, come together, and lie side by side on the midplane or metaphase plane of the spindle. This physical pairing of homologous chromosomes is one of the key events in the meiotic process, and does not occur in mitosis. The phenomenon is called *synapsis* and involves the coming together of chromosomes in such a way that their linear order of equivalent genes match. Because of this close physical contact, any break that occurs in the DNA threads can result in the exchange of homologous units. This exchange of parts of one homologous chromosome with another during synapsis is referred to as *crossing-over* (Fig. 4-7). As a result, the characteristics represented by each chromosome of the homologous pairs are juggled, and when they separate, they are no longer "pure" maternal or "pure" paternal chromosomes, but a mixture of each. As indicated in Chapter 1, this potential for genetic variation is important in the operation of natural selection and the adaptation of particular populations to environmental change.

The mechanics of meiosis (Fig. 4-8) may be more readily understood by focusing attention for the moment on the centromeres, rather than on the chromosomes themselves. A centromere is an integral part of each chromosome and appears under the light microscope as a definite structural entity, often as a constriction. It can be located centrically, acentrically, or almost terminally, and is involved in the proper orientation of the chromosome on the spindle and its movements to the poles.

At the time of synapsis each chromosome has duplicated itself (each strand of DNA has separated and formed its complement). When the pairing of like chromosomes occurs, there are actually four chromatids present, each pair held together by one centromere. This group of four chromatids makes up one tetrad, and there will be as many tetrads as there are homologous pairs. For example, the human has 46 chromosomes, 23 homologous pairs; so at synapsis there will be 23 tetrads.

Once synapsis has occurred and the tetrads have formed, the next step of meiosis is the separation of the tetrad into four chromosomes.

This is accomplished by two meiotic divisions, giving rise to four cells. The first divides the tetrads into *dyads* (halves of a tetrad), and the second separates dyads into *monads* (individual chromosomes). At the first division the centromeres do not separate (Alston, 1967) but move apart to the opposite poles, taking with them the two chromatids joined by the single centromere. These chromatids make up the dyads. During the second meiotic division the chromosomes again line up at the metaphase plate, but this time the centromeres divide and pass to the opposite poles. As a result of the two divisions, each nucleus contains only one type of each chromosome rather than two.

When the egg undergoes meiotic division, the

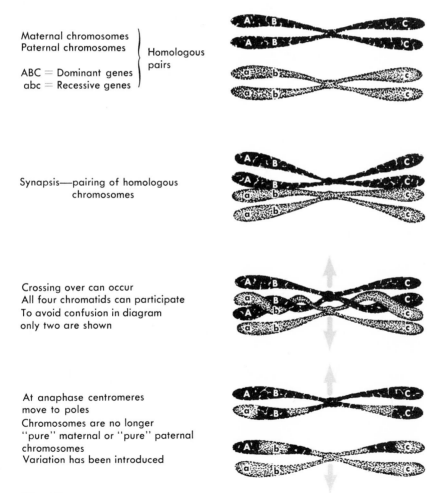

Maternal chromosomes
Paternal chromosomes ⎫ Homologous pairs

ABC = Dominant genes
abc = Recessive genes

Synapsis—pairing of homologous chromosomes

Crossing over can occur
All four chromatids can participate
To avoid confusion in diagram
only two are shown

At anaphase centromeres move to poles
Chromosomes are no longer "pure" maternal or "pure" paternal chromosomes
Variation has been introduced

Fig. 4-7
Diagram illustrating crossing over between homologous pairs of chromosomes.

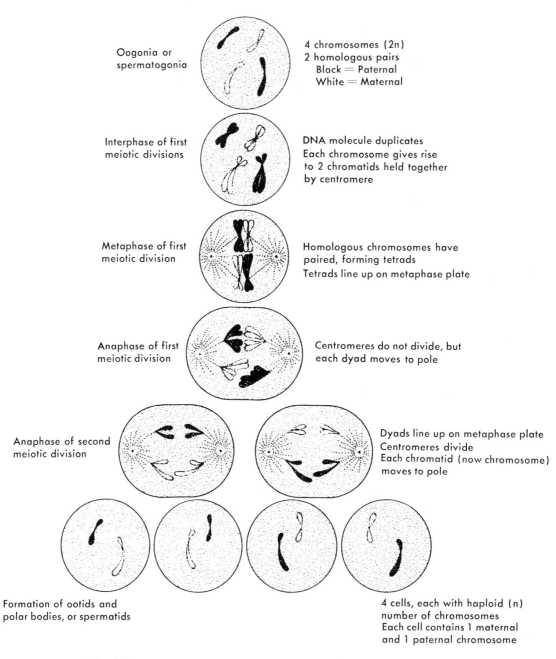

Oogonia or
spermatogonia

4 chromosomes (2n)
2 homologous pairs
    Black = Paternal
    White = Maternal

Interphase of first
meiotic divisions

DNA molecule duplicates
Each chromosome gives rise
to 2 chromatids held together
by centromere

Metaphase of first
meiotic division

Homologous chromosomes have
paired, forming tetrads
Tetrads line up on metaphase plate

Anaphase of first
meiotic division

Centromeres do not divide, but
each dyad moves to pole

Anaphase of second
meiotic division

Dyads line up on metaphase plate
Centromeres divide
Each chromatid (now chromosome)
moves to pole

Formation of ootids and
polar bodies, or spermatids

4 cells, each with haploid (n)
number of chromosomes
Each cell contains 1 maternal
and 1 paternal chromosome

Fig. 4-8
Simplified scheme of meiosis as illustrated by the fate of the centromere.

axis of the spindle in many cases is at right angles to the surface of the egg and nearer to one surface than to the other. When the cytoplasm divides in oogenesis, most of it remains with the chromosomes at the inner pole of the spindle. Only a small amount of cytoplasm pinches off with the outer chromosomes (Fig. 4-9). This unequal cytoplasmic division produces a large daughter cell and a small cell known as the polar body; both contain the same number of chromosomes. The chromosomes behave in the same fashion in spermatogenesis, but the small amount of cytoplasm present is divided equally at the first meiotic division. As a result two cells that are smaller than the primary spermatocytes form.

The cells resulting from the first meiotic division give rise to either secondary oocytes and polar bodies or secondary spermatocytes. There is no resting stage between this division and the next as in mitosis; instead a new spindle forms, and dyads move to the metaphase plate. The dyads then split, and each chromosome moves to the respective poles of the spindle.

Again the egg cytoplasm divides unequally (second meiotic division), but the primary spermatocyte separates into equal parts. Each cell formed now contains only half of the original number of chromosomes for the particular species; this is the *haploid* number.

Through oogenesis each primary oocyte produces a large haploid cell. This ootid has the obvious advantage of concentrating most of the cytoplasm and yolk into one cell. The first polar body may also divide and give rise to another

polar body, but eventually all the polar bodies degenerate. However, in the case of spermatogenesis four spermatids form from a primary spermatoctye, each containing an equal amount of cytoplasm and the haploid number of chromosomes. A member of each pair of chromosomes must be incorporated in the ootid or spermatid. When fertilization occurs, the full complement is returned to the zygote, and the individual cell again contains the diploid number consistent with the species.

Comparison of spermatogenesis and oogenesis
Time sequence of meiotic stages

Although one may distinguish three phases, proliferation, growth, and nuclear maturation, leading to the maturation of the ova or sperm, these events do not occur in the same order in the two kinds of gametes. Spermatogenesis takes place in the seminiferous tubules before any cytoplasmic differentiation of the sperm. After cell division has ceased and the chromosome number is reduced to half, the spermatids become attached to the Sertoli cells where they undergo *spermiogenesis*, or transformation, and complete their differentiation into mature spermatozoa. Actually, in the case of the sperm, there is a drastic change in shape and characteristics of the spermatozoon and a loss, rather than a differentiation, of their cytoplasm.

In the oocyte the reverse is true. The egg accumulates reserve food material and enters a period of growth in the ovary. When the oocyte starts to grow, the nucleus enters the prophase stage. Only after growth is completed does the

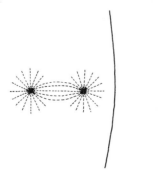 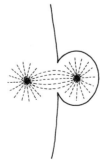

Fig. 4-9
Unequal cell division in oogenesis.

egg continue its meiotic divisions, which eventually give rise to the ootid and the three polar bodies. In the frog, for example, this growth period lasts for 3 years, since 1- and 2-year-old frogs do not have mature eggs. In the mammal, the growth period is correlated with the reproductive cycles. The nucleus remains in the prophase stage of the first meiotic division from birth until the preovulatory phase. According to Hadek (1965) the meiotic division resumes 4 to 15 hours before ovulation in the mouse and immediately preceding ovulation in the rabbit. As the cytoplasm of the oocyte increases in size, the nucleus produces large amounts of nuclear sap, giving it a bloated appearance. This enlarged oocyte nucleus is referred to as the *germinal vesicle.*

Evidence of nuclear activity in oocyte

Unlike the sperm that becomes specialized for motility, the egg must set up the machinery for maintaining the embryo after fertilization. During the prophase stage, the oocyte of certain animals with large eggs (newts, for example) contain chromosomes that have peculiarly shaped loops that appear to be thrown out at right angles to the central axis of the chromosomes. These loops give the chromosomes a fuzzy appearance. They look like lampbrushes and are known as *lampbrush chromosomes.* These loops may represent an unwinding of sections of DNA molecules, allowing them to come into intimate contact with the nuclear sap contents. From this pool of raw materials they are able to synthesize messenger RNA, which presumably leaves the nucleus by way of the nuclear pores and passes out into the cytoplasm of the cell. Studies of newly fertilized sea urchin eggs using actinomycin D (which blocks synthesis of new RNA) and of enucleated fragments of cells indicate that in this species at least it is the *RNA synthesized during the growth of the egg in the ovary* that is responsible for the manufacture of proteins during early stages of development. It is not until the late blastula or early gastrula state that the hereditary material

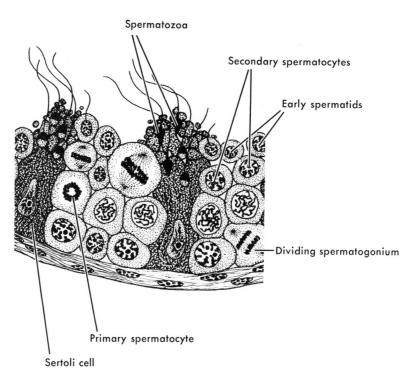

Fig. 4-10

Diagram of part of seminiferous tubule showing heads of spermatozoa embedded in the pockets of Sertoli cells.

carried by the sperm starts to express itself and influences the synthetic activities of the developing embryo.

Speed of meiotic process

The length of time it takes for the meiotic process to go to completion in the body also differs between the male and female animals. In the males, spermatogenesis occurs in the seminiferous tubules, since the sperm remain in contact with the Sertoli cells until their maturation is completed. After their release, they travel down the male reproductive duct and are ready to fertilize the egg.

In the female, oogenesis may be completed in the ovary, and when ovulated, the ovum contains the haploid number of chromosomes. In most vertebrates, however, only a part of the process has been accomplished by ovulation. The first meiotic division has occurred with the resulting formation of the first polar body, and the spindle is formed for the second division. The chromosomes (dyads) remain lined up on the equatorial plate at metaphase and remain this way *until the sperm penetrates the egg.* Thus the completion of the second meiotic division is among the many other reactions that are initiated by sperm penetration, in many vertebrate animals.

CYTOPLASMIC DIFFERENTIATION
Spermiogenesis

As indicated in Chapter 3 the sperm performs two functions: it penetrates and activates the egg to start developing, and it contributes the male hereditary characteristics to the zygote (fertilized egg). Previous to these events, the final stage of spermatogenesis transforms the haploid spermatid into a mature spermatozoon. As shown in Fig. 4-10, this process, *spermiogenesis,* takes place while the spermatids are embedded in the pockets of the Sertoli cells. Spermiogenesis involves complex changes in the cytoplasmic content of the cell, and shrinkage and loss of fluid from the nucleus (Fig. 4-11). Spermatozoa of vertebrate animals show a remarkable uniformity in overall construction. The exceedingly small, elongated sperm consists of a *head, neck, body* or middle piece, and a *tail*

or flagellum. Most of the cytoplasm is eliminated from the sperm as it becomes specialized for motility and egg penetration. Its motility, however, is not realized until it comes in contact with secretions from the accessory glands.

The elongated head of the vertebrate sperm varies from almond shaped (human) to oval, rod, cone, spiral, etc., and houses the haploid, tightly packed chromosomes, which contain the genes. The nucleus loses fluid and the chromatin material becomes so condensed that it does not appear in the form of distinct chromosomes even under the electron microscope. The nucleus may make up the entire length of the sperm or be restricted to one area. An anterior cap, or *acrosome,* produced by the Golgi apparatus, covers the head, and functions in penetrating the egg and making contact with the egg cytoplasm. An acrosomal vesicle forms. In some instances it contains a supply of lytic enzymes that dissolve the egg membranes during the fertilization process.

A short area known as the "neck" connects the head to the body of the sperm. Its anterior end contains the *proximal centriole,* which fits into a depression of the nucleus and is believed to help initiate cell division in the zygote. The *distal centriole,* which becomes the axial filament, is located in the posterior end of the neck. The body of the sperm consists of the filament and the enveloping mitochondria, arranged in a spiral pattern around the filament. These mitochondria, the "powerhouses" of the sperm, carry the oxidative enzymes responsible for supplying the necessary energy for motility.

The tail, or flagellum, is the longest part of the sperm and is responsible for propelling it forward through its liquid environment. In cross section the tail, under the electron microscope, is seen to consist of a pair of longitudinal tubules along its middle, surrounded by a ring of nine pairs of longitudinal tubules. This pattern is typical of such organelles of motility as cilia and flagella. An extra outer ring of nine more fibers is present in the sperm of mammals. These tubules seem to be responsible for the cell's cytoskeleton, but may participate also in cell movement. The exact mechanism responsible for sperm motility still remains a mystery,

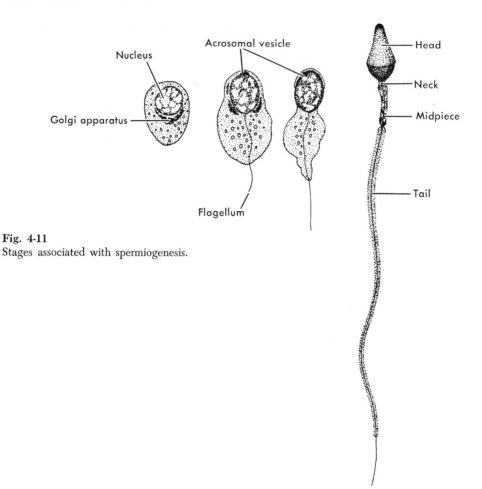

Fig. 4-11
Stages associated with spermiogenesis.

despite the fact that the subject is intriguing to a number of scientists from various areas of biology. Recent investigations suggest that the protein of cilia and flagella resemble the proteins of muscle fibrils. The tubules may contain adenosine triphosphatose, the enzyme associated with contraction. Perhaps at this time all we can do, in trying to emphasize the similarities among biological phenomena, is to suggest that there may be certain likenesses between the two contractile processes.

Most of the cytoplasm of the sperm is discarded. As the acrosome forms at the anterior end, the cytoplasm flows backward, leaving a thin film of cytoplasm covering the acrosome, nucleus, midpiece, and much of the flagellum. The terminal segment of the tail often lacks the cytoplasmic membrane, and consists only of the axial filament. The excess cytoplasm is cast off and eliminated, leaving no reserve food stores for the sperm, thus making it dependent on the environment for its nutrition.

Cytoplasmic maturation of egg
Formation of yolk

It is from the cytoplasm of the ovum that the new individual develops after the two gametes fuse. However, in many vertebrates the embryo must have a source of food reserves that will tide the animal over until it can acquire its own external supplies. Thus, the increase in egg size is primarily attributable to the synthesis of this food reserve or yolk. In the frog, a young oocyte of approximately 50 microns in diameter will grow over a 3-year period to about 1500 microns, with most of the growth occurring in the third year. The chick egg increases about 200 times in the 1 or 2 weeks before ovulation. The mammalian oocyte does not undergo extensive growth when compared with the ova of other vertebrates. A mouse egg is much smaller than a frog's egg and only increases about 43 times as it matures. The diameter of a mammalian egg is around 100 microns, and it contains little reserve food materials since the embryo will be supplied with its nutritional requirements from the mother by way of the placenta. The variation in yolk content is considered an adaptive feature of the vertebrates and can be associated with the particular developmental state of the animal. The animals that begin feeding early (frog) or that have food supplied to them (viviparous mammals) store little yolk in their eggs. Its presence or absence does not alter the basic structure of the egg, the cytoplasm that is responsible for the embryo's body; but the amount of yolk will affect future cleavage planes as well as rates of cleavage.

Most young vertebrate oocytes contain few of the complex structures found in adult cells. The granular cytoplasm is rich in nucleic acids, primarily RNA, which is associated with protein synthesis, but it contains few mitochondria and lacks a typical endoplasmic reticulum. Lipids, lipoproteins, and glycogen appear, but mainly yolk accumulates in the cytoplasm as its future energy supply. Yolk is a general term given to the material stored as food in the egg. It is not a definite chemical entity but varies from one type of egg to another. The general components are proteins, phospholipids, and neutral fats; and the final product, the yolk, ranges from fine granules to large, flat granules described as yolk platelets (in amphibian eggs).

Yolk granules may be sparse but evenly dispersed throughout the cytoplasm, as in amphioxus and the human egg. Such an egg is known as an *isolecithal egg*. In some vertebrates the granules are unevenly distributed in the cytoplasm. Located primarily in the vegetative region, they leave the animal pole relatively free. These eggs are referred to as *telolecithal*. This type of egg ranges from those of the frog in which stratification of the yolk platelets occurs, with few yolk platelets at the animal pole and densely packed granules at the vegetal pole, to the egg of the reptile or chick in which the entire egg is composed primarily of yolk. In these latter examples the cytoplasm forms only a thin disk on the upper side of the egg. The fish egg is somewhat similar to that of the bird, although in some cases, rather than a disk of cytoplasm, a thin surface layer of cytoplasm surrounds the entire yolk. In any case, the nucleus is always restricted to the cytoplasmic portion of the egg.

Evidence for the site of yolk formation in the egg is somewhat contradictory. It may be synthesized by the endoplasmic reticulum, the Golgi apparatus, or mitochondria of the developing egg. However, the site of yolk synthesis (or certain of its components) in most vertebrates appears to be the liver of the adult female. Proteins and phospholipids transported by the bloodstream pass to the follicle cell, which deposits the material in the oocyte. The injection of a vital dye (trypan blue for example) into the bloodstream of a bird allows visualization of this function of the follicle cell. The blue dye passes to the follicular cells and then into the oocyte.

Establishment of egg organization

As the oocyte matures, an organization is set up in the egg that will affect the future development of the embryo. This organization occurs on both the macroscopic level and on the microscopic and submicroscopic or molecular levels. Polarity of the egg is established early and is one of the main results of oocyte differentiation. Almost nothing is known of its origin. In isolecithal forms where little yolk is present, the site of polar body formation is a good indicator of the *animal pole*. Most of the cytoplasm will be at this pole in the telolecithal eggs. On the other hand, yolk granules concentrate at the opposite or *vegetal pole*. This stratification of cytoplasmic substances produces polarity in the mature oocyte. Pigment granules are visible examples of materials distributed in a stratified manner. In the frog, dark brown to black pigment granules, located at the animal pole, concentrate primarily in the cortical region of the egg. They cover the surface of the egg to a point slightly below its equator. The egg axis, therefore, is established as a line connecting the two poles and results from the stratification of materials accumulating in the ooplasm.

The animal pole contains the germinal vesicle, small granules, and a higher content of respiratory enzymes than does the vegetal pole. It is considered the most active part of the egg. The vegetal pole is more sluggish physiologically and marks the location of the nutritive materials of the future embryo. The two poles are destined to become specific sites of the embryo. For example, the animal pole will become the cephalic or head end of the future tadpole. In those eggs with a large amount of yolks (chick, for example) the high concentration of yolk becomes the ventral side of the animal.

The establishment of the *egg cortex,* consisting of the thin outer layer of cytoplasm and the cell membrane, is one of the most important changes that occurs in the oocyte on the submicroscopic level. It differs from the rest of the cell in that most of the egg cytoplasm is a sol with the various inclusions (mitochondria, ribosomes) distributed at random in the continuous liquid phase. The cortex, however, is a gel whose viscous consistency holds its components in place. In several vertebrates, but not all, this surface layer of the egg contains granules that play an important part at the time of fertilization. The granules are located next to the cell membrane in a mature oocyte and are composed of acid mucopolysaccharides. There is evidence that the cortex has some kind of organizing ability. When a newly fertilized egg is centrifuged and the contents are displaced, if there is enough time before the first cleavage furrow forms, the internal constituents return to their normal position in relation to the cortex. The cortex remains fixed during centrifugation and gives a stability to the location of various surface areas as development is initiated. Recent experiments indicate that the cortex may contain regions with special inducing properties, for example, the gray crescent area whose significance is discussed in a later chapter.

EGG MEMBRANES

By the time the vertebrate egg reaches maturity, egg envelopes or membranes, which pro-

tect it from chemical or physical injury, develop. In some animals they act as barriers to multiple sperm penetration. Not all vertebrates have the same type of egg membranes. They vary according to the class of animal and reflect the adaptations made by the animal in order to ensure development of the young in its particular environment. There are several ways of classifying these membranes, but the simplest way is to group them according to their origin. Those membranes formed in the ovary and laid down between the plasmalemma and the follicular cells are considered to be *primary membranes.* The follicular cells produce *secondary membranes.* However, it is difficult if not impossible always to determine whether the egg cytoplasm, the follicular cells, or the cooperative efforts of both produce the membranes. *Tertiary membranes* are secreted by the cells of the oviduct as the egg travels down the duct toward the cloaca.

Membranes produced by ovary or follicular cells

Eggs, like all living cells, have a plasma membrane around their surface that holds the yolk and cytoplasm together as an entity and functions osmotically to control the egg contents. The membrane is the *plasmalemma.* A noncellular, transparent *vitelline membrane* forms on the outside of the plasmalemma, but is given different names in different animals. In amphibia and birds it is in close contact with the ooplasmic surface until the egg is fertilized, at which time it separates from this surface, forming a tough fertilization membrane. In fish this membrane is referred to as the *chorion,* and in reptiles and mammals it is given the name *zona pellucida.* It usually remains intact through several stages of cleavage where it appears to help hold the dividing cells together.

External to the primary membrane are the follicle cells. Microvilli from the follicle cells and from the plasmalemma surface of the oocyte often interdigitate at the zona pellucida giving it the appearance of a radially striated zone under the light microscope. This striated zone is known as the *zona radiata* (Fig. 4-12). When the graafian follicle of the mammal ruptures

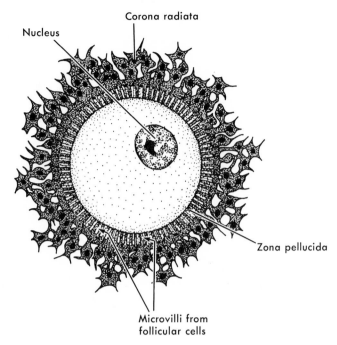

Nucleus

Corona radiata

Zona pellucida

Microvilli from
follicular cells

Fig. 4-12

Section through a young mammalian oocyte surrounded by follicle cells. The electron microscope reveals the cytoplasm of the follicle cells to be drawn out into fingerlike projections between the oocyte and follicle cell. These microvilli contact the surface of the oocyte and, under the light microscope, appear as radiating lines. In the mammal, this area is known as the zona radiata.

and releases the mature ovum, the egg carries with it, for some distance down the fallopian tube, a layer of follicular cells. These cells are columnar in shape and arranged radially in a single layer around the ovum. They are known as the *corona radiata* and should not be confused with the unfortunate similar term, zona radiata, which refers to the interdigitating microvilli.

Membranes produced by oviduct

The tertiary membranes involve albumen layers, shell membranes, and the shell itself. As the egg of the amphibian spirals down the oviduct, three rather uniform layers of albumen (jelly) are deposited around it. The inner layer is a thin one and most viscous; the outer, wide and more fluid; the middle layer, intermediate. The jelly envelopes hold the eggs together in masses or strands, protect the eggs from infections, insulate the eggs, make them unappetizing to predators since they are tasteless, and anchor the eggs to twigs and plants. Besides these physi-

cal functions, the jelly coats apparently also help to make the frog's egg fertilizable, since up to now no egg taken directly from the body cavity has been induced to develop into an embryo.

Five membranes make up the envelopes of the chick egg. External to the vitelline membranes are added the white of the egg (albumen), two shell membranes, and a porous shell (Fig. 4-13). As the egg begins its spiral pathway down the oviduct, albumen is secreted around the vitelline membrane of the egg. The rotation of the egg in the oviduct twists the albumen that projects from the yolk and forms what is known as the *chalaza*. As the egg proceeds down the duct, concentric layers of egg white are added around the yolk. The chalaza helps anchor the egg in the center of the albumen, which is an additional nutritional reserve for the developing embryo and which has bactericidal qualities. Inner and outer shell membranes are secreted around the egg white and are in contact with one another except at the blunt end of the egg. In this area one can see that the inner mem-

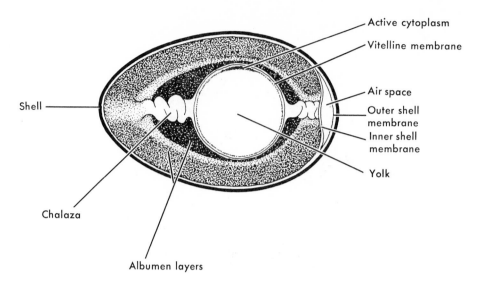

Fig. 4-13
Diagram of the five membranes enveloping the chick egg.

brane remains with the egg white, while the outer membrane becomes associated with the shell of the egg.

SUGGESTED READINGS

1. Alston, R. E.: Cellular continuity and development, Chicago, 1967, Scott, Foresman & Co.
2. Austin, C. R., and Short, R. V.: Germ cells and fertilization, Cambridge, 1972, University Press.
3. Bishop, D. W.: Biology of spermatozoa. In Young, W. C. (editor): Sex and internal secretions, Baltimore, 1967, The Williams & Wilkins Co., pp. 707-795.
4. Blackler, A. W.: Contributions to the study of germ-cells in the Anura, J. Embryol. Exp. Morphol. **6:** 491-503, 1958.
5. Blandau, R. J.: Biology of eggs and implantations. In Young, W. C. (editor): Sex and internal secretions, Baltimore, 1967, The Williams & Wilkins Co., pp. 797-882.
6. Fawcett, D. W.: The structure of the mammalian spermatozoon, Int. Rev. Cyt. **7:**195-234, 1958.
7. Hadek, R.: The structure of the mammalian egg, Int. Rev. Cyt. **18:**29-71, 1965.
8. Mazia, D.: The cell cycle, Sci. Am. **230:**54-64, 1974.
9. Steward, F. D., Mapes, M. O., Kent, A. E., and Holsten, R. D.: Growth and the development of cultured plant cells, Science **143:**20-27, 1964.
10. Taylor, J. H. (editor): The organization and duplication of genetic material. In Selected papers on molecular genetics, New York, 1965, Academic Press Inc., pp. 296-311.
11. Watson, J. D.: Moving toward the clonal man, The Atlantic **227:**50-53, 1971.
12. Weismann, A.: The continuity of the germ-plasm as the foundation of a theory of heredity, 1889, Reprinted in Gabriel, M. L., and Fogel, S. (editors): Great experiments in biology, Englewood Cliffs, N. J., 1955, Prentice-Hall, Inc.

CHAPTER 5

FERTILIZATION

FUNCTION OF FERTILIZATION

Fertilization is the union of the male and female gametes and the formation of a single group of chromosomes. It is usually irreversible. This fusion establishes in the zygote the diploid condition characteristic of the species involved. The genetic sex of the individual is also determined at this time; the individual is male or female depending on whether the egg is fertilized by a sperm carrying a Y or an X chromosome. When the sperm unites with the egg, the egg becomes activated and the zygote begins a series of cleavages that lead to the development of the embryo. The spermatozoon normally contributes the centrosome, which organizes the necessary machinery for cell division. In some cases the point at which the sperm enters the egg establishes the plane of bilateral symmetry in the future embryo.

In describing fertilization, the sequence of events leading to the union of the two gametes is usually considered a part of the process and involves the following steps:

1. Activation of the spermatozoon, referred to as *capacitation*
2. Approach of the spermatozoon to the egg and its contact with the egg membranes
3. Penetration of the membranes surrounding the ovum
4. Activation of the egg
5. Syngamy or fusion of the pronuclei, and the establishment of the first cleavage spindle

Fertilization has greater significance, however, than the union of the sperm with the egg and the production of a new individual. When it involves the union of chromosomes from unrelated groups, it also ensures the distribution of genes throughout the population. It is a method of gene dispersal that introduces variety, offering greater combinations for natural selection. At this level of interpretation, fertilization is a phenomenon that aids in adaptive variation, and is one of a series of nuclear changes that leads to the evolution of the species.

Certain marine invertebrates, particularly the sea urchins, are the subjects of most of the studies of fertilization. Their eggs are readily available, relatively large, lack obscuring yolk granules, and can be maintained with ease in their normal physiological medium, seawater. Observation of the steps leading to the fusion of the egg and sperm is less difficult than in other forms. Among the vertebrates, fish and amphibian eggs provide good investigative material for analytical studies, but there are few extensive descriptions of fertilization of mammalian eggs. Not only are these eggs difficult to obtain but there are also many problems in establishing and maintaining an environment suitable for the continued viability of the gametes (Marx, 1973).

The factors involved in the successful fertilization of the egg by the sperm have not all been defined. In fact, the whole subject is somewhat controversial, with no general agreement as to the essential requirements or the steps involved in the fertilization reaction. There is a tendency, therefore, to extrapolate and assume that the processes that occur in one form of animal life (marine invertebrates) take place in the mammals as well. This may not be true. The generalized picture of fertilization presented in this chapter is a composite one and all events may not occur in all animals. If we recognize the danger of overgeneralization, the stepwise pattern of fertilization described offers insight into an extremely complex process. Many features remain unknown, and many species need to be investigated, before a specific picture of fertilization can be detailed for any one group of animals.

The understanding of fertilization is further complicated by the fact that although normally the penetration of the egg by the sperm triggers egg activation and the subsequent events leading to development, the same reaction can be induced by other means. In nature, the eggs of a few animals, bees and wasps for example, usually develop without fertilization. Activation of the egg, then, does not depend on some unique property of the spermatozoon, since a variety of agents are effective in initiating changes in the egg cytoplasm. Such a phenomenon (that is, the development of an egg without fertilization) is known as parthenogenesis, and when it occurs in nature it is referred to as *natural parthenogenesis*. When experimentally induced in the laboratory, it is *artificial parthenogenesis*. For many years this phenomenon has intrigued biologists trying to gain insight into the problems of fertilization by inducing development through artificial parthenogenesis. By this experimental technique they hope to separate those factors of development that are indigenous to the egg from those introduced by the sperm.

CONTACT OF EGG BY SPERM
Meeting of gametes

For fertilization to occur successfully, the male gamete first must find the female gamete; the ripe sperm must be delivered at the right time to the vicinity of the ripe egg. Fertilization does not occur at the same stage in the life cycle of all unfertilized eggs. The eggs of various animals differ in their stage of nuclear maturation at the time of fertilization. In some animals the germinal vesicle is still intact and sperm penetration initiates the meiotic process. In others, the second polar body has formed and the female pronucleus is ready to fuse with the male pronucleus. The majority of vertebrate eggs are ovulated when they are in the second meiotic metaphase.

As can be seen in Fig. 5-1, the sperm can enter the egg anytime between the germinal vesicle stage (oocyte) and the stage when both polar bodies have formed (ootid). The stage of nuclear maturation, however, at which a particular egg can be fertilized is specific for the animal involved.

Several devices have evolved in vertebrates to ensure encounter between these two germ cells. The reproductive patterns of most animals involve the use of at least one such device. Light and environmental temperature affects the sexual maturation of many marine invertebrates, sea urchins for example. As stated in Chapter 3, breeding cycles of vertebrates are under the control of hormones that direct the simultaneous maturation of the gametes and bring about their synchronous release. In many cases intricate patterns of mating behavior that bring the adult female and males together at the proper biological time have evolved. In terrestrial animals copulatory organs facilitate

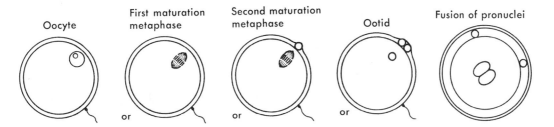

Oocyte	First maturation metaphase	Second maturation metaphase	Ootid	Fusion of pronuclei
	or	or	or	

Fig. 5-1

Stages of egg maturation and fertilization. Sperm can enter the egg any time between oocyte stage and completion of meiosis. The stage of nuclear maturation at which a particular egg can be fertilized is specific for the animal involved.

the delivery of sperm into the female reproductive tract near the site of egg release.

The timing of gamete release is a critical one. Once ejaculated or ovulated, in general, the life-span of the sperm or ova is short, ranging from a few minutes to a few days. The ova of many fish and amphibia, unless protected in some way, lose their ability to be fertilized within seconds or minutes after their release into the water. For example, those amphibia that deposit their sperm in packets (spermatophores) provide an environment in which the sperm remain viable outside the reproductive tract of the male for a long period of time. Sperm released into pond water have a shorter functional life-span than do those shed in the more physiological saltwater. Gametes deposited in the female reproductive tract (internal fertilization) remain fertilizable for an even longer period of time. The ovulated human egg remains fertilizable for about 24 hours. The sperm also remains active for about that length of time.

The fact that the sperm is so tiny, contains little or no energy stores, and expends energy as it moves about definitely limits its functional life. There are exceptions to this; for example, during hibernation, the spermatozoa of the bat may survive in the reproductive tract of the female for several months. In the hen the sperm migrate the length of the oviduct where they collect in the ostium. A hen can lay fertile eggs for as long as 3 weeks after insemination, demonstrating that the life-span of spermatozoa in this species is longer than in many vertebrates.

Man also manipulates the life-span of sperm by preserving them, usually under low pressure in sperm banks. This has been done for many years by livestock breeders who collect semen from prize studs for artificial insemination of breeding females. Only recently has the idea of sperm banks for storage of human sperm been accepted, although the suggestion was made many years ago by Mueller who was concerned about the survival of the human population in an atomic age. Now the idea is correlated with the ban on population growth. Some males who plan to undergo vasectomy store their sperm in sperm banks. A reservoir is thus provided for their genetic material in case they change their minds about the number of children they wish to father.

Eggs also can become overripe and unfertilizable. They can remain in the uteri of the frog from 4 to 10 days and still be fertilized, but they lose this ability as the time increases. The complete degeneration of the eggs of most mammals follows ovulation without fertilization. They apparently undergo fragmentation and are absorbed by the cells of the reproductive tract or are expelled through the vagina. Such factors as concentration of sperm, anaerobic or aerobic conditions, presence of glycolyzable substrates in the semen, and pH of the environment affect the life of the gametes. For these reasons it is extremely difficult to find an artificial medium that simulates the normal environment of the reproductive tract, one in which the eggs can be fertilized and their developmental stages followed in vitro.

Animals shed astronomical numbers of eggs and sperm if the gametes are merely released near one another into the surrounding water. It is estimated that the bullfrog, *Rana catesbeiana,* may lay as many as 20,000 eggs at a time. Even in more protected environments the male releases excessive numbers of spermatozoa compared to the number of eggs ovulated. In a single ejaculation the human male may produce several million motile sperm, but only one sperm penetrates the plasma membrane of one egg. These large numbers of male gametes appear to be essential for successful fertilization.

Even the female reproductive tract is a hostile environment for the migrating sperm. Several barriers interfere with the progress of the sperm toward the *ampulla* of the *fallopian*

tubes, where the union of gametes ultimately takes place. Cilia lining the tubes (as shown in Fig. 5-2) beat in the opposite direction, toward the uterus. The lumen size progressively decreases from the uterus to the *ostium* of the fallopian tube, making it more difficult for sperm migration. The mucous secretions of the reproductive tract dilute the sperm; many are lost on the surface of the mucous lining. As a result, despite the excessive numbers produced, few sperm actually make their way to the site of fertilization. Austin (1965) reports that he was able to recover only less than 100 sperm

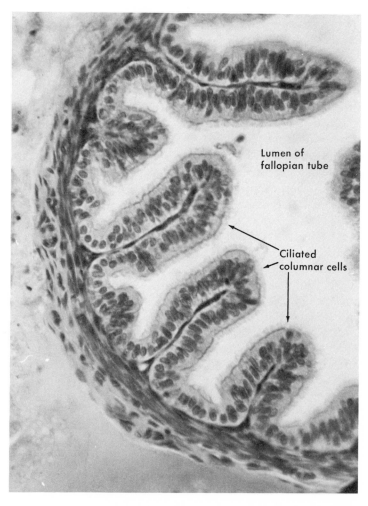

Lumen of
fallopian tube

Ciliated
columnar cells

Fig. 5-2
Transverse section of fallopian tube showing the epithelial lining composed of ciliated columnar cells. Cilia beat toward the uterus. (× 450.)

in the fallopian tubes of the rat, mouse, and hamster, about 200 in the field vole, and less than a thousand in the rabbit, dog, and sheep.

Although copulatory organs develop in terrestrial animals, the distance covered by the sperm before they reach the immediate environment of the egg is very great, considering the size of the gamete. The contractions of the muscles in the wall of the ductus deferens and urethra aid the deposition of sperm into the female genital tract of mammals. The human sperm travels from 3 to 6 mm. per minute. It takes 3 to 4 hours for human and rabbit sperm to reach their destinations. In general, sperm move at a faster rate than can be accounted for by the simple movements of their flagella. Contractions of the muscular wall of the female reproductive tract propel the sperm forward. It has been suggested that the downward beating of the cilia in the tubes aids the sperm ascent by creating currents in the lumen of the tube. The contents of the tube flow down the sides and then circulate up through the center, presumably moving the sperm along with it. Apparently, spermatozoa use their flagella only when they have reached the vicinity of the egg. Random movements and chance dictate which sperm comes in contact with which egg.

Since most sperm are motile, they must be deposited in an aquatic medium in order for them to reach the egg. Aquatic animals merely release their sperm in the water over the eggs at the time they are spawned, or soon after. The right environmental conditions stimulate large numbers of sea urchins to shed their eggs or sperm into the water at one time, forming clouds of gametes. Fertilization takes place on a grand scale. Insemination of frog eggs occurs as the female lays her eggs during *amplexus*, sexual embrace of the female by the male. The sperm must be in the immediate vicinity since the eggs are encased in jelly-like envelopes that absorb water. As soon as they reach the water, the jelly rapidly swells and is a handicap to further sperm penetration. As was pointed out earlier, some amphibians protect their sperm by packaging them in protective, moisture-conserving capsules that the female picks up by her *cloacal lips* and retains until needed. Vertebrate animals, engaging in internal fertilization, substitute semen for the water medium. It also supplies an energy source for the almost cytoplasmically naked spermatozoa.

In many vertebrates the union of sperm and egg is further complicated by the various membranes that surround the egg. They must be pierced if the sperm is to make contact with the cytoplasmic surface. In many invertebrates and a few vertebrates (such as teleosts and sturgeons), several small holes or micropyles in the membrane allow the sperm to pass through the thick outer covering of the egg, as seen in Fig. 5-3. The lamprey egg has a small tuft of material at the animal pole and the chorion in this region lacks a thick jelly coat. It is at this point that sperm penetrate the chorion. In some manner the micropyles attract the sperm as shown by their increase in motility as they approach the egg. For the majority of the vertebrates, however, micropyles do not exist and the sperm must penetrate the jelly coats or other investing membranes. Follicle cells still cling to the *zona pellucida* after ovulation of the mammalian egg and the minute spermatozoon must penetrate all layers.

Interacting substances of sperm and eggs

Most investigators agree that there is no definite evidence of chemotaxis in animals. Chemotaxis is usually defined as the ability of the sperm to detect a difference in concentration of some substance released into the water by the egg and to move from an area of lower to one of greater concentration of that substance. Apparently, such a chemical attraction of the male gamete operates only in the plants, mosses, and ferns. There is a suggestion, however, that fish may have such a factor. The spermatozoa of these vertebrates become increasingly active as they approach the micropyle of the chorion, and they gather about its opening as if attracted specifically to its location. An isolated bit of chorion containing a micropyle also attracts sperm. On the other hand the vitelline membrane of the egg alone does not stimulate the sperm to greater activity or cause them to move toward the piece of tissue. The chorion, specifically the walls of the micropyle, appears to release some kind of substance that aids the spermatozoa in finding the opening leading to the egg. However, the substance has not been chemically identified.

We have known for many years that the eggs and sperm of some animals are chemically attracted to one another. They release into the surrounding medium substances that bring about agglutination of the sperm and the adherence of the sperm to the egg. These substances are considered to be more of a trapping agent for the sperm than a chemotaxic factor. In some cases they appear to act by preventing penetration of the egg by more than one sperm. Studies

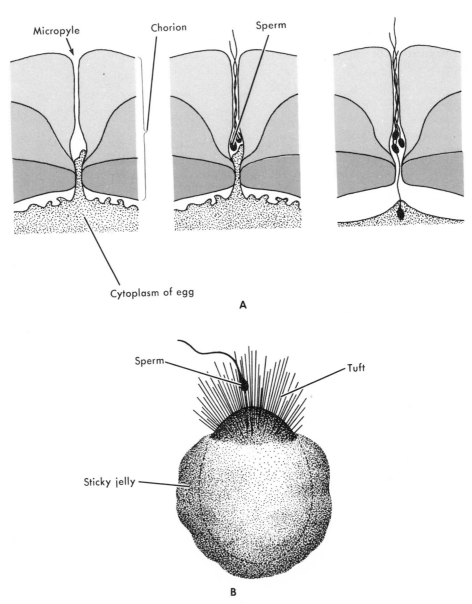

Fig. 5-3
Thick membranes complicate the union of sperm and egg. **A,** Small holes, or micropyles, allow the sperm to pass through the outer covering of some teleost and sturgeon eggs. **B,** A sperm penetrates the chorion of the lamprey egg at region of tufts.

of these interacting substances have been carried out mostly on the sea urchin, but the eggs of vertebrates probably induce a similar agglutinating effect. Such substances have been described for the cyclostomes, fish, and amphibians.

F. R. Lillie (1919), one of the pioneers in the field of fertilization, studied the process in sea urchins and concluded that the jelly coats of the egg did more than protect. He found them to be saturated by an active material that he believed was released by the egg. This material stimulated sperm motility and brought about a clumping of the sperm, usually head to head. If ripe unfertilized sea urchin eggs were allowed to remain in seawater for a time and then the eggs were removed and sperm added, the spermatozoa became sticky and adhered to one another. Lillie called the material located in the jelly coat *fertilizin*. A protein substance extractable from the surface of the spermatozoa was given the name *antifertilizin*. According to Lillie's fertilizin theory, presented in diagram form in Fig. 5-4, fertilizin present in the cortex

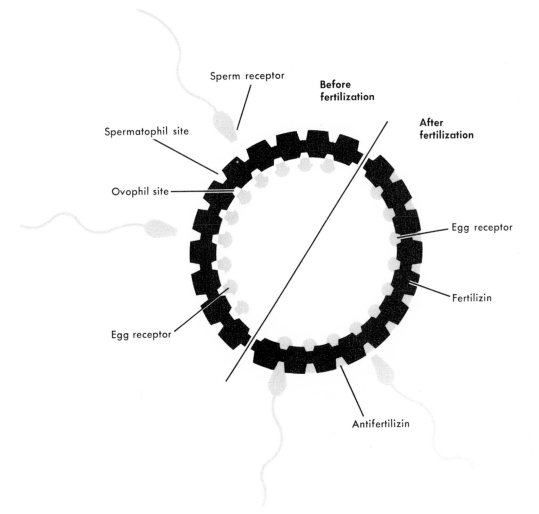

Fig. 5-4
Schematic presentation of Lillie's fertilizin theory. Fertilizin present in cortex of egg contains an ovophilic and a spermatophilic binding site. At fertilization the receptor on sperm surface combines with spermatophil site, somehow blocking all other sperm-binding sites.

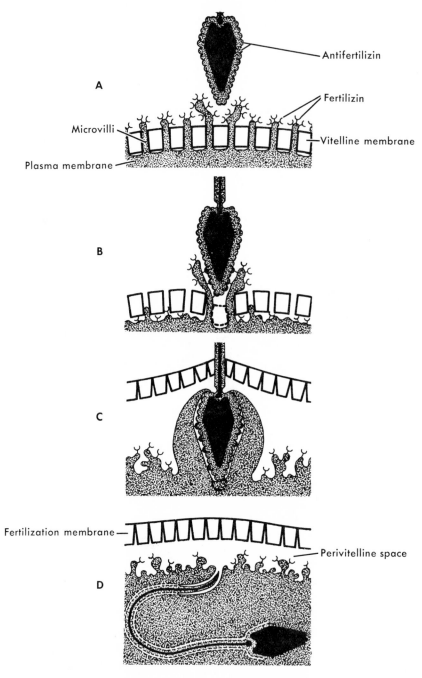

Fig. 5-5
Scheme for sperm penetration. **A,** Fertilizin is located on tips of microvilli, extensions of plasma membrane that perforate the vitelline membrane. **B,** Antifertilizin of sperm reacts with fertilizin when sperm contacts egg surface and (**C** and **D**) sperm is drawn inside vitelline membrane. All other microvilli (**B** and **C**) are retracted and no other sperm can enter egg cytoplasm.

of the egg contains two active binding sites. One is an ovophil group, the other a spermatophil. At fertilization the receptor on the sperm surface combines with the spermatophil site. Lillie hypothesized that when this happens all the rest of the sperm-binding sites somehow become blocked and penetration of more than one sperm is thus prevented. The ovophil groups, in turn, react with the egg causing it to become activated.

Although all of Lillie's conclusions are no longer acceptable, his work stimulated many investigations in the field. A more modern interpretation of Lillie's interacting substances has been offered by Tyler (1963). According to him, fertilizin is definitely located in the plasma membrane of eggs, extending into the egg's gelatinous coats (if present). Antifertilizin can be detected in the membrane of the sperm. Both substances are specific receptor substances that interact in an antigen-antibody–like fashion. The reaction depends on the spatial arrangement of the atoms, in that one molecule fits the surface of another something like a key in a lock.

Tyler suggests a scheme for sperm penetration, shown in Fig. 5-5, in which the interacting substances aid in the incorporation of the sperm into the egg cytoplasm. As detected in electron micrographs, many microvilli, extensions of the plasma membrane, perforate the vitelline membrane. Fertilizin located on the protruding tips of the microvilli reacts with the antifertilizin of the sperm. After this initial contact with the fertilizing sperm, the microvilli retract drawing the sperm into the egg. Other sperm are unable to penetrate the vitelline membrane and enter the egg cytoplasm, since the receptors on the plasma membrane are inaccessible to them.

Fertilizin is a glycoprotein that is probably synthesized in the gonad during meiosis, rather than by the egg as Lillie believed. It composes the jelly coat; it actually is the jelly coat and dissolves in the seawater after the eggs are laid. Since it is multivalent, it can link several spermatozoa together, resulting in the clumping reaction of sperm, possibly as shown in Fig. 5-6. Fertilizin consists of a number of amino acids and monosaccharides that vary from one species

of animals to another and that are responsible for the species specificity of the material. The reactions between fertilizin and antifertilizin are stronger when they involve egg and sperm from the same species, although related species give weak reactions. The specificity of the reaction helps ensure the fertilization of the egg by the same species of spermatozoon and not some other.

One theory suggests that the fertilizin molecules on the egg surface trap the sperm and hold it at its surface, making penetration easier. However, this is difficult to prove. All investigators do not agree that the fertilizin molecule is located on the egg surface as well as on jelly coats. Others believe that the reaction between the two molecules merely traps the sperm in the vicinity of the egg, inhibiting polyspermy and allowing one sperm to penetrate the egg surface.

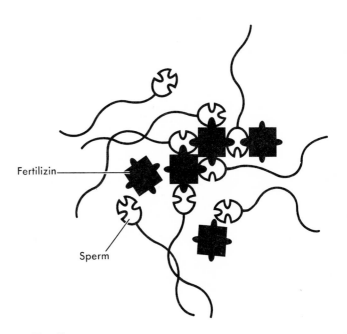

Fig. 5-6
Suggested action of sea urchin fertilizin. Multivalent fertilizin can link several sperm together, producing clumping reaction.

Although most of the investigations have been carried out on invertebrates, there is evidence that the jelly coats of frog and toad eggs contain interacting substances that are both species-specific and shared (between species) and that they play a role in the penetration of the egg by the sperm. The cells in the various regions of the frog's oviduct are responsible for secreting the jellies, with the upper third responsible for the jelly containing antigens shared by more than one species, and the lower levels of the oviduct producing species-specific antigens. The species-specific antigens then would be present in the outer jelly coat, since it is the last to be added. Shaver, in 1966, suggested a scheme of sperm penetration in which a reaction occurs between the species-specific molecules of the sperm and those in the outer jelly coat of the frog's egg, that is, the union of combining sites on the sperm surface with the jelly molecules. This helps to ensure interbreeding by the same species. As a result the sperm is activated, or *capacitated,* a reaction described more fully later in this chapter. As the sperm increased its penetration distance through the jelly envelope, other combining sites on its surface would react with jelly molecules common to other species and the final reaction between complementary sites on egg and sperm would allow the last step in sperm penetration to occur.

There are some reports of the presence of interacting substances present in the eggs of rabbits, mice, and cows where the zona pellucida is evidently responsible for the production of the material. In general, interacting substances in the gametes of mammals have not been studied in any detail.

SPERM PENETRATION

The actual penetration of the egg by the spermatozoon can be separated into three general steps.

1. The sperm must penetrate the membranes that surround the egg. These vary from the thick tough chorion or vitelline membrane of some fishes, to the jelly layers of the amphibian, and to the zona pellucida and attached corona radiata of the mammals.

2. When the spermatozoon contacts the egg surface, its membrane fuses with the plasma membrane of the egg.

3. The sperm nucleus along with its middle piece is drawn into the cytoplasm of the egg. The tail may or may not be left outside the membrane or trapped in the perivitelline space.

The egg water of sea urchins not only brings about the agglutination of the spermatozoa, but it also causes the sperm to undergo a structural change known as the *acrosomal reaction.* Whether fertilizin is the responsible agent for all the changes associated with this reaction is not known. The acrosomal reaction takes a variety of forms in different animals, but the end result is the release of materials, usually in the form of the acrosomal filament, and the secretion of lysins. The filament aids the sperm in penetrating the membrane barriers of the egg, and the lysins dissolve away parts of the membrane, providing a pathway for the entering spermatozoon. The solvent action of these enzymes provides the mechanism for sperm penetration.

Capacitation

Before the acrosomal reaction can take place, however, the sperm must undergo some kind of physiological change that increases its ability to penetrate the egg. The general term *capacitation* is given to this change. The egg water initiates this sperm activation in the sea urchin, and a similar process occurs in the amphibian when the spermatozoon comes in contact with the jelly coats. Removal of the jelly coats from the egg before they come in contact with the sperm inhibits fertilization. On the other hand, eggs taken from the body cavity, which lack jelly coats and normally cannot be fertilized, may be penetrated by the spermatozoon if they are first exposed to jellied eggs. Obviously the spermatozoa and the jelly coat somehow interact and increase the fertilizing capacity of the gamete (Shaver, 1966).

The environment of the female genital tract induces capacitation in the sperm of those animals that practice internal fertilization. In mammals freshly ejaculated sperm transferred to the ampulla region of newly ovulated eggs fertilizes few eggs. On the other hand, insertion of the sperm into the genital tract before ovulation occurs, activates the sperm in some way and enhances their capacity to fertilize the egg.

Acrosomal reaction
Membrane fusion

Once the spermatozoa are activated, the series of events described as the acrosomal reaction may be followed by electron microscopy. Prior to the 1960s researchers believed that the plasma membrane of the egg elevated and phagocytized the sperm, drawing it inside the egg. Although this may occur in some instances, electron microscopic studies reveal that in general the penetration of the egg by the sperm involves a fusion of their membranes. In this process the shape of the acrosome is altered. The successive stages in the acrosomal reaction in the invertebrate *Hydroides hexagonus* is depicted in Fig. 5-7. The acrosomal vesicle (the covering over the acrosome) splits, the acrosomal granule disappears (apparently releasing lysin), and the one or more filaments contact the plasma membrane. Invagination occurs in the plasma membrane at the points of contact with the filaments, and fusion of the two membranes takes place at these areas of interdigitation. These and other detailed studies of the acrosomal reaction have been carried out by the Colwins, who investigated this process in the annelid worm *Hydroides* and in the protochordate *Saccoglossus*. According to the Colwins, "the major role of the acrosome is apparently to deliver the sperm plasma membrane to the egg plasma membrane" (Colwin, 1963).

A similar series of acrosomal events have been observed in the toad, chicken, hamster, rabbit, guinea pig, and man; so it appears that the *Hydroides-Saccoglossus* pattern of gamete membrane fusion described by the Colwins also occurs in the chordates. Few complete studies, however, have been made on the vertebrates. Mammalian spermatozoa recovered after they have penetrated the zona pellucida lack an acrosome. This loss is usually interpreted as analogous to the splitting of the acrosomal vesicle when the invertebrate sperm contacts the egg. The acrosomal granules released apparently aid the sperm in penetrating the thick pellucida.

One of the most detailed studies of sperm penetration in the mammal was made by Szollosi and Ris (1961). They followed later stages in the fertilization process in the rat and described the penetration of the plasma membrane by the sperm of this animal. Their electron micrographs showed that after the sperm penetrated the ovum it had no plasma membrane, although one was present before and during the process of fertilization. They suggested that contact between the sperm head and the plasma membrane of the egg brought about a rupture of the two membranes. As a result, the egg membrane fused with the sperm plasma membrane at the point of contact and formed a continuous membrane around the egg and outer surface of the sperm. At first a deep fold of membrane forms around the sperm (Fig. 5-8). Eventually, as fusion of membranes proceeds toward the tail of the sperm, the entire naked sperm is drawn into the egg, leaving its plasma membrane to be incorporated into the egg membrane.

These investigations by the Colwins and by Szollosi and Ris demonstrate the importance of egg and sperm plasma membranes in the actual entrance of the sperm into the egg cytoplasm. It is possible that the acrosome of both invertebrate and vertebrate sperm undergoes similar changes. However, at the present time insufficient evidence on enough species prevents us from making a generalized statement concerning acrosomal structure, sperm activation, and egg membrane penetration.

Once the acrosomal filaments contact the plasma membrane, the cytoplasm flows up inside the filament membrane, covering the sperm head, midpiece, and possibly the tail (Fig. 5-7 G to I). This cytoplasmic elevation is the *fertilization cone*. The type of acrosomal filament varies from animal to animal, ranging from one in *Arbacia* to many in the annelid *Hydroides hexagonus*. The shape of the fertilization cone differs according to the form of the acrosome filaments. In mammals, it has been described as a small mound at the site of sperm contact. The fertilization cone may be of short duration, lasting only 20 seconds. In some invertebrate eggs the cone forms before fertilization; thus doubt

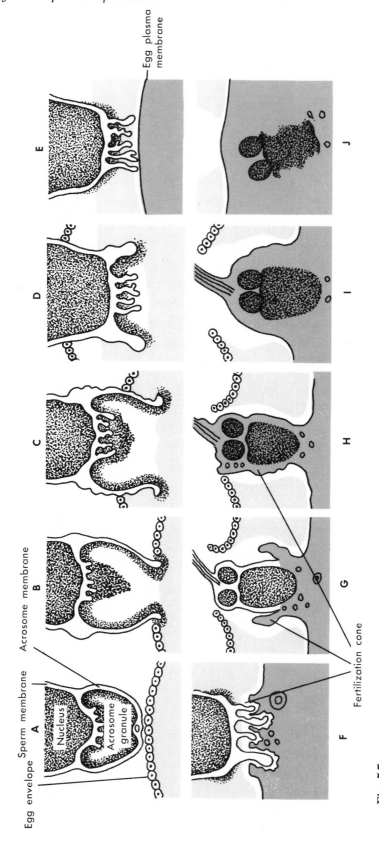

Fig. 5-7

Sperm penetration in the marine annelid *Hydroides*. The acrosome membrane of the unactivated acrosome, **A**, splits when the sperm contacts the egg envelope, **B**. The acrosome granule breaks down, apparently releasing lytic enzymes and dissolving the egg envelope in contact with the acrosome. The sperm then penetrates the egg envelope, **C** and **D**. The acrosomal membrane gives rise to fingerlike projections that contact the egg plasma membrane, **E**. As a result, the egg cytoplasm is stimulated to form the cytoplasmic cone that surrounds the sperm and evidently aids in drawing it into the egg cytoplasm, **F** to **I**. The acrosomal and egg membranes fuse, **G**. The sperm is completely drawn into the egg where the internal parts of the sperm merge with cytoplasm of the egg, **J**. (Courtesy Colwin, A. L., and Colwin, L. H.: J. Biophys. Biochem. Cytol. **10**:231-254, 1961.)

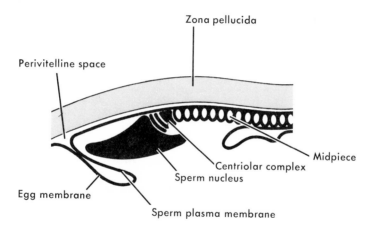

Fig. 5-8

Sperm penetration in rat. Sperm has penetrated zona pellucida, and sperm plasma membrane can be seen to be continuous with egg plasma membrane. Naked sperm is drawn into egg. (From Szollosi, D. G., and Ris, H.: J. Biophys. Biochem. Cytol. **10**:275-283, 1961.)

is cast on its function. In other examples the sperm appears to penetrate the membrane by undulating movements of the tail and no cytoplasmic cone forms at all.

Release of lysins

The spermatozoa of most vertebrates contain a substance that enables them to penetrate the various layers around the egg. The material dissolves a localized pathway through the membranes enabling the acrosomal filament to reach the egg surface. The Colwins have depicted this lytic activity in Fig. 5-7, *B*. This substance is enzymic in nature and known by the general name of *sperm lysins*. Lysins differ from one species to another and are released when the acrosomal granule disappears. Attempts to extract the lysins and identify them chemically have not been too successful because of the small amount of material available. They are protein in nature according to chemical analysis, but the specific class of enzymes has not been identified. Some investigators feel that the sperm may release more than one kind of enzyme.

According to recent studies, the jelly layers of certain amphibian eggs depend on the presence of disulfide bonds for maintaining their structure. It has been suggested that the lysins of this group of animals may utilize a disulfide bond as a substrate. According to these workers (Gusseck and Hedrick, 1971), the fusion of the egg

plasma membrane and sperm membrane occur by a sulfhydryl-disulfide bond interchange. They believe that fertilization should be explained on a molecular basis.

The mammalian egg offers a unique problem of sperm penetration, since at ovulation it is surrounded by the zona pellucida, the corona radiata, and various numbers of cumulus cells. It is very difficult to pull away the cumulus oophorus from a newly ovulated rodent egg although the sperm must penetrate this barrier. Its entrance is made easier by a lysin, a cumulus-dispersing factor, identified as hyaluronidase, present in living rabbit, rat, and mouse sperm suspensions or extracts. This dispersing factor acts upon the intercellular cement of the follicular cells by depolymerizing and hydrolyzing the *hyaluronic acid* cement that holds the cells together.

In vitro studies show that the concentration of the enzyme is proportional to the number of sperm present, since it is associated with the sperm itself rather than the semen. After some hours in the female reproductive tract the spermatozoa undergo capacitation and release their enzymes into the seminal fluid. Researchers assumed that the concentration of the enzyme was high to be effective in denuding the ovum, but they later learned that the sperm of the dog contains no hyaluronidase. This enzyme, then, is not the total answer to sperm penetration. It is now believed that the sperm probably contains sufficient enzyme to make a pathway for itself through the various layers. Narrow slits in the zona pellucida appear after the sperm penetrates this membrane and offer visual evidence of a lytic substance.

Microvilli anchor the cells of the corona radiata to the zona pellucida of the ovum. The two cannot be mechanically separated without injury to one of the membranes. The sperm may release more than one enzyme to act on the two layers. The cells fall apart after contact with sperm or contents of the oviduct for a few hours. Some investigators suggest the possibility that a tubular factor that acts on the cells of the corona radiata is also secreted. Apparently after contact with the contents of the fallopian tube, the microvilli are retracted and free the ovum. Possibly the ciliary and muscular movements of the oviduct may mechanically remove the coronal cells as the egg makes its way down the tubes to the uterus.

EGG ACTIVATION

The sperm always enters the animal hemisphere of the amphibian egg, but in amphioxus penetration occurs at the vegetal pole. In other animals there are no restrictions. Sperm may enter the human ovum, for example, at any site on its surface. Once the sperm penetrates the egg membranes and deposits the compact nucleus inside the egg by the acrosomal tube, the male nucleus undergoes several changes. The compact nucleus becomes hydrated and forms the male pronucleus, which is larger than the female pronucleus in several forms studied. The head of the sperm usually rotates 180 degrees so that the centrosome of the midpiece leads the way when the male pronucleus migrates toward the female pronucleus. The centrosomes duplicate as the sperm head becomes hydrated and astral rays develop in the egg cytoplasm around the sperm aster. It is the sperm centriole that must organize the mitotic spindle if the egg is to cleave in its normal manner. In those eggs in which the maturation process was completed by the time the sperm penetrates the egg, the sperm immediately moves to meet the female pronucleus. However,

in those in which the completion of meiosis is a part of the activation process, the sperm remains quiescent, once it enters the ooplasm, until the second polar body forms. Evidently some change occurs in the cytoplasm (reflecting the stage of nuclear maturation) that signals hydration of the sperm and the appearance of sperm asters.

At the time the eggs are shed, regardless of the stage of nuclear maturation, they usually become quiescent and enter developmental arrest. There is no new synthesis of RNA, and no other developmental changes occur unless the egg is penetrated by a sperm. The arrest appears to be of a chemical nature since no new proteins are synthesized. The release of this arrest by the entrance of a sperm or by artificial means is referred to as egg *activation*. We do not know whether activation is caused by mechanical or chemical stimulation by the sperm. Once activated, however, the egg embarks on a series of changes that leads to the development of an embryo. These changes involve the cortex as well as the more internal regions of the egg and are both structural and functional in nature. The immediate effect of sperm entrance is the completion of meiosis, if this has not yet occurred. The end result of egg activation is the fusion of the male and female pronuclei and the reestablishment of the diploid state characteristic of the species involved.

Completion of meiosis

Usually the formation of the second polar body must be completed, since in most vertebrates arrest of the meiotic process occurs while the eggs are still in the ovarian follicle. Ovulation usually begins after the spindle forms for the second meiotic division, and the dyads arrange themselves on the metaphase plate. The penetration of the sperm stimulates the chromosomes on the maturation spindle to pass into the anaphase stage. The completion of nuclear maturation immediately follows the fertilization process. Little information is available concerning the details of the extrusion of the second polar body. We do know, however, that in the rabbit, as long as 45 minutes may elapse between sperm penetration and completion of the second polar body. It may take 2 hours for the mouse, and 4 hours for the rat to complete the meiotic process.

Cortical reaction

The penetration of the egg by the sperm produces an almost instantaneous reaction in the cortex of the egg. These changes start at the point of sperm contact and pass over the surface of the egg; the exact changes that occur vary from animal to animal. In the past most of our information was based on microscopic examinations with dark-field illumination or polarized light. Studies show that the interference color changes at the time of fertilization, indicating a dispersion of material at the egg surface, possibly lipids. Often there is streaming of cytoplasm toward the point of sperm entrance and rearrangement of cytoplasmic constituents within the egg. Cortical granules visible at the surface of the egg disappear, and a membrane, the *fertilization membrane,* lifts off the egg surface.

Not until the electron microscope became available was it possible to obtain more precise information. These new studies reveal that the surface of the sea urchin egg consists of two membranes, an outer vitelline membrane and an inner plasma membrane. At fertilization the inner membrane remains on the egg and a space, the *perivitelline space,* develops between the two. Granules enclosed in membranes and closely associated with the egg membrane are located in the cortex of the egg. These cortical granules explode and disappear at the time of fertilization. Electron micrographs reveal that both the granule membrane and the egg plasma membrane rupture at the point of contact and the two membranes then become continuous as shown in Fig. 5-9, *B.* As a result the granules are ejected into the newly established perivitelline space where they line up and become attached to the vitelline membrane (Fig. 5-9, *C*). The vitelline membrane and the material of the cortical granules contribute to the fertilization membrane in these animals (Fig. 5-9, *D*).

Cortical granules or vacuoles that disappear after fertilization have been reported in the eggs of teleostean fishes, amphibians, hamsters, and rabbits. The granules of the fishes and amphibians contain a polysaccharide, similar to that identified in the sea urchin egg. A lack of sufficient information prevents us from defining their specific role in the fertilization process. However, the inference can certainly be drawn that the activity of the granules at the time of

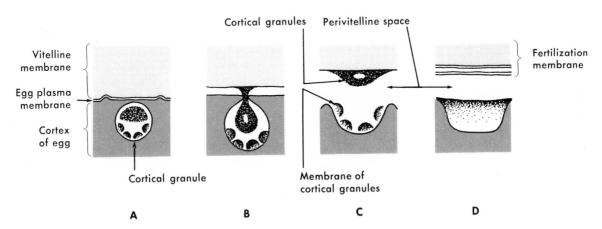

Fig. 5-9

Formation of fertilization membrane in sea urchin. **A,** Surface of egg consists of an outer vitelline membrane and an inner egg plasma membrane. Membrane-enclosed cortical granules are located in cortex near egg plasma membrane. **B,** At fertilization cortical granules explode. **C,** Membrane of cortical granule is added to egg plasma membrane and cortical granules line up with vitelline membrane. **D,** Vitelline membrane plus the material of cortical granules form fertilization membrane.

fertilization is an integral part of egg activation.

Fertilization membranes similar to those described for the sea urchin have been studied in the protherian mammals, the frog, and the trout. The vitelline membrane contributes to the fertilization membrane in the frog; a similar membrane, the chorion, helps form the fertilization membrane in the trout. Instead of a vitelline membrane or chorion, it is the zona pellucida that surrounds the eggs of higher mammals. There is little evidence that the mammalian membrane actually elevates at fertilization although the egg shrinks and a perivitelline space is established. However, it does undergo certain structural changes that can be correlated with entrance of the first sperm and that make it less permeable to other spermatozoa. After fertilization, the egg's surface becomes smooth, and the microvilli of the corona radiata are no longer visible. Regardless of the specific type of outer membrane (vitelline, chorion, or zona pellucida), the surface of the fertilized egg and the unfertilized egg differ structurally from one another.

We do not understand the mechanisms involved in the formation of the fertilization membrane. It has been suggested that the "exploding" granules release substances into the perivitelline space to cause an influx of water, an osmotic phenomenon that might explain the growth of this space. As the material leaves the cortex of the egg, some shrinkage in ooplasm occurs and this, too, could contribute to the formation of the space. The lifting of the vitelline membrane from the egg surface and the explosion of the cortical granules are energy-requiring reactions and thus can be prevented by inhibitors of oxidative phosphorylation.

Polyspermy block

When a sperm penetrates an egg, certain physiological changes occur that can be correlated with the structural changes at the egg's surface. Once the sperm enters the egg, the egg surface becomes refractory to other sperm. The condition whereby the egg is penetrated by more than one sperm is known as *polyspermy* and is usually lethal to the cleaving egg. If two sperm with their centrioles enter the egg, a triaster or

tetraster forms, which directs the formation of two or more spindles. The chromosomes become distributed unequally on the spindles, and cell division soon comes to a halt. Therefore, after the penetration of one sperm a barrier, which restricts the entrance of another sperm, usually develops. In the sea urchin this polyspermy-preventing barrier appears to reside in the fertilization membrane, since its mechanical removal allows multiple sperm entry.

In other animals the egg surface acts as the barrier, but in many mammals it is the zona pellucida that becomes impermeable to more than one sperm. This reaction is known as the *zona reaction*. If polyspermy does result, the sperm usually remain in the perivitelline space. The presence of the sperm in the space seems to indicate that the plasma membrane acts as a secondary barrier. In a few cases polyspermy is normal. More than one sperm enter the eggs of certain insects, amphibians, reptiles, and birds. In these animals, however, only one sperm develops into the male pronucleus and, therefore, only one cleavage spindle forms.

The precise polyspermy-blocking reaction is not understood. Since it is correlated with changes in the cortical region of the egg, the molecular rearrangement occurring at the surface of the egg at the time of fertilization may be responsible in some way in preventing entrance of more than one sperm. The perivitelline fluid that is formed, partially at least, from the discharged cortical vacuoles, appears to be effective also in blocking the entrance of more than one sperm. Vacquier et al. (1973) recently demonstrated the presence of a protease in the cortical granules of sea urchin eggs. The protease hardens the vitelline membrane and lytically releases supernumerary sperm bound to the egg before the cortical reaction. The protease thus prevents polyspermy by this dual action.

Parthenogenesis

Activation of the egg does not depend on some unique property of the spermatozoon, since a number of agents are also effective in initiating changes in the egg cytoplasm. The fact that an egg can be stimulated artificially indicates that it contains all the essentials for the developing embryo. In a number of organisms, eggs normally develop without fertilization, by natural or spontaneous parthenogenesis. Aphids, wasps, and the male honeybee are examples. Most eggs, however, can be stimulated in the laboratory to undergo cleavage or *artificial parthenogenesis,* but only a few of these eggs complete their development. A large variety of substances can trigger the activation mechanism. The eggs will react to chemical treatments, temperature shocks, pH, puncture with a fine needle that introduces foreign proteins, vibrations, and ultraviolet radiation. This long list of agents capable of inducing development indicates that no one common feature brings about the stimulus, but that the controlling factor rests in the egg cytoplasm itself.

The initial response of these artificial stimuli is the cortical reaction, and it can be obtained by many of the stimuli. This first response is followed by a second reaction, from the nucleus. Cleavage is more difficult to obtain. If cleavage follows the stimulation, some kind of substitute must be made for the centriole since it is usually contributed by the sperm and is responsible for formation of the cleavage spindle. In some cases the spindle that has formed for the second meiotic division becomes more centrally located and serves as a cleavage spindle. In other cases the spindle appears to form spontaneously.

One would expect that animals that result from artificial parthenogenesis would be haploid. Although this is true for many of them, the diploid state is established in several of the more viable forms. The egg employs a variety of techniques to produce diploidy. One method involves a lack of cytoplasmic cleavage after the chromosomes have duplicated. A new nuclear membrane forms around the duplicated set of chromosomes and thus gives rise to an egg with a diploid nucleus. In some cases the fusion of female pronuclei with the polar body establishes the diploid state.

SUGGESTED READINGS

1. Austin, C. R.: Fertilization, Englewood Cliffs, N. J., 1965, Prentice-Hall, Inc.
2. Blandau, R. J.: Biology of eggs and implantation. Vol. II. In Young, W. C. (editor): Sex and internal secretion, Baltimore, 1961, The Williams & Wilkins Co.
3. Colwin, A. L., and Colwin, L. H.: Role of the gamete membranes in fertilization in *Saccoglossus kowalevskii* (Enteropneusta), J. Cell Biol. **19**:447-500, 1963.
4. Gusseck, D. J., and Hedrick, J. L.: A molecular approach to fertilization. I. Disulfide bonds in *Xenopus laevis* jelly coat and a molecular hypothesis for fertilization, Devel. Biol. **25**:337-347, 1971.
5. Lillie, F. R.: The mechanisms of fertilization, Science **38**:524-528, 1913. Reprinted in Willier, B. H., and Oppenheimer, J. (editors): Foundations of experimental embryology, Englewood Cliffs, N. J., 1964, Prentice-Hall, Inc.
6. Marx, J. L.: Embryology: Out of the womb—into the test tube, Science **182**:811-814, 1973.
7. Monroy, A.: Chemistry and physiology of fertilization, New York, 1965, Holt, Rinehart & Winston, Inc.
8. Rothschild, Lord N. M. V.: Fertilization, New York, 1956, John Wiley & Sons, Inc.
9. Szollosi, D. G., and Ris, H.: Observations on sperm penetration in the rat, J. Biophys. Biochem. Cytol. **10**:275-283, 1961.
10. Tyler, A.: The manipulations of macromolecular substances during fertilization and early development of animal eggs, Am. Zool. **3**:(2):109-126, 1963.
11. Vacquier, V. D., Tegner, M. J., and Epel, D.: Protease released from sea urchin eggs at fertilization alters the vitelline layer and aids in preventing polyspermy, Exp. Cell Res. **80**:111-119, 1973.

CHAPTER 6

CLEAVAGE

Biologists have demonstrated again and again the uniformity of living things. The morphologists point out common building plans; the biochemists describe similar metabolic cycles; the geneticists unravel common pathways in the transcription and translation of genetic information. The embryologists also show uniformity in the developmental processes of animals. The maturation of the gametes in the gonads as well as those processes leading to the establishment of a basic embryonic form, follow similar developmental pathways in all vertebrate animals. The resulting body plan of one animal resembles that of another. The primordia (rudiments) of future organs develop and are arranged in a similar pattern.

During evolution of the vertebrates, the hereditary factors controlling the generalized pattern of development have been retained. After the establishment of general structures, more specific ones that express the diversity of the species follow. Development always proceeds from the general to the specific. The formation of a *blastula* by all vertebrates is an example of this generalized type of development. Although the specific size and shape may vary, all vertebrates form a blastula as the next stage after fertilization.

The development of a normal, adult animal from a zygote involves a series of distinct steps in which specific tasks are accomplished. *Cleavage,* the mitotic division of the egg, is the first step after fertilization and is a universally occurring phenomenon among metazoan animals. A series of rapid cell divisions enables a fertilized egg to develop into a complex multicellular animal, perfect in every detail. Penetration of the plasma membrane by the sperm normally activates the egg and stimulates it to start dividing.

Fertilization removes the block to cellular division that existed in the egg prior to fertilization, and initiates a type of mitosis. As a result, cleavage brings about:

1. Partition of the cytoplasm into smaller units, *blastomeres*
2. Replication and distribution of nuclear genes throughout the cytoplasmic substances

3. A *blastula stage* consisting of groups of geographically segregated cells surrounding a cavity, the *blastocoel*

MECHANICS OF CLEAVAGE

As early as the late nineteenth century Boveri suggested that the sperm centriole controlled cleavage and that fertilization introduced the centriole into the egg. Under the light microscope the centrioles appear as granules or rods located in the center of a clear area of cytoplasm, the centrosome. In electron micrographs, however, instead of single granules, they are shown to exist in pairs, with the long axis of one centriole of each pair perpendicular to the other. At present there is no explanation for the right-angle arrangement. The centrioles are hollow cylinders, 1500 Å in diameter and 3000 to 5000 Å in length (DuPraw, 1968). Nine sets of triple tubes, extending the length of the cylinder, compose their walls.

There is no evidence that the centrioles arise by division, or budding, of preexisting ones, or that they have genetic continuity as stated in the older literature. Instead, they appear to be self-duplicating bodies that form anew from precursor molecules in the surrounding cytoplasm. However, the daughter centrioles always assemble in close relationship with the mother centriole. During the interphase, or possibly as early as the end of the preceding telophase, the centrioles replicate; they then take up their position on each side of the nucleus, where radiating, tubular, astral rays develop about them. Each cell at metaphase, therefore, contains four centrioles, two at each pole, with each member of the pair oriented at right angles to the other (Fig. 6-1).

Embryologists generally agree that the centrioles organize the asters and mitotic spindle of the fertilized egg. As the centrioles migrate to the opposite side of the nucleus, a fiberlike connection appears between the two centrioles— the beginning of the spindle. The synthesis of the microtubules composing the spindle fibers of the mitotic apparatus is the essential activity of sperm centrioles. These fibers, or microtubules, extend from pole to pole. Electron micrographs also confirm the attachment of spindle filaments to the centromeres (or kinetochores) of the chromosomes. At the end of the telophase most of these tubules disappear.

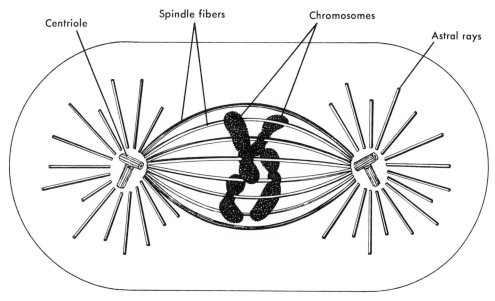

Fig. 6-1

Schematic representation of cell at metaphase showing two centrioles at each pole, with each member of the pair oriented at right angles to the other. Some spindle fibers pass from pole to pole, others from pole to centromere of chromosome.

Early cytologists suspected that the formation of the cleavage furrows and the division of the cell were under the control of chromosomes, since their movements were closely coordinated with the events of cell division. However, it now appears that the mitotic apparatus controls both the movement of chromosomes and the formation of the cleavage furrow. Surgical removal of the chromosomes does not inhibit blastomere division. So, obviously, the chromosomes themselves do not control furrow formation.

When the cell is about to divide, the cortex becomes progressively stiffer, and furrows tend to form between each pair of centrioles. These are especially evident when the egg cleaves unequally, for example, when the polar bodies split off from the egg. The furrow forms between the two centers even though the centrioles and their spindles are near the surface of the egg. As a result of this eccentric location, the cytoplasm divides into a large cell and a small polar body. It is possible with modern techniques to move the metaphase spindle around inside the egg. Movement of the spindle more centrally results in a much larger polar body. By moving the mitotic apparatus about, a furrow can be induced to form at any point on the egg surface.

Although the centrioles induce the furrow to form at a specific location, we do not understand the exact mechanism by which this is accomplished. It may vary with different species. One theory suggests that the spindle and the cell surface interact, inducing the cortex to become activated, that is, to actually grow and form a contractile ring in the region of the furrow. The spindle can be removed once the ring is established, provided that mid-anaphase has been reached, and cleavage will continue according to the original orientation of the spindle. Removal of the spindle before mid-anaphase, in the sea urchin egg, inhibits division. The relationship between spindle and cortex may be an actual physical one. The astral rays in the *Crepidula* egg (a mollusk), for example, are physically attached to the plasma membrane. Some evidence suggests that the influence exerted by the spindle may be attributable to diffusion of some substances from it to the cortex of the cell.

PARTITIONING OF CYTOPLASM

The fertilized egg rapidly divides into smaller and smaller units or cells, usually referred to as *blastomeres*. Cleavage produces hundreds or thousands of blastomeres. The rapidity with which one cell division follows another is a major difference between this type of cell division and ordinary mitosis. The mitotic cycles of cleavage have a much shortened interphase. During the period of cell division, there is little or no increase in total cytoplasmic mass. The cells actually decrease in volume with each division until they reach the size of the normal adult cell characteristic of the particular species. This lack of growth after cellular division is a second difference between cleavage and ordinary mitosis. In normal mitosis, after the cells divide, a period of growth occurs. There is replication of chromosomes as well as synthesis of cytoplasmic materials. As a result, the newly formed cells regain the size of the original mother cell. In cleavage, on the other hand, nuclear synthesis goes on, but little or no cytoplasmic growth occurs. For example, the blastula, consisting of thousands of cells, is usually only slightly larger than the unfertilized egg. Thus, cleavage can be looked upon in part as a mechanism whereby the cell returns to the normal size for a particular species.

The fact that no cytoplasmic growth occurs does not mean that the cytoplasm is synthetically inactive. Fertilization (which marks the zero time of embryonic differentiation) releases the inhibition of the egg, probably by unmasking messenger RNA stored in the cytoplasm. There is evidence that during maturation, the oocyte manfactures and stores in its cytoplasm information on how to synthesize the proteins required by the cell during cleavage. These proteins are needed for a variety of reasons. Cell membranes must be manufactured to cover the newly exposed cell surfaces formed by cleavage. It is estimated that the first division increases the surface area by as much as 28% over that of the uncleaved egg. New proteins are also needed to construct the microtubules of the spindles. Further, some proteins, nuclear proteins for example, are apparently incorporated into the nucleus as histones (basic proteins linked to

DNA) and RNA polymerase (responsible for mediating the transcription of genetic information from DNA to RNA).

The removal of the zygote nucleus from sea urchin eggs or the addition of actinomycin D (which inhibits the synthesis of RNA) to egg suspensions, does not prevent fertilized (or artificially stimulated) eggs from synthesizing new proteins through the blastula stage (Denny and Tyler, 1964; Gross, Malkin, and Moyer, 1964). These experiments strongly suggest that the manufacture of new RNA does not occur during this period. Instead, stable RNA molecules stored in the cytoplasm during the maturation process carry the embryo through the cleavage stages. About the time the embryo reaches the blastula or gastrula phase of development, the diploid nucleus directs the synthesis of messenger RNA (mRNA), and it is this new mRNA that will lead the embryo through differentiation. Two kinds of proteins, therefore, are synthesized by the cytoplasm, and their production follows a time sequence. The first proteins relate to cleavage, whereas the later ones involve embryonic differentiation.

As indicated in Chapter 4, during cytoplasmic maturation the oocyte synthesizes and incorporates many materials into its organization. Modern biologists believe that the egg establishes the foundations of the future embryo while still in the ovary. It contains a variety of materials that in some way determines the development of the embryo. It manufactures glycogen, lipids, proteins, and nucleoproteins. It takes up the precursors for future synthetic processes from the environment and stores them in the cytoplasm.

The contents are not distributed uniformly within the egg but are arranged in an organized and specific manner in layers or regions. The cytoplasm is thus heterogenous (Smith and Ecker, 1970). This stratification of materials within the egg endows it with a *polarity*, since the materials are usually more concentrated at one pole than the other. The submicroscopic structure of the cortex differs from that in the interior of the cell; the yolk becomes concentrated at one area of the cell more than at another. Different organelles are located in different parts of the cell. The egg with its mosaic of organized substances becomes partitioned through cleavage and gives rise to cells containing different types of cytoplasm as indicated in Fig. 6-2, *B*, which shows the eight-cell stage of amphioxus. Obviously the cells formed from the yolk-rich *vegetal pole* of the frog's egg contain more yolk than those formed from the *animal pole area*. The mass of cells resulting from cleavage are not duplicates of one another except genetically, but each cell has its own individuality, since each contains a nucleus, nucleoli, cell organelles, and a specific volume of the original cytoplasm surrounded by a cell membrane.

The packaging of the cellular materials does not go on at random, however. Cellular division occurs in such a manner that by the time the blastula stage is reached the cells are grouped together into geographic areas. These areas can be marked, identified, and followed through the subsequent stages of development. Nontoxic vital dyes or particles, such as carbon, embedded on the surfaces of the cells visualize cellular movement. In some cases advantage can be taken of naturally occurring markers, such as pigment granules. As the embryo develops, the tagged cells migrate to various areas of the body and differentiate into tissues and organs.

Eventually, a depletion of reserve cytoplasmic materials brings cleavage to a halt. The synthetic processes associated with chromosome duplication, spindle-fiber formation, and membrane construction diminish. Each blastomere contains its specific quantity of cytoplasm and the cell attains its adult size.

DISTRIBUTION OF NUCLEAR GENES

Since each new blastomere contains its own diploid number of chromosomes, a doubling of chromosomal material (DNA and accompanying protein) occurs with each cleavage, just as in adult mitosis. The chromosomes contributed by the male as well as those of the female replicate and distribute themselves to each blastomere. Cleavage is a time of great synthetic activity as far as the nucleus is concerned and results in hundreds of blastomeres, all with identical nuclei. In some animals (sea urchin, for example)

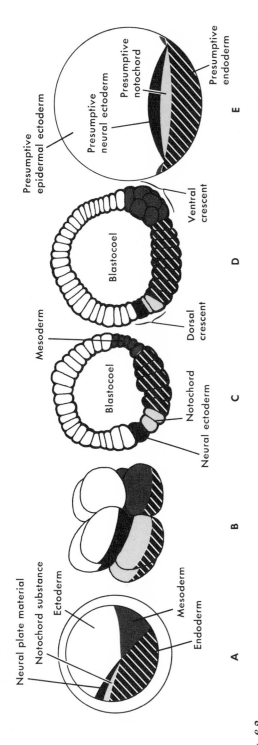

Fig. 6-2
Diagram showing distribution of presumptive organ forming areas during cleavage and blastulation in amphioxus. **A**, Uncleaved egg. **B**, Eight-cell stage. **C**, Section through early blastula showing blastocoel. **D**, Section through late blastula showing dorsal and ventral crescent, blastocoel, and elongation. **E**, Posterior view of dorsal crescent.

synthesis of DNA is one of those processes stimulated by fertilization. It goes on at the expense of materials stored in the egg. In some invertebrate animals, even before the pronuclei fuse, the pronuclei start their synthetic activities as shown by the uptake of thymidine. Replication begins during interphase and the chromosomes double before mitosis starts.

If the eggs are divided into nucleated and nonnucleated halves by centrifugation, both parts of the egg undergo division. Obviously the nucleus is not necessary for cleavage. In these cases centrioles apparently appear anew and induce furrow formation. Nevertheless, the nonnucleated half does not continue through many divisions, usually not past the blastula stage. Thus, the nucleus appears to be essential if the zygote is to differentiate into a normal animal.

At fertilization the ratio of nucleus to cytoplasm is abnormally small when compared to adult cells. As cleavage continues, this ratio increases. According to Brachet (1950), in a mature sea urchin egg the ratio $\frac{\text{volume of the nucleus}}{\text{volume of the cytoplasm}}$ is 1/550. By the time the blastula stage is reached, the ratio has changed to 1/6.

The duplication of chromosomes during cleavage gives rise to nuclei that are equivalent in every way. This has been demonstrated many times. In 1928 Spemann devised a simple but elegant experiment to test this idea. He tied hairs around the fertilized eggs of *Triturus* (newts) as they were about to cleave. This famous experiment is illustrated in Fig. 6-3. As a result, the cytoplasm of one half of the egg lacked a nucleus but was connected by a narrow bridge of cytoplasm to the half that still contained a nucleus (Fig. 6-3, *A*). When the egg nucleus divided, the cytoplasm on that side of the ligature cleaved; the other side did not. Spemann allowed the cleaved side to reach the 16-blastomere stage and then released the hair loop so that one of the nuclei could pass through the cytoplasmic bridge to the uncleaved side (Fig. 6-3, *C*). When this happened, this side also started to cleave. Eventually, Spemann completely separated the two halves of the egg and in several instances obtained two complete embryos (Fig. 6-3, *D*). He concluded that the nuclei from a 16-cell stage were similar if not identical to the original zygote nucleus and were capable of directing normal development (Spemann, 1962). It was inferred that cleaving nuclei of early embryos are completely equivalent to the fertilized nuclei and to one another.

The concept of the equivalency (or potency) of nuclei was retested with more modern techniques. Nuclei from cells in different states of development were transplanted into enucleated eggs (Briggs and King, 1952; Gurdon, 1968). These investigators demonstrated that in an amphibian the nucleus of a differentiated cell retains the ability to direct embryonic development, although it may be highly abnormal. The nucleus of an unfertilized egg is located near the surface of the egg. One can, with the aid of a microscope, remove it with a needle or (in *Xenopus laevis*) kill it with pinpointed ultraviolet radiation. As a result, one obtains an enucleated egg with intact cytoplasm. Gurdon then removed the diploid nucleus from a differentiated somatic cell, in this case a cell from the intestine of a feeding tadpole, and inserted this nucleus back into the ennucleated frog's egg. He postulated that if the nucleus of a differentiated cell were combined with egg cytoplasm and brought about normal embryonic development, that is, an embryo containing all cell types, then the nucleus did not lose genes during cell differentiation. In a few cases frogs developed that were normal in all respects. The development of these normal frogs showed that the specialized somatic cell had, in fact, retained a copy of every different gene and was capable of differentiating cells, not just intestinal epithelium. When inserted into the cytoplasmic environment of an egg, the nucleus of a differentiated cell, like the original nucleus of a germ cell, carried out the various processes involved in development.

Gurdon also made serial nuclear transplantations, using the same procedure described above with one exception. A larva that itself resulted from nuclear transplantation (rather than from fertilization of an egg) donated the nucleus from one of its differentiated cells. When this procedure was repeated several times, the nu-

cleus of a larva several generations later still retained its ability to direct normal development. The resulting population is called a *clone*, a population consisting of individuals that are genetically identical. The concept of serial transplantation is illustrated in Fig. 6-4. It is a technique that enables one to test the potency of the genes. If genes are lost or altered in the blastomere nucleus during cleavage, normal development of the egg does not occur.

Nuclei obtained from early cleavage stages,

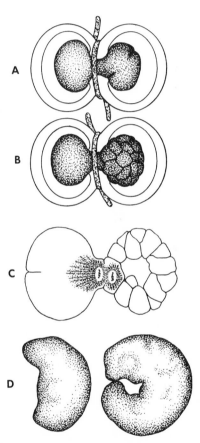

Fig. 6-3
Spemann's experiment proving that the duplication of chromosomes during cleavage gives rise to nuclei that are equivalent. **A,** Hair tied around a fertilized *Triturus* egg separated it into one half with a nucleus and one half without. **B,** Right half with a nucleus continued to divide, the left side did not. **C,** At the 16-blastomere stage the hair was released and a nucleus was allowed to pass through the cytoplasmic bridge to uncleaved side. The left side then started to cleave. Twin embryos developed, although development of left embryo lagged behind the right one.

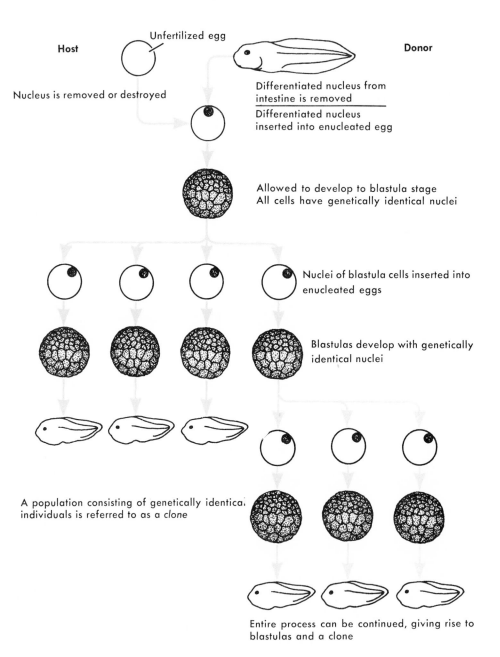

Unfertilized egg

Host

Donor

Nucleus is removed or destroyed

Differentiated nucleus from
intestine is removed

Differentiated nucleus
inserted into enucleated egg

Allowed to develop to blastula stage
All cells have genetically identical nuclei

Nuclei of blastula cells inserted into
enucleated eggs

Blastulas develop with genetically
identical nuclei

A population consisting of genetically identical
individuals is referred to as a *clone*

Entire process can be continued, giving rise to
blastulas and a clone

Fig. 6-4
Drawing of serial transplantation.

the morula, blastula, gastrula, and differentiated organs were tested. Gurdon (1968) removed the nuclei from some specialized cells—intestinal cells with brush borders—from tadpoles that had begun to feed. He inserted these diploid nuclei into eggs from which the nuclei had been removed. In most cases abnormal development occurred, but a few of the eggs cleaved and grew into normal adult frogs. Spemann showed that nuclei from early cleavage stages (16-cell stage) brought about normal development. Gurdon and Briggs and King carried the problem a little further. They demonstrated that nuclei from differentiated cells in a certain small percentage of cases, retained their ability to direct the egg through normal development. In general however, as development continued, the nuclei from the more differentiated cells became progressively restricted.

Evidence, then, supports the idea that the genes of the nuclei of early developing cells are not permanently changed during development, at least when transfers are made *between closely related species* and subspecies. They retain the capacity for directing the development of the zygote to normal maturity.

INTERACTION OF NUCLEUS AND CYTOPLASM

Although the nucleus is an important factor in embryonic growth, the cytoplasm also influences the developmental processes. The interaction between nucleus and cytoplasm plays a significant role. We have seen how the process of cleavage results in the progressive segregation of the cytoplasmic components. The genetically identical genes are thus distributed to cells with different types of cytoplasmic components. According to Moore (1962) "the action of genes is a function of their location in a specific cytoplasm." The restricting properties of the cytoplasm was particularly evident when he transferred nuclei to enucleated ova of a different species. The arrested development at the blastula stage aptly demonstrated the importance of cytoplasmic influence.

Sally Hennen (1961) undertook similar studies but carried the work a little further. She inserted nuclei of *Rana pipiens* into foreign cytoplasm, the enucleated eggs of *Rana sylvatica*. After several apparently normal cleavages, she transferred the *pipiens* nuclei back into enucleated *pipiens* ova. As a result of this back-transfer, she produced abnormal and incomplete development. In most embryos the arrest of development occurred before the midlarval stage. Careful chromosomal analysis of the back-transferred nuclei revealed abnormal chromosomal numbers and types. The chromosomes had been altered when they replicated in the foreign cytoplasm of *sylvatica*. These chromosomal changes were irreversible and prevented the direction of normal development when returned to their own type of cytoplasm.

FACTORS INFLUENCING CLEAVAGE
Influence of yolk on cleavage
Total or holoblastic cleavage

Food is usually stored in the egg in the form of inert yolk granules or platelets. In those eggs in which there is little yolk, dispersion of granules is at random in the cytoplasm. As described earlier, eggs with a homogenous cytoplasm, such as those of amphioxus and mammals, are considered isolecithal. The sparcity of yolk offers little impediment to the cleavage furrow and the egg divides completely into two blastomeres. Complete or total cleavage is referred to as *holoblastic*. In the telolecithal eggs of amphibians and certain other vertebrates, the yolk is in the form of large yolk platelets concentrated at one pole, the vegetal pole. Although the dense platelets retard the furrows, they do not inhibit them. This type of egg is also completely divided (holoblastic cleavage).

Two "laws" based on observations of early biologists predict cleavage planes.

1. In most spheroidal eggs the nucleus lies in the center of the protoplasmic mass. The mitotic spindle tends to elongate and orient in the direction of the greatest protoplasmic mass. The plane of cell division divides the long axis of the spindle transversely.
2. The second cleavage "law" states that each cleavage furrow tends to bisect the previous furrow thus dividing the egg into equal parts.

In a typically holoblastic cleavage the first furrow is meridional, that is, it tends to bisect both poles of the egg and passes through the center of the egg as demonstrated in Figs. 6-5 and 6-6. The second cleavage plane is also meridional but at right angles to the first. In general, in this type of cleavage the blastomeres formed are equal, and the second cleavage results in four equal blastomeres. The third cleavage conforms to the second cleavage law. It is latitudinal; it bisects the median axis somewhere between the two poles. In those eggs with little yolk, the plane of the third cleavage approaches the equatorial plane. However, even in isolecithal eggs there is usually enough yolk to displace the third cleavage plane slightly toward the animal pole.

In the telolecithal eggs of the frog, the unequal distribution of yolk displaces the third horizontal cleavage even further from the equator. As a result of this third cleavage, unequal blastomeres are produced: the larger cells at the vegetal pole are referred to as *macromeres* and the smaller ones at the animal pole, *micromeres*. The fourth cleavage plane in holoblastic cleavage is again meridional, bisecting the third. Two furrows, passing from pole to pole, synchronously divide the eight cells into sixteen blastomeres. After the fourth cleavage, synchrony is lost in many vertebrate eggs. Blastomeres containing the heavy yolk platelets divide at a slower rate than those at the animal pole. The larger, yolk-laden cells lag behind. While a new cleavage plane bisects the micromeres, the previous furrow completes the division of the macromeres at the vegetal pole. As a result of continued cleavage, more micromeres than macromeres form (Fig. 6-5).

The blastomeres flatten along the surface in contact with one another but round on their free surface. At first they form a closely packed ball held together by the vitelline membrane. Later, the cells adhere to one another on their own. At this stage the embryo resembles a mulberry and is referred to as the *morula stage*.

Narrow spaces appear between the cells after the third cleavage. They eventually coalesce, forming a space in the center of the morula. This cavity increases in size as cleavage continues. The morula is replaced with the next stage of development, the blastula. This hollow ball of cells is composed of a layer of cells, the blastoderm, surrounding the cavity, or *blastocoel*. The blastocoel, resulting from cleavage of isolecithal eggs, is more or less centrally located in the blastula as indicated in Fig. 6-7. Cleavage of the

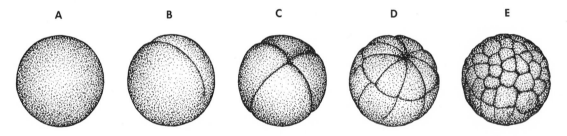

Fig. 6-5
Cleaving frog egg demonstrating holoblastic cleavage.

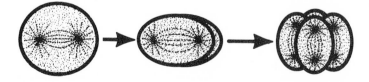

Fig. 6-6
Diagram demonstrating the laws of cleavage. Mitotic spindle orients itself so that its long axis is parallel to that of cytoplasmic mass. Each furrow bisects the previous cleavage furrow. As a result of holoblastic cleavage the blastomeres tend to be equal in size. Diagram shows spindle orientation as the cell prepares for the next cell division.

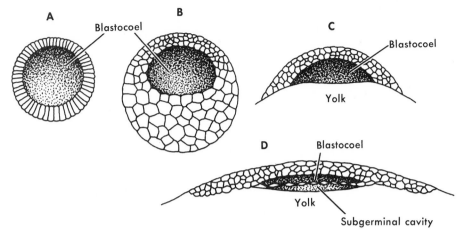

Fig. 6-7
Comparison of, **A**, amphioxus, **B**, frog, **C**, fish, and, **D**, chick blastulas.

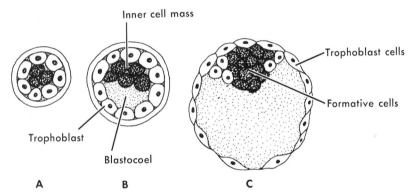

Fig. 6-8
Cleavage of mammalian egg gives rise to formative cells of embryo and trophoblast, or nutritive cells.

telolecithal egg gives rise to an eccentrically located cavity. Heavy yolk-laden cells form the floor of the blastocoel and two to three layers of small micromeres compose the roof.

Mammalian eggs cleave in a rather specialized manner. With the exception of the monotremes, mammalian eggs are isolecithal and cleavage is holoblastic. However, in most animals the first two blastomeres produced are of unequal size. In some mammals these first two blastomeres are destined to form two different types of tissue. For example, in the pig, the smaller blastomere will give rise to the *formative cells* of the embryo but the larger blastomere will become the *trophoblast,* or nutritive cells. Unlike the lower animals, cleavage is not always synchronous. The larger blastomere produced by the first

cleavage often divides first, resulting in a three-blastomere stage. Five-, six-, seven-, and even eight-cell stages have been observed. By the 16-cell stage, the morula formed in most mammals contains centrally placed cells (the *inner cell mass*) and an envelope of smaller outer cells, which will give rise to the trophoblast cells as shown in Fig. 6-8, *A*. In subsequent cleavages these smaller cells divide at a faster rate than do the centrally located cells. The blastocoel begins to form by the 32-cell stage.

By the morula stage the embryo enters the uterine cavity and fluid from this cavity passes through the trophoblastic layer, (the outer cells of the morula) and accumulates in the spaces between the cells of the inner cell mass. As a result of the increased fluid, the whole embryo

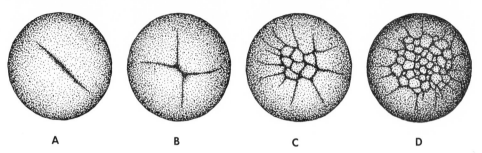

Fig. 6-9
Top view of chick blastoderm illustrating meroblastic cleavage pattern. **A,** First plane meridional. **B,** Second cleavage furrow forms at right angles to first. **C,** About 32-cell stage. **D,** About 64 cells. Note central and marginal cells.

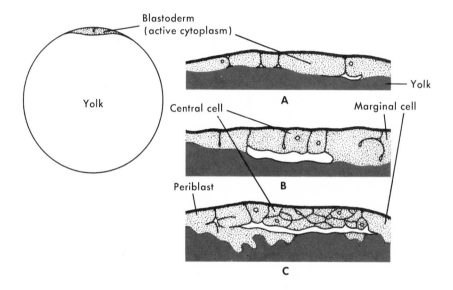

Fig. 6-10
A, Section through blastoderm showing furrow bisecting upper portion of blastodisk and producing central cells with top and side surfaces but open to yolk below. **B** and **C,** The marginal cells are continuous with peripheral cytoplasm and yolk; horizontal cleft separates central cells from yolk.

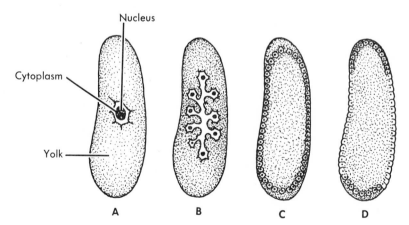

Fig. 6-11
Superficial cleavage occurs mainly in insect eggs. See text for description.

appears bloated and the outer cells become flattened and lifted off the inner cells. This inner cell mass remains attached at only one point to the inner surface of the outer flattened cells (Fig. 6-8, *C*). The cavity formed by the surrounding cells is considered the blastocoel. The mammalian embryo is now called the blastocyst.

Incomplete or meroblastic cleavage

Further accumulation of yolk occurs in the eggs of sharks, birds, and reptiles. In these eggs the yolk consists of a compact mass surrounded by a thin film of cytoplasm. A disk or cap of cytoplasm (*blastodisk*) forms at the animal pole of the egg and is the only part of the egg that is partitioned. Cleavage is said to be incomplete, or *meroblastic,* when the cleavage furrow cannot bisect the whole egg.

The first cleavage furrow is considered meridional in incomplete cleavage. The furrow bisects the upper portion of the blastodisk but does not divide the more yolk-laden cytoplasm of the lower portion of the disk. In other words, the furrow penetrates only about half the thickness of the disk. The second furrow consists of two furrows, one on each side and at right angles to the first (Fig. 6-9). The third set of furrows is vertical, bisecting the plane of the second cleavage, and therefore parallel to the first; the plane of the fourth cleavage is considered to be vertical also. In Figs. 6-9 and 6-10, meroblastic cleavage results in a cluster of centrally located cells that have top and side surfaces but lack a floor and are continuous with the yolk below. The peripheral or *marginal cells* surround the *central cells*. These cells are incomplete since the furrows do not extend to margins of the disk. They lack a floor and have only two sides (formed by the furrows); their outer edges are continuous with the peripheral cytoplasm (Fig. 6-10, *C*). Up to this point all blastomeres lie in one plane. As cleavage continues, more and more marginal cells develop sides and become part of the central cells. Eventually either a cleft separates the nucleated part of the cell from the rest of the yolk or there is a horizontal cell division (Fig. 6-10, *C*). In either case, central cells become surrounded by cell membranes and are complete cells, no longer continuous with the

yolk. These central cells form a superficial layer above the cleft; on the other hand, the marginal areas and the area beneath the cleft consist of incomplete cells, or *periblast.*

In the fishes (Fig. 6-7, *C*) this superficial layer composes the roof of the cavity, considered to be the blastocoel in these forms. In most reptiles and birds only some of the central cells are incorporated into the superficial layer, which becomes designated as the *epiblast.* A few blastomeres remain in the space between the epiblast and yolk; these cells later unite into a thin layer, the *hypoblast.* The hypoblast may also form by delamination from the upper layer or possibly by the addition of cells from the posterior thickened area where epiblast joins the peripheral area. In any event, the cavity becomes divided into two parts. The space between the epiblast and the newly formed hypoblast is referred to as the blastocoel and is considered homologous to that of the amphibian. The area between the hypoblast and the yolk is usually called the subgerminal space (Fig. 6-7, *D*).

It is the central cells that will give rise to the embryo and the periblast that will function in a nutritive manner. The cavity, which is limited to a space under the central area, causes these central cells to take on a more transparent appearance as compared with the more peripheral cells. These latter cells rest on the yolk and appear more opaque. The blastodisk therefore becomes subdivided into two areas. The centrally located transparent cells constitute the *area pellucida* and the more opaque peripheral area composes the *area opaca.*

Superficial cleavage

A third type of cleavage (Fig. 6-11) should be mentioned although it occurs only in invertebrate eggs, mainly insects and other arthropods. In the insect egg the yolk content is high and is more or less segregated from the cytoplasm. The cytoplasm forms a thin coat around the ovum and surrounds the nucleus in the form of a small island within the yolk-laden insect egg (Fig. 6-11, *A*). This type of egg is known as *centrolecithal* and its cleavage, as *superficial cleavage.* The nucleus in the island of cytoplasm first undergoes a number of divisions while the cytoplasm remains uncleaved (Fig. 6-11, *B*). After several mitotic divisions, each nucleus becomes surrounded by a small amount of cytoplasm and migrates to the surface of the egg (Fig. 6-11, *C*). A syncytium, consisting of several nuclei in a ring of undivided cytoplasm, develops. After the migration of the nuclei, there are formed many furrows, which pass from the surface inward, dividing the cytoplasm into cells whose inner surface is continuous with the yolk. Eventually the cytoplasm is separated from the yolk, and the cells, now with complete surfaces, arrange themselves in a layer around the compact central mass of yolk as in Fig. 6-11, *D*.

Influence of cytoplasm on cleavage

Factors other than the amount of yolk deposited in the egg determine pattern of cleavage. The organization of the cytoplasm itself, which was laid down in the ovary, influences the orientation of the spindle within the egg. This, in turn, determines the type of cleavage that will follow. Three main categories (Fig. 6-12) are usually described: *bilateral, radial,* and *spiral.* Radial and spiral cleavages occur in the eggs of invertebrates. Bilateral cleavage is usually associated with vertebrate eggs.

In bilateral cleavage the spindle is oriented in such a way that the first furrow usually coincides with the median plane of the embryo and separates the right side from the left. In radial cleavage the furrows bisect the egg and are at right angles to one another. The blastomeres are thus arranged in a radially symmetrical pattern around the polar axis. After the horizontal cleavage, the blastomeres of the upper tier lie over the corresponding blastomeres of the lower tier. In spiral cleavage the spindles become tipped and divisions occur in an oblique direction. As a result the blastomeres of the upper tier shift so that they come to lie over the junction of the blastomeres in the lower tier rather than over the cells themselves. This is especially obvious at the third cleavage in which an unequal division of cytoplasm occurs, producing micromeres and macromeres.

The spiral may turn in either a clockwise or counterclockwise direction, referred to as *dextral* or *sinistral,* respectively. The coiling of the shells

of gastropod mollusks reflect this type of cleavage. The direction of coiling demonstrates the importance of the maternal genes during these early stages of development. If cleavage spindles are oriented so that division is clockwise (dextral), the shell of the adult snail coils dextrally. On the other hand, the shell coils sinistrally when cleavage occurs in the counterclockwise direction. In one species of snail some individuals are dextral and some are sinistral. A single gene determines the direction of cleavage in these snails. The allele for dextral coiling (L) proved dominant over the recessive sinistral (l) allele. If the eggs of a sinistral female (ll) are fertilized by sperm from a homozygous male (LL), the resulting offspring all cleave sinistrally, despite the fact that the F_1 genotype is Ll. This cross is diagrammed in Fig. 6-13.

If F_1 individuals are crossed (Ll × Ll), the second generation are all dextral. The usual phenotypic segregation does not occur according to normal Mendelian inheritance since three fourths would be expected to spiral according to the dominant pattern and one fourth sinistrally. Actually, the genes do segregate according to normal rules of inheritance (LL, Ll, ll; 1:2:1), but they do not express themselves since the direction of coiling was determined by the *maternal* genotype, in this case Ll.

A different result occurs if the original parents have a different genotype. If the eggs of a dextral female is fertilized by a sinistral male, all of the F_1 snails demonstrate dextral spiraling, dictated by the genotype (LL) of the mother. The coiling in the F_2 generation would also give rise to dextral spiraling as described above. It is not until the third generation that the three-to-one segregation expresses itself. In this case, eggs obtained from LL or Ll individuals all produce dextral spiraling, but ll genotypes give rise to sinistral (Fig. 6-13).

The results of these crosses depend on the organization of the egg. The establishment of this organization occurs in the oocyte while the egg is in the ovary undergoing cytoplasmic maturation (Fig. 6-14). The spiraling of the zygote, therefore, is under the control of maternal genes. At the time of fertilization, the genotype of the sperm does not influence the deter-

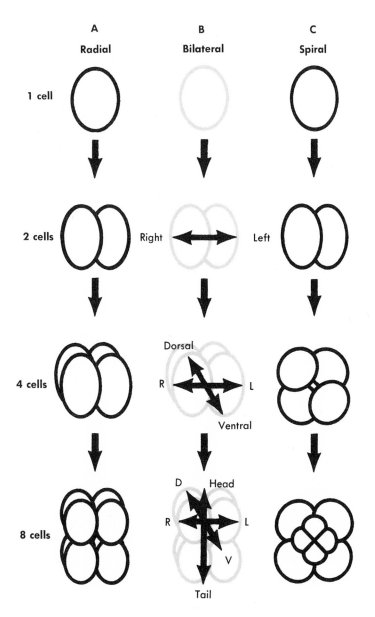

Fig. 6-12

Diagram illustrating three main types of cleavage. **A,** In radial cleavage, furrows bisect egg and are at right angles to one another. Blastomeres are arranged in radially symmetrical pattern around polar axis. **B,** In bilateral cleavage, first furrow usually divides embryo into right and left sides. **C,** In spiral cleavage the spindles are tipped and are arranged in a spiral. The blastomeres of the upper tier are shifted so that they lie over the junction of blastomeres of the lower tier. Four- and eight-cell stages of spiral cleavage shown from top view.

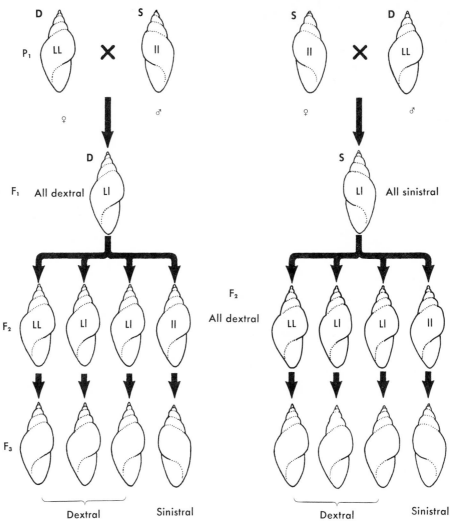

Fig. 6-13
Inheritance of coiling in snails illustrating the influence of maternal genotype.

mination of the cleavage pattern. It will be expressed, however, in next generation.

Rate of cleavage

In most vertebrate eggs, the first cellular division occurs at a definite rate in relation to the time of sperm penetration. This rate of cleavage is definitely affected by temperature, which influences the rate of all chemical and physical processes. If a batch of frog eggs are fertilized and all are maintained at the same temperature, the time of the first cleavage furrow can be predicted. For example at 18° C the first cleavage furrow will divide the egg into two blastomeres in about 3½ hours, but at 25° C, the furrow appears in 2½ hours. At 25° C the second furrow forms an hour later, the third forms a half hour later, and the fourth, in 20 minutes. As each cleavage occurs, the time between formation of successive furrows decreases. In general, at each division all vertebrate blastomeres are divided, resulting in a doubling of the total number: 2, 4, 8, 16, 32, etc. This rule, however, does not hold for mammalian eggs in which, as pointed out earlier, synchrony is lost and cells divide on an individual basis.

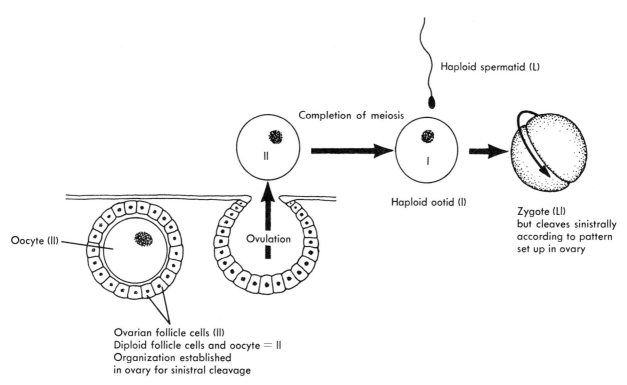

Haploid spermatid (L)

Completion of meiosis

Haploid ootid (I)

Zygote (LI)
but cleaves sinistrally
according to pattern
set up in ovary

Oocyte (II)

Ovulation

Ovarian follicle cells (II)
Diploid follicle cells and oocyte = II
Organization established
in ovary for sinistral cleavage

Fig. 6-14
Schematic drawing illustrating the determination of egg organization in the ovary.

Although temperature is an important factor, the rate of cleavage is specific for a particular species and is under cytoplasmic rather than nuclear control. Different species have different rates of cleavage and these rates have been programmed into the cytoplasm of the egg synthesized in the ovary. The fact that the maternal genes determine the rate of cleavage may be demonstrated by fertilizing an egg of one species with the sperm of another species, whose cleavage rate is different. If cleavage occurs in this type of experiment the rate is always characteristic of the mother species.

RESULTS OF CLEAVAGE
Beginning of vertebrate body plan

As stated in Chapter 2, the vertebrate body plan is bilaterally symmetrical, has an anteroposterior axis, and a dorsal ventral surface. This basic plan is established early in development. Just how early seems to depend upon the specific vertebrate under consideration.

As indicated in Chapter 4, the synthesis of yolk is a definite feature of cytoplasmic maturation. The polarity of the egg is usually determined in the ovary and the yolk accumulates at one end of the egg, the vegetal (or vegetative) pole. However, sometimes this localization of yolk does not occur until fertilization (such as in many teleost fish). The nucleus of the unfertilized egg (the germinal vesicle) migrates away from the yolk to the opposite end of the egg, marking the animal pole for isolecithal eggs. The cytoplasm of the egg is not homogeneous. The potential for greater activity rests with the cytoplasm of the animal pole and decreases in gradient fashion to the vegetal pole.

Polarity of the egg is usually explained as quantitative or qualitative differences in the cytoplasmic substances of the egg and involves more than just the deposition of yolk. These differences have a definite relationship to the organization of the embryo and the establishment of the adult vertebrate plan described above. The area of the animal pole, that region shown to be most physiologically active, usually becomes the anterior end of the embryo, and the material at the vegetative pole lies in the future ventral region of the embryo (Figs. 6-15 and 6-18, *B*). Apparently the polarity of the cytoplasm assumes a definite relationship to the future embryonic axis and body organization.

The majority of animals, including all vertebrates, are *bilaterally* symmetrical; that is, they possess only one pair of symmetrical sides. If a median longitudinal or sagittal plane passes along the anteroposterior axis, it divides the animal into two symmetrical halves that are mirror images of one another. In some cases, the first cleavage furrow divides the egg into right and left sides and establishes the future symmetry of the vertebrate body (Fig. 6-12, *B*). Bilateral symmetry is believed to have adaptive value for the animal that moves forward on a substratum. It contributes to cephalization and helps orient the individual in directional movement.

The question arises, as it does for all vertebrate structures, whether bilateral symmetry preexists in some manner in the egg or whether it depends on the influence of other factors, such as the environment. The subject has been stud-

ied mostly in amphibians and birds, and in these animals the plane of symmetry is not definitely preformed in the egg, (Clavert, 1962) but is imposed at a later date.

The amphibian sperm penetrates the cortex of the egg at any point around its circumference, approximately 20 or 30 degrees down from the midregion of the animal pole. As it enters the egg, it carries with it a trail of pigment granules from the surface of the egg, marking what is known as the *penetration path*. Since the pigment granules are concentrated in the outer cortical region, they can be used to visualize this superficial layer. Extensive movements of the surface layers occurs at the time of fertilization. The granules are seen to migrate over the animal pole toward the site of sperm entrance as shown in Fig. 6-16. As a result of sperm penetration and cortex migration, in 30 to 60 minutes (depending on the temperature of the water) the area opposite the sperm entrance contains less pigment granules, is gray in color, and assumes a crescent shape. This area is known as the *gray crescent*. It is located in the marginal area where the yellowish material of the vegetal pole meets the darkly pigmented cytoplasm of the animal pole. The plane that passes through the point of sperm entrance and

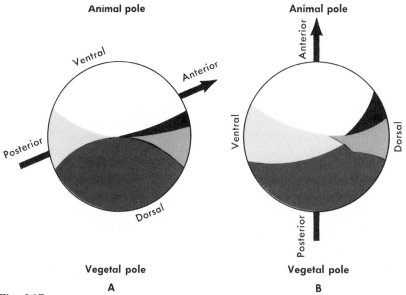

Fig. 6-15

Diagram showing polarity of two chordate eggs: **A**, amphioxus and, **B**, frog.

through the egg's axis divides the gray crescent into two equal halves and determines the bilateral symmetry of the egg and of the future tadpole.

The entrance of the sperm determines the site of the gray crescent, and once the crescent is formed, the plane of symmetry is fixed once and for all. In the majority of cases it is the first cleavage furrow that passes through the gray crescent and determines the right and left side of the individual. The site of sperm entrance becomes the future anterior end of the embryo. The material of the gray crescent gives rise to the posterior region.

The determination of symmetry does not appear to be rigidly fixed but remains labile during the earliest stages of development. In the majority of cases the first cleavage furrow divides a urodele egg into right and left halves, but if the first two blastomeres are separated, each blastomere is capable of developing into a smaller but normal embryo with its own bilateral symmery. One can conclude, therefore, that the factors normally responsible for bilateral symmerty are established early in the egg but can be modified by external factors. The eggs of amphibian, chondrostean fish, and prototherian mammals established bilateral symmetry before

cleavage begins by the rearrangement of ooplasmic materials at the time of fertilization. On the other hand, the eggs of teleosts, birds, and reptiles are retarded in symmetrization. In these animals with meroblastic cleavage, bilateral symmetry depends on the position of the egg in the uterus, that is, whether the pointed or blunt end faces the cloaca, and how the egg axis orients in space. According to a recent report the rotation of the egg, as it moves down the oviduct, forces the chick blastodisk into an oblique position; the force of gravity determines the bilateral plane. The anterior end always develops at the lowest point of the blastodisk and the posterior part of the embryo at the highest point (Kochav and Eyal-Giladi, 1971). Regardless of the precise mechanisms involved, authorities usually agree that by the time the area pellucida forms, the final plane of bilateral symmetry is established.

The moment when bilateral symmetry is fixed in mammals is uncertain. According to Rugh (1964) after 6½ days of gestation the dorsoventral axis of the mouse develops perpendicularly to the long axis and perpendicularly to the ligament supporting the uterus. The formation of the primitive streak indicates the posterior end of the embryo.

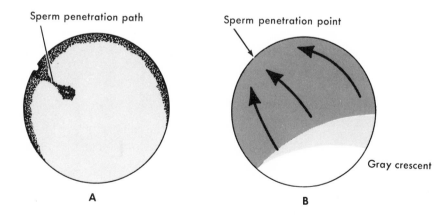

Fig. 6-16

A, When sperm penetrate an amphibian egg, pigment granules on the surface of the egg are carried inside, marking the penetration path. **B,** Entrance of the sperm stimulates cortical movements and granules migrate to sperm penetration point. Gray crescent is established opposite site of sperm entrance.

Formation of blastula
Types of chordate blastulas

As a result of cleavage a cluster of cells forms, the *blastula*, which assumes different shapes depending on the species involved. A diagrammatic comparison of different blastulas is presented in Fig. 6-7. If cleavage is holoblastic, the mass of cells takes the form of a hollow ball, but if cleavage is incomplete (meroblastic), cells assume the shape of a disk (blastodisk). Both holoblastic and meroblastic cleavage give rise to blastulas that can be classified into two types.

1. In one type of blastula all the cells become incorporated into the body of the embryo. The zygotes of amphioxus and amphibians form blastulas of this type.

2. Two kinds of cells compose the second type of blastula. One cell type gives rise to the embryo proper and the second type of cell forms auxiliary cells. The latter cells function in implantation, nutrition, respiration, and excretion and play no part in forming the body of the embryo. Elasmobranchs and teleost fishes, reptiles, birds, and mammals possess this type of blastula.

The blastula plays an important role in the development of the individual and represents the first embryonic stage after fertilization. A blastular stage must be formed before the embryo can follow the sequence of steps leading to the establishment of the normal adult animal.

The techniques of vital staining or marking of blastomeres enables biologists to construct maps of the prospective areas of the embryo. The labeled cells can be traced as the embryo develops and the fate of various areas followed. The mapping process reveals that certain cells give rise to certain germ layers, which, in turn, make up specific tissues and organs within the embryo. They have a predetermined destiny and under normal conditions give rise to specific major organ-forming areas of the future adult. These germ layers are the *ectoderm, mesoderm,* and *endoderm,* terms that mean outer, middle, and inner skins and refer to their position within the embryo. Since the cells of the blastula are located on or near the surface of the embryo and as yet do not exist in layers, the area of the future germ layers during the blastula stage is referred to as *presumptive*. For example, that area of the blastula destined to form the neural ectoderm is called the *presumptive neural ectoderm.*

The early biologists constructed maps of the blastulas based on the trajectories of tagged cells. They showed the fate of any region in the blastula under normal developmental conditions and were referred to as *fate maps.* According to these maps (see Figs. 6-2, 6-17, and 6-18), similar patterns exist in all vertebrates. Regardless of the specific shape of the blastula (round or disk-shaped), the organ forming areas are arranged in a pattern around the presumptive notochordal region.

The following general description of four different types of vertebrate blastulas emphasizes the similarity of this basic plan. This pattern is established despite the fact that the eggs contain varying amounts of yolk and employ different types of cleavage patterns.

PROTOCHORDATE BLASTULA. An understanding of blastulation in amphioxus demonstrates this fundamental developmental process in its simplest form, since the egg of this protochordate contains little yolk. As a result of cleavage the cells arrange themselves in the form of a hollow, pear-shaped structure as shown in Fig. 6-2, *D*. The blastoderm forms a single layer around the cavity or blastocoel. Since holoblastic cleavage divides the egg more or less equally (it is never entirely equal), the resulting blastomeres are of approximately the same size. Consequently, the cavity is centrally located within the ball of cells (Fig. 6-2, *D*). The cells from the vegetal pole of the egg will become the floor of the blastula, or *hypoblast,* and are the future endoderm of the embryo. Those cells from the region of the animal pole will form the roof over the hypoblast, the *epiblast,* and will give rise to the epidermis, the neural cells, and notochordal and mesodermal cells.

Most of the cells of the composite epiblast will give rise to epidermal ectoderm. Some small epiblast cells with special staining affinities located at the margins of the prospective endoderm layer, form a ring around the blastula. Fig. 6-2, *D*, shows that this ring of cells consists of two general areas, the dorsal and ventral crescents.

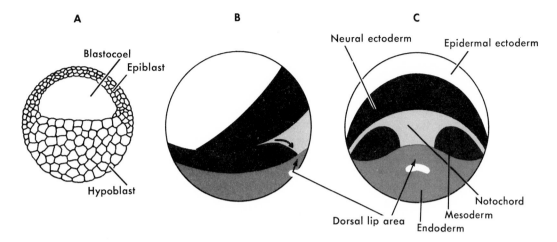

Fig. 6-17
Fate map of amphibian late blastula and early gastrula. **A,** Section showing eccentrically located blastocoel, small epiblast cells, and larger hypoblast cells. **B,** Side lateral and, **C,** posterior views indicating location of presumptive organ-forming areas. Epiblast is composed of presumptive ectoderm (epidermal and neural), presumptive mesoderm, and presumptive notochordal cells. Hypoblast contains cells of presumptive endoderm.

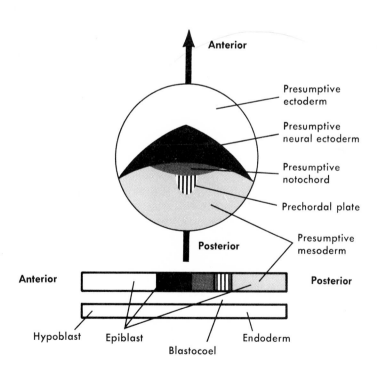

Fig. 6-18
Fate map of avian blastula. **A,** Surface view illustrating location of presumptive organ-forming areas of epiblast. **B,** Early chick blastoderm sectioned through the median axis in an anteroposterior plane demonstrating epiblast (and presumptive layers), blastocoel, and hypoblast.

The cells of the dorsal crescent give rise to the presumptive notochord and neural plate cells (Fig. 6-2, *E*). The ventral crescent contains the cells that make up the presumptive mesoderm.

AMPHIBIAN BLASTULA. The blastula of the amphibian embryo is also a round structure that can be roughly divided into three regions as shown in Fig. 6-17. They are similar but not identical to those of amphioxus. The amphibian egg contains a greater amount of yolk than an amphioxus ovum. As a result the cells formed from the vegetative pole of the egg, the hypoblast, lack pigmentation and are much larger than those at the animal pole. They push into the blastocoel (Fig. 6-17, *A*) causing this cavity to become eccentrically located. The large yolk-filled cells become the endoderm and will turn up later in the gut region.

The rest of the cells compose the epiblast layer, but unlike the blastula of amphioxus, the epiblast of the amphibian is several cells thick. In the frog, the darkly pigmented cells, derived from the animal pole of the egg, give rise to the future ectoderm of the animal. Further division of the ectodermal regions provide cells for the epidermis and the nervous system of the embryo.

The third area of the blastula consists of a ring of cells around the equator. Most of these cells occupying the equatorial region are presumptive mesoderm. Unlike the amphioxus blastula in which the presumptive mesoderm cells occupied approximately half of this marginal zone (ventral crescent) (Figs. 6-2, *E*, and 6-15, *A*), the presumptive mesoderm cells of the amphibian almost encircle the blastula. The notochord material, wedged between the tapering edges of the mesoderm, can best be seen in dorsal view (Fig. 6-17, *C*). It is located just dorsal to those cells that will first migrate into the interior of the blastula. Just above the notochordal cells is a crescent-shaped area, the presumptive neural ectoderm mentioned above. These cells will give rise to the brain and spinal cord of the individual.

AVIAN BLASTULA. The area pellucida, consisting of the central cells freed from yolk (see Fig. 6-10), contributes to the formation of the embryo. It is the part of the chick blastoderm included in the fate map. It consists of two layers of cells (Fig. 6-18, *B*)—those cells exposed to the surface, the epiblast, and those cells located below the cleft in the area pellucida, the hypoblast. As in lower animals, the blastula is bilaminar (2 layers). Instead of having a rounded appearance it may be thought of as being flattened, as if the epiblast of the amphioxus blastula were flattened against the hypoblast, changing the blastocoel into a slit-like cavity as shown in Fig. 6-18, *B*. The blastodisk (the flattened blastula) rests on a bed of undivided yolk. Since the avian blastula includes the blastomeres located on each side of the cleft, the fate map must treat each layer (epiblast and hypoblast) separately.

The formation of the embryo proper involves only a limited portion of the area pellucida. Some of it contributes to the formation of extraembryonic membranes. Since the shell limits the environment of the developing chick embryo, these necessary membranes function in respiration, excretion, and nutrition—physiological processes that are easily handled when the embryo develops in an aquatic medium.

As in the other blastulas studied so far, the marking of the cells during cleavage reveals that the cells of the epiblast are organized around the notochord (Fig. 6-18). The cells in the anterior part of the area pellucida form the ectoderm and embryonic membranes. The posterior half of the area pellucida gives rise to mesoderm of the body proper and to the extraembryonic mesoderm of the membranes. In the middle of the area pellucida the presumptive neural plate cells take the form of a transverse crescent-shaped mass. Posterior to the presumptive neural plate cells, near the middle of the area pellucida, lies the presumptive notochord material. The lateral edges of these two areas do not extend to the edges of the area pellucida.

In general, the hypoblast, those cells below the cleft, are destined to form the endoderm. The gut incorporates some of these cells into its wall, but most of them will form the lining of the yolk sac. Fig. 6-18, *B*, is a schematic drawing of an early chick blastoderm sectioned through the median axis in an anteroposterior plane.

MAMMALIAN BLASTULA. It is almost impossible to mark or stain the cells of the mammalian embryo and follow their path through the sequence of developmental phases. The rat, mouse, rabbit, pig, and monkey are the eutherian mammals most studied, and much of our knowledge is based on these forms. Only a few human embryos are available for examination, but one can assume that their development parallels that of the monkey.

Despite the fact that the mammalian egg undergoes holoblastic cleavage, the cells composing the inner cell mass spread out and form a plate or disk resembling the blastodisk of the bird and reptile. The mammalian blastodisk becomes divided into epiblast and hypoblast as in the chick and reptile, but there is no consensus as to how this occurs. A flattened layer of cells become distinguished from the rest of the inner cell mass and lines the interior surface of the blastocoel as indicated in the schematic drawing of the blastodisk of the monkey (Fig. 6-19). This layer of cells, considered to be the hypoblast, is formed either by the splitting of cells from the lower aspect of the inner cell mass or by the migration of some of the enveloping cells from the edges of the inner cell mass along the internal surface. The specific source of these cells varies with the specific mammal involved. Regardless of its origin, the hypoblast will give rise to the endoderm as in other animals.

The cells that remain in the inner cell mass are considered to be the epiblast and will give rise to the epithelium, neural ectoderm, notochord, and mesodermal components of the embryo. The mammalian fate map resembles that of the reptile and bird. The mammalian blastula, however, is composed of cells destined to fill two different functions. Together, the hypoblast and epiblast cells are considered to be the *formative cells* of the embryo, those cells destined to give rise to the embryo proper. The envelope of cells surrounding the inner cell mass will become the nutritive cells, or *trophoblast* (Fig. 6-8). The lack of yolk in the mammalian egg forces the embryo to find a nutritive source early in development. The trophoblast cells function to establish a relationship with the maternal body—source of the necessary nourishment.

The dichotomy of function in the cells of the mammalian blastula can be traced back to the first cleavage division, although little qualitative difference can be determined between these first two blastomeres. In fact one of the first two mouse blastomeres can be destroyed, and under certain controlled conditions the other will develop into a smaller but normal mouse. The fact that the two blastomeres can be separated and each give rise to a complete individual indicates that all the nuclear and cytoplasmic factors necessary for normal develop-

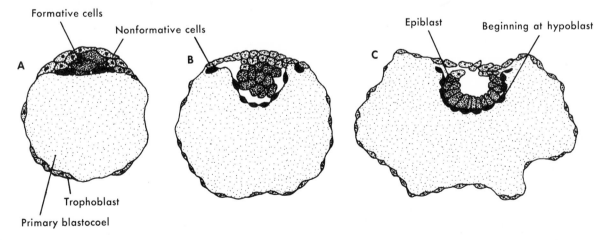

Fig. 6-19
A and **B**, Inner cell mass of developing blastocyst of monkey becomes divided into formative and nonformative cells. Trophoblast cells will become the nutritive cells. **C**, Formative cells separate into epiblast and hypoblast layers.

ment are contained within each cell. As discussed in Chapter 4, a blastomere that is capable of developing into a complete individual is said to be *totipotent*.

Significance of blastula stage

There is great uniformity in the early stages of development of vertebrate animals. The essential similarities of gametogenesis and fertilization have been stressed. The blastula and gastrula are the next stages in development that are fundamentally similar in all animals. Actually one stage merges into another in a continuous process, but it is convenient to classify them for clarity of discussion.

A summary of the steps leading to the formation of the blastula can be enumerated; the particular shape of the blastula is not important:

1. The cytoplasm is cleaved by a series of rapid mitotic divisions into a number of small blastomeres.
2. The packaging of the heterogeneous cytoplasm results in no two blastomeres necessarily having an identical cytoplasmic content.
3. At each cleavage the chromosomes with their genes are replicated and distributed to the blastomere. The nuclei of all the blastomeres are identical.
4. General areas of the blastula are destined to give rise to certain structures, and the segregation of these *major organ-forming areas* is an important function of blastulation.
5. Regardless of whether the areas are to form internal or external organs, most of the blastomeres are arranged on the surface of the embryo surrounding a cavity, the blastocoel.
6. For comparative purposes the blastula is considered to be a two-layered structure composed of an upper epiblast and a lower hypoblast.
7. The major organ-forming areas become arranged in a particular pattern that apparently facilitates their rearrangement during the next step in development.
8. By the time the late blastular stage is reached a physiological center, which will organize and direct the migration of the major organ-forming areas, is established.
9. The rearrangement of the blastomeres through morphogenetic movements (gastrulation) will give rise to the three germ layers out of which the future organs are constructed.

SUGGESTED READINGS

1. Brachet, J.: Chemical embryology, New York, 1950, Interscience Publishers.
2. Briggs, R., and King, T. J.: Transplantation of living nuclei from blastula cells into enucleated frogs eggs, Proc. Nat. Acad. Sci. **38**(5):455-463, 1952.
3. Clavert, J.: Symmetrization of the egg of vertebrates. In Abercrombie, M., and Brachet, J. (editor): Adv. Morphog. **2**:27-60, New York, 1962, Academic Press Inc.
4. Denny, P. C., and Tyler, A.: Activation of protein biosynthesis in non-nucleate fragments of sea urchin eggs, Biochem. Biophys. Res. Commun., vol. 14, no. 3, 1964. (Reprinted in Flickinger, R. A. (editor): Developmental biology, New York, 1966, William C. Brown Co., Publishers.)
5. DuPraw, E. J.: Cell and molecular biology, New York, 1968, Academic Press Inc.
6. Gross, P. R., Malkin, L. I., and Moyer, W. A.: Templates for first proteins of embryonic development, Proc. Nat. Acad. Sci. **51**(3):407-414, 1964.
7. Gurdon, J. B.: Transplanted nuclei and cell division, Sci. Am. **219**(6):24-35, 1968.
8. Hennen, S.: On the capacity of *Rana pipiens* nuclei to promote development in their own cytoplasm after replicating in *Rana sylvatica* cytoplasm, Genetics **46**:869-870, 1961.
9. King, T. J., and Briggs, R.: Serial transplantation of embryonic nuclei, Cold Spring Harbor Symposia on Quantitative Biology **21**:271-290, 1956.
10. Kochav, S., and Eyal-Giladi, H.: Bilateral symmetry in chick embryo determination by gravity, Science **171**:1027-1029, 1971.
11. Moore, J. A.: Nuclear transplantation and problems of specificity in developing embryos, J. Cell. Comp. Phys. **60**:19-34, 1962.
12. Rugh, R.: Vertebrate embryology, New York, 1964, Harcourt, Brace & World, Inc.
13. Smith, L. D., and Ecker, R. E.: Regulatory processes in the maturation and early cleavage of amphibian eggs. In Moscona, A. A., and Monroy, A., editors: Current topics in developmental biology, vol. 5, New York, 1970, Academic Press Inc.
14. Spemann, H.: Embryonic development and induction, New York, 1962, Hafner Publishing Co.

CHAPTER 7

GERM LAYER FORMATION

GASTRULATION

Cleavage slows down as blastulation is completed. Cell divisions continue, but a period of growth occurs after each mitosis, restoring the size of the individual cells. The cells of the blastula destined to form the basic layers of the embryo, segregate into areas on the surface of the blastula, as described in Chapter 5. They must regroup for further development to occur. New associations form as the cells migrate to new locations in the embryo. For example, the presumptive notochord cells move from the surface of the blastula and line up underneath the medullary plate (neural ectoderm) in the gastrula. In this position the presumptive notochord influences further development of the neural ectoderm. These new cellular interactions appear to be necessary for differentiation to take place; differentiation is necessary for subsequent organogenesis.

Gastrulation is the process that brings about the reorganization and displacement of organ-forming areas. The resulting embryo changes from a diploblastic blastula to a triploblastic *gastrula* composed of the three primary germ layers (referred to in the previous chapter). Important dynamic and irreversible changes occur as the embryo develops from an early gastrula (crescent blastopore stage of amphibia) to a late gastrula (yolk-plug stage of amphibia). Gastrulation does not consist of random movements but, like most developmental processes, is a series of orderly and integrated steps. The organizational center established by the late blastula stage directs the cellular migration during this period. The cells normally migrate to the inside of the embryo along predetermined routes predictable for each species. This highly complex, sequential, process is so organized that it results in a basic body form common to all vertebrates. Organogenesis proceeds after the establishment of this basic form.

Morphogenetic movements

Cells migrate either individually or in sheets from one area of the blastula to another in the resulting gastrula. This migration, referred to collectively as *morphogenetic movements*, is one of the basic procedures necessary for the construction of the primitive embryonic form. The coordination of all these movements is extremely important in gastrulation, since it results in the creation of new shapes and structures. The presumptive notochord and presumptive mesoderm move from the surface of the blastula to the interior of the embryo. Once initiated, these movements are irreversible. Once the mesoderm leaves the surface of the embryo, it cannot return to its original location.

Certain general types of cell movements convert the blastula into a gastrula. Depending on the amount of yolk present, some species employ more of one type of movement than another in constructing their gastrula stage. The infolding, or *invagination,* of one portion of the blastula is an essential morphogenetic movement, illustrated by gastrulation in amphioxus. The lack of heavy yolk permits the entire vegetal half of the blastula to push inward, eventually obliterating the blastocoel. *Involution,* the inward turning of cells over a rim, is found in those blastulas containing moderate amounts of yolk (frog blastulas). The heavy yolk-filled cells at the vegetal pole do not move at all: instead, cells move around them. Cells on the surface of the frog's blastula migrate toward the margins of the blastopore *(converge),* move over its lips to the inside of the blastula *(involute),* and once inside, undergo *divergent* streaming and take up their future position in the gastrula. *Epiboly,* usually defined as an "extending upon," involves movements that cover other inward-moving cells and result, in the amphibian, in ectoderm covering the entire surface of the gastrula. As a result of epiboly there is anteroposterior extension of the embryo as well as peripheral expansion. *Cell proliferation* and *delamination* (the splitting of blocks of tissues into layers) are not types of morphogenetic movements, but also contribute to the formation of the gastrula stage.

The ability to carry out these movements appears to rest with the cells themselves. For example, the initiation of gastrulation in the amphibian is marked by the formation of elongated bottle cells that disappear inside the embryo. These cells, described in more detail later in the chapter, actually change shape, a shape

they retain even when the embryo is torn apart and the cells become isolated from one another. Actively elongating microtubles and microfibrils in the cytoplasm of the cells are mainly responsible for their changing shape.

Individual cells also have the ability to recognize one another. The modern use of tritiated thymidine as a method of labeling cells enables investigators to trace cells in mixed culture. Since the cells possess independent movement, they sort themselves out according to "like" cells. Cells have specific affinities. As early as 1939 Johannes Holtfreter discovered that exposure of amphibian embryos to solutions of high pH, caused the cells to lose their cohesiveness and to dissociate. However, when returned to a physiological medium, they reconstruct the tissue of origin. If more than one type of cell is excised and dissociated together, medullary plate and epidermis, for example, the clump of dissociated cells will sort themselves out according to specific cell type. The medullary plate cells come together and take up an internal position and the epidermal cells cover them. Cells have a tendency, then, to arrange themselves in a definite histotypic (tissue-type) pattern (Moscona, 1957), indicating that during normal development some kind of cell-to-cell relationship exists. It may be that the various types of cells segregate according to the positive or negative affinities of the cells. Weiss and Taylor (1960) suggest that cells recognize one another because of reactions of specific molecules at the cell surface or interphase. They compare such reactions with an antigen-antibody reaction.

GASTRULATION IN AMPHIOXUS

Gastrulation in vertebrate animals (like blastulation) is easiest understood when studied in amphioxus. In Chapter 6 we followed the formation of the blastula and identified the presumptive major organ-forming areas, geographically isolated on its surface (Fig. 6-2). The arrangement of the cells into a cup-shaped gastrula is the next step in development.

As gastrulation begins, the cells in the region of the dorsal crescent (presumptive notochord and neural plate cells) and ventral crescent (presumptive mesodermal cells) increase their mitotic activity. The prospective endodermal cells at the vegetal pole do not divide, but form a flat plate that gradually folds inward, invaginating into the blastocoel. This endodermal plate leads the way and eventually becomes apposed to the presumptive ectoderm (as shown in Fig. 7-1) forming a cuplike structure with an outer and inner wall. The endodermal cells that push inward will eventually give rise to the primitive gut. The cavity of the gut is known as the *archenteron,* or *gastrocoel,* and communicates to the outside by an opening, the *blastopore.* Since the blastopore marks the entrance of the cells into the gut, it is often referred to as a mouth. The rim of the blastopore, therefore, becomes the lips of the blastopore, distinguishable as dorsal, lateral, and ventral lips.

The notochord cells, which originally make up a part of the rim of the cup, roll inside (involute) along with the endodermal cells, and come to lie in the middorsal area of the developing embryo. The presumptive mesoderm cells of the blastula form a continuous layer with the endodermal cells. As the endodermal plate continues to invaginate, the presumptive mesoderm cells converge dorsally toward the roof and take up a position on either side of the notochord cells. As a result of the archenteron formation, the blastocoel becomes obliterated.

Fig. 7-1 should help to visualize this process. As the mesodermal and notochordal cells move inside the gastrula, the lips of the blastopore contract and the opening grows smaller.

The embryo elongates in an anteroposterior direction as the prospective epidermal and neural plate cells actively divide. The anteroposterior extension of the embryo causes the presumptive neural ectoderm, originally crescent-shaped in the blastula, to be pulled into an elongated strip on the middorsal surface. At the end of gastrulation, the outer shell of the embryo consists of the neural ectoderm cells, covering the dorsal surface of the gastrula, and epidermal ectoderm, composing the remaining portion of the shell. The presumptive notochordal cells lie in the middorsal region under the neural ectoderm cells. Lateral to the notochord are the presumptive mesodermal cells, completing the roof of the archenteron. The presumptive endodermal cells compose the sides and floor of the archenteron and make up most of the gut. This is best seen in a cross section of the gastrula (Fig. 7-2, A). The only entrance into the interior of the gastrula is by way of the blastopore.

The third germ layer forms in amphioxus when the notochord, mesoderm, and endoderm separate from one another. Crevices appear at

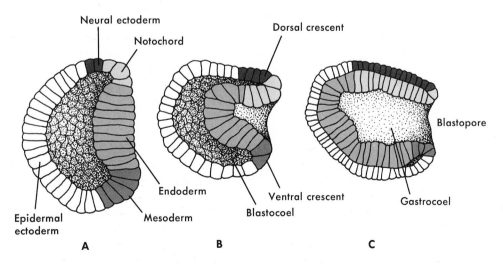

Fig. 7-1

Longitudinal hemisection showing gastrulation in amphioxus. **A,** Prospective endodermal cells form a flat plate that, **B,** gradually folds inward, invaginating into blastocoel. **C,** Endoderm becomes apposed to presumptive ectoderm. Cavity of cup-shaped structure, the gastrocoel, communicates with the outside by an opening, the blastopore.

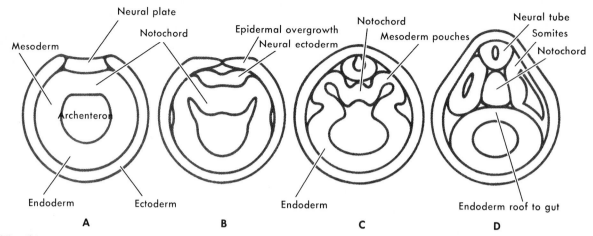

Fig. 7-2
Drawing of cross sections through amphioxus gastrulas showing location of presumptive organ-forming areas. See text for details of development.

their junctions, separating presumptive noto-chord from presumptive mesoderm and meso-derm from presumptive endoderm. They become three distinct entities. The presumptive noto-chordal cells round up and become a discrete rodlike structure running the length of the embryo in the middorsal region. It is considered a notochord at this stage, although differentia-tion must occur before it is identical to the noto-chord found in the adult. The presumptive meso-derm, which runs the length of the animal on either side of the notochord, pushes outward toward the ectoderm, forming pouchlike struc-tures. The anterior portion contains a narrow cavity continuous with the archenteron (Figs. 7-2, *B* and *C*). No pocket forms in the more posterior part of the mesoderm material.

After the mesoderm separates from the noto-chord and endoderm cells, transverse crevices form along the bilateral strips of mesoderm. These crevices divide the strips into a longitu-dinal series of blocks or somites located on each side of the notochord. In the anterior region, each block of mesodermal cells still contains a cavity. The solid blocks of mesoderm in the posterior end eventually acquire cavities. These cavities will contribute the body cavity of the adult. After the separation of the notochord and mesoderm from the rest of the cells, the freed dorsal edges of the presumptive endodermal

layer (originally lateral and ventrally located) move up and fuse beneath the notochordal rod. The endoderm thus completes the roof of the primitive gut (Fig. 7-2, *D*).

Significance of amphioxus development

The study of embryology, along with paleon-tology, offers an insight into the history of animals. Animals now living have become so modified that it is difficult to follow their descent from common ancestral types. As emphasized in Chapter 2, it is especially difficult to trace the evolution of protochordates, since their bodies were soft and rarely fossilized. Paleon-tology, therefore tells us little about the phy-logeny of the chordates, a story that man in his egocentric way finds most intriguing. On the other hand, the study of the embryology of liv-ing organisms reveals basic patterns of develop-ment. Those animals that follow similar path-ways are believed to be related, since these similarities suggest development from common ancestoral types.

The formation of the blastopore and its posi-tion in the developing embryo are characteristics that divide bilateral animals into two main evolutionary groups. In one group the blastopore marks the area of the mouth. These animals are referred to as *Protostomia* and include the flat-worms, annelids, mollusks, arthropods, and

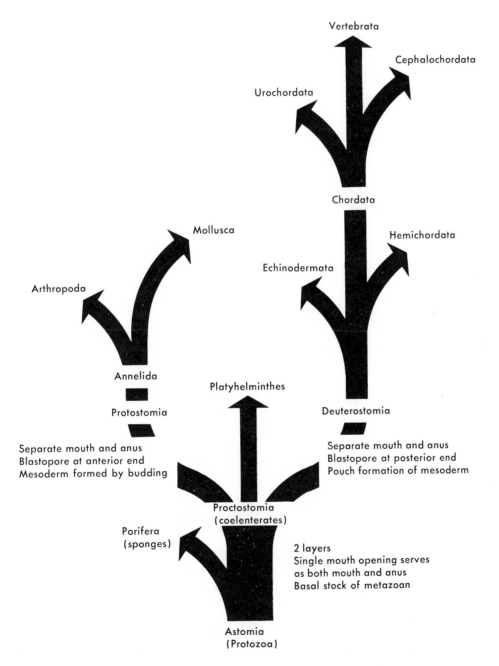

Fig. 7-3
Phylogeny of the animal kingdom suggesting the possible lines of evolution of the vertebrates.

other smaller related groups. In the other group, the blastopore identifies the posterior region of the animal. The anus arises from or near the blastopore, and a new mouth forms at the anterior end by the invaginating ectoderm. This branch of animals, known as the *Deuterostomia* ('second opening'), embraces the echinoderms, the chordates, and several smaller phyla. Both groups evolved from a common coelenterate stage in which neither anterior nor posterior ends were determined. However, the development of the animals in each of these two main branches differs considerably and indicates two main evolutionary lines.

A second main difference between groups of animals is seen in the way they form mesoderm. Triploblastic animals, that is, those that have a third layer located between the "skin" and "gut," use two different embryonic pathways to form this third layer. In one group, the mesoderm arises as solid masses of cells derived from the posterior regions of the embryo. Cavities form in these solid masses and give rise to the body cavity. In the second type the mesoderm arises in the form of pouches. These pouch cavities become the body cavities of the adult. The first method of mesoderm formation is found in the annelid worms, mollusks, and arthropods. The second is found in the echinoderms and amphioxus.

Although the pouchlike formation of mesoderm never occurs in the vertebrates, mesoderm formation is comparable in the Hemichordata and in the invertebrate phylum Echinodermata. This similarity of mesoderm formation has led many biologists to relate the origin of the chordates to the echinoderms (see Chapter 2). Mesoderm forms in the vertebrate by a modification of the echinoderm and amphioxus pattern. The mesoderm of the vertebrates pushes out as a sheet between ectoderm and endoderm and only later shows segmentation and cavitation.

Based on the location of the blastopore and manner of mesoderm formation, as well as certain other factors such as larval types, muscle chemistry, and similarity of sera proteins, most biologists agree that, above the coelenterates, two stocks of invertebrates arose forming a

Y-shaped "tree." The ancestors of present-day echinoderms are located at the base of one branch with most of the invertebrates on the other. The best clues relate the chordates to the branch originating with the echinoderms. Figs. 2-9 and 7-3 present a simplified version of this "tree." Amphioxus is usually acknowledged as a representative of a primitive type of chordate. As stated in Chapter 2, it is of special interest, since it apparently links the chordates to the invertebrates and therefore indicates the pathway of evolution followed by the vertebrates.

GASTRULATION IN AMPHIBIA

The sparsely scattered yolk in the egg of amphioxus enables those cells that give rise to muscle, notochord, and gut to invaginate and migrate anteriorly. Invagination appears to be the primary process responsible for gastrulation in these embryos. In contrast, the yolk-laden, vegetal cells of the frog fill much of the interior of the blastula and react passively. It is mechanically difficult for them to move about as in amphioxus. Consequently, the process of gastrulation is modified in those animals possessing moderately telolecithal eggs, for example, the amphibians.

However, the end result of gastrulation remains the same. Areas on the surface of the blastula destined to become internal organs move to the interior where they arrange themselves in a proper relationship to each other and to the embryo as a whole. Involution plays a larger role in the gastrulation of amphibians than that of amphioxus. Cells enter the interior of the blastula by involution and circumvent the yolk-filled endodermal cells, gaining their proper position in the gastrula.

Presumptive endoderm

Those endodermal cells of the marginal zone, destined to form the foregut, are among the first cells to move inside the frog blastula. They lie below the gray crescent, in the center of the area, and on the axis of bilateral symmetry (Fig. 7-4). The cells elongate and actually push inward (invaginate), forming a dark cleftlike depression or groove about halfway between the equator and the vegetal pole. This inward move-

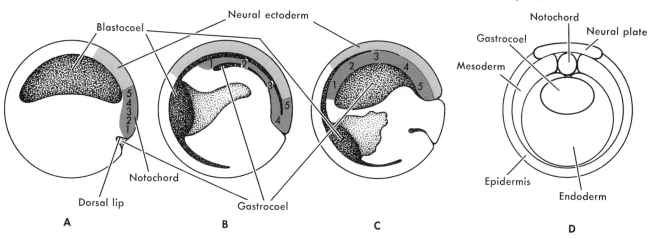

Fig. 7-4

Gastrulation in amphibian shown in sagittal section. Cells involute over rim of dorsal lip and migrate anteriorly under neural ectoderm, eventually obliterating blastocoel and forming a new cavity, the gastrocoel or archenteron. See text for details of cell migration.

ment of cells toward the blastocoelic space can best be seen in sagittal section (diagrammed in Fig. 7-4, *A* to *C*, and photographed in Fig. 7-5). As gastrulation continues, the groove enlarges and forms a cavity leading into the interior. This new cavity, surrounded by the invaginated cells, is the *archenteron,* or *gastrocoel,* of the amphibian gastrula. As the cells continue to migrate toward the cephalic end of the embryo, the archenteron increases in size and crowds the blastocoel to one side, as shown in Fig. 7-4, *B* and *C*, with Fig. 7-5, *C* and *D*, showing the eventual obliteration of it. The rim of the groove (Figs. 7-4, *A,* and 7-5, *A*) marks the beginning of the dorsal lip of the blastopore stage or early gastrula.

These first invaginating endodermal cells enter the blastula by actually changing their shape. The surface cells located near the prospective blastopore become bottle-shaped. One end of a cell remains attached to the surface of the blastula while the cell itself becomes extended inward and the bulk of the cell mass shifts into the deep endoderm. This process is shown in Fig. 7-6. As a result of this inward pull, the blastula becomes indented where the cells cohere at one end. This indentation pulls other endoderm cells inside and is the beginning of the blastopore. If blastoporal endodermal cells are

dissected away and placed on an explant of blastocoelic endoderm, they immediately cohere at the surface of the explant and sink into the deeper endodermal cells. According to Trinkaus (1965) the bottle cells apparently initiate gastrulation by invaginating at the region of the presumptive blastopore.

The shape of the blastopore changes as gastrulation proceeds. If the cells of the blastula are marked and their migration is followed, one can see that the stained areas stretch toward the small crescent-shaped groove; the cells migrate to the rim of the blastopore, roll over its surface, and disappear inside the embryo. Once inside, the cells continue to push in an anterior direction away from the blastopore.

The prechordal plate cells are the next cells to involute. They pass into the interior and, in turn, are followed by the presumptive notochordal cells. All of the marginal zone, previously identified on the fate map as the presumptive notochordal and persumptive mesodermal regions, eventually migrate to the blastopore and disappear inside the embryo.

At first the blastopore is a crescent-shaped structure (Fig. 7-7, *B*). But as cells converge from more lateral positions, the crescent-shaped opening lengthens to a horseshoe shape (Fig. 7-7, *C*). The last cells to involute are those on

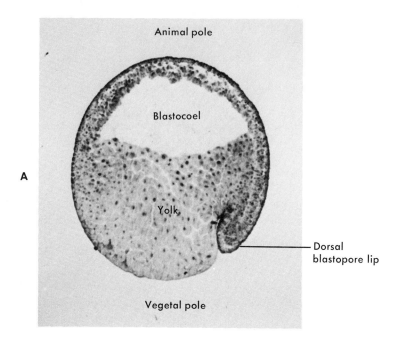

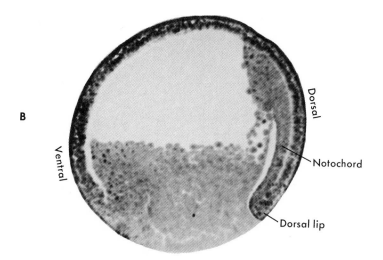

Fig. 7-5
Sagittal views of gastrulation in four frog embryos. The invagination of endodermal cells is the first indication of gastrulation. The horseshoe-shaped blastopore appears as a notch halfway between the equator and vegetal pole, **A**. Involution of notochordal, somitic, and lateral mesoderm around the dorsal and lateral lips of the blastopore follows. The slitlike cavity, the archenteron, expands dorsally and laterally. About half of the notochordal cells are inside the embryo, **B**. When the ventral lips form, the blastopore is ring shaped. The archenteron expands, pushing the blastocoel to the side, **C**, and eventually obliterating it **D**. (× 4.)

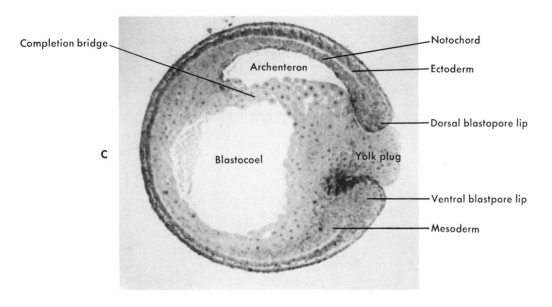

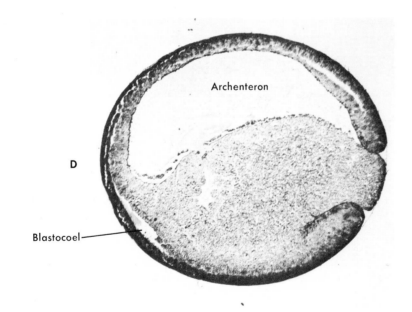

Fig. 7-5, cont'd
For legend see opposite page.

the opposite side of the blastula from the dorsal crescent. As they pass inside the embryo, the ventral lips of the blastopore form and the blastopore now resembles a ring, enclosing the yolk plug (Fig. 7-7, *D*). This stage of development in the frog, therefore, is referred to as the *yolk-plug stage* or the late gastrula. More material passes over the dorsal lips than over the lateral ones, and more over the lateral lips than the ventral. As these presumptive layers move to the inside, the expanding ectodermal cells replace them on the surface. The position of the blastopore is not fixed, but as the cells migrate to it and then involute, the blastopore moves away from the animal pole toward the vegetative pole.

By the end of gastrulation the vegetal region of the blastula is drawn inside the embryo. In its new location it is in a position to give rise to the gut and its derivatives. As a result of the formation of the archenteron and the obliteration of the blastocoel, the force of gravity causes the embryo to rotate and the endodermal cells take up a ventral position as represented in Figs. 7-5, *D*, and 7-8, *B*. Those cells that were originally located at the vegetal pole (marked X on the diagram) are now located on the surface of the archenteron floor in the midgut region. Those endodermal cells, destined to form the foregut and the first to invaginate, are now located properly at the anterior end of the gut (Fig. 7-8). As gastrulation continues, the em-

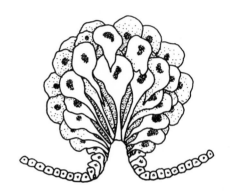

Fig. 7-6
Section of frog gastrula, blastopore view, showing bottle-shaped cells. One end of cell remains attached to surface of the early gastrula while the cell itself becomes extended inward.

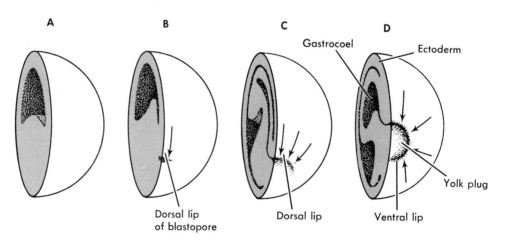

A   B   C   D

Gastrocoel   Ectoderm

Dorsal lip of blastopore   Dorsal lip   Ventral lip   Yolk plug

Fig. 7-7
Formation of germ layers in frog embryo. Hemisections showing development of **A,** blastula stage. **B,** Notochord cells involute forming crescent-shaped blastopore. **C,** Lateral lips added by involution of mesoderm. **D,** Ventral lips of blastopore formed when mesoderm opposite dorsal crescent involutes.

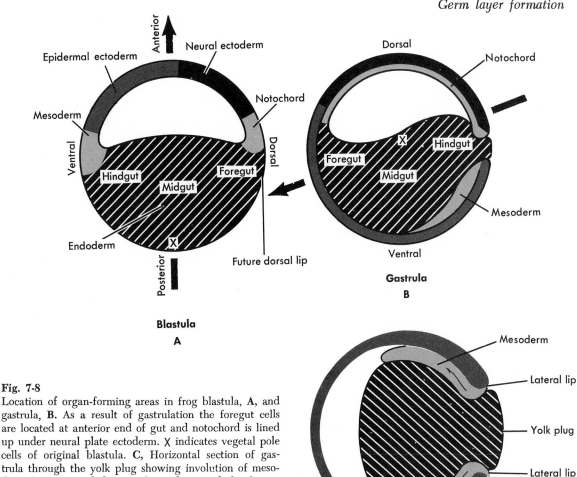

Fig. 7-8

Location of organ-forming areas in frog blastula, **A**, and gastrula, **B**. As a result of gastrulation the foregut cells are located at anterior end of gut and notochord is lined up under neural plate ectoderm. Χ indicates vegetal pole cells of original blastula. **C**, Horizontal section of gastrula through the yolk plug showing involution of mesoderm between endoderm and ectoderm and the formation of lateral lips.

bryo loses its spherical form and under the influence of the archenteron elongates, establishing the anteroposterior and dorsoventral axes of the embryo. The formation of the gray cresent determined bilateral symmetry at the time of fertilization, as indicated in Chapter 6.

Presumptive notochord

The endodermal cells, followed by prechordal plate cells, continue to push forward in the middorsal line toward the animal pole, along the inner surface of the presumptive ectoderm (Figs. 7-4 and 7-5). They are succeeded by the presumptive notochordal cells, which do not become bottle shaped as did the earlier endodermal cells but, rather, orient the larger mass

of their cells toward the exterior of the embryo surface.

The migration of the presumptive notochord cells can be compared to movement of a ribbon-like structure. The anterior end of the ribbon leads the way inside the embryo and the rest of the ribbon follows. As some cells closest to the forming blastopore involute and follow the prechordal plate cells inside the embryo, the next cells move to the blastopore on the outer surface layer and then roll over the rim to the inside. There is a point in gastrulation at which some notochordal cells are inside the embryo traveling toward the animal pole region, some are involuting at the dorsal lip, and some remain on the surface of the embryo (Fig. 7-4, *B*).

Eventually all of the presumptive notochordal cells will be "pulled" inside and none will be left on the surface of the gastrula. These cells take up a position in the midline below the neural plate, forming a middorsal strip in the roof of the archenteron. Later these cells will give rise to the notochord, a transient embryonic structure. As the notochordal cells disappear inside the embryo, the neural ectoderm cells are pulled in an anteroposterior direction. They form an elongated plate, the medullary plate, on the surface of the embryo.

Presumptive mesoderm

The mesodermal cells located in the marginal zone of the blastula also converge toward the blastopore, involute over its edges, and disappear within the embryo. These movements are synchronized with those of the presumptive endoderm, prechordal plate cells, and presumptive notochordal cells. The "wings" of mesoderm, destined to form the somites of the individual, are located in the blastula on either side of the presumptive notochord. They migrate in a lateral direction toward the blastopore and involute over the lateral lips as indicated in Figs. 7-7, *C*, and 7-13, *A*. That part of the somitic mesoderm located closest to the blastopore in the early gastrula is the first to reach the blastopore and roll over its rim. These mesodermal cells then migrate in an anterior and dorsal direction where they give rise to the most anterior blocks of mesoderm (somites).

More laterally placed somitic mesoderm involutes later and forms the somites in the posterior region of the embryo. In this way the consecutively arranged, presumptive somites involute, one after the other, and take up their position along the notochord in an anteroposterior orientation. The mesoderm located laterally to the somitic mesoderm converges and passes interiorly through the lateral lips; the most ventral presumptive mesoderm, located in the opposite side of the embryo from the gray crescent, involutes over the ventral blastoporal lips. Fig. 7-7, *D*, is a map of the trajectories of these cells.

Once inside the embryo, the mesoderm inserts itself between the outer shell of presumptive ectoderm and the inner layer of endoderm, and moves away from the blastopore in an anterior direction (Fig. 7-8, *B* and *C*). It does not remain in a position comparable to its site in the blastula, that is, in the marginal zone, but migrates dorsally up the sides of the gastrula, eventually establishing a close association with the notochord. The combined sheet of notochordal and mesodermal cells is known as the *chorda-mesodermal mantle*. Because of this dorsal migration, the mesodermal layer is much thicker in the dorsal region of the embryo where it forms the roof of the archenteron. This relationship can be seen in a cross section of the late gastrula (Fig. 7-4, *D*). Laterally, the mesodermal layer is less thick toward the more ventral areas of the embryo. Although the mesodermal sheet migrates anteriorly, it does not reach the most anterior regions of the embryo (Fig. 7-8, *C*). Later, the mouth will form in this area.

Presumptive ectoderm

As the cells on the surface of the early gastrula migrate to the blastopore and roll over the lips to the inside, they are replaced on the outside by the spreading presumptive epidermal cells. The stretching and thinning of the epidermal and nervous layers compensate for this increase in surface area. Several layers of cells compose the presumptive ectoderm in early gastrulation but only two layers of cells remain by late gastrulation.

In the process of covering the surface of the gastrula, the neural crescent becomes elongated in an anteroposterior direction and decreases in width. It remains on the dorsal surface of the embryo and assumes the shape of a shield, with the broad end of the shield directed anteriorly.

As the inward migration of the marginal zone draws to a completion, the epidermal ectoderm approaches the edges of the blastopore until finally, when all mesodermal and notochordal cells disappear inside, ectodermal cells compose the lips of the blastopore. After about 36 hours, only a small area of endodermal cells surrounded by blastopore remains visible. This stage of development, identified as the yolk-plug stage, was previously described and diagrammed in Fig. 7-7, *D*.

Closure of blastopore

When the material of the marginal zone finally disappears from the surface of the gastrula, the blastopore closes. The yolk plug withdraws inside the gastrula and the lateral lips come together. The closing of the blastopore marks the termination of the gastrula stage. The neurula stage follows as the various regions of the gastrula begin to differentiate.

GASTRULATION IN CHICK

The chick egg is usually studied as the representative type of an extreme telolecithal egg, since it has practical convenience, is easily handled, and available in any season of the year. Its development was studied as far back as Aristotle, Harvey, Malpighi, Wolf, Pander, and von Baer, and the sequence of its events is better known than that of any other vertebrate. The large amount of yolk modifies not only cleavage but also the morphogenetic movements involved in the organization of the germ layers. Various other animals, such as elasmobranchs, bony fishes, and reptiles, also have heavily yolked eggs, but the chick represents the climax of yolk accumulation that started in the chordates with the isolecithal egg of amphioxus. Thus we shall use it as our example and limit our discussion to those processes involved in the formation of the germ layers in the chick.

The same basic processes occur in the flattened blastoderm of the chick as in the rounded gastrula of the frog. Certain cells on the surface of the blastodisk move inside and establish correct spatial relationships. Interactions then take place between the cells; the organ primordia form and begin to differentiate. In the bird there is so much yolk present that the cells make no attempt to move around it, as they do in the frog. Instead, all cellular activities occur in the small disk of cytoplasm that sits on top of the yolk. It is in this cap that morphogenetic activities take place and the cells undergo convergent and divergent streaming, involution, invagination, and epiboly.

At the end of blastulation, the blastodisk consists of two layers, epiblast (prospective ectoderm and mesoderm) and the beginnings of the hypoblast (endoderm) next to the yolk (Fig. 6-18, *B*). The flattened space between the layers is considered the blastocoel. Gastrulation begins in the chick soon after the egg is laid. After 3 to 4 hours of incubation, there is the suggestion of a thickening of the blastoderm in the posterior region of the epiblast in the area pellucida. By 8 hours the thickening has lengthened and broadened as a result of the convergence of surface cells to the area. This densely packed area of epiblast cells marks the caudal end of the animal. The epiblast also extends over the area opaca, but it contributes to extraembryonic membranes and will not be considered in the discussion of the development of the embryo itself.

The cells composing the epiblast, destined to become mesoderm, migrate to this posterior region of the area pellucida, pile up, finally involute, and then spread anteriorly and laterally between the epiblast and hypoblast layers. This concentration of cells at the surface (the formation of the thickening described above) occurs because the cells migrate and proliferate faster in that area than they can spread out under the epiblast.

Spratt (1946) grew the developing chick blastoderm on a plasma clot and studied the cellular migrations by placing carbon particles on the epiblast. He followed the path of migration of the carbon-marked cells. As shown in Fig. 7-9, the particles moved posteriorly and toward the midline as gastrulation proceeded. The elongated thickening produced in the posterior region of the area pellucida by the sixteenth hour of incubation is identified as the *primitive streak*. This stage of development is the *primitive-streak stage* (Fig. 7-10).

Since the cells move toward the primitive streak and disappear from the surface of the blastodisk at this point, the formation of the streak is a progressive affair. The cells composing it constantly change. Although in general, the cells of the streak contribute to the middle layer of mesoderm, they are also the source of ectoderm and endoderm. In the early stages of gastrulation the streak is a small thickened region in the posterior part of the area pellucida. However, as more cells migrate to the area, it

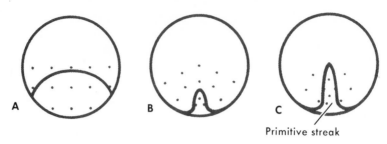

Primitive streak

Fig. 7-9
Formation of primitive streak in chick. Diagram showing movement of carbon-marked cells to midline of epiblast.

grows anteriorly and posteriorly. Also, according to mitotic counts, cell proliferation goes on at a higher rate in this region than in others of the area pellucida. The primitive streak grows, therefore, because of the proliferation of cells as well as of the addition of cell that migrate to it.

After about 20 hours of incubation, the streak stretches two thirds to three fourths the distance of the area pellucida. Different regions can be identified after 12 hours. The anterior end terminates in the *primitive pit*, a funnel-shaped structure surrounded by a cluster of closely packed cells termed *Hensen's node*. The streak itself consists of a central furrow, the *primitive groove* (the site of cellular invagination and involution), flanked on either side by a ridge, the *primitive folds*. As the body of the embryo forms, the area pellucida stretches in an anteroposterior direction, becoming more elliptical or pear shaped. The long axis of the primitive streak is thus parallel with the long axis of the future embryonic body.

Migrating epiblast cells converge along the entire length of the primitive streak, including the primitive pit and Hensen's node (Fig. 7-11). As in the amphibian, the prechordal plate cells are among the first to travel inside. They migrate over Hensen's node, involute at the funnel-shaped pit, and then move in a direction that is anterior to the streak. They are followed (as in the amphibian gastrula) by the presumptive notochordal cells from the notochordal crescent. Once inside, the presumptive notochordal cells migrate anteriorly and eventually establish the rodlike notochord lying in the area pellucida, anterior to the streak and in the midline of the future embryo.

On the fate map (Fig. 6-18), the presumptive mesodermal cells occupy approximately the posterior half of the area pellucida. They must migrate from the surface of the blastodisk to its interior and insert themselves between the endoderm and ectoderm. They converge from either side of the epiblast to the primitive streak, involute, and then diverge anteriorly and laterally to form the broad middle layer. An examination of cross sections of the area anterior to Hensen's node shows the notochord flanked on either side by the mesoderm (Fig. 7-12).

As a result of gastrulation the entire posterior area of the blastoderm, the one identified as presumptive mesoderm, disappears from the surface. The remaining cells of the epiblast (presumptive ectoderm) follow the migrating presumptive mesoderm as it moves toward the primitive streak, but do not themselves involute. Eventually when all the cells destined to form the notochord and mesoderm have made their way inside the embryo, there are no more cells on the surface to replace them. Then the streak starts to regress.

According to Spratt, the carbon-marked cells of Hensen's node migrate posteriorly as more and more notochordal cells move inside. As the streak regresses, cells destined to give rise to the embryo are left behind. They increase in mass and give rise to that part of the embryo located anterior to the streak. For example, the marking of cells shows that as the anterior part of the streak regresses, cells are added to the notochord. The notochord does not grow forward but, rather, grows posteriorly as the streak shortens. The primitive streak continues to shrink in size until, by 48 hours of incubation, the

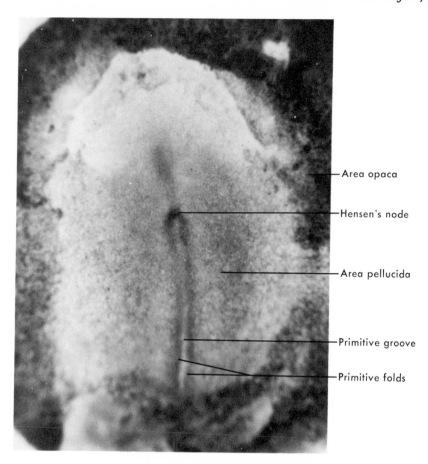

— Area opaca

— Hensen's node

— Area pellucida

— Primitive groove

— Primitive folds

Fig. 7-10
Dorsal view of primitive streak stage (approximately 18 hours) of chick embryo. (× 4.)

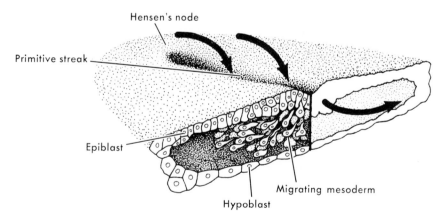

Hensen's node

Primitive streak

Epiblast

Hypoblast

Migrating mesoderm

Fig. 7-11
Transverse section through primitive streak showing *(arrows)* convergence of epiblast cells to primitive streak, movement inside, and divergent migration between epiblast and hypoblast.

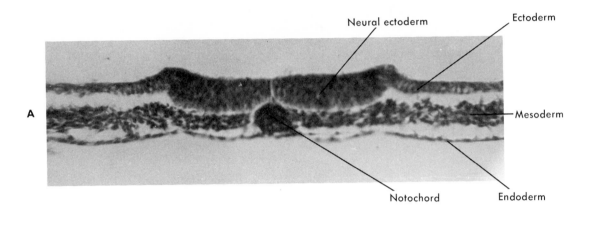

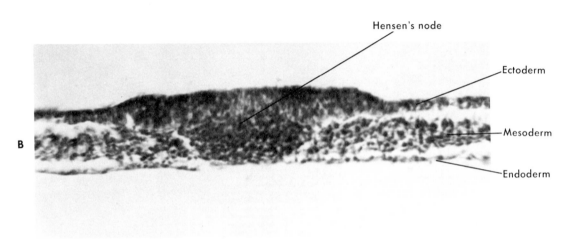

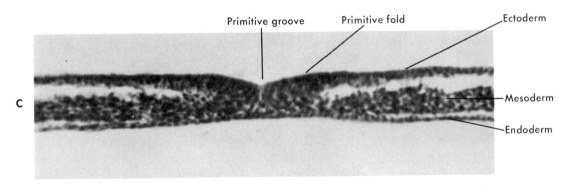

Fig. 7-12
Transverse sections through early chick embryo and primitive streak. (× 40.) **A,** Section anterior to Hensen's node showing notochord, mesoderm, endoderm, neural plate, and epidermal ectoderm. **B,** Section through elevated Hensen's node. **C,** Section through primitive streak, posterior to Hensen's node, showing primitive folds, primitive groove, and mesoderm.

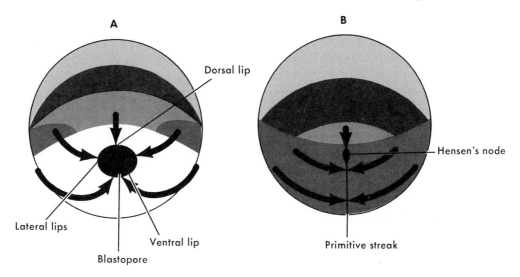

Fig. 7-13
Comparison of frog blastopore with chick primitive streak. Notochord cells involute over the dorsal lip of the frog, **A**, and Hensen's node in the chick, **B**. Mesoderm involutes over lateral and ventral lips in the frog and through primitive streak in the chick. In both examples, surface cells undergo convergent streaming, disappear at blastopore or streak, and take up a position inside the embryo between the epiblast and hypoblast, establishing the third germ layer.

posterior end is incorporated into the tail bud of the developing chick. The embryo is said to be in the *head-process stage* when the notochord takes up its position inside the embryo, anterior to the streak, and the streak, itself regresses.

Comparison of blastopore and primitive streak

Many biologists consider the primitive streak of the chick and the blastopore of the frog to be homologous structures with comparable functions. The movement of cells toward the blastopore in the frog resembles the migration of chick cells toward the primitive streak, as demonstrated in Fig. 7-13. The cells of the frog involute through the lips of the blastopore; the cells of the chick move into the interior through the primitive groove. In both cases, surface cells undergo convergent streaming, disappear at the streak or blastopore and then take up a position inside the embryo between the epiblast and hypoblast, establishing the third germ layer.

The large amount of yolk in the chick egg is responsible for the main difference between the two structures, that is, the blastopore and the primitive streak. The primitive streak is

never open as in the frog, but is comparable to the fused lips of the blastopore. Unlike the frog blastopore, it never communicates with the archenteron. The dorsal lip of the amphibian gastrula and Hensen's node appear to correspond to one another, since it is in these respective areas that the notochordal material makes its way inside the embryo. The presumptive mesoderm of the frog involutes over the lateral lips of the blastopore; the presumptive mesoderm of the chick converges to the primitive streak.

The regression of the primitive streak can be compared with the closure of the amphibian blastopore. When the amphibian blastopore closes, the less active regions of morphogenetic activity, that is, lateral and ventral lips, close first, whereas the dorsal lips, the most active site of cellular activity, close last. A comparable situation occurs in the chick as the primitive streak regresses. Regression occurs faster in the posterior portions of the streak. Hensen's node remains functional until the end.

GASTRULATION IN MAMMALS

Since there is a lack of yolk in the eggs of viviparous mammals, food must be supplied to the embryo. It depends on the mother for food, oxygen, and the elimination of wastes. An early differentiation of tissues in the developing ovum of mammals (including man) gives rise to fetal membranes. These will function in intimate contact with the maternal tissue and carry out the vital functions of the embryo. By the time implantation occurs two of these fetal membranes, the amnion and the yolk sac, have started to develop. But gastrulation lags behind. There is a precocious appearance of extraembryonic mesoderm in the human embryo before intraembryonic mesoderm forms; in fact, even before the appearance of the primitive-streak stage. Essentially, the developing egg first establishes the mechanics for maintaining the embryo before it constructs its body form.

Instead of following a chronological description of mammalian development, we shall continue, as in the frog and the chick, with a discussion of the development of the embryo proper, specifically the differentiation of the germ layers. The membranes that form early in development are associated with viviparity and are adaptive structures. They do not contribute to the definitive body form. The description of these membranes is delayed until a later chapter.

Differentiation of inner cell mass

The blastocyst stage of the mammal is complete when the cells divide into the inner cell mass and trophoblast cells (Fig. 6-19). This sorting of cells according to their future function occurs during the 3 days it takes the egg to travel down the fallopian tube. The blastocyst is an adaptive structure; it makes possible intrauterine development in the mammal. However, during the first few days, it is still enclosed by the zona pellucida. In mice, the blastocyst expands, thinning and rupturing the zona. Also, a lytic agent, probably emanating from the uterus, lyses the membrane. Loss of the zona pellucida allows the mouse blastocyst to "hatch" and exposes the trophoblast cells to the uterine wall (McLaren, 1970). They are free to attach to the uterine mucosa.

Gastrulation begins in the mammal when cells on the undersurface of the inner cell mass ap-

parently segregate and arrange themselves in a layer of cuboidal cells, the endoderm (Fig. 6-19, *B*). The formation of the endoderm in the mammal is reminiscent of its formation in the bird; in both examples the endoderm migrates or delaminates from the epiblast layer. No one has been able to mark the cells of the human embryos; therefore, the details of early development in these forms are tentative.

Around 7 days the human ovum starts to implant into the uterine wall. At this time there develops a cavity that separates the upper surface of the inner mass cells from the outer wall of trophoblast cells. Fig. 7-14 is a schematic representation of this stage. This cavity is destined to become the amniotic cavity. It fills with fluid and bathes the embryo as it develops. The trophoblast cells, usually considered to be of ectodermal origin, form the chorion, one of the embryonic membranes, and contribute to the development of the placenta.

The endoderm cells not only cover the lower surface of the inner cell mass, they also extend beyond the margins of the disk. Here they become continuous with cells believed to be of trophoblast origin, the cells of Heuser's membrane. As a result, endoderm cells and the cells of Heuser's membrane line the large cavity of the blastocyst. This cavity is known as the *primary yolk sac*, although no yolk is present. Once the endoderm differentiates and the amniotic cavity forms, the inner cell mass flattens and forms a bilaminar disk. This disk consists of columnar epiblast cells closely applied to endodermal cells. This two-layered disk is circular in outline and gives rise to all the tissues of the embryo.

The endodermal cells form the roof of the yolk sac (Fig. 7-14). Some of the cuboidal endodermal cells in the anterior regions become more columnar and mark the site of the future *prechordal plate*. It, in turn, determines the cephalocaudal orientation of the embryo. As the cephalic end of the embryo continues to develop, the prechordal plate marks the anterior limits of the foregut and eventually contributes to the formation of the oral plate.

Increasing amounts of precociously developed mesoderm appear between the trophoblast cells

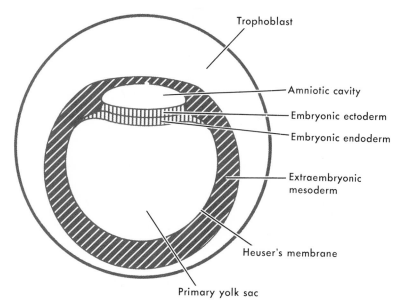

Fig. 7-14
Drawing showing formation of amnion and yolk sac in the human embryo.

and the endoderm that lines the primary yolk sac. It is referred to as extraembryonic mesoderm. Appearing in this mesoderm are spaces that merge and give rise to the extraembryonic coelom. The coelom expands, crowding up around the embryo and leaving only a small stalk of cells effectively suspending the embryo from the chorion (mesoderm plus trophoblast), as shown in Fig. 7-15. This remaining mesodermal condensation will become the body stalk of the embryo, connecting its caudal end to the chorion. The mesoderm next to the trophoblast cells is considered somatic (parietal) mesoderm and that covering the yolk sac is splanchnic (visceral) mesoderm. This extraembryonic mesoderm does not contribute to the formation of the embryo, but to the membrane composing the chorion and yolk sac. It is only after the inner cell mass and trophoblast cells have developed to this point that the primitive streak forms in the bilaminar disk and the body of the embryo begins its differentiation.

Differentiation of germ layers

During the third week of human development, cells segregate into germ layers in a manner similar to that of lower animals. By the fifteenth day cells accumulate in the posterior region of the disk. This phenomenon distinguishes the caudal end of the embryo and initiates the beginning of the primitive streak. The primitive streak of the mammal, like that of the chick, consists of a primitive groove, primitive folds, Hensen's node, and the primitive pit. Cells from the surface of the disk migrate to the primitive streak, move inside, and take up a position between the endoderm and ectoderm. A transverse section through the 16-day-old human embryo shows the mesoderm as a definite layer between the ectoderm and endoderm. This mesoderm contributes to the formation of the embryo proper and is referred to as the intraembryonic mesoderm, to distinguish it from the extraembryonic that will form the membranes. The intraembryonic mesoderm, once inserted as a third layer, spreads anteriorly and laterally until it becomes continuous with the extraembryonic mesoderm of the amnion and yolk sac. It also spreads caudally and contributes mesoderm to the connecting stalk. The formation of the intraembryonic mesoderm transforms the embryo to a trilaminar structure. It now contains three germ layers.

As the intraembryonic mesoderm forms, Hen-

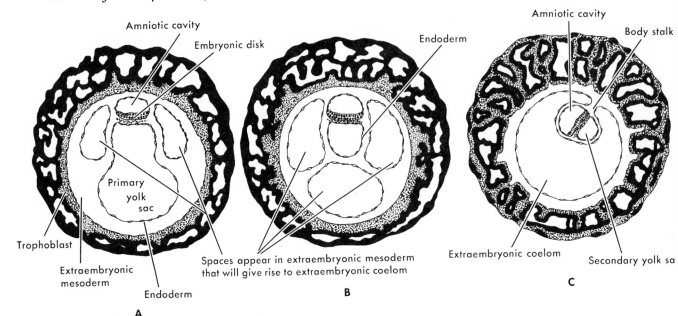

Fig. 7-15
Drawing illustrating the formation of extraembryonic coelom and body stalk. **A** and **B**, Primary yolk sac is partially filled in with mesoderm. Spaces appear in the mesoderm that merge to form the extraembryonic coelom. **C**, Extraembryonic coelom expands, crowding up around the embryo, until only a small stalk of cells is left suspending the embryo from the chorion. A secondary yolk sac is established.

sen's node appears as a thickening in the cephalic end of the primitive streak. The primitive pit, as in the chick, probably represents the dorsal lip of the blastopore described for the lower animals. The presumptive notochordal cells pass through the pit. They then migrate anteriorly to a position intermediate between the ectoderm and endoderm to form the head process of the embryo.

As the presumptive mesodermal cells move inside, the ectodermal cells immediately over the notochord and to each side of it, arrange themselves in an elongated ectodermal band. This band of cells extending in an anteroposterior direction is the neural plate. Immediately surrounding the plate, separating it from the rest of the ectoderm, is an area of special cells, the *neural crest cells*. The remaining ectoderm gives rise to epidermal ectoderm and provides the external surface of the embryo, as it did in the lower forms previously described.

Once the mesodermal cells move inside the embryo, they concentrate on either side of the notochord. The thickened mesoderm thins out

as it extends laterally and merges with the extraembryonic mesoderm. Somites begin to form in the mesoderm adjoining the notochord, during the third week of human development. The most anterior somite is located at about the cephalic tip of the notochord. Their appearance marks the *somite stage* of development. This stage lasts until about the thirtieth day, at which time approximately 42 to 44 pairs of somites are present in the human embryo. The *lateral plate* mesoderm remains unsegmented (as in lower animals) and is attached to each somite by the *intermediate mesoderm*. The lateral plate mesoderm splits and gives rise to the *intraembryonic coelom*.

When the endodermal cells separate from the rest of the inner cell mass, they form the embryonic gut. Cuboidal endodermal cells compose the roof of the primary yolk sac and Heuser's membrane composes the walls (Fig. 7-14). Mesoderm, proliferated by the inner surface of the trophoblast, surrounds the original primary yolk sac; the spaces within the mass of embryonic coelom are described above. The pri-

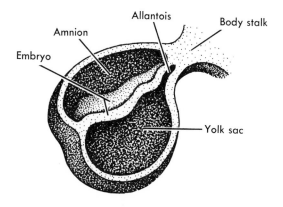

Fig. 7-16
Small diverticulum, the allantois, grows out from yolk sac into body stalk.

mary yolk sac decreases in size as a result of the mesodermal proliferation and the extraembryonic coelom expansion. The endodermal cells rearrange themselves and line the much smaller secondary yolk sac (Fig. 7-15, *C*), which still adjoins the embryonic disk.

At this stage the extraembryonic coelom of the human embryo surrounds the embryonic disk and amnion except at one point, the body stalk, which attaches the caudal end of the disk to the trophoblast. A small diverticulum (pocket) from the yolk sac (as shown in Fig. 7-16) grows into the connecting stalk. This small extension of the yolk sac is the *allantois*. It never expands in the mammalian embryo as it does in the chick and reptile but will contribute to the formation of the urinary bladder of the adult. Its blood vessels, on the other hand, will be important when the fetal tissues make contact with the uterine wall. It is these fetal allantoic arteries and veins that will carry the substances to and from the maternal vascular system.

GERM LAYER CONCEPT AND ITS LIMITATIONS

Construction of the organs of the body from the germ layers is an old concept. Von Baer (1792-1876), often referred to as the father of comparative embryology, spoke of the "layers" of the embryo. He believed that there were four instead of three, since he considered the middle layer to be divided into two parts. As originally conceived it was a rigid concept and specified that certain cells of the blastula were destined to

form specific (germ) layers. A germ layer, in turn, could contribute only to certain tissues. Epidermal or nervous tissues were limited in origin to the ectodermal layer; endodermal tissue could arise only from the endoderm, and mesodermal tissue from the mesodermal germ layer. This belief in absolute specificity of tissue origin was held by embryologists for many decades.

The concept was questioned when new data became available because of the advent of experimental embryology and the application of these techniques to the study of gastrulation. Until the embryo reaches the late gastrula stage, the destinies of cells can be altered by experimentally changing their location within the embryo. Each cell has the potential of forming more than one specific layer. The ultimate fates of the cells were not as *predetermined* as previously assumed. The presumptive epidermal ectoderm cell of the early blastula is destined to give rise to the epidermis of the individual. However, if it is transplanted at the early gastrula stage to another location near the dorsal lip, it will involute and be carried inside the gastrula where it can give rise to kidney, muscle, or skeletal structures usually associated with other germ layers.

The germ layer concept can be used in generalizing the structure of the embryo, but we now know that similar structures do not always arise from corresponding germ layers. Cartilage, for example, usually forms from mesoderm, but in some animals, neural crest cells, considered to be ectoderm, contribute to the cartilage of the visceral arches. Teeth have both endodermal and ectodermal origins. The thymus may also develop from both of these layers, adding further evidence to the idea that the potencies of the germ layers are not as fixed as supposed by the early embryologists.

The important factor in determining the fate of a cell may be the type of cell involved and the sphere of influence in which it becomes located. The interaction between a cell and its environment is believed to determine the direction of its differentiation. The idea that cell potency can be influenced by the cell's microenvironment is generally accepted by today's embryologists. The accumulation of such information shattered the faith of some biologists in the germ layer concept and they discarded it as meaningless. Others, placed it in a new, more modern perspective, since under normal developmental conditions cells of the blastula do follow established pathways of migration, take up regional positions within the gastrula, undergo mitosis, and then differentiate into predictable tissues and organs.

Modern embryologists consider that the germ layer theory says nothing about the potentialities of cells within the embryo or about their reactions to different environments. It is purely a morphological concept. However, it certainly remains a useful means of categorizing development and is of value when one discusses morphology. The concept is used in this manner in these chapters, and the origins of structures of the body are traced to one or more of the three germ layers.

SUGGESTED READINGS

1. Costello, D. P.: Cleavage, blastulation and gastrulation. In Willier, B. H., Weiss, P., and Hamburger, V. (editors): Analysis of development, Philadelphia, 1955, W. B. Saunders & Co.

2. Holtfreter, J.: Tissue affinity, a means of embryonic morphogenesis, 1939. Reprinted in Willier, B. H., and Oppenheimer, J. M. (editors): Foundations of experimental embryology, Englewood Cliffs, N. J., 1964, Prentice-Hall, Inc.

3. McLaren, A.: The fate of the zona pellucida in mice, J. Embryol. Exp. Morphol. 23:1-19, 1970.

4. Moscona, A.: The development *in vitro* of chimeric aggregates of dissociated embryonic chick and mouse cells, Proc. Nat. Acad. Sci. 43:184-194, 1957.

5. Spratt, N. T.: Formation of the primitive streak in the explanted chick blastoderm marked with carbon particles, J. Exp. Zool. 103:259-304, 1946.

6. Symposium on factors controlling cell shape during development, Am. Zool. 13:937-1135, 1973.

7. Trinkaus, J. P.: Mechanisms of morphogenetic movement. In DeHaan, R. L., and Ursprung, H. (editors): Organogenesis, New York, 1965, Holt, Rinehart & Winston.

8. Weiss, P., and Taylor, A. C.: Reconstitution of complete organs from single-cell suspensions, Proc. Nat. Acad. Sci. 46:1177-1185, 1960.

CHAPTER 8

BASIC EMBRYONIC FORM

EARLY EMBRYONIC STATE

Developmental changes continue throughout the life of the individual (ontogeny), but those that are carried out before hatching or birth (prenatal) occur faster and involve greater architectural molding than those that continue into the posthatching or postnatal period. These early embryonic stages can be further divided into *prefunctional* and *functional periods*. The prefunctional state implies a lack of cellular or organ structure necessary to carry out the specialized physiological activities. The initiation of function must await the completion of basic embryonic structure, which for many organs is established about the end of the neurula stage. All organs do not begin to function at the same time. For example, the heart of the chick starts pumping blood after 40 hours of incubation have passed, and the blood circulates in the human embryo by the fourth week of gestation, but the development and differentiation of skeletal muscle and the initiation of its contraction begin later.

The greatest structural changes occur during the earliest embryonic stages (prefunctional) and result from differentiation and growth of the embryo as the fertilized egg develops into the multicellular and multilayered organism. These changes depend on morphogenetic movements of cells or layers of cells. The formation of the germ layers and the establishment of the basic body form (with all its organ primordia) limit further drastic changes in structure. In the human embryo the major organs and systems form by the end of the eighth week. Once established, further development primarily involves continued differentiation and growth. Those animals that undergo metamorphosis are exceptions, however, since there is a new wave of developmental processes that induces further remodeling of structure and form.

Structural development occurs in an orderly stepwise manner under the control of genes. Gene activity covers the spectrum. They act singly to produce a variety of effects (pleiotropism), or they cooperate with other genes to produce a singe effect. Most of the genes of the multicellular animal are in a repressed state until gastrulation. After gastrulation further development of the embryo results as the genes become sequentially derepressed.

We have stressed the orderliness of developmental procedures several times in this book. Development is an extremely complex process, however, and can be better described and understood if broken down into some of its components. For convenience of discussion we shall divide the processes responsible for establishing body form into the following three areas: (1) growth, (2) differentiation, and (3) morphogenesis.

BASIC PROCESSES OF DEVELOPMENT
Growth

Growth is an important process in development and concerns the permanent enlargement of parts of the organism or of the whole. Although it is a difficult word to define, it refers to the increase in cell size and number, or total mass. In general, an increase in protoplasm produces growth, but the nonliving materials manufactured by the cells and deposited in the form of fibers, ground substances, or jelly also contribute to the mass. Growth is more than cell division. For example, the oocyte of *Rana pipiens* over a period of 3 years increases in size by a factor of 27,000. In fact, cleavage is usually not considered as growth since the mass of the fertilized egg is merely subdivided into smaller and smaller units.

Growth is a regulated process; it does not continue unchecked. Many years ago Mendel crossed dwarf and giant varieties of pea plants and demonstrated the importance of inherited factors in determining their size. These genetic factors control the metabolic processes of the cell, which in turn affect cell division and synthesis of new materials. In general, giantism and dwarfism result from an increase or decrease in cell numbers rather than cell size, since the size of cells in plants and animals is limited. Growth of cells, organs, or organisms also reflect the conditions of their surrounding environment. The available space, the proper mixture of nutrients, including oxygen, and the accumulation of cell products are important factors. For example, maternal malnutrition limits the size of the fetus. Hormones also play a role in regulating growth.

Hormones released by the pituitary, thyroid, adrenal glands, and gonads stimulate or inhibit cell proliferation in developing organs.

There are several ways of measuring growth. Cell division is a part of growth and is demonstrated by merely counting the increase in cell numbers of a measured sample. Growth is also associated with the synthesis of new protoplasm. Protein growth can be calculated by measuring the increase in protein nitrogen per unit of DNA. A third way of measuring growth is by weighing the organism at certain regular intervals over a period of time. The shape of the growth curve plotted from such data is usually a sigmoid curve, i.e., it resembles the letter S as shown in Fig. 8-1. Growth starts out very slowly, increases rapidly in the midperiod, slows down again, and then essentially stops. When cell death equals cell growth, no further increase in overall growth occurs, stabilizing the weight of the organism.

The growth of the organism is an expression of the total growth of the individual parts. Individual organs grow by increasing their cell numbers. Although growth curves are similar for all organs, each organ does not necessarily grow at the same rate or at the same time. The change in position and shape of the various organs during development reflects this differential growth rate. For example, the proportions of an organism constantly change. Fig. 8-2 shows the alterations in the form of the human body as it develops from embryo to adult.

Growth and differentiation may or may not go on at the same rate at the same time. A certain antagonism exists between cell division and cell differentiation in some cells. For example, after myoblasts fuse to form the myotube, they do not normally divide. Further, a highly differentiated cell, such as a nerve cell, cannot undergo cell division, yet it increases in size. It is capable of limited growth as evidenced by the regeneration of a cut nerve fiber. On the other hand, the cloning and subcloning of retinal pigment cells and cartilage cells, both considered differentiated phenotypes, provide evidence that these specialized cells, after dividing several times, still retain their specialized characteristics. In a few cases, only some of the cells composing an organ undergo differentiation and enter the functional

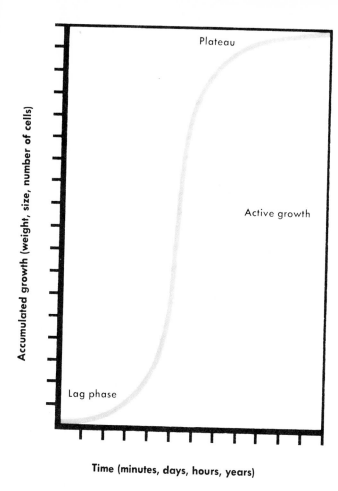

Time (minutes, days, hours, years)

Fig. 8-1
Growth curve of cells, organisms, or populations is S shaped. The abscissa is an expression of time, and the ordinate is some measurement of growth. Growth starts out slowly, enters a period of rapid increase, and then reaches a plateau.

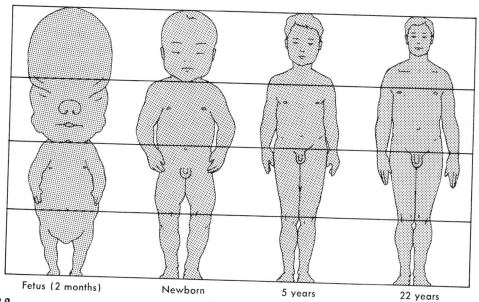

Fetus (2 months)   Newborn   5 years   22 years

Fig. 8-2
Alterations in form of human body as it develops from embryo to adult.

state. A few remain in the prefunctional state in the adult and continue to grow. The cells composing the germinativum layer of the epidermis are examples of undifferentiated cells in the adult. They undergo mitosis and replace the layers of the integument above them throughout the life of the individual. The undifferentiated cells in adult bone marrow that constantly divide provide a second example; some bone marrow cells eventually differentiate (become functional) and replace the worn-out red blood cells of the organism.

Differentiation

The cells of the early embryo look much alike although they differ in size, amount of yolk present, and amount of pigment granules. According to electron micrographs, embryonic cells contain few organelles; the various membrane systems of the endoplasmic reticulum are often absent in the embryonic or undifferentiated cell. As development continues, the cells become *differentiated*. They become different from one another and from the state in which they previously existed.

The establishment of the germ layers by the end of gastrulation gives rise to layers of cells that are differentiated but remain prefunctional. For example, the cells that make up the neural plate at this time are different from the surrounding epidermal ectoderm and from their previous state of presumptive nerve ectoderm. They are still unable to function, however. They cannot carry out physiological activities until they undergo a second more special type of differentiation, *histological differentiation*. As a result of this second level of differentiation, new proteins appear in the cell and a specialized cell results. These special proteins allow certain cells to perform one function and not another. Muscle cells contract, nerve cells conduct, and gland cells secrete.

Induction

By the end of gastrulation, cells have moved to new locations within the embryo and established new relationships. No cell exists in isolation but is in intimate association with other cells. These new relationships apposed new cell surfaces and allowed new exchanges between cells, new stimulations, and new inhibitions. This interrelationship plays a major role in development as groups of cells become more restricted and give rise to tissues and organs (Ebert, 1970).

During normal development, the chorda-mesoderm cells, those that form the dorsal lip of the blastopore of the early animal, line up beneath the neural plate and influence the formation of the brain in the anterior region. The surgical removal of the dorsal lip cells so that they cannot occupy this position beneath the neural plate prevents the formation of the brain. Normally, the presumptive neural ectoderm cells become determined and give rise to nerve cells; under the conditions described, when not in contact with the chorda-mesoderm cells, they remain in an undifferentiated state. The term *induction* is used to describe the influence of a group of cells on the morphogenetic development of an adjacent group of cells. It is the primary event in embryonic differentiation. The response of the neural plate to the chorda-mesoderm is considered a classical example of embryonic induction. It is through the inductive process that cells lose their lability and become determined.

The specific influence exerted by the roof of the archenteron (chorda-mesoderm cells) on the neural plate to form brain vesicles is called *primary induction*. It occurs not only in the frog, but in amphioxus, fishes, and other amphibians. In amniotes, the anterior part of the primitive streak, considered homologous to the dorsal lip, produces similar responses. Induction is a part of a continuum that releases certain reactions inherent in a cell. It results in the induced cell's ability to synthesize specific proteins, which, in the case of nerve cells, would be nerve-specific proteins.

Not only must the chorda-mesoderm cells have the ability to induce changes in the neural ectoderm, but the neural ectoderm must be able to respond to the inductive stimuli. This ability to react is referred to as *competence* and the condition exists for only a certain period of time. Transplantation experiments show that the competence of neural ectoderm decreases from the blastula to neurula stage. At the late gastrula stage, ectoderm that comes in contact with the inductor for the *first time* lacks competence to form brain structures. By the late neurula stage, the ectoderm is unable to form neural tissue at all, and once the ectoderm has become epidermis, it remains epidermis.

The cells of the dorsal lip of the blastopore responsible for bringing about embryonic induction in the amphibia are often referred to as the *organizer*. This term, coined by Spemann, refers to the ability of these cells to organize a regionalized central nervous system. Spemann and his student, Hilde Mangold (1924), transplanted the dorsal lip of one salamander embryo to the lateral surface of another and induced a second embryo to form at the site of the transplant. The second embryo had axial organs that were more or less complete and that were formed partly from grafted tissue and partly from host. This experiment is diagrammed in Fig. 8-3. It was the

first clear demonstration of a primary induction, and Hans Spemann was awarded the Nobel Prize in 1935 for developing his concept of the organizing effects of the dorsal lip.

The cells that make up the dorsal lip of the frog can be traced back to the gray crescent. If the two blastomeres formed at the end of the first cleavage are separated, each will develop into a smaller but complete individual, provided that the first cleavage bisected the gray crescent. When this happens, the inductive material is present in sufficient amount in each of the separated blastomeres to bring about normal development. If the first cleavage furrow divides the egg so that only one blastomere receives the gray crescent material, as in Fig. 8-4, then only this blastomere has the potential of developing into a whole individual. The blastomere that lacks a significant portion of gray crescent substance is unable to complete its development.

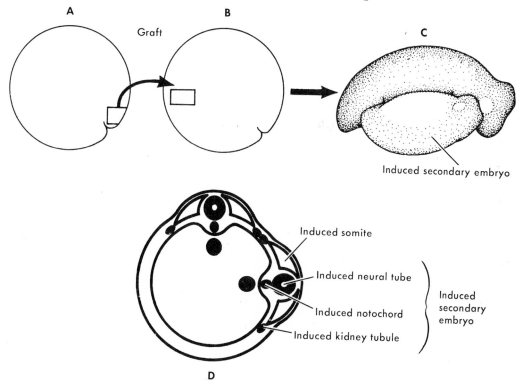

Fig. 8-3

Diagram showing the results of Spemann's and Mangold's experiment. The dorsal lip of embryo **A** was transplanted to a second embryo, **B**. In **C**, the transplanted dorsal lip induced formation of a second embryo on the lateral surface of **B**. Cross section through the resulting embryo **D** shows normal development of host and the development of the induced secondary embryo.

The chemistry and mechanisms of embryonic induction have been the subject of much research since the time of Spemann's experiments. A great deal of frustration resulted from these studies, which often yielded contradictory results. We still do not completely understand the exact nature of inductors, and the role of the tissue responding to the induction is even more of an enigma. Only a few systems have been defined and their timing and spatial arrangements described.

Investigators agree that the influence occurs over a period of time and in a stepwise manner. Jacobson (1966) describes a succession of inductive systems (at least three) that express their influence over a period of time and bring about the determination of the lens in *Taricha torosa*, a West Coast newt. In the early gastrula stage, the endodermal wall of the future pharynx underlying the head ectoderm acts as the first inductor of the lens. Removal of this endodermal wall prevents lens formation. Later in gastrulation after the mesoderm involutes and migrates anteriorly in the embryo, its anterior edge acts as the second inductor of the lens. Its removal also inhibits lens formation. Finally after neurulation, the optic vesicles bulge out from the brain and the future retina contacts the future lens. This retinal contact results in the third induction, which continues until the adult stage.

In order for induction to occur, actual physical contact is not necessary, but the cells must be in the same microenvironment. Induction involves some kind of morphological or chemical communication between cells. There is evidence that induction is attributable to the release of some chemical by one group of cells that causes another group to differentiate, but the molecule involved may not be the same for all inductions. The effective substance can pass through filters. Since its activity is destroyed by such protein-destroying enzymes as trypsin, pepsin, and chymotrypsin, it is likely that some type of protein is the responsible agent.

Despite the fact that the mechanism of induction is not understood at the molecular level, induction should be considered a basic mechanism in the development of the embryo. It is

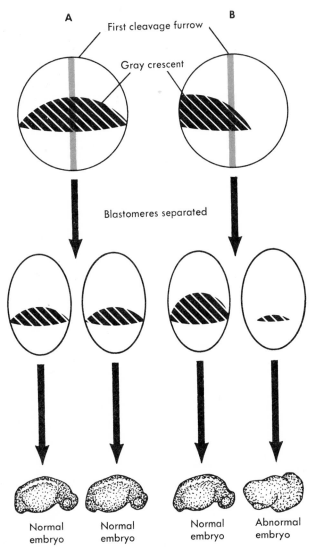

Fig. 8-4
A, If the first cleavage furrow bisects the gray crescent and the resulting blastomeres are separated, two small but normal individuals will develop. **B,** If the first furrow divides the egg so that only one blastomere receives most of the material of the gray crescent, only this blastomere will give rise to a normal individual.

specific and sequential, since more than primary induction is involved. A hierarchy of organizers are presumed to exist, leading to the development of the final embryonic form.

Restriction of cell potency

The restriction of cell potency *(determination)* is associated with the gastrulative process (Needham, 1942) and leads to cell differentiation. It limits the pathways of differentiation open to a cell or a population of cells. The older concept of differentiation was based on the idea that development occurred as a result of a series of restrictions on cell capacity. These restrictions led the cell down a narrowing pathway that eventually allowed it to form only a specific structure. The more modern concept of differentiation rests on a molecular basis. It recognizes the appearance of new macromolecules (nucleic acids, protein, etc.) in the cytoplasm of the cell. It is the interaction of these different macromolecules with similar hereditary machinery that causes the cells to become progressively determined, eventually bringing about a fully differentiated cell.

When cells become determined, areas of the embryo differ visibly from other areas. As a result, organ rudiments or organ primordia form. Certain chemical changes occur within the cell, however, before any external difference is apparent. The basis of differentiation is chemical (for example, the appearance of fetal hemoglobin or myosin), but the ability to perform special functions depends on the presence of cytoplasmic mechanisms. The nerve cell develops long processes. Myofibrils appear in muscle cells.

The cells in the middorsal area of an early gastrula give rise to neural ectoderm. The neural ectoderm differentiates (in the prefunctional sense) into neural plate cells. As development proceeds, the neural plate cells differentiate histologically into nervous tissue. The nervous tissue in the anterior region of the embryo gives rise to the brain, and in the more posterior region, to the spinal cord. This is the normal destiny of neural ectoderm cells brought about by a series of determinative steps. Once the highly specialized nerve cell forms, it can no longer express the complete potential contained within the nucleus of the cell. That is, although presumably endowed with identical genomes of other cells, its developmental pathway is restricted and it can only form nervous tissue. It is determined. Once an embryonic cell becomes determined, under normal circumstances the process is irreversible.

By carrying out a simple transplantation experiment we can show that the determination of neural ectoderm occurs over a brief period of time. A group of the neural ectoderm cells are surgically removed from an early unpigmented gastrula and reinserted into a new, more ventral location on the surface of a second pigmented gastrula of the same stage. The donor cells can be distinguished from the host cells on the basis of their pigmentation and their activities followed. The embryo of the newt is quite often used in such experiments since there are pigmented *(Triturus taeniatus)* and nonpigmented *(Triturus cristatus)* species available for study. If nonpigmented donor cells, which normally give rise to neural ectoderm, are transplanted to this new location in a pigmented host, as shown in Fig. 8-5, the pigmented cells become epidermal ectoderm. The transplanted cells conform and develop into whatever the surrounding cells become. Although the normal destiny of these cells is to form neural ectoderm, they can be influenced by their surrounding environment to give rise to something else. As a matter of fact, if the presumptive neural ectoderm cells are placed close to the dorsal lips of the early gastrula, they involute with the other cells and give rise to chordamesoderm.

At this stage of development, that is, early gastrula, the cells composing the neural ectoderm have the ability to develop into other types of cells, which, in the above examples, are epidermal ectoderm and chorda-mesoderm. This labile characteristic is not limited to neural ectoderm but includes other cells as well.

If the transplantation experiment is carried out at the *end* of gastrulation, the results differ. A change has occurred. If some neural plate cells of the late gastrula or early neurula (the next stage of development) are inserted into the host of the same stage, as in the previous experiment, the cells of the neural plate follow their own

A Early gastrula stage

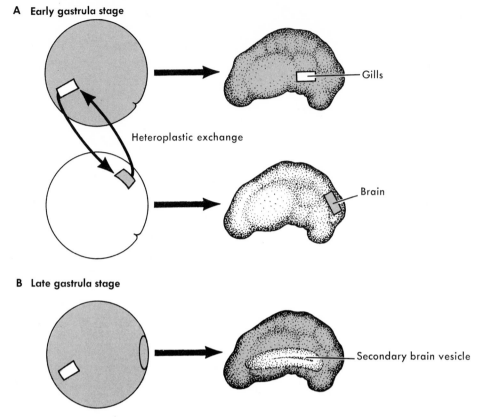

Gills

Heteroplastic exchange

Brain

B Late gastrula stage

Secondary brain vesicle

Fig. 8-5

A, In early gastrula stage, if presumptive neural ectoderm (unpigmented) is exchanged with presumptive epidermis (pigmented), the unpigmented neural ectoderm develops into epidermis and the presumptive epidermal ectoderm becomes a part of the brain. **B,** If the experiment is carried out at late gastrula stage and the nonpigmented neural ectoderm is transplanted to epidermal layer of pigmented host, the neural ectoderm continues to develop into brain vesicles. It has become determined. (Based on experiments by Spemann, 1921).

destiny and form only brainlike structures. They can no longer give rise to epidermal ectoderm. The cells are said to be determined; they have started down a developmental pathway that is irrevocably fixed.

Gene activation

PROTEIN SYNTHESIS. A cell differs from its neighbor, that is, it is differentiated, because of the presence of its particular proteins. These proteins either give rise to the structure of the body or form enzymes that direct the synthetic activities of the cell. Some of the enzymes of a liver cell are the same as the enzymes of, for example, a pancreas cell, but some are different. It is the appearance of these unique substances in the developing cell that indicates the beginning of its histological differentiation. Since the genetic composition of a liver cell and a pancreas cell in the same animal is identical the synthesis of different proteins is believed to occur when certain parts of the chromosome are turned, "on" or "turned off." An understanding of protein synthesis, which eventually is expressed morphologically, involves an understanding of gene regulation.

The control of gene action in the synthesis of proteins has been explored primarily in bacteria and viruses. Beadle and Tatum were the first to show that genes control protein synthesis. They suggested the one gene–one enzyme hypothesis. They worked with the relatively simple bread mold *Neurospora,* which is able to synthesize all of its purines, pyrimidines, and vitamins. They irradiated the spores of *Neurospora* and were able to demonstrate a mutant that synthesized a defective enzyme. As a result of the mutation, the mold was unable to synthesize vitamin B_6, pyridoxine. Only recently have investigations been expanded to explore protein synthesis in the more complex embryo of a multicellular animal. However some of the information obtained from bacterial studies is believed to be basic to all types of cells (Ursprung, 1965).

INFLUENCE OF MALE GENES. During gastrulation the nuclear genes of the diploid cell begin to express themselves. If the egg of one species is fertilized by the sperm of another species, cleavage often goes on but the interspecies hybrid cannot carry out the gastrulative process. This has been interpreted to indicate that the mRNA stored in the egg was capable of synthesizing the proteins needed for cleavage, but could not satisfy the needs for differentiation. Apparently newly synthesized proteins are essential for gastrulation because there is an increase in mRNA synthesis by the end of blastulation, especially in the presumptive endoderm and mesodermal cells. This lack of synthetic ability in the hybrid is caused by some nuclear genetic incompatibility of the foreign genes of the sperm that prevents their expression at late blastulation.

Sometimes, the appearance of new proteins in the embryo can be traced directly to the influence of the paternal genes. If sea urchin eggs of *Paracentrotus lividus* are fertilized with sperm of *Psammechinus microtuberculatus,* there result true hybrids that contain the maternal cytoplasm, a haploid set of maternal genes, as well as a haploid set of paternal genes. According to immunological techniques, proteins (antigens) unique for the male species appear in the hybrid sea urchin embryos about the time of gastrulation. These proteins were not present in the egg and, therefore, must have been synthesized under the influence of the sperm genes.

The formation of *andromerogons* is another way of demonstrating the influence of the male genes. In this case the female pronucleus is removed immediately after fertilization before it

has time to fuse with the male pronucleus. If the sperm is from a species different from that of the egg, the resulting zygote is said to be a hybrid andromerogon. As a result of this technique the zygote formed has the maternal cytoplasm and paternal nucleus. No maternal nuclear material is present. Thus, these individuals are usually haploid. Any new protein synthesized must be the result of the cooperation between the cytoplasm and the nucleus. In those viable embryos (the hybrid andromerogons are extremely fragile) cleavage patterns are always from the maternal side, but the characteristics of the larva, pigmentation, for example, are intermediate between the two species, indicating that these factors are under the control of the male genes.

There is much more evidence available that demonstrates the importance of gastrulation as a time in which new structures are formed. The above two examples, however, are sufficient to show that at gastrulation the two sets of chromosomes (maternal and paternal) brought together at the time of fertilization, start to cooperate with one another in the production of the characteristics associated with the next generation.

CONSTANCY OF GENETIC INFORMATION. For many years differentiation was considered attributable to one of two processes. Either each cell received a different genetic endowment (genome) from its parent, which accounted for its differentiation, or the genetic endowment remained the same in each cell and the environment with which it interacted changed.

Around 1900, A. Weismann suggested that when a fertilized egg cleaved, each daughter cell did not receive identical genetic information. He called the hereditary material determiners. According to him, the egg contained all the determinants (or determiners) necessary to make a complete embryo. With each cleavage they were parceled out in such a manner that different cells received different determinants. As a result of this sorting out of the hereditary material, different cells differentiated along different lines and developed into distinct cell types, depending on the types of determinants they received. This hypothesis was tested by separating cells at the various cleavage stages.

These experiments showed that at the two-cell stage each blastomere (of certain animals) was capable of developing into a complete individual; each cell had received all the necessary instructions or determinants. Weismann's hypothesis, therefore, was not upheld by experimental evidence.

In Chapter 4 in the discussion about mitosis we emphasized that from its parent each cell received intact and unchanged genetic information encoded in DNA. Differentiation must be attributable then to the second process suggested above; that is, it is the environment in which the genetic material resides that determines the outcome of its activities. As pointed out earlier, the third cleavage divides the cytoplasm of a telolecithal egg in such a way that the blastomeres of the animal pole contain much less yolk than those of the vegetal pole. Although the genetic endowment of each blastomere remains the same, the environment provided by each blastomere is different. The synthetic process that goes on because of the interaction between the hereditary material and substrate provides different metabolites, and these, in turn, are believed to result in different morphological expressions.

We reviewed the composition of the chromosomes in Chapter 4 and noted that they consisted of a double spiral of linearly placed nucleotide units. Deoxyribose sugar, phosphoric acid, and nitrogen bases (Fig. 8-6) compose these units. The specificity of the hereditary information contained in the chromosome depends on the sequence of the nitrogenous bases, since the "backbone" of the molecule, the deoxyribose sugar and phosphoric acid, is the same for all animals and plants. The sequence of bases in the DNA molecule codes for the sequence of amino acids in proteins. Three bases (a triplet), referred to as a *codon*, are always necessary to code for one amino acid. A gene responsible for protein synthesis must consist of a sequence of codons (triplets).

During cell division (see Chapter 4) the chromosomes replicate. As a result, an exact copy of the code is distributed to each daughter cell. However, when protein synthesis occurs, instead of replicating as in mitosis, the DNA

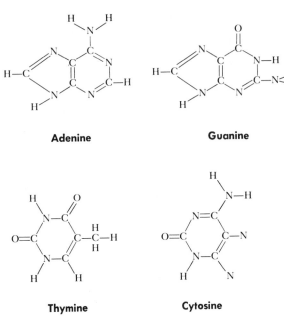

Adenine   **Guanine**

Thymine   **Cytosine**

Fig. 8-6
Structural formulas of the four different nitrogenous bases composing genes. The specificity of the hereditary information contained in the chromosome depends on the sequence of these bases.

molecule containing the necessary code separates into two strands and serves as a template for the synthesis of another molecule, RNA. This process is referred to as *transcription*. The fact has been shown experimentally that only one of the strands of DNA codes for the amino acid sequence. The other strand lacks the code.

As a result of transcription, long chains that lack double spirals make up the RNA molecule. It is similar in composition to DNA, with the exception that the sugar molecule involved is ribose instead of deoxyribose. The nitrogenous bases remain the same as those in DNA with one exception. Instead of thymine, uracil is found in its place. The new nucleic acid is called messenger RNA (mRNA), since it then leaves the nucleus, passing into the cytoplasm where it becomes associated with several particles called ribosomes. These form complexes known as polyribosomes. The total number and sequence of the codons in the RNA molecule corresponds to those on the DNA molecule, and its base triplets are in the same order (although complementary). Therefore, in microorganisms it carries the code for the protein to be synthesized.

Two other types of RNA aid in the synthesis of proteins: ribosomal RNA and transfer RNA. Ribosomal RNA is in the form of particles, the ribosomes. The ribosomes are the actual sites of synthesis of protein but, in bacteria at least, do not themselves specify an amino acid sequence. Transfer RNA, also called soluble RNA (sRNA), acts as an adapter molecule. It is able to pick up specific amino acids, with the help of enzymes and link them to their codons. These small molecules of transfer RNA are specific for each of the 20 amino acids. In a key location on the molecule, the transfer RNA for a particular amino acid contains a sequence of bases complementary to a specific triplet on the mRNA. Each molecule of transfer RNA, therefore, attaches to an amino acid and its codon in messenger RNA. It is the "pairing" attraction between the triplets of tRNA and mRNA that is responsible for holding specific amino acid–tRNA complexes in specific places long enough for the amino acids to react and hook together. Of course, these reactions are speeded up by enzymes. When the bond between tRNA and amino acid is broken, the energy released is used to form peptide bonds between the amino acids. The sequence of amino acids is ultimately dictated by the base sequence of the original DNA molecule in the nucleus of the cell.

PROTEIN SYNTHESIS IN HIGHER ANIMALS. The synthesis of proteins in metazoan animals is less clear, since the specificity of RNAs has not been defined. Although we are certain that RNA acts as a template for protein synthesis, we have no evidence that mRNA actually carries a message. For example, mRNA is synthesized at the puffs of dipteran giant chromosomes. However, it is not possible to prove that the mRNA contains a message that can be identified with the final product. We know little or nothing about the RNA of higher organisms, but the biochemical mechanism of mRNA formation is believed to differ radically from that of bacteria. RNAs are identified primarily on the basis of their size and base composition. We are not even certain of the source of RNA; not only nuclear DNA but cytoplasmic DNA or cytoplasmic RNA have been suggested as possibilities.

The problem of determining the source of RNA in the cells of higher animals lies in a lack of a nuclear precursor for a specific mRNA functioning at the ribosomal level. It has been suggested that the RNA present in the cytoplasm may be a part of a high molecular weight nuclear RNA molecule, designated heterogeneous nuclear RNA (HnRNA) (Darnell, Jelinek, and Molloy, 1973). Biochemists are in the process of trying to match the existence of sequences of nucleotides in HnRNA with a specific sequence in a specific RNA. One such sequence discovered many years ago is now known to be shared by both HnRNA and mRNA. This sequence, consisting of about 200 nucleotides containing adenylic residues, is termed "poly (A)." Its presence in both HnRNA and mRNA (but not in rRNA and tRNA) strengthens the idea that mRNA in eukaryotic cells is derived from a modification of a larger RNA-precursor molecule.

An alternative hypothesis (Bell, 1971) suggests that an informational transfer occurs between the nucleus and cytoplasm. He suggests that small segments of nuclear DNA gene copies (I-DNA) pass out of the nucleus into the cytoplasm in the form of I-somes of different sizes. There is evidence, for example, that DNA constantly turns over in eukaryotic cells, even in nondividing cells. Also, DNA has been identified in the cytoplasm. According to the I-some theory of information transfer, the I-somes in the cytoplasm are transcribed to yield an RNA template for protein synthesis. During differentiation copies of genes necessary for each phase of development are excised from the nuclear genome and pass out into the cytoplasm where they carry out their specific tasks. To prove this hypothesis correct, the next step obviously is to isolate these genes in the cytoplasm of the cell.

GENE REGULATION. The next important problem concerns the selectivity of protein synthesis. How are the activities of the various genes coordinated? What determines what gene will be activated and consequently what protein will be synthesized? All cells possess common enzymes for catalyzing common metabolic pathways, but

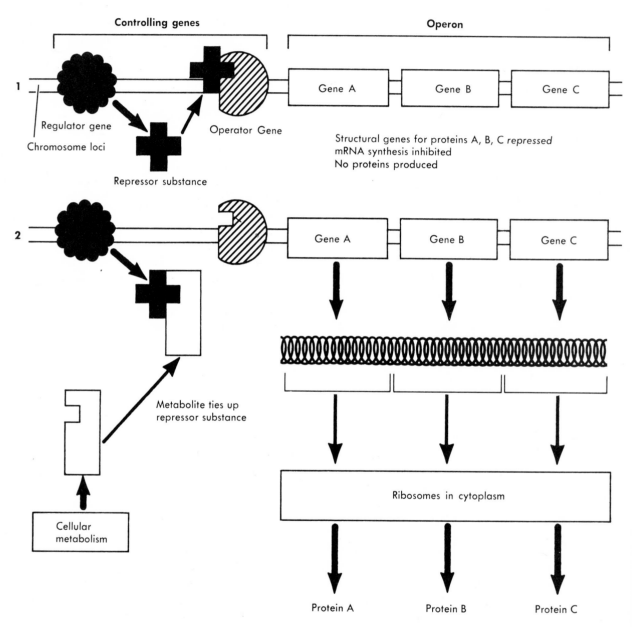

Fig. 8-7

Conceptual scheme explaining the regulation of specific protein synthesis in the colon bacillus, *Escherichia coli*. Two general types of genes are postulated: controlling genes and structural genes. At least two different genes belong to controlling group: regulator gene and operator gene. **1**, Regulator gene releases a repressor substance that reacts with the operator gene "turning off" its activity. As a result the structural genes for proteins A, B, and C are repressed and mRNA synthesis is inhibited. **2**, When a cellular metabolite reacts with the repressor substance, the operator gene becomes active. As a result the structural genes are stimulated to produce mRNAs that will give rise in the cytoplasm to synthesis of specific A, B, and C proteins.

different cells in higher organisms possess also unique enzymes. There is general agreement that the differentiation of a cell depends on its ability to synthesize these unique proteins. The synthesis of a specific protein depends in turn on the gene transcribing its code to mRNA, which carries the message out into the cytoplasm and directs the synthesis. Obviously all genes do not synthesize all proteins in all cells all the time. For example, probably all the cells in the body contain the genes for making myosin, but only the genes of a muscle cell are turned on and direct its synthesis. There must be some kind of a programmed mechanism to coordinate and regulate the thousands of chemical reactions that go on in the body. The kind and amount of protein must be programmed, as well as the time and sequence of its appearance.

Much of our present knowledge of the regulation of protein synthesis is based on genetic studies of bacteria. A conceptual scheme was worked out by Jacob and Monod (1961), attempting to explain the regulation of specific protein synthesis in the colon bacillus, *Escherichia coli*. This scheme, known as the regulator-operator-operon hypothesis, is diagrammed in Fig. 8-7. Apparently, in bacteria most of the genes would be active at one time if they are not repressed. This repression is brought about by the interaction of several genes. Two general types of genes have been postulated. One codes for the specific mRNA. This gene, which functions in the synthesis of the protein, is called the *structural gene*. The other general type of gene controls the turning on and off of the structural gene. At least two different genes belong to this controlling group; the *operator gene* controls the structural and, in turn, is controlled by the *regulator gene*. When the operator gene is active, mRNA is produced according to the structural gene. The regulator gene controls the operator gene by releasing a product known as a *repressor*. This substance turns off the operator gene. The structural gene is derepressed when and if some specific metabolite of the cell reacts with the repressor product of the regulator gene and blocks its effect on the operator gene. The operator gene can then become active. When this occurs, the structural gene is free to begin transcription again.

The operator gene apparently controls more than one structural gene so that if its block is removed, several structural genes are derepressed (activated). This allows the production of several different mRNAs that will give rise to the synthesis of several proteins. Such a set of genes controlled by one operator gene is referred to as an *operon*.

At the present time, we do not know if the control of gene activity in higher organisms resembles that in microorganisms. There is scattered evidence that induction and repression of enzymes that occur in bacteria also take place in vertebrates, for the most part in the liver. One may logically assume this function for the liver, since it is the organ subjected to a varying supply of nutrients. It helps to maintain a constant environment for such organs as muscles, brain, and heart. Undoubtedly, gene control would be more complex in a metazoan animal and must be modified. For example, the genome of multicellular animals is much larger than in microorganisms and differentiation requires the cooperation of nonadjacent genes. Also, a large amount of repetitive nucleotide sequences (redundancy) occurs scattered through the genome. Only a small portion is active at any one time.

A modification of Jacob and Monod's scheme for gene regulation was suggested by Britten and Davidson (1969). According to their model, sensor and integrator genes substitute for regulator genes of bacteria. They stress the multiplicity of changes in gene activity that can result from a single initiatory event. Their model includes a highly integrative system in which certain genes are sensitive to the products of other genes. A single event may activate several controlling genes, which, in turn, activate a vast number of structural (producer) genes. They speak of a magnitude of batteries of genes that may be necessary for the maintenance of the cell state, and they point out that there must be precise coordination of these batteries of structural genes if the differentiated state is reached.

Probably the most universal control of gene regulation occurs at the level of transcription. However, we do not understand how it occurs. Certain proteins associated with DNA may "mask" it in some way and inhibit it from transcription. Histones, proteins manufactured in the cytoplasm, are closely associated with the chromosomes and have been implicated in the control of gene activity. For example, addition of histones in vitro to nuclear preparations represses gene activity. Removal of histones caused de-repression. There is also evidence that nonhistone proteins may move from the cytoplasm into the nucleus and also act to repress gene activity.

Certain hormones increase the rate of transcription and therefore the amount of RNA synthesized. Administration of estrone and estradiol to ovariectomized rats induces in the uterus a considerable increase in protein synthesis, which is blocked by administration of actinomycin D. Some biologists suggest that the hormone reacts with a protein receptor and that the complex in some way releases a repressed state of an operon. Hormones may also exert their influence by changing cell permeabilities. The influx of various ions in some way may regulate the activity of the gene.

Gene regulation, however, occurs at many more levels than the operon. In some instances differential gene replication is correlated with certain stages in the development of the embryo. For example, in *Xenopus*, 28S and 18S ribosomal RNAs (designated according to their size) are synthesized during the early stages of the developing egg (oogenesis). Their synthesis ceases when the egg matures and does not begin again until the initiation of development. The synthesis of rRNA apparently occurs in the nucleoli and during oogenesis extra chromosomal nucleoli form. The result of molecular mapping demonstrates that the genes for rRNA are redundant; that is, there are repeated sequences. The oocyte has many more genes for rRNA than does the nucleus of a somatic cell—some 1000 times more. During oogenesis the oocyte of *Xenopus* makes extra copies of genes for rRNA and stores them in the nucleoli. Presumably they are used as templates to support the increased rate of synthesis of rRNA that occurs during oogenesis, since they become nonfunctional at later stages of development. According to Brown and Dawid (1968) the immature oocyte of *X. laevis* synthesizes rRNA at a rate comparable to the equal weight of liver tissue, comprising some 2000 cells.

There is biochemical evidence that the type of chromatin varies among cells. Chromatin is the term given to the complex of DNA with protein and RNA. It exists in a condensed state during most of the mitotic cycle and in the extended state during the interphase. It is during the extended state that transcription occurs. Different cells transcribe different amounts of the genome, and the transcribable DNA may differ from cell to cell. For example, the transcribable DNA from liver cells is organ specific and differs from that extracted from bone marrow or kidney.

The control of gene activity in multicellular organisms remains largely speculative. Most investigators believe that transcription and translation of genetic information follow pathways similar to those of microorganisms. However, we still do not understand the genetic mechanisms that ensures the progressive, sequential, programmatic reading of the genetic code over defined time intervals.

EVOLUTIONARY SIGNIFICANCE. One can see from this brief and necessarily superficial review that the transmission of hereditary material from parent to offspring implies the constancy of the double-stranded DNA molecule in the nucleus of the cells. The correct duplication of this material, its passage to the next generation in the egg or sperm, the new gene combinations occurring at fertilization, and the activity of the various types of RNA result in the appearance of parental characteristics in the offspring.

The mechanisms of DNA transcription and RNA activity are remarkably similar not only in all vertebrates and invertebrates, but in all living things. The DNA always consists of the same four nucleotides. Multitudes of different proteins are assembled from the same 20 amino acids because of the activity of RNA. It has even been shown that under circumstances the purified RNA of one organism (polio virus) can direct the protein-synthesizing system of another organism (*E. coli*) to synthesize protein.

However, diversity is obvious when the living organisms of the world are considered. Diversity appears among organisms and in the parts of the organisms. It is this diversity or variation among organisms at the anatomical, physiological, and behavioral levels that allows them to adapt to different environments. Charles Darwin realized that animals produce many more offspring than could survive. While some animals flourish, others are eliminated. Those that could best adapt to their environment continued to produce offspring whereas those that could not were "weeded out." As stated in Chapter 1, this process is referred to as *natural selection* and depends on the great diversity among animals.

The deviation of animals from this basic biological uniformity can be explained by turning once again to the DNA molecule. It is here that any alteration must express itself if it is to be passed to the next generation. If a change occurs in the sequence or composition of the base triplets of a cell's DNA, then the code is changed and results in a different amino acid being incorporated into a particular spot in the assembled protein. This change in synthesized protein expresses itself in the function or structure of the cell. Alteration of the code on the DNA molecule is referred to as a *mutation*. Mutation is the basis for evolution, because it is the only means of producing new genes. If the alteration is great, such as if it affects some vital process in the cell, then the mutation is usually lethal to the organism. Obviously only slight changes can be tolerated by an organism at any one time. Spontaneous mutations occur very rarely, but over a period of geological time mutant genes accumulate within a natural population and result in gradually altered form (phenotype). The process of evolution selects those geneotypes that can live most successfully under the conditions prevalent at the time.

The early developmental processes of all vertebrates are conservative and follow known pathways that produce successful results. Over the ages, mutations must have occurred during the early stages of development but proved lethal. For example, a mutation at the gastrula stage could place the foregut in positions that would not allow further development. On the other hand, at later stages of development, there probably occurred mutations that caused the gut of one embryo to develop into a crop and a gizzard, and the gut of another to develop into the mammalian stomach. These modifications introduced at a late stage of development gave rise to organisms that have different survival values. The crop and gizzard of the grain-eating bird enable it to cope with one type of environment much better than if its gut were of the mammalian type.

The similarity of embryonic form was observed by the embryologists over a century ago. They noted that all embryos start out as an egg, undergo cleavage, form a blastula, and then form a gastrula in which the germ layers are established, before developing further to the neurula and transforming to the adult form. Many years before the theory of evolution became popular and before knowledge of the gene and its activity was accepted, von Baer noted that the more general characteristics of the embryo are established before the more specific features become apparent.

The acceptance of Darwin's theory of evolution in the mideighteenth century focused attention on the embryo from an evolutionist's viewpoint. It seemed obvious to the biologists of the day that the basic similarity in vertebrate embryonic form was attributable to the fact that all were related in some way. They had evolved one from another. Those characteristics held by a large group of animals must have been held by a common ancestor.

Ernst Haeckel, a prominent German morphologist of this period, was convinced that the development of the individual (ontogeny) passed through the various stages of adult ancestors (phylogeny) and suggested what has become the aphorism, the "biogenetic law." The law is usually expressed as "ontogeny recapitulates phylogeny," or in more general terms, the embryo repeats in its development the evolutionary stages of its adult ancestors. It climbs its own family tree. Fig. 1-1 demonstrates the obvious similarity of comparable embryonic stages of vertebrates The embryos closely resemble one another in stage I when the pharyngeal arches form. It is difficult to tell the examples of one class from another. By the time the embryos reach stage III the more specialized characteristics that allow them to be categorized into the various classes appear. Haeckel believed that evolution occurred by the addition of new stages at the end of certain life histories. Therefore, the developmental history of any animal included all the previous stages of development.

Time has proved Haeckel's theory to rest on false premises. Gill pouches, produced by the outpocketing of the pharynx, are found in all chordate embryos from fish to man. The pouches either remain intact or they become perforated to form gill slits. In the aquatic animals, vascular lamellae develop on the sides of the pouches and function in the exchange of gases in respiration. These become the gills of the aquatic animal. Human adults, of course, have no gills and neither do human embryos. In the embryo the pharyngeal pouches do appear but are transitory structures. Similarities are present, therefore, only in the embryonic stages. The embryo of a mammal passes through stages that resemble the embryos of the lower forms, but it never passes through stages that resemble the adults of these forms.

BASIC EMBRYONIC PLAN

At the end of gastrulation epidermal ectoderm covers the cylindrically shaped embryo. The

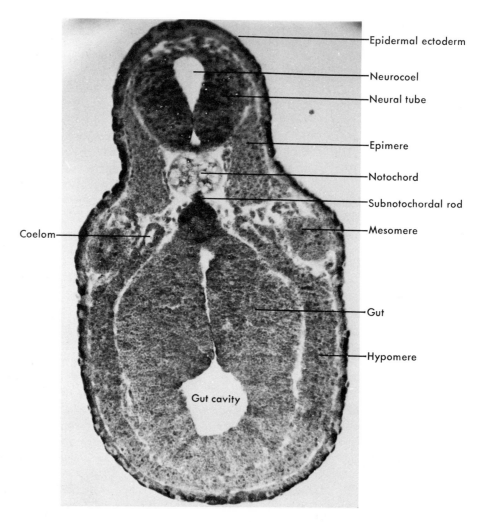

Fig. 8-8
Transverse section through the 4 mm. frog tadpole demonstrating the basic body form. The notochord extends as a rod-shaped structure down the length of the embryo. The neural tube, gut, and mesoderm are arranged around it. Epidermal ectoderm covers the embryo. (× 100.)

neural plate lies in the middorsal region with the prechordal plate cells lined up beneath its anterior regions. By the end of the gastrulation stage the mesoderm takes up a position between the ectoderm and endoderm. At first the mesoderm, closely associated with the notochord, is known as the *chorda-mesodermal mantle.* In the next developmental step the notochord segregates itself, forming a rod-shaped structure that extends as an axis down the length of the embryo in the middorsal region under the neural tube (Fig. 8-8).

When the notochord material separates from the mesoderm, the mesoderm disassociates itself from the endoderm. Only in amphioxus does the mesoderm originate as a pouchlike structure; in all vertebrates it is a solid band, which later delaminates or splits to form a lumen.

The gut of the embryo, composed of endodermal cells, extends from the head to the tail regions. Once the blastopore fuses in the amphibians, the gut is a closed cavity. In meroblastic animals the ventral area of the gut is open and rests on the yolk. Subcephalic and

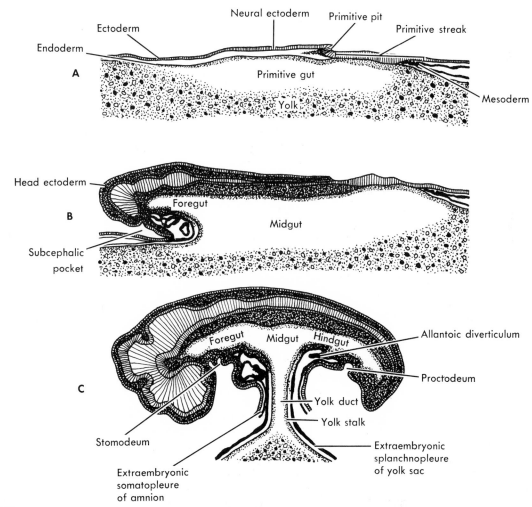

Fig. 8-9
Schematic drawing (sagittal view) showing stages in the formation of the body of chick embryo. **A,** Chick body develops anterior to the area of primitive streak. **B,** Folds roll under head process, separating it from underlying yolk by a subcephalic pocket. Floor to foregut is established. **C,** As a result of subcephalic, lateral, and subcaudal folds, the body of the embryo becomes defined and separated from extraembryonic regions.

subcaudal folds progressively undercut the anterior and posterior ends of the body until eventually most of the gut of the flattened blastula contains a floor open to the yolk only in the region of the umbilicus (Fig. 8-9). Regardless of the type of gastrula formed (round or flattened), the gut is properly oriented; the region that gives rise to the foregut is located in the anterior region of the embryo, and the part that forms the cloaca is positioned posteriorly. Thus, dorsoventral, anteroposterior axes are established by this time in the body of the embryo.

In summary, all vertebrate embryos continue to follow generalized pathways at this stage of development, and as a result establish similar, basic, embryonic forms. This general arrangement exists in all vertebrate embryos by the end of gastrulation, regardless of their phylogenetic status, and regardless of the amount of yolk present in the original egg or of the types of morphogenetic movements utilized to bring about the architectural structure. From this basic generalized plan, organ primordia develop. For example, the liver forms in all embryos as a diverticulum from the gut. The eyes develop as extensions of the brain.

The basic embryonic form of all vertebrates consists of five tubes that eventually differentiate and give rise to the adult structures. They are present in both rounded and flattened gastrulas. These tubes are oriented around the solid, rodlike notochord, which forms the axis of the body. This relationship is shown in Fig. 8-10, a cross section through the embryo. The neural tube

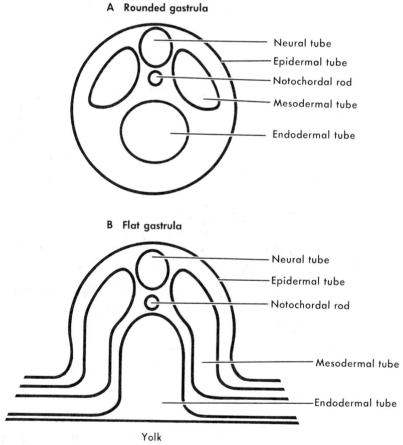

Fig. 8-10
Comparison of basic embryonic forms of animals developing from round blastulas, **A,** and flat blastulas, **B.** Both types of gastrulas are composed of five "tubes" oriented around the solid notochord.

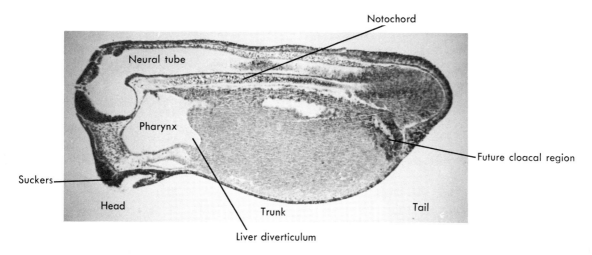

Fig. 8-11
Sagittal section of a 4 mm. frog embryo showing the differentiation of head, trunk, and tail regions. Notochord extends the length of the body and is located beneath neural tube. Enlarged anterior end of the neural tube develops into the brain. (× 4.)

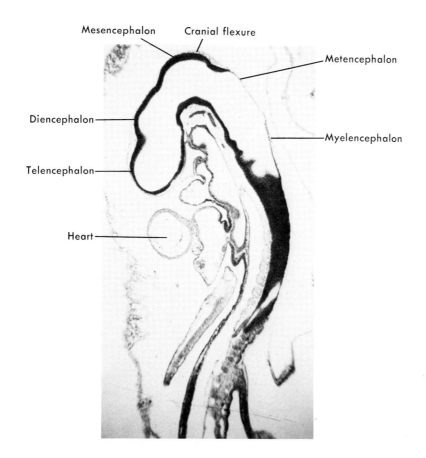

Fig. 8-12
Sagittal section through 48-hour chick embryo showing the cranial flexure at midbrain region. (× 4.)

forms dorsally to the notochord and the endoderm tube ventrally to it. Two mesodermal tubes are located one on each side of the notochord and endodermal tubes. The epidermal tube encases the entire embryo.

As the late gastrula stages develop into the neurula, the body of the embryo flattens laterally and extends in an anteroposterior direction. The dorsal region of the body arches, pushing the neural tube, notochord, and somites (mesoderm) more dorsally in the body. The anterior extension of the embryo is known as the *cephalic* or *head region;* a similar projection in the posterior region becomes the *caudal* or *tail* outgrowth. The remainder of the embryo is designated as the *trunk* area. These relationships are shown in Fig. 8-11, a sagittal view of a 4 mm. tadpole.

Associated with the differentiation of general body regions is the overall positional change of the body. Except in the fish, the anterior region of the neural tube becomes bent or flexed toward a ventral position. This flexure involves the midbrain and results in its growth perpendicular to the axis of the notochord. The midbrain bends toward the cardiac region in what is known as the *cephalic* or *cranial flexure,* readily observable in the 48-hour chick embryo (Fig. 8-12). The cervical flexure appears in the region of the hindbrain at a later stage of development. Associated with the flexures is a general bending or twisting of the body region of most vertebrates, beginning at the head end of the embryo and progressing posteriorly until the anterior and posterior regions become curved ventrally toward one another, producing a comma- or C-shaped embryo. The embryos of higher vertebrates, those enclosed within extraembryonic membranes, also undergo rotation or *torsion.* As a result, the embryo comes to lie on its side, usually the left one. This rotation occurs in chicks, as well as in pigs and other mammals.

MORPHOGENESIS

Morphogenesis is the result of cell differentiation and growth. The term refers to the formation of new structures and the establishment of body form unique for the animal under consideration. It begins with the next stage in development after gastrulation.

Neurulation

As the migrating cells reach their various positions in the embryo during gastrulation, the neural ectoderm layer is one of the first to begin differentiation. In some animals the neural plate gives rise to the neural tube within 24 hours. The separation of the plate from the surrounding epidermal ectoderm, the formation of a tubular structure lying beneath the epidermal layer and the segregation of neural crest cells is referred to as *neurulation.* The embryo is considered to be in the *neurula stage,* a term especially applied to the amphibian, when the neural plate can be identified. In the chick it is defined as the stage immediately following the definitive primitive streak stage. The neural tube forms on the dorsal surface and extends the length of all chordate embryos. The formation of a single, dorsal, hollow neural cord separates the chordates from the invertebrate animals, whose neural cord is solid, ventrally located, and sometimes double.

As gastrulation ends, the cells of the oval area of neural ectoderm elongate because of the presence of microtubules and form a flat neural or medullary plate. The neural plate divides into several presumptive areas that develop into certain defined structures, provided that the necessary induction takes place. The anterolateral regions of the neural plate form the olfactory area. Posteriorly, the plate divides into the presumptive forebrain and optic area, midbrain, and hindbrain, respectively. The epidermal ectoderm over the hindbrain eventually forms auditory vesicles, and this region of the plate develops into the auditory area.

The cells of the neural plate become flask-shaped and differentiate from the more squamous (flat) cells of the epidermal epithelium. The plate extends from the dorsal lip of the blastopore, in those animals with round gastrulas, and from Hensen's node anteriorly in those embryos with a disk-shaped blastoderm. There are two general procedures by which vertebrates bring about tubulation of the neural tissue; the neural-fold method and the thickened-keel method. Although we can describe neurulation, we do not understand all the forces responsible for the formation of the neural tube.

In the majority of vertebrates the basic process

of neurulation is one of folding. This folding is caused by the apical constriction of the neural plate cells, probably brought about by a microfilament that encircles the apex of the neural cell in purse-string fashion (Burnside, 1973). As a result, in the middorsal region of the medullary plate a longitudinal depression forms, flanked by lateral neural folds. The folds are the result of the upward movement of the epidermal ectoderm at the margins of the plate. As the folds push upward and toward the midline, the depression deepens and a neural groove forms. The neural folds appear in the amphibian soon after closure of the blastopore and are first evident in the cephalic end of the chick around the three-somite stage (approximately 21 to 23 hours of incubation). Neural folds are definitely identified in the human embryo at the seven-to-eight-somite stage (18 to 20 days after fertilization).

Differential growth causes the lateral folds to move toward one another where a double fusion takes place, as illustrated in Fig. 8-13. The margin of the neural ectoderm detaches from the epidermal ectoderm and fuses to form the neural tube, first in the midbody region, and then continues in either direction zipper-fashion. At the same time the lateral epidermal ectoderms also fuse with one another, filling the spot once occupied by the nerve ectoderm. As a result, the neural tube comes to rest *under* the external surface of the embryo. For a time the neural tube is open to the outside at its anterior and posterior ends, but these openings eventually close. The neural tube is hollow from the beginning, with its lining consisting of some of the original surface cells of the blastula. The cavity of the neural tube is larger at the anterior end and develops into the vesicles of the brain. The smaller more posterior extension of the hollow tube is destined to form the spinal cord, with its cavity becoming the central canal of the cord.

The thickened-keel method is the second method by which vertebrates, primarily certain fish, achieve neurulation. The material composing the medullary plate is in the form of a rod or keel running down the length of the animal. This keel detaches itself from the surrounding epidermal ectoderm and sinks down into the dorsal area of the embryo. The epidermal ecto-

derm covers the surface where it was located. Eventually a cavity forms in the keel, transforming it into a longitudinal nerve tube.

As neurulation continues, the embryo stretches along its anteroposterior axis, with the neural tube participating in the elongation process. The stretching that occurs in the posterior region of the embryo causes the body to extend beyond the blastopore into what is known as the *tail bud.*

Formation of neural crest cells

After the neural tube separates from the epidermal ectoderm, certain other ectoderm cells collect in the midline in the space between the tube and epidermal surface. These are the *neural crest cells,* which are neither part of the epidermal ectoderm nor included in the neural tube. As soon as the crest cells form, they migrate to various parts of the body where they play a definite role in specific organogenesis. If they are surgically removed from the embryo, those structures to which they normally contribute do not form. Such excising techniques reveal that normally they contribute spinal ganglia, sensory nerves, sheath cells, and sympathetic neurons to the nervous system. They may also give rise to some of the color-bearing cells of the body (chromatophores), the medulla of the adrenal gland, and the muscles and cartilage.

Differentiation of epidermal ectoderm

The ectoderm makes a major contribution to body structure by forming the nervous system. In addition, the part of the ectoderm that is neither neural ectoderm nor neural crest cells becomes the epidermis of the skin. In the early embryo it consists of two layers, an outer layer (periderm), which develops into certain sensory organs in the amphibian and is shed by the birds and mammals, and an inner layer, which becomes the stratum germinativum of the epidermis. These cuboidal cells retain the ability to divide during the life of the organism and replace those layers of the skin that are sloughed off or worn away. The epidermis in combination with the dermis (mesoderm) composes the integument of the organism. It is from the epidermis and dermis that certain accessory struc-

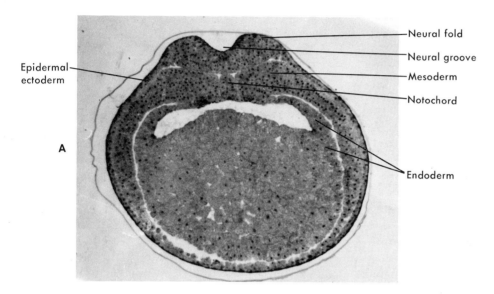

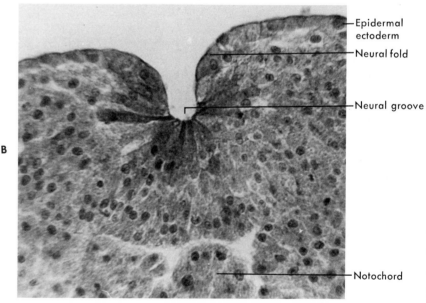

Fig. 8-13

A, During neurulation the neural plate of a frog embryo begins to form neural folds and a neural groove. **B,** Cells of neural plate become flask shaped and differentiate from the more squamous cells of epidermal epithelium. **C,** Margins of the neural ectoderm detach from epidermal ectoderm and fuse to form the neural tube. The notochord is beneath the neural tube. (× 40.)

tures (glands, hair, horns, feathers, etc.) develop and certain outgrowths (limb buds, fins, and external gills) form.

The ectoderm eventually also gives rise to platelike thickenings of the epidermal epithelium, called *placodes*. They are associated with certain sensory organs and are discussed in greater detail when we describe the histogenesis of specific organs. However, there are five or six placodes that can be mentioned appropriately at this time because they are involved in organogenesis. In the anterior end of the animal, thickenings form the olfactory placode, which will give rise to the olfactory sacs. The forebrain induces the cells of the lens placode to elongate and form the lens of the eye. The thickenings associated with the hindbrain become auditory placodes, which eventually convert to auditory vesicles. Aquatic animals have lateral-line organs stretching from the anterior to the posterior end of the body. Other thickenings appear in the head region and give rise to certain cranial nerves.

Differentiation of mesoderm

As neurulation proceeds, the mesoderm is the second area to differentiate actively. It contributes much to the growing embryo. The thickened mass of mesoderm adjacent to the notochord becomes transversely divided into a number of segments, as described for the human embryo in the previous chapter. Each segment is referred to as a *somite* or *epimere* and consists of a block of cells on each side of the notochord; that is, there is always a pair of somites in each segment (Fig. 8-14, *B*). *Segmentation* or *metamerism* is a basic characteristic of the invertebrate phyla, especially of the Annelida and Arthropoda, in which there is obvious serial repetition of body parts. Vertebrates also show segmentation, but in a much more limited fashion. Neither the skin nor gut are segmented, but the mesoderm is. This characteristic is best evident in the embryonic stage. The blocks of mesodermal material give rise to the early segmentation of muscles and vertebrae.

Although the dorsal mass of mesoderm divides

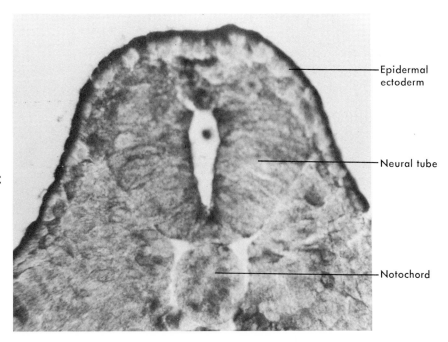

C

Epidermal ectoderm

Neural tube

Notochord

into blocks of cells, the more lateral extension of the mesoderm remains unsegmented, as indicated in Fig. 8-14, *B*. It spreads laterally and ventrally as *lateral plate mesoderm*, the *hypomere*. Each somite remains attached to the lateral plate by way of a stalk, the *intermediate mesoderm* or *mesomere*, which will form the urogenital system of the embryo. The lateral plate, or hypomere, separates into two layers, best seen in a cross section of the embryo (Fig. 8-14, *C*).

The layer closest to the endoderm becomes the *visceral layer*, or *splanchnic mesoderm*. Both the cardiac muscles and the smooth muscles of the gut develop from the splanchnic mesoderm. It is usually closely applied to the endoderm and together with this layer makes up the *splanchnopleure*. The layer nearest the epidermis gives rise to *parietal* or *somatic mesoderm*. Along with the ectoderm layer it is known as the *somatopleure*. The cavity formed by this mesodermal

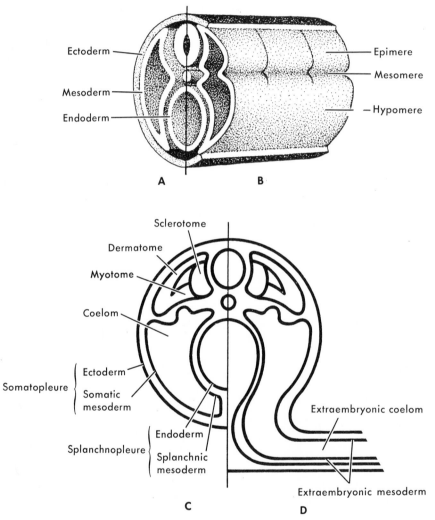

Fig. 8-14
The mesoderm inserts itself between the ectoderm and endoderm in the early gastrula, **A.** As development continues, the mesoderm divides into three areas: epimere, mesomere, and hypomere, **B.** These, in turn, undergo further differentiation as shown in **C** and **D.** Rounded gastrula, **C,** and flat gastrula, **D,** differ since extraembryonic mesoderm is present in the flat gastrula and will split to form the extraembryonic coelom and give rise to the extraembryonic membranes.

splitting is the *coelom,* which will become the peritoneal cavity, the body cavity of the adult. In those forms that have the flattened gastrula, the lateral mesoderm continues to extend outside the embryo proper where it is known as the *extraembryonic mesoderm* (Fig. 8-4, *D*). It will contribute to those structures that are not a part of the embryo proper, the extraembryonic membranes. When this extraembryonic mesoderm splits into two layers, the cavity (the extraembryonic coelom) remains continuous with the coelom inside the embryo for many hours.

During later development each somite or epimere separates from the intermediate mesoderm and differentiates into three areas destined to form specific areas in the adult. The inner portion of mesodermal block gives rise to loose aggregates of migrating cells known as *mesenchyme cells,* which take up positions around the notochord and neural tube. These cells become known as the *sclerotome* and give rise to the vertebral column. The remaining block of cells further differentiates into *dermatome* and *myotome.* The more lateral dermatome cells migrate outward and cover the inner surface of the ectoderm, where they become the dermis of the skin in the dorsal and dorsolateral areas of the body. The myotomes give rise to the voluntary skeletal muscles of the body. In the adult amphioxus (Fig. 16-8) the myotomes remain as segmented, V-shaped muscle blocks arranged from the anterior end to the posterior end of the body on each side of the animal. In higher animals a lateral longitudinal septum divides the myotomes into the dorsal *epaxial muscles* and the *ventral hypaxial* group. The longitudinal septum and the two muscle groups are easily seen in the adult shark.

Differentiation of endoderm

The method by which the endodermal material is converted into a primitive gut tube varies among the different animals and depends on the type of cleavage involved. However, regardless of the mechanism involved, the resulting tube-like structure soon divides into three unequal portions: the foregut, midgut, and hindgut regions. Various evaginations or diverticula form from this endodermal tube and give rise to organ

primordia. The thyroid, trachea, liver, pancreas, and urinary bladder are examples of structures originating from the primary endoderm. As development continues, mesoderm usually combines with the endoderm and the splanchnopleure contributes to the histological pattern of the adult structure. Endoderm lines the gut, and the splanchnic mesoderm contributes the connective tissue, smooth muscles, and serosa (peritoneal lining) of the gut.

By the neurula stage, the chordamesodermal mantle of amphibians separates into its respective units and the mesoderm extends ventrally between the ectodermal and endodermal layers to the midventral line. The segregation of the mesoderm leaves the edges of the endoderm free to migrate dorsally, completing the roof to the archenteron (Fig. 8-8). As a result, yolk-filled endoderm cells compose the walls, floor, and roof of the archenteron. By the neurula stage these yolky cells move inside the embryo and the yolk plug diminishes in size. Finally, the lateral lips of the blastopore fuse, obliterating the blastopore, and the endodermal cells are no longer visible from the outside.

In birds and mammals the gut tube arises in a different manner. The formation of the head process in the anterior end of the embryo elevates the flat sheet of endoderm, resting on the yolk, along with the ectoderm. The formation of the head process is the beginning of the separation of the embryo from the yolk. The development of the head process involves both an upward and anterior projection of the two layers off the blastoderm as well as a caudal movement. The inner surface of the fold that undercuts the head process forms the lining of the gut, and the outer surface contributes to the yolk sac as illustrated in sagittal view, Fig. 8-9. As a consequence of the undercutting, a space forms between the head fold and the blastoderm, the subcephalic pocket, which results in the cephalic region of the embryo projecting free from the blastoderm. Since the head fold is lined with endoderm, an anterior chamber forms the *foregut,* consisting of a roof, sides and a floor. The rest of the endoderm rests on the yolk. Eventually a similar elevation and undercutting in the caudal end of the embryo produce a hindgut and leave only the midgut open to the cavity of the yolk sac. The folds undercutting the embryo in the anterior and posterior ends move closer together during development, diminishing the space between the foregut and hindgut regions. Finally, only a yolk stalk connects the embryo to the yolk sac.

In the posterior area the walls of the hindgut project to various degrees into the extending tail region as the *tailgut*. Ventral to the tailgut the endoderm approaches the epidermal ectoderm. An invagination of the ectoderm, the *proctodeum*, becomes associated with the endoderm to form the *proctodeal* or *anal plate*. Eventually this plate ruptures and the *anus*, the posterior passageway of the gut to the outside, forms.

A similar plate forms somewhat earlier in the anterior end of the animal. The cephalic regions of the foregut extend anteriorly as the embryo elongates. It extends into the head as the *head gut* and expands toward the ectoderm beneath the brain as a large chamber, the *pharynx*. In the anterior end of the embryo, an epidermal invagination, the *stomodeum*, approaches the endodermal cells. As in the posterior region of the embryo, a plate forms, the *stomodeal* or *oral plate*.

Histogenesis

After gastrulation and neurulation the embryo enters the next phase of its development, *organogenesis*. The cells of the embryo's three undifferentiated germ layers undergo mitotic divisions and differentiate into four fundamental tissues of the adult organism. These are usually classified as (1) epithelial, (2) nervous, (3) connective, and (4) muscle tissue. *Histogenesis* is the name given to the process by which the undifferentiated or prefunctional cells of the germ layers differentiate into specialized or functional cells of the body. Histogenesis can be considered as the first step in organogenesis.

Each *tissue* consists of a group of similar cells that carry out comparable functions united by intercellular substances. The cells of the tissues are specialized cells, but epithelial and connective tissues are considered less specialized than ner-

vous and muscle tissues. Their general form and internal structure are modified during development in such a way that each tissue can carry out a particular function. The appearance of myosin, for example, responsible for a cell's ability to contract, is the first discernable difference in the cells of future muscle tissue. Pepsin starts to accumulate in the gastric cells of the digestive tract.

The formation of an intercellular substance, usually secreted by the cell and often referred to as the *matrix* of the tissue separates each cell from a neighboring cell. Epithelial cells, which are closely associated with one another in lining external and internal surfaces, have little intercellular substances. In some cases, however, it is the matrix that is important in giving form and function to the body. The intercellular substances of bone and cartilage are examples of this type of tissue. Blood is a unique tissue in which the cells, the formed elements of the blood, are suspended in a fluid matrix (the plasma).

As we begin our study of organogenesis, a brief summary of the contributions made by each germ layer to specific tissues may be of value. The ectoderm gives rise to the nervous tissue and the outer epithelial covering of the body. The endoderm forms the gut epithelium and all its derivatives. The mesoderm contributes to the organs located between the other two layers, that is, muscles, blood, skeleton, and organs of excretion and reproduction.

Following is a more detailed list of the specialized cells derived from the germ layers:

Ectodermal layer

Epithelium of the skin and its derivatives hair, feathers, nails, scales, sweat glands, sebaceous glands, and mammary glands; primary dental laminae, which give rise to enamel organs of teeth; lens of the eye, part of cornea, tympanic membrane, and pituitary gland

Nervous system, consisting of brain, spinal cord, peripheral nerves, ganglia, rods and cones of eye, various receptors of skin, auditory and taste receptors

Neural crest cells, which give rise to pigment

cells of the hair, feathers, and skin; cartilages in some animals, adrenal gland medulla

Mesodermal layer

Skeletal, cardiac, and smooth muscle, components of the circulatory system, connective tissue, lymphatic organs, lining of pleura, pericardium and peritoneum, adrenal cortex, and epithelium of urogenital system

Endodermal layer

Epithelium of digestive tract and its derivatives, the liver, pancreas, and gallbladder; epithelial lining of respiratory tract (larynx, trachea, bronchi, and probably alveoli of lungs); primordial germ cells of some animals; epithelium of tympanum and eustachian tube; thyroid, parathyroid, and thymus glands

Organ systems

Groups of specialized cells (tissues) can function independently, but usually the four fundamental tissues combine to form the *organs* of the animal. An organ (kidney, heart, or stomach) is a large functional unit whose combination of tissues enable it to carry out some general function. Certain organs, in turn, cooperate with other related organs to constitute *organ systems.* This level or organization is of interest to the comparative anatomists and comparative physiologists. The organ systems carry out the main functions of the body, such as respiration, excretion, and reproduction. The gonads and the combination of ducts discussed in Chapter 3 constitute an example of an organ system, the reproductive system.

The organ systems of the adult vertebrate body (which is emphasized in the remaining chapters) may be categorized by the following scheme, reflecting their general germ layer derivation:

1. Ectodermal layer
    a. Integumentary system
    b. Nervous system
2. Endodermal layer
    c. Digestive system
    d. Respiratory system
3. Mesodermal layer
    e. Muscular system
    f. Skeletal system
    g. Circulatory system
    h. Reproductive system
    i. Excretory system

SUGGESTED READINGS

1. Beadle, G. W., and Tatum, E. L.: Genetic control of biochemical reactions in *Neurospora,* 1941. Reprinted in Peters, J. A., editor: Classic papers in genetics, Englewood Cliffs, N. J., 1959, Prentice-Hall, Inc.
2. Bell, E.: Information transfer between nucleus and cytoplasm during differentiation. In Control mechanisms of growth and differentiation. Symposia of the Society for Experimental Biology, No. 25. New York, 1971, Academic Press Inc.
3. Britten, R. J., and Davidson, E. H.: Gene regulation for higher cells: A theory, Science **165**:349-357, 1969.
4. Brown, D. D., and Dawid, I.: Specific gene amplication in oocytes, Science **160**:272-280, 1968.
5. Burnside, B.: Microtubules and microfilaments in amphibian neurulation, Am. Zool. **13**(4):989-1006, 1973.
6. Darnell, J. E., Jelinek, W. R., and Molloy, G. R.: Biogenesis of mRNA: Genetic regulation in mammalian cells. Science **181**:1215-1221, 1973.
7. Ebert, J., and Sussex, I. M.: Interacting systems in development, New York, 1970, Holt, Rinehart and Winston, Inc.
8. Jacob, F., and Monad, J.: On the regulation of gene activity, Cold Spring Harbor Symposium, Quant. Biol. **26**:193-211, 1961.
9. Lerner, I. M.: A concept of natural selection: A centennial view, Proc. Am. Phil. Soc. **103**:173-182, 1959. Reprinted in Laetsch, W. M.: The biological perspective, introductory readings, Boston, 1969, Little, Brown & Co.
10. Needham, J.: Biochemistry and morphogenesis, New York, 1942, Cambridge University Press.
11. Spemann, H.: Embryonic development and induction, New York, 1938, Hafner Publishing Co., Inc.
12. Ursprung, H.: Genes and development in organogenesis, DeHaan, R. L., and Ursprung, H., editors, New York, 1965, Holt, Rinehart and Winston.
13. Weismann, A.: The continuity of the germ-plasm as the foundation of theory of heredity, 1889. Reprinted in Gabriel, M. L., and Fogel, S., editors: Great experiments in biology, Englewood Cliffs, N. J., 1955, Prentice-Hall, Inc.

CHAPTER 9

EMBRYONIC ADAPTATIONS

Before we pursue the study of adult structures further, we should pause and consider those transitory organs that allow embryos to adapt successfully to various environments. They do not contribute to the morphogenesis of adult organs, but protect the embryo or satisfy its needs for food, oxygen, and the elimination of wastes. They form outside the body of the embryo and therefore are considered *extraembryonic*.

In general, extraembryonic membranes do not develop if there is only a small amount of food (yolk) present (such as in the fish and amphibian egg). Instead, the young of these forms hatch at an early age and forage for themselves as free-swimming larvae. The young of higher mammals develop from yolkless eggs and, of course, are an exception since the mother retains them in her body for varying periods of time. The deposition of a large amount of food in a yolk sac allows a longer developmental period within a protected environment (that is, within the confines of a shell). Consequently the young hatch at a more advanced stage. Terrestrial animals, therefore, usually have longer developmental periods than do aquatic ones.

The closed environment presents certain problems. In order to move successfully onto land, higher animals must have eggs that not only contain food for the developing embryo but also provide for the elimination of metabolic wastes, for protection against desiccation, and for an exchange of respiratory gases. These functions all occur with ease in a watery environment and aquatic animals have no need for auxiliary structures. The metabolic wastes diffuse or are released into the surrounding water.

Certain membranes develop inside the shelled egg. They are the *amnion, yolk sac, allantois,* and *chorion*. The development of these fetal membranes follows similar patterns in reptiles, birds, and monotreme mammals. They enable the embryo to maintain its vital functions despite its confinement within a shell, thereby freeing the vertebrate animal from an aquatic environment and making terrestrial life possible. The amnion first appears in the class Reptilia and is retained by its two derivative classes, Aves and Mammalia. Consequently, the term *amniotes* refers to these three groups of animals. The fishes and amphibians lack this membrane and are known as the *anamniotes*.

The eggs of higher mammals lack yolk. Correlated with this loss is a physiological dependence on the mother. She retains the young within her body where an elaboration and modification of the reptilian membranes give rise to certain adaptations in the pouched animals (marsupials, or Metatheria) and a definitive placenta in the higher mammals (placentals, or Eutheria).

Conservative developmental mechanics have survival value for the very early embryo, as emphasized in Chapter 8. However, the appearance of these new structures, extraembryonic membranes, during evolutionary development allowed higher vertebrates to eliminate the vulnerable larval stages from their life cycle thereby ensuring the survival of the adult. The adaptive embryonic structures perfected in the reptiles, birds, and mammals are relatively recent additions (evolutionarily speaking). They evolved in association with already established structures: the yolk sac and allantois with the embryo's gut, and the amnion and chorion with its external surface.

EXTRAEMBRYONIC MEMBRANES OF ANAMNIOTES

In general, the anamniotes (fish and amphibia) do not have extraembryonic membranes. They hatch in prodigious numbers into the water where their problems of respiration, excretion, and protection against dessication are minimal. Yolk, in the form of yolk platelets stored in the cells of the gut, is available during early development in such forms as the amphibian tadpole. These animals, therefore, store their food intracellularly and the embryos do not have true yolk sacs. The young vertebrates soon hatch and forage for themselves as their yolk supply dwindles.

Some anamniotes, however, retain their young in the uterus until time of hatching. There are a few examples of placental relationships, but as a general rule, during cytoplasmic maturation the egg manufactures and stores food for the developing embryo. In the meroblastic fishes a syncytium forms from the ectodermal and meso-

dermal layers of the blastodisk and spreads over the segregated yolk. In the teleosts there is no constriction separating the yolk from the rest of the body and it remains as a bulge on the ventral surface of the embryo. It gradually diminishes as the vitelline circulation absorbs the yolk and carries it to the body of the embryo. By the time the young fish is ready to feed on its own, the formerly extended ventral wall is flat and continuous with the body wall. Strictly speaking, therefore, the teleost does not have an extraembryonic yolk sac.

Three layers form the yolk sac of the elasmobranchs. The blastodisk extends peripherally over the yolk and gives rise to the walls of the sac. The surface next to the yolk differentiates into endoderm, the outer surface the ectoderm, and in between the mesoderm. A true umbilicus divides the sac from the body proper and the yolk sac dangles by a narrow stalk from the ventral surface of the body. This type of yolk sac is obviously extraembryonic. Enzymes secreted by the yolk sac digest the yolk and the vitelline circulation, located in the walls of the sac, absorb the product. Or the yolk may pass up through the opening of the stalk into the intestine where digestion and absorption proceed in the usual manner.

EXTRAEMBRYONIC MEMBRANES OF AMNIOTES
Evolution of shelled or cleidoic egg

The reptile, the first truly terrestrial animal, evolved from the amphibian. This latter group, represented today by frogs, toads, and salamanders, arose from fish ancestors and took the first steps toward dry land. These early amphibians, however, were not completely free to explore the terrestrial environment. The adults might roam, but they needed to return to the water during their breeding periods to deposit their eggs.

During their evolution the body of the amphibians underwent several changes from that of their fish ancestors. The reptiles retained these structures and elaborated upon them. Many of them (limbs, muscles, lungs, heart, and kidney) allowed the animal to leave the aquatic environment and move to a terrestrial one. These struc-

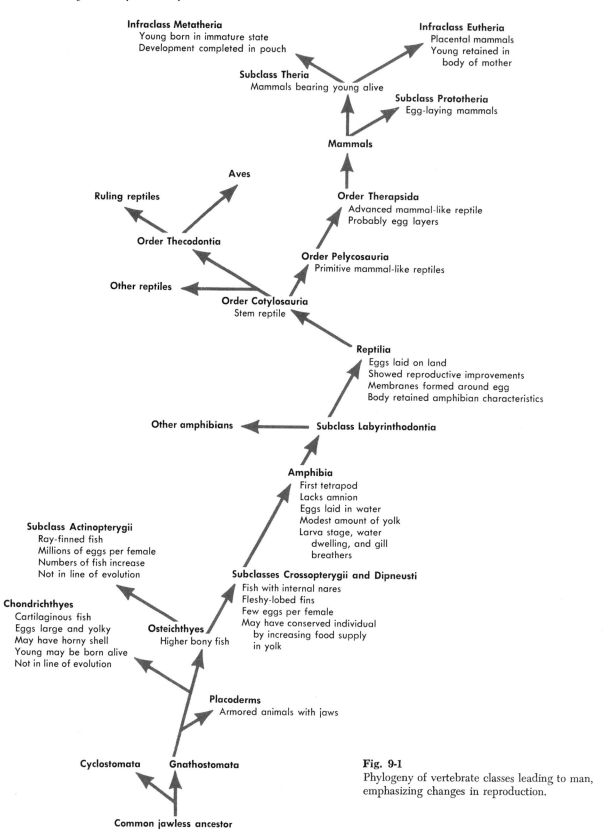

Infraclass Metatheria
Young born in immature state
Development completed in pouch

Infraclass Eutheria
Placental mammals
Young retained in
body of mother

Subclass Theria
Mammals bearing young alive

Subclass Prototheria
Egg-laying mammals

Mammals

Aves

Ruling reptiles

Order Therapsida
Advanced mammal-like reptile
Probably egg layers

Order Thecodontia

Order Pelycosauria
Primitive mammal-like reptiles

Other reptiles

Order Cotylosauria
Stem reptile

Reptilia
Eggs laid on land
Showed reproductive improvements
Membranes formed around egg
Body retained amphibian characteristics

Other amphibians

Subclass Labyrinthodontia

Amphibia
First tetrapod
Lacks amnion
Eggs laid in water
Modest amount of yolk
Larva stage, water
dwelling, and gill
breathers

Subclass Actinopterygii
Ray-finned fish
Millions of eggs per female
Numbers of fish increase
Not in line of evolution

Subclasses Crossopterygii and Dipneusti
Fish with internal nares
Fleshy-lobed fins
Few eggs per female
May have conserved individual
by increasing food supply
in yolk

Chondrichthyes
Cartilaginous fish
Eggs large and yolky
May have horny shell
Young may be born alive
Not in line of evolution

Osteichthyes
Higher bony fish

Placoderms
Armored animals with jaws

Cyclostomata

Gnathostomata

Common jawless ancestor

Fig. 9-1
Phylogeny of vertebrate classes leading to man,
emphasizing changes in reproduction.

tures are discussed later when we consider the adult organism. From the standpoint of development, under consideration in these early chapters, possibly the most important evolutionary step was the evolution of the "closed" or "locked-up" (cleidoic) egg. It was laid on land and may have been the first terrestrial adaptation to appear.

According to Romer (1957), the egg first came ashore, followed later by the adult reptile. The new egg probably developed long before the animal who laid it was equipped for terrestrial living. There was a survival value in depositing the egg on land since it offered protection not only from predators but, most of all, from droughts. Some believe that heavy rains during the late Paleozoic days alternated with seasonal droughts. The long larval stage of the amphibian takes place in the water since the young are gill breathers. Periods of dryness threatened the completion of these embryonic stages. An egg equipped to survive periods of droughts had definite survival value.

Fossils of shelled reptilian eggs exist from the lower Permian period (Table 9-1, Fig. 9-1). The eggs, preserved because of their shells, appear early in the history of the reptiles. They belonged to those recently evolved reptiles that

TABLE 9-1. Phylogeny of vertebrate classes correlated with geological periods

Era	Duration	Period	Predominant vertebrates	Evolution of vertebrates
Cenozoic	65 million years	Quaternary Tertiary	Age of mammals	Dominance of man
Mesozoic	150 million years	Cretaceous		Oldest remains of true mammals
				Oldest known true birds
		Jurassic	Age of reptiles	Mammals probably gave up egg laying and bore young alive
				Animals closest to reptiles and mammals found in late Triassic rocks
		Triassic		Birds probably originated from thecodont stock, continued to lay eggs
Paleozoic	350 million years	Permian		Therapsida developed Shelled reptilian eggs present (fossilized) Cotylosauria (stem reptiles) well established; Amphibians in decline
		Carboniferous	Age of amphibians	Traces of Cotylosauria first noted
		Devonian	Age of fishes	Evolution of amniote egg; many labyrinthodont fossils and amphibians at their peak Labyrinthodont fossils first noted
				First tetrapod; beginning of change from water to land Invasion of freshwater by fish
		Silurian		Oldest jawed vertebrates, the placoderms
				Oldest known vertebrate; traces of ostracoderms first noted
		Ordovician		No known vertebrates; all invertebrate groups present
		Cambrian		

left their watery homes probably in pursuit of primitive insects that arose during the time of the coal swamps.

According to Romer the reptile was little more than an amphibian living in the ancient streams. Its short, stubby legs were still sprawled out sideways in an amphibian manner. In fact, the whole reptilian skeleton resembled that of the oldest amphibian. By the end of the Paleozoic era, however, many of the reptiles took advantage of the cleidoic egg and left the water for the land. During the Mesozoic era the great radiation of the reptiles began that lasted for 100 million years. So great was their domination that this era became known as the "Age of the reptiles" (Table 9-1). Since fossil remains offer no evidence that the anatomy of the early reptile differed greatly from that of the amphibian, apparently the development of the "closed" egg was the important factor that enabled the evolution of higher animals to occur.

Soon after the reptile evolved, two distinct lines of descent gave rise to birds and mammals. These two groups continued to evolve through parallel evolution and have many traits in common. The term "glorified reptiles" often applied to birds, describes them best when their feathers are removed. The adult structure of the bird, as well as its embryonic development, reflects its relationship to the reptile.

Birds and mammals are active land animals, as compared with the reptiles, and have a higher metabolic rate. They are *homoiothermic,* that is, they have an internally controlled body temperature. Unlike the reptiles they can inhabit cold, temperate, and polar zones. Although the egg and its mode of development are similar in both bird and reptile, the egg of the bird demands a higher temperature for its development. The egg, laid at the gastrula stage, can remain in this state for as long as 2 or 3 weeks at air temperature. During the developmental period the bird sits on the eggs incubating them with body heat. Apparently the nest not only protects the young but also is an adaptation that aids in the maintenance of temperature as well. Obviously, the female mammal provides this controlled environment necessary for development by retaining the young within her body.

Developmental changes associated with amniote egg

There is no direct evidence of developmental changes during the evolution of land animals. However, a comparison of modern reptiles with modern amphibians points out developmental differences between the two groups as well as some of their similarities.

1. The amount of yolk in the reptilian egg increases significantly, affecting a change in the pattern of cleavage. Meroblastic cleavage replaces the holoblastic division found in the amphibian egg.

2. A longer period of reptilian development follows the incorporation of large amounts of food material into the embryo's developing environment (the environment within the shell). Conversely, amphibian larvae hatch and seek their own food at a much earlier developmental stage.

3. Although the amount of yolk present in the egg differs, the process of ovulation remains the same in amphibians, reptiles, and birds.

4. As the egg passes down the upper portion of the oviduct, the duct secretes albumen around the yolk. In the fish and amphibian the jelly layers of albumen act as cushions or as adhesive, anchoring the eggs to vegetation, preventing them from washing away in the river currents. In the closed egg, the albumen wraps around the yolk, suspending it from the egg membranes and protecting it from shocks. It becomes a reservoir of water (perhaps its greatest contribution) and possibly additional food for the developing embryo.

5. The oviduct of higher vertebrates secretes two thin shell membranes around the egg. In some species they separate at one end and become filled with air as shown in Fig. 4-13. In more posterior portions, the oviduct deposits a porous shell, which allows the exchange of gases to take place.

6. Fertilization occurs in the upper regions of the oviduct before deposition of the shell. Copulatory organs develop in the higher vertebrates.

A closer scrutiny of the amphibian indicates that, although these points of difference separate modern amphibia from the reptiles, many of the characteristics attributed to reptiles are already present in some of the amphibians. As an illustration, the amphibian oviduct also secretes albumen around the egg as in the higher vertebrates. In some species of frogs, the albumen hardens and functions as a shell. In the shell-less eggs of *Gymnophiona* a chalaza holds the eggs together in a mass.

Land animals evolved by way of a series of steps that aided them in adapting to terrestrial conditions. Each change (storage of additional food material, storage of water supply, reservoir for collecting waste materials within a closed environment, etc.) led to a longer protected developmental period. Consequently the young amniote hatches as a replica of the adult, eliminating the more vulnerable larval form.

Characteristics of cleidoic egg

The majority of modern amphibia still rely upon water for their developmental medium; the modern reptile often lays its eggs in moist places. Only the birds perfected cleidoic development.

The characteristics of the cleidoic egg may be summarized as follows:

1. A shell forms about the egg. In reptiles the shell is soft and allows the passage of water. However in the bird, the deposition of calcium in the shell makes it impervious to water. The duckbill platypus, one of the primitive mammals, surrounds its egg with a leathery shell similar to that of the reptile.
2. The egg stores water in the form of a thin, gelatinous material known as egg white. In those eggs with impervious shells, the egg white, or albumen, is the main source of water supply. It is completely absorbed by the end of growth.
3. Four extraembryonic membranes develop in the cleidoic egg and allow it to be deposited on land. The *yolk sac* contains the yolk, the food for the developing embryo. The *chorion* acts as a protective membrane and, in combination with the *allantois*, functions in gas exchange. The amniotic cavity fills with a watery fluid that bathes the developing embryo. Thus, literally, the embryo did not leave the aquatic

environment at all, but carries its "pond" with it in the form of amniotic fluid. The fourth membrane, the vascular *allantois*, functions in gas exchange, and absorption of water and albumen. Within the confined space of the egg, the allantois also stores metabolic wastes. The kidneys of these embryos transform the wastes into nontoxic, insoluble uric acid, which the bird deposits in the allantoic sac and leaves behind in the shell at the time of hatching.

Formation of extraembryonic membranes in reptiles and birds

The embryo, perched on the top of a large mass of yolk, develops from the pellucida region of the blastoderm. The area opaca of the blastoderm continues to spread peripherally over the yolk mass. The three germ layers delineated in the region of the embryo continue to differentiate laterally in the area opaca. Here they form the extraembryonic somatopleure and splanchnopleure. These layers give rise to the embryonic membranes of the amniotes. The amnion and chorion form from the extraembryonic somatopleure; the yolk sac and allantoic sac develop from the extraembryonic splanchnopleure. The membranes of all amniotes form in essentially the same way and carry out the same functions.

Yolk sac

The yolk sac is the first membrane to form. The gut region of the early embryo (Figs. 8-9 and 9-2, *A* and *B*) has a dorsal roof and sides, but no floor. The ventrally open gut rests on the yolk mass. The extraembryonic mesoderm accompanied by extraembryonic endoderm closely applied to the yolk, extend peripherally, eventually surrounding the yolk.

As the body of the embryo grows, in the anterior region folds that roll under the head area appear, separating it from the underlying yolk and forming a subcephalic pocket (Fig. 8-9, *B*). Eventually, similar folds develop on either side of the body, undercutting it laterally as shown in cross section in Fig. 9-2, *B*. Posterior limiting folds form about the third day of incubation and lift the tail region from the surrounding yolk

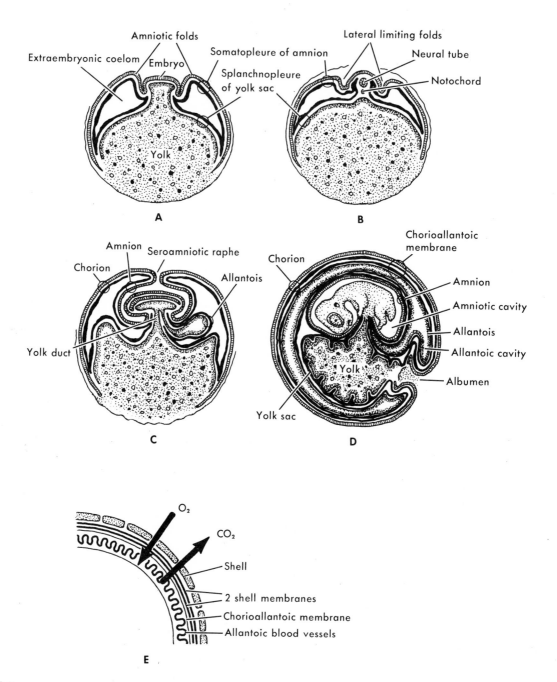

Fig. 9-2

Drawings illustrating the formation of extraembryonic membranes in the chick. **A,** Sagittal view showing developing yolk sac and amnion. **B,** Transverse section through **A. C,** Sagittal section showing beginning of allantois. **D,** Sagittal view showing chorion, allantois, amnion, and yolk sac. **E,** Diagrammatic section through chick membranes showing layers through which the exchange of gases occur.

area. As a result, the subcephalic, lateral, and subcaudal folds define the body of the embryo and separate the embryonic from the extraembryonic regions. As these undercutting folds move toward one another, they establish a floor to the gut except for a small region of the midgut. These folds do not completely merge, but a small aperture (the yolk duct) remains, opening into the yolk sac. This relationship is shown in Figs. 8-9, *C*, and 9-2, *C*. The yolk stalk connects the body of the embryo with the yolk sac and consists of an inner layer of endoderm and an outer layer of splanchnic mesoderm, the same combination of layers comprising the yolk sac.

The constriction of the yolk stalk region brings together the omphalomesenteric blood vessels (arteries and veins) located in the splanchnic mesoderm of the embryo. They continue in the walls of the yolk sac as vitelline vessels, with their arteries and veins composing the *vitelline arch*. The yolk sac with its richly enmeshed circulatory system suspends the yolk from the body. As the embryo ages, the lining of the yolk sac develops folds, considerably increasing its surface area (Fig. 9-2, *D*). The endodermal cells lining the yolk sac secrete digestive enzymes that break the yolk down into soluble form. It is then absorbed into the vitelline veins and carried by their embryonic continuations, the omphalomesenteric veins, into the body proper. From here, the general circulatory system carries the soluble food material to all parts of the embryo for its metabolic use. As absorption of the yolk continues, the yolk sac shrivels and withdraws into the body and disappears completely by the time of hatching.

Amnion and chorion

The origins of these two membranes are considered together since they form simultaneously from the extraembryonic somatopleure. The *amnion* encloses the embryo in a sac, which fills with fluid, the "ancestral pond" referred to earlier. The amniotic fluid not only protects the embryo from desiccation but also acts as a watery cushion, shielding it from mechanical injury. The contraction of smooth muscle fibers in the wall of the amnion circulates the fluid that moves the parts of the embryo about and

prevents them from growing together. The chorion, closely applied to the inner surface of the shell, and the allantois function in the respiratory exchange of the embryo.

Anterior to the chick's head region, the extraembryonic somatopleure forms a fold after about 30 hours of incubation. As viewed from the dorsal surface, this crescent-shaped thickening grows progressively backward over the head of the embryo. It is essentially a sheet of somatopleure folded back upon itself, seen best in a diagrammatic sagittal view (Fig. 9-2, *A* and *C*). The wall of ectoderm and mesoderm next to the embryo becomes the amnion; the outer layer gives rise to the chorion. As the embryo develops, it pushes forward into the fold at the same time the fold itself grows posteriorly. The anterior amniotic fold fuses with the lateral ones, covering much of the anterior and middle regions of the body. On about the third day of incubation, a posterior tail fold forms, similar to the one in the anterior region. It grows anteriorly, where it fuses with the anterior and lateral folds, completely encasing the embryo in a double-walled pocket. The point of fusion leaves a scar, the *seroamniotic raphe* (Fig. 9-2, *C*).

The fusion of the fold produces two sac-like membranes and two cavities. The cavity formed between the embryo and the first fold, the amnion, becomes the *amniotic cavity*. Ectoderm lines its inner surface, the embryo side, and somatic mesoderm, its outer surface. The outer layer of the original fold gives rise to the chorion, with an inner surface of mesoderm and an outer surface of ectoderm. The cavity between the chorion and the amnion is the *seroamniotic cavity*, or extraembryonic coelom. Somatic mesoderm, derived from the inner wall of the chorion and the outer wall of the amnion, lines the coelom. As the chorion and amnion form, the somatopleure continues to grow peripherally and laterally, as shown in Fig. 9-2, *C*, until it completely covers the embryo and all the other membranes that are forming at this time (Fig. 9-2, *D*).

Allantois

By about the sixtieth hour of incubation, an outpocketing of endoderm appears in the floor of the hindgut. The pocket, which is the beginning of the allantois, continues to grow into the extraembryonic coelom, eventually filling it (Fig. 9-2, *C* and *D*). This endodermal evagination of the gut carries with it the closely associated splanchnic mesoderm. The combination of these two layers, splanchnopleure, as in the example of the yolk sac, forms the wall of the allantois. As the pocket enlarges and spreads outward, the splanchnic mesoderm comes in contact with the somatic mesodermal lining of the chorion. These two mesodermal layers fuse and form a single membrane, the *chorioallantoic membrane*, which becomes highly vascularized.

The growing membranes rupture the vitelline membrane (which still surrounds the egg) and continue to expand outward toward the shell membranes. They push the albumen to one side, where a pocket of the allantois envelops it. The blood vessels that cover the allantoic walls absorb the water and albumen. These vessels form in the splanchnic layer of the allantois and consist of two allantoic arteries and two allantoic veins. The highly vascular chorioallantoic membrane expands, eventually assuming a position adjacent to the shell membrane. It functions as the primary respiratory organ until hatching. Oxygen passes through the porous shell and diffuses through the shell membranes, the chorioallantoic membrane, and the walls of the allantoic blood vessels, as in Fig. 9-2, *E*. Carbon dioxide moves in the opposite direction. The allantoic sac is also an excretory organ. The relatively insoluble uric acid, deposited in the sac, remains with the shell at the time of hatching. This process represents another evolutionary modification that made it possible for animals to move permanently from an aquatic to a terrestrial environment.

Formation of extraembryonic membranes in mammals
Amnion

Because of their intimate relationship with germ-layer formation, the development of the amnion, allantois, and yolk sac in the human embryo was discussed in Chapter 7. The amnion is essentially the same in all mammals, although it arises by several different mechanisms. In some animals, such as the marsupial, the pig, and most insectivores, the amnion forms after gastrulation by folding in much the same way as in the chick and reptile. Many gradations exist between the fold method and that employed by the human embryo. In the monkey or man, the amniotic cavity develops precociously and a space appears by *cavitation* in the inner cell mass between the future embryonic disk and trophoblast cells, as shown in Fig. 7-14. Except in the area of the future body stalk, amniogenic cells of the human embryo eventually separate from the inner layer of the chorion and form a distinct amniotic membrane. Apparently there is a correlation between the method of amnion formation and the time of implantation; embryos of those animals utilizing the somatopleure-fold method tend to implant later than those in which cavitation occurs.

Regardless of how the amnion forms, the mammalian embryo lies bathed in the fluid of the amniotic cavity like the embryos of the reptiles and birds. At first the amniotic cells secrete the fluid of the cavity, but later the fetal urine also collects in it. Human fetuses swallow their amniotic fluid, which the cells of the gut then absorb. The fluid with its dissolved materials eventually enters the fetal circulation and passes into the mother's bloodstream via the placenta. Her kidneys eliminate both her metabolic wastes and those of the fetus.

Yolk sac

Evidently the mammals evolved early from the stem reptile since their first traces appear in the late Triassic rocks (Table 9-1). At this time the mammalian egg, no doubt, resembled the reptilian egg and contained a large supply of yolk. However, sometime during the Triassic and Jurassic days some of the mammals became viviparous, and the mother supplied the necessary food to her young while she carried them in her uterus. Apparently, during the early part of the Mesozoic era, a reduction of the yolk occurred and the yolk finally disappeared in the advanced subclass of the mammals, the Eutheria, or placental mammals. Although no yolk remained in the egg, the yolk sac continued to form when the ectoderm and endoderm differentiated. Since it is an organ that was more fully developed and functional at an early stage of evolutionary development, the yolk sac is considered a *vestigial* structure.

The vitelline blood vessels develop in the walls of this vestigial secondary yolk sac in much the same way that they did in the functional sacs of the reptiles and birds. The blood cells in the very young embryos arise in the walls of the yolk sac from mesenchyme cells probably derived from the splanchnic mesoderm. In man, during the second month of gestation intraembryonic organs, especially the liver and spleen, assume the function of blood cell formation.

Allantois

The allantois, which forms from the hindgut of all amniote embryos, probably evolved from the amphibian bladder. It is essentially an extraembryonic respiratory and excretory organ in the reptile and bird. In the mammal, it also functions in absorption.

As in the reptile and bird, splanchnopleure composes the mammalian allantois. The amount of endoderm present in the splanchnopleure varies among the mammals. It ranges from a large endodermal sac in the dog and pig to a much reduced structure in the monkey and man. In some rodents it is entirely absent. However, the mesoderm component remains very important in all forms. The mesodermal layer contributes to the formation of the umbilical blood vessels of the mammals. These vessels are homologous with the allantoic vessels of reptiles and the chick and are the only vessels found in the body stalk, or umbilicus, of the human embryo. The allantois is important since the allantoic mesoderm and its umbilical vessels fuse with the chorionic mesoderm and its trophoblast covering to produce the fetal portion of the mammalian placenta.

Trophoblast and chorion

The trophoblast is considered a primary fetal membrane of the mammal. Its origin traces back to the superficial layer of the morula. It functions in implantation. Later when mesoderm lines its cavity, it becomes the chorion and contributes to the formation of the placenta.

IMPLANTATION. Since the mammalian egg lacks yolk, the embryo has no immediate source of food. As the morula makes its way down the uterine tube and into the uterus, it obtains some nutritive materials from the fluids that fill the cavity of these organs. This material is usually called *embryotrophe,* or uterine milk. It is secreted by the uterine glands and is rich in mucopolysaccharides, glycogen, and lipids. Before substantial growth can occur, however, the blastocyst must attach to the uterus and establish the nutritional supply to the embryo. This process of attachment is known as *implantation.* The intimacy of this attachment differs among the various species of mammals. In most mammals the blastocyst remains in the cavity of the uterus in close contact with the endometrium. But in other mammals, such as man, chimpanzee, and certain bats, the blastocyst actually penetrates the endometrium, eroding its tissues as it becomes embedded in the endometrial wall. Two types of implantation are compared schematically in Fig. 9-3.

As a result of implantation the fetal membranes and the endometrial mucosa of the uterus come into sufficiently intimate contact that a physiological exchange can occur between them. Both the endometrium and the embryo contribute to the process of implantation. The zona pellucida, which surrounds the egg since its ovulation from the ovary, must be removed before the blastocyst can implant. This membrane holds the cells together during cleavage and prevents the morula from sticking to the endometrial wall on its journey down the tubes. Once it disappears, the freed trophoblast cells contact the uterine wall and attach to it. In those cases in which it actually penetrates the endometrium, the trophoblast destroys and ingests the endometrium, apparently by the secretion of cytolytic enzymes. However, these enzymes, although postulated, have yet to be identified.

The active secretion of progesterone by the corpus luteal cells of the mother makes the endometrium receptive for implantation and prepares it for maintenance of the blastocyst, as described in Chapter 3 (Blandau, 1961). The hormonally primed endometrium becomes highly sensitive to either foreign localized pressure or some

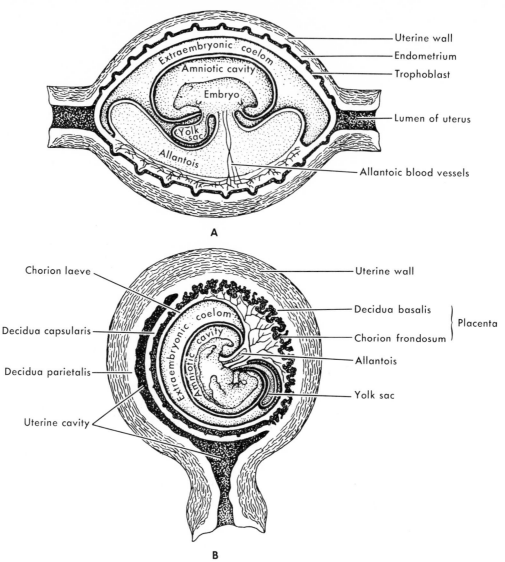

Fig. 9-3

Comparison of two types of mammalian implantation. **A,** Diagram showing implantation in the pig. Chorionic sac expands until it fills the uterine cavity but does not penetrate the uterine epithelium. **B,** Implantation of human embryo. The blastocyst penetrates the uterine endometrium where it becomes embedded. The decidua capsularis of uterus covers the developing embryo.

chemical secreted by the egg. This condition, known as the *decidual reaction,* actively contributes to implantation.

Implantation does not occur immediately after fertilization of the egg. Instead, the egg travels down the fallopian tube and floats free in the uterus for several days. This free uterine period ranges from 3 to 3½ days in the mouse, 9 to 10 days in the dog, and 4 to 6 days in man.

The orientation of the blastocyst with respect to the uterus and its supporting mesometrium is relatively constant within a species but varies considerably between different species (Mossman, 1937). The inner cell mass orients toward the mesometrium, on the opposite side from it, or lateral to it. The implantation site of multiple young as well as single embryos appears regulated. Implantation does not occur randomly. In those animals with multiple young, the first blastocyst implants in the uterus near the fallopian tube junction. Apparently some kind of refractory zone forms around the implanting blastocyst, possibly because of the cytolytic activity of the trophoblast cells. The second blastocyst implants farther away toward the cervix and is also surrounded by a refractory zone. Embryos closest to the uterotubal junction have been reported furthest along in development in comparison to those closest to the cervix. If reabsorption occurs, the embryos nearest the cervix are usually the ones affected.

PLACENTATION. The development of the placenta, a temporary organ that aids in the nourishment, respiration, and excretion of the mammalian embryo, is associated with viviparity. It makes possible the extension of the ancestral environment and, through its relationship with the mother, maintains the vital functions of the embryo until it assumes an independent existence. Strictly speaking, the placenta is not a "membrane" at all, but an organ, since at full term the human placenta, for example, has the shape of a flattened cake and weighs about 1 pound. It is between 6 and 8 inches in diameter and is about 1 inch thick. However, the placenta is an extraembryonic structure, and convention usually allows its consideration along with the fetal membranes.

During the course of their evolution viviparous fish and reptiles experimented with a placental type of relationship. In some of these animals the yolk sac comes in contact with the vascular uterine wall and some exchange of materials occurs between the two organs. A true placenta, however, does not exist. Mammals demonstrate a wide range in fetal-to-maternal relationships. They vary from the egg-laying monotremes (subclass Prototheria), whose embryo needs no close maternal relationship, through the marsupials (an intermediate condition), to the truly placental eutherian animals. Fossil evidence indicates that these last two divisions (infraclasses Metatheria and Eutheria) were separate groups as far back as the Cretaceous period, 135 million years ago.

The marsupial young, of which the opossums and kangaroos are representatives, are born in a partly developed state, after as little as 8 days of development. They crawl into the pouch, or marsupium, of the mother, become attached to a teat, and complete their development in the pouch. Before birth the allantois of the marsupial is undeveloped, and therefore there is no chorioallantoic membrane. That part of the smooth-walled chorion containing the yolk sac makes contact with the uterine wall instead. Probably some exchange of substances occurs between these membranes and the uterus of most pouched animals. Many biologists consider the marsupials, along with the monotremes, aplacental mammals; however, some acknowledge that the inefficient apposition of fetal yolk sac and chorion with maternal tissue functions as a kind of placenta. Since the vitelline blood vessels of the yolk sac carry materials to and from the fetus, the placenta is referred to as a *choriovitelline placenta* (Fig. 9-4, *A*). In the eutherian animals it is that part of the chorion lined with the allantois that becomes intimately associated with the uterine wall during the gestation period. In this type of definitive placenta the umbilical (allantoic) vessels transport the materials. For this reason the placenta of higher mammals is known as the *chorioallantoic placenta* (Fig. 9-4, *B*).

The placenta is a structure of dual origin since both the fetus and mother contribute tissues to its formation. In the human female the maternal component consists of that part of the uterine wall (endometrium referred to in Chapter 3) that sloughes off at the termination of pregnancy. The name "decidua" (meaning 'to shed') refers to the pregnant endometrium, with different regions of the decidua assigned different names depending on their relationship to the implantation site, as indicated in Fig. 9-3, *B*. *Decidua basalis* refers to that part of the endometrium beneath the blastocyst that contributes to the placenta. The thin portion of the endometrium on the lumen side of the uterus that covers the implantation site is the *decidua capsularis*, and the endometrium lining the uterus other than at the implantation site is the *decidua parietalis*.

The fetal component of the placenta consists essentially of highly branched, fingerlike pro-

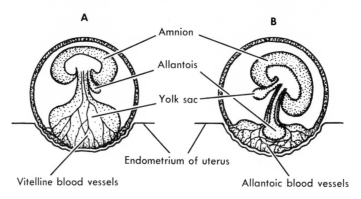

Fig. 9-4

Comparison of two types of mammalian placentas: **A,** choriovitelline placenta and, **B,** chorioallantoic placenta. See text for description.

cesses, the villi, covered by the trophoblast layer. The villi contact the decidua basalis. Embryonic blood vessels form in the core of each villus. The umbilical circulatory system, which carries blood from the fetus to the villi and back again to the body of the fetus, develops. At first the chorionic villi are established equally well around the surface of the chorion; later they form a pattern characteristic of the species involved. Fetal and maternal tissues demonstrate different relationships in different animals as pregnancy continues. In the human, after the third month those villi facing the decidua capsularis degenerate. As a result, this area of the chorion surface, the *chorion laeve,* becomes very smooth (Fig. 9-3, *B*). On the other hand, those villi adjacent to the decidua basalis continue to grow and branch. The chorionic membranes and villi in this area form the *chorion frondosum.* It is the chorion frondosum and the decidua basalis that give rise to the *definitive placenta* of the human being. As the embryonic body develops, it separates from the various membranes until only the *umbilical cord* connects the fetus with the placenta.

One classification of mammalian placentas depends on the arrangement of the villi on the chorion. It is possible to recognize four different types as shown in Fig. 9-5. Primates (including man) and rodents have a *discoidal placenta* since the location of the villi is in one disk-shaped area of the chorion. In some cases, however, the distribution of the villi occurs over the chorion in random tufts. These placentas are the *diffuse*

placentas found in pigs and horses. In the third type of placenta the villi gather in clusters known as cotyledons. Ruminants (cattle, sheep) usually have *cotyledonary placentas* (Fig. 9-7, *A*). The *zonary placenta* is the fourth type of placenta present in cats, dogs, and other carnivores. In these animals encircling bands of villi appear in different zones of the chorion.

The condition of the uterine endometrium at the time of birth constitutes another basis for classifying placentas. In some animals the relationship of fetal chorion to maternal endometrium is one of apposition of fetal-to-maternal tissue, a kind of finger-in-the-glove relationship. At birth (parturition) the chorionic villi pull away from the endometrium; there is no damage to the uterine wall and consequently no loss of blood. Since there is no "shedding" of the endometrial wall (the decidua), the placenta of animals such as pigs and cattle is referred to as *nondeciduate.* A more intimate relationship of chorion to maternal endometrium forms in some animals. In these examples, the blastocyst erodes away the decidua and embeds in the wall. The chorionic villi grow and branch in the endometrium like the roots of a tree. Obviously, when the chorion is expelled at parturition, a part of the wall is also lost (shed) and bleeding occurs. This type of placenta is known as a *deciduate placenta.*

The degree of intimacy between fetal tissues and maternal tissues provides still another characteristic for categorizing placentas. Fig. 9-8

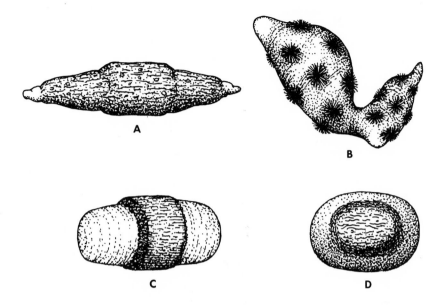

Fig. 9-5
Diagrams of chorionic sacs showing gross forms of placentas. **A,** Diffuse placenta (pig). **B,** Cotyledonary placenta (sheep, deer, cow). **C,** Zonary (dog, cat, and raccoon). **D,** Discoidal placenta (man, monkey, bear).

schematically shows two types. This relationship is an intimate one in primates and rodents since there is an erosion of maternal tissues consisting of the epithelial lining, the connective tissue, and the endothelial cells that form the blood vessels. As a result the maternal blood that fills the sinusoids bathes the fetal villi. Such a placenta, classified as *hemochorial,* is the most intimate type of mammalian placenta (Fig. 9-8, *B*). Some textbooks list another type in which the epithelium and connective tissue of the villi are also lost. If this actually occurred, it would leave the naked fetal blood vessels bathed with maternal blood. According to recent electron micrographs, however, trophoblastic layers remain around the endothelium of the blood vessels, in some cases at least. Thus naked blood vessels lying in a pool of maternal blood is probably a nonexistent condition.

The human embryo most often implants near the midline in the posterior wall of the uterus. The trophoblast separates at an early stage into two distinguishable layers, an inner more cellular layer, the *cytotrophoblast,* and an outer syncytial layer (devoid of cell boundaries according to electron micrographs) known as the *syncytio-*

trophoblast. These two layers persist for the first half of pregnancy; during the last part, the rate of mitotic divisions in the cytotrophoblast layer decreases.

The actively proliferating trophoblast cells apparently release enzymes that aid in their invasion of the maternal tissue. By the ninth day, the embedded blastocyst forms only a slight bulge covered by the uterine epithelium. The trophoblast layer does not develop uniformly around the implanted blastocyst. Only a thin layer of trophoblast cells covers the blastocyst on the uterine lumen side; extensive development occurs on the interior surface in contact with the richly vascular decidua basalis. The continued development of the trophoblast cells at this latter site gives rise to the disk-shaped, or discoidal, placenta described for man. At this time, however, the fingerlike projections of the chorion (the villi) have not yet formed, nor have the spaces (lacunae) appeared in the syncytiotrophoblast layer.

About the tenth day, the syncytiotrophoblast undergoes changes and vacuoles appear. These vacuoles eventually coalesce and give rise to larger spaces or *lacunae.* See Fig. 9-6, *A*. As a

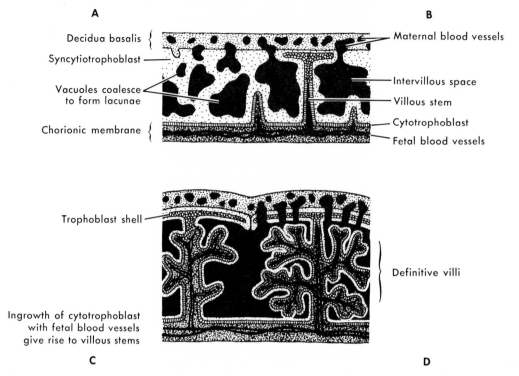

Fig. 9-6

Drawings illustrating the development of placenta. **A,** Vacuoles in the syncytiotrophoblast layer coalesce to form lacunae. **B,** Lacunae merge to form intervillous spaces that become filled with maternal blood. Cytotrophoblast forms villous stems in which fetal blood vessels develop. **C,** Growth of villous stem and formation of trophoblast shell. **D,** Definitive villi in intervillous space.

result, the syncytiotrophoblast contains a system of communicating spaces, with strands of tissue separating one lacuna from another. The irregular lacunae fill with blood and exudate from the maternal tissues, broken down by the invading trophoblastic cells. The various changes represent steps in the formation of the placenta. The period of placental formation between the sixth and thirteenth day of human development is often referred to as the *previllous period* (Wilkin, 1965).

The villous period of placenta organogenesis begins with the fourteenth day. The lacunae merge with one another and form the *intervillous space* into which the villi will grow (Fig. 9-6, *B*). The intervillous space becomes a large blood sinus that separates the placenta in such a way that it basically consists of the chorionic membrane on one side of the space and a parallel decidua basalis on the other.

The villi are the most essential structures of the definitive placenta, since it is through the villi that the interchange of material between fetus and mother takes place. As growth and differentiation of the chorion (somatic mesoderm and trophoblast) continues, the syncytial trabeculae take on a radial orientation. Active proliferation of the inner layer of trophoblast, the cytotrophoblast cells, follows, and the cells of this layer invade the syncytial trabeculae and form villous stems (Fig. 9-6, *B*). These stems acquire mesoderm cores from the extraembryonic somatopleure mesoderm. The mesoderm forms arterioles, venules, and capillaries that later anastomose with the umbilical arteries and veins. The circulation of the fetal part of the placenta functions around the twenty-first day. The establishment of these blood vessels in the mesodermal core of each cytotrophoblast ingrowth produces the *definitive villi*. As a result, a layer of

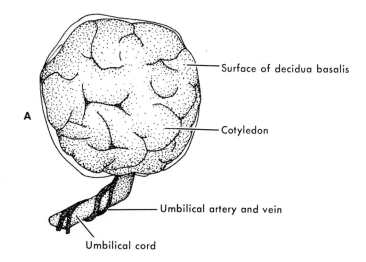

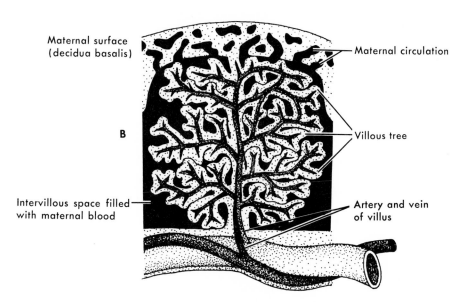

Fig. 9-7

A, Drawings of cotyledonary placenta at term. **B,** Drawing of villous structure of one cotyledon. Fetal circulation forms in mesodermal core of villous stem. Maternal blood "percolates" through the irregular spaces of intervillous space where physiological exchanges occur between fetus and mother. See text for more detailed discussion.

syncytiotrophoblast covers each cytotrophoblast villus, and somatic mesoderm forms its core.

Some of these villi project into the sinus where they *float free,* but others stretch across the intervillous space until they reach the decidua. They then spread tangentially, meeting and fusing with adjacent villi to form a shell around the chorion, as may be seen in Fig. 9-6, *C* and *D.* These villi are the *anchored villi.* Fingerlike projections from the villous stems grow laterally in

the intervillous space, like branches of a tree. They fuse with similar branches of other villous stems as gestation advances, creating a sponge-like structure, limited to the disk-shaped area covering the embryonic pole. Maternal blood percolates through the irregular spaces of the "sponge" that now makes up the intervillous space (Fig. 9-7, *B*). In the early embryo a layer of syncytiotrophoblast, cytotrophoblast, mesoderm of the villous core, and the fetal capillary wall (endothelium) separate the blood of the intervillous space from that of the fetus. By midpregnancy these layers thin and the efficiency in transfer of materials between the maternal blood and the fetal blood increases. The cytotrophoblast disappears, the syncytiotrophoblast thins, and the endothelium of the fetal blood vessels mingle intimately with the villous surface.

The relationship between maternal and fetal tissue is not always as intimate as that described for the hemochorial placenta of man as shown in Fig. 9-8, *A*. Basically, the placenta consists of two separate bloodstreams, fetal and maternal, separated by various cell layers. In some animals there are as many as six layers of tissue interposed between the fetal and the maternal circulations. Of course, such a placental relationship

is nondeciduate. If all layers are present, the placenta is referred to as *epitheliochorial* (Fig. 9-8, *A*). But many examples exist in which one or more layers are lacking. The following layers of tissue compose the placenta of such animals as the pig and horse:

1. An endothelial layer lines the maternal blood vessels.
2. A layer of connective tissue supports the maternal blood vessels.
3. Epithelium lines the surface of the uterus.
4. A layer of trophoblast cells covers the surface of the chorion.
5. Connective tissue forms the core of each villus.
6. Endothelium lines the fetal blood vessel embedded in the connective tissue core of each villus.

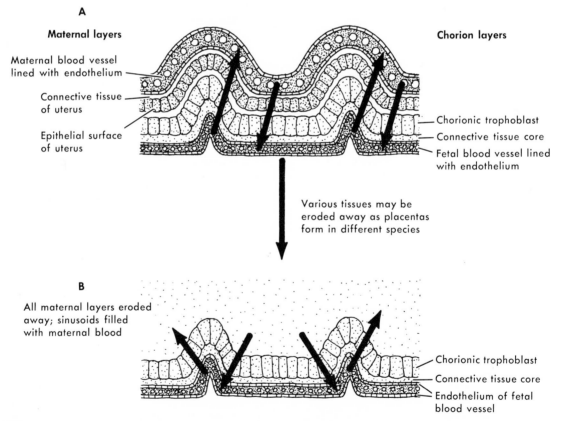

Fig. 9-8

Drawing illustrating the relationship of maternal and fetal circulatory systems. Placenta consists of fetal and maternal bloodstreams separated by various cell layers. When all six layers are present, the placenta is referred to as epitheliochorial, **A.** Erosion of maternal tissue allows the chorionic trophoblast to be bathed by maternal blood, and diffusion occurs through three layers. This type of placenta is considered a hemochorial placenta, **B.**

If erosion occurs to only the epithelial surface of the uterus and the remaining five layers are left intact as occurs in the sheep and cow, the placenta is classified as *syndesmochorial*. In the cat and dog, a second layer is lost. In these animals the embedded chorion takes up a position adjacent to the endothelium of the maternal blood vessels. This type of placenta is called *endotheliochorial*.

In summary, mammalian placentas can be classified in several ways, with gradations existing within each category. The classification may be based on the type of blood vessels involved, the shape of the placenta, whether or not the endometrium is shed at parturition, and the degree of intimacy between chorion and the decidua basalis. Returning to man as our example, we can classify the human placentas as chorioallantoic, discoidal, deciduate, and hemochorial, respectively.

Placental barrier. Hormones induce increased vascularity and prepare the uterus for implantation. The coiled arteries of the endometrium drain into capillaries and veins. As the blastocyst implants in primate and human females, the blood vessels break down under the stimulation of the hormone, progesterone; the spaces coalesce; and sinusoids form in the endometrial wall of the uterus. The syncytiotrophoblast cells invade these sinusoids. As a result, the maternal blood fills the intervillous space and surrounds the developing villous system, providing nourishment for the developing blastocyst. Although the maternal blood bathes the villi of the human chorion, it does not actually merge with the fetal blood, because of the layers of cells, the *placental barrier*, that normally separate the two.

The placenta acts like a semipermeable membrane, and most small molecules cross this barrier according to the ordinary laws of diffusion. This "membrane" prevents the transmission of most microorganisms to the fetus. Some exceptions exist, since the maternal rubella virus (German measles) passes during the first 3 months of pregnancy and causes blindness and certain congenital heart defects in the embryo. Also, during the second half of pregnancy, syphilitic spirochetes cause congenital syphilis in the fetus. There is evidence that Rh-positive fetal erythrocytes pass into the maternal circulation at the time of abortion or parturition. When this happens, if the mother is Rh-negative, she produces antibodies against the Rh-positive antigen. These antibodies may cross the placental barrier during the next pregnancy and destroy the red blood cells of the fetus, producing the hemolytic disease erythroblastosis fetalis in the newborn infant. Since the antibodies are known to be gamma globulins, and therefore large molecules, many biologists question the supposed selectivity of the placental barrier.

Carbohydrates, proteins, fats, water, and inorganic salts pass from the mother's blood system to that of the fetus. Certain drugs and small, soluble molecules also penetrate the placental barrier. If the molecule happens to be heroin, the child is born already addicted to the drug. The metabolites pass from the maternal blood through this barrier to the embryonic circulation, and excretory products move in the opposite direction. The kidneys of the mother eliminate the waste products of fetal metabolism along with her own waste products. The placenta also acts as a lung; the oxygen carried in the bloodstream of the mother diffuses into the fetal blood, and the carbon dioxide diffuses in the opposite direction.

Not only does the placenta take over vital embryonic functions, but it also acts as an endocrine organ. Once established, the placenta assumes hormonal control, maintaining the pregnant state of the body. The placenta secretes both estrogen and progesterone. Apparently, the chorion or trophoblast cells specifically secrete the gonad-stimulating hormone. The term *chorionic gonadotrophin* differentiates it from the gonadotrophin secreted by the pituitary, *hypophyseal gonadotrophin*. This latter hormone controls the normal reproductive cycles of the female.

SUGGESTED READINGS

1. Blandau, R. J.: Biology of eggs and implantation. In Young, W. C., and Corner, G. W. (editors): Sex and internal secretions, Baltimore, 1961, The Williams & Wilkins Co.
2. Carter, G. S.: Structure and habit in vertebrate evolution, Seattle, 1967, University of Washington Press.

3. Hamilton, W. J., Boyd, J. D., and Mossman, H. W.: Human embryology, Philadelphia, 1962, The Blakiston Co.

4. Hertig, A. T., Rock, J., and Adams, E. C.: A description of 34 human ova within the first 17 days of development, Am. J. Anat. **98**:435-493, 1956.

5. Mossman, H. W.: Comparative morphogenesis of the fetal membranes and accessory uterine structures, Contrib. Embryol. Carnegie Institute Washington **26**:129-296, 1937.

6. Patten, B. M.: Human embryology, Philadelphia, 1946, The Blakiston Co.

7. Romer, A. S.: Man and the vertebrates, Chicago, 1941, University of Chicago Press.

8. Romer, A. S.: Major steps in vertebrate evolution, Science **158**:1629-1637, 1967.

9. Romer, A. S.: The procession of life, Cleveland, 1968, World Publishing Co.

10. Wilkins, P. G.: Organogenesis of the human placenta. In DeHaan, R. L., and Ursprung, H. (editors): Organogenesis, New York, 1965, Holt, Rinehart & Winston.

11. Williams, P. L., Wendell-Smith, C. P., and Treadgold, S.: Basic human embryology, Philadelphia, 1966, J. B. Lippincott Co.

12. Witschi, E.: Development of vertebrates, Philadelphia, 1956, W. B. Saunders Co.

PART THREE

ORGANOGENESIS OF VERTEBRATE SYSTEMS

Section A
ORGANS DERIVED FROM ECTODERM

Section B
ORGANS DERIVED FROM ENDODERM

Section C
ORGANS DERIVED FROM MESODERM

CHAPTER 10

SKIN AND ITS ACCESSORY STRUCTURES

ORGANS OF ECTODERMAL DERIVATION

By the time the primitive body form develops, the neural ectoderm segregates from the epidermal ectoderm by a process called neurulation, described in Chapter 8. It lies along the dorsal surface of the embryo as a primary organ rudiment, the neural tube, where it undergoes extensive differentiation, described in detail in Chapter 12.

Epidermal ectoderm forms a continuous covering over the surface of the cylinder-shaped embryo. This ectodermal layer is only one cell thick in such animals as the shark, chick, pig, opossum, or human, but is two cells thick in the fish and amphibian. The one-celled epidermis soon divides into two layers so that the epidermal layer of all vertebrates eventually consists of two layers: an inner one, the *stratum germinativum*, that has the ability to proliferate, and an outer transitory, protective layer referred to as the *periderm*. The periderm first appears in the human embryo at 1½ months of age.

In general, the ectodermal layer gives rise to the skin. The vertebrate skin, including all its accessory structures, is defined as the *integument* or covering of the organism. Its functions are obvious, since it separates the internal environment of the individual from its surrounding environment. It protects the body from physical injury, acts as a barrier to microorganisms, insulates the body, and aids in the maintenance of its temperature. It may also act as an organ of excretion and respiration. It helps the individual to find food, or a mate, and to escape from predators by means of mechanoreceptors, radioreceptors, and chemoreceptors located either over the entire integument or in localized areas (see Chapter 11).

As the members of the various chordate classes adapted to the diverse niches available to them, the adult integument also changed. It varies from a one-cell-thick covering in amphioxus to a stratified layer of several cells in those terrestrial animals in which desiccation presents a threat to survival. The multilayered skin of land animals is more impermeable than that of animals bathed by an aquatic medium. In any case, the surface cells of the vertebrate skin are not exposed to the environment, but are protected by some kind of seal. A cuticle or a layer of mucus covers the body of aquatic animals; keratin, deposited in the cells of land animals, protects the surface of terrestrial forms. The accessory structures of the integument develop mainly from ectoderm, but often a papilla of mesoderm is present. Such accessory structures include unicellular and multicellular glands, scales, nails, beaks, horns, antlers, feathers, and hair and reflect the adaptation of the organism to its environment. This chapter is limited to a discussion of the skin and its accessory structures.

Specialized structures such as the lens of the eye, the cornea, and certain cranial ganglia also form from epithelium. Thickenings, called *placodes*, develop into the organs of special senses: the olfactory organ, the ear, and the lateral-line organs. The morphogenesis and histogenesis of these specialized epithelial structures are described in Chapter 11.

Epidermal ectoderm also gives rise to the lining of the orifices of the body and to some of the structures located within the cavities. After the formation of primary organ rudiments in the embryo, the mouth and anus form. The ectoderm gives rise to a depression, the *stomodeum*, in the anterior region of the embryo near the cranial tip of the notochordal process. When the stomodeum contacts the endoderm, an oral plate forms and soon ruptures, giving rise to a mouth and an oral cavity. In the human embryo this occurs about the twenty-sixth day. After the rupture of the oral plate, it is difficult to determine the depth of stomodeal ectoderm penetration. Since it is almost impossible to distinguish the exact boundary line between ectoderm and endoderm, the specific embryonic origin of some of the structures located in the oral cavity cannot be described with certainty. In general, most embryologists agree that ectoderm contributes to the lips, cheeks, gums, teeth, tongue, palate, and salivary glands, although the endoderm may also contribute to these same structures. Since these organs are usually discussed in most anatomy books as part of the digestive system, for the sake of convenience and conformance with the generally accepted policy, we shall delay the discussion of the morphogenesis of these structures until Chapter 13.

In some holoblastic vertebrates a part of the blastopore becomes the anal opening. In others, it forms in a similar fashion to that of the mouth. The skin ectoderm in the posterior region forms a depression, referred to as the *proctodeum*. A proctodeal plate results when the cells forming the depression come in contact with the hindgut endoderm. The further development of this plate in the mammal is intimately related to the division of the cloaca into the dorsal rectum and ventral urogenital sinus. Eventually the plate breaks down, establishing continuity between those structures derived from the cloaca and the outside. It is as difficult to distinguish germ layer boundaries in the formation of the cloacal cavity as it was with the mouth. The ectoderm, however, is acknowledged to contribute to the lower part of the anal canal and to the terminal portions of the genital and urinary tracts. Since the development and evolution of the cloaca is usually considered a part of the urogenital system, discussion of the cloaca is continued in Chapter 18.

SKIN
Development of skin

The adult skin is composed of three layers: a superficial stratified epithelium, the *epidermis;* a dense fibrous *dermis;* and beneath these layers, a loose, fatty *subcutaneous layer.* The skin has a dual origin and any discussion of it must include not only its ectodermal but its mesodermal component as well.

The stratum germinativum forms directly from ectoderm and gives rise to the epidermis, but the dermis differentiates from a layer of mesodermal tissue. The origin of the dermis is not always clear but seems to vary, depending on the species involved. It may arise from head mesenchyme, from dermatome, possibly from neural crest cells, or from mesenchyme derived from the more lateral and ventral somatic mesodermal regions of the body. In general, the vascular dermis supports, cushions, and nourishes the avascular epidermis. Neural crest cells, considered ectodermal in origin, invade the epidermis and dermis and give rise to certain pigment-containing cells referred to as *chromato-phores.*

The formation of the integument is an excellent example of tissue interaction during development since the ectoderm depends on the mesoderm for the direction of its differentiation (Rawles, 1955). If the epidermal cells are separated from the underlying mesodermal cells and grown in tissue culture, the germinativum layer loses the ability to divide. If dermis is then added to the culture, cell proliferation begins again. When undifferentiated epidermis is combined experimentally with different types of dermal cells, it will respond according to the type of dermis present (McLoughlin, 1963). For example, it is possible to induce beaks, feathers, scales, or mucus secretions to form from the epidermis by placing the appropriate dermis adjacent to the maturing epidermal cells. Thus, the dermis determines whether the epidermis clears and forms the cornea of the eye, becomes keratinized and gives rise to the skin, or whatever.

However, the presence of mesoderm is probably not the only answer to epidermal differentiation. Further studies indicate that some kind of substratum also appears necessary for epidermal development. On the other hand, although it needs the contact of a substratum on one of its surfaces, the outer surface of the ectoderm must be free of cellular contact for it to develop normally.

The differentiation of vertebrate skin is a very complex subject and involves many factors, some of which we do not understand at the present time. As is true of most organs, at an early stage of development the ectoderm has greater developmental potentiality than at later stages. It acquires specialized characteristics about the time of gastrulation and begins to show regional specialization. The fates of the different areas become definitely determined at various times depending on the organ and the species involved. Usually this occurs soon after gastrulation, when new interrelationships established by the tissues play a vital role in their further organization.

As is true for most inductive interactions, we do not understand the exact mechanisms by which the various dermas influence the epidermis. Presumably the dermis acts either by affecting the genes of the ectodermal cells directly or by influencing the cytoplasm of the epithelial cells. In any event, in vitro studies demonstrate that *isolated* epidermis eventually becomes necrotic (dies).

Evolution of vertebrate skin

The skin of amphioxus is an example of a chordate covering in its simplest form, probably representing the state of the early chordates living 400 million years ago in the Silurian period. It is similar to the skin of some invertebrates. It differs from the skin of all other chordates since the ectoderm in the adult animal develops into a single layer of ciliated columnar cells. These cells rest on a thin layer of mesodermal tissue, the basement membrane or cutis. A noncellular cuticle containing many pores and presumably secreted by the epidermal cells covers their outer surface. Amphioxus has only a very thin dermal layer and no epidermal derivatives. This thin barrier, no doubt, allows some exchange of materials between the blood and the aquatic medium.

There is a large gap in our knowledge between the present day protochordates, of which amphioxus is an example, and the earliest known vertebrate fossils, the ostracoderms, since the ostracoderms were heavily armored with bone, a dermal (mesoderm) derivative. One theory postulates that the invertebrates of the period, the eurypterids, preyed upon the tiny ostracoderms, and the presence of a bony armor offered the ostracoderms definite survival value.

A second theory attempts to associate the presence of a bony armor to a seal of the body. The earliest vertebrates left the saltwater of their origins and invaded the freshwater streams and ponds where absorption of water became a problem unless kept out by some kind of a seal. The kidneys of these animals, evolved to handle saltwater, are believed to have been incapable of coping with the hypotonic pond water. The bony armor of the ostracoderms may have helped in keeping the pond water on the outside of the animal.

The dermal portion of the integument gave rise to bony plates of the ostracoderms and placoderms and should not logically be discussed in a chapter devoted to ectoderm. However, it is impossible to gain an insight into the structure of the vertebrate skin without some knowledge of its evolutionary development. This, of course, includes a consideration of the mesodermal component, the dermal contribution to the integument, so important during the early days of vertebrate history. Table 10-1 summarizes some of the changes that occurred in the epidermis and dermis of vertebrates as they evolved.

Many biologists consider the presence of a bone-filled dermis in fossil vertebrates to represent the vertebrate primitive state. The mesodermal component of the dermis of these animals apparently formed bone, a type of connective tissue, which was covered by a thin layer of epidermis. Later in evolutionary history, as the kidneys and an impervious skin evolved along with a biting mouth, the animal changed from a sedentary to a predacious animal. The lack of a cumbersome armor and an increase in motility were a definite advantage.

Mesenchyme cells are capable of differentiating into a variety of tissues as indicated in Chapter 15. Under normal circumstances they give rise, not only to bone, but also to different types of connective tissue. It is not a great change, therefore, for mesenchyme to stop forming bone and start forming dermis. For example, instead of producing a bony matrix in which salts are deposited, the mesenchyme probably

TABLE 10-1. Evolution of skin

	Class	Epidermis	Dermis	Glands	Function
Anamniote	Ostracodermi		Heavy dermal armor		Protection Bony seal
	Petromyzontes and Myxini	Thin, nonkeratinized cells alive	Lacks bony scales	Many mucous glands	Protection
	Placodermi		Heavy dermal armor		
	Chondrichthyes and Holocephali		Thin dermal scales cover epidermis or penetrate through it (placoid scales)	Mucous and serous glands	Seal against water entrance to body
	Osteichthyes		Thin bony scales	Mucous glands	
	Amphibia	Superficial cells keratinized Rest of epidermis thin	Vascular and fibrous dermis	Multicellular gland present	Protection Respiration
Amniote	Reptilia	Epidermis keratinized Epidermal scales present	Thin and compact	Glands scarce Restricted to mouth and cloaca	Protection against desiccation and abrasion
	Aves	Generally thin epidermis Beaks, feet, and combs thicker Scales on feet Feathers present	Dermis vascular	Few glands	Protection against desiccation and abrasion
	Mammalia	Reptilian scales on legs and tails of some mammals Hair present Epidermis thick	Generally thick	Diverse integumentary glands: sebaceous, sweat, mammary	Control of body heat

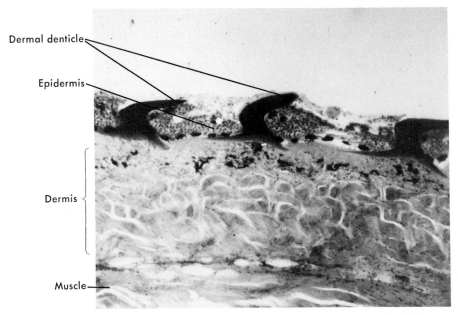

Dermal denticle

Epidermis

Dermis

Muscle

Fig. 10-1
Placode scales in shark skin. (× 100.)

differentiated into a tissue whose matrix lacked a deposition of salts. As a result, the dermis evolved, consisting of fibers of different types intertwined in different degrees of denseness and producing the leathery types of integument associated with modern animals.

Dermal degeneration (that is, the absence of bone in the integument) is almost complete in modern animals. The skin of most cyclostomes lack bone, and only dermal denticles, toothlike projections known as placoid scales, remain on the surface of sharklike fishes. Fig. 10-1 shows these scales projecting through the epidermal layer. Bony fishes retain dermal scales, but they are lost in most land animals, with the exception of the abdominal ribs (gastralia) of lizards, crocodiles, and sphenodon, the bony plates of the turtles, and the flat bones of the vertebrate skull, which are described in Chapter 15.

In summary, when one considers the integument from an evolutionary standpoint, a decrease in ossification and a decrease in thickness of the skin occurs as anamniotes evolved. On the other hand in land forms the epidermal layer and especially the dermal component increase in thickness. These changes prevent the evaporation of water and help to maintain body temperature.

Basic integument

The basic integument of vertebrates consists of an epithelium of several layers (a stratified epithelium) resting on a dermal layer. It ranges from the simple, thin skin of the cyclostomes to the thick hides of mammals. In cyclostomes, all cells remain alive covered by a thin, nonliving cuticular layer. On the other hand, in mammals several layers of cells compose the skin, with the outer layer consisting of dead keratinized cells (Patt and Patt, 1969).

In fish, the basal layer (stratum germinativum) of the epidermis contains three different cell types. They differentiate into mucus-secreting cells (the major cell type), club cells, and granular cells containing some keratin filaments (Flaxman, 1972). However, the stratum germinativum of most vertebrates above the fish appears to be morphologically uniform and to consist of only one type of cell. It gives rise to cuboidal cells that are the only cells in the epidermis to undergo mitosis. Cell division occurs in the stratum germinativum either continuously or periodically in all vertebrate classes. It may go on at a fast or slow rate; in either case, after they divide, the daughter cells follow one of three alternatives. Either they both migrate to the surface of the integument, both remain in the basal layer where they act as reserve cells giving rise to future skin cells, or one daughter cell remains and one moves toward the surface.

During their migration to the surface of the integument, the cells usually become keratinized, a process that involves the stepwise deposition in the cell of a number of fibrous proteins all loosely referred to as keratin. Keratinization occurs when the proteins are cross-linked through disulfide bridges; however, because of its insoluble properties, the characterization and identification of the specific protein composition of keratin is incomplete. The cells of fish lack morphologic keratinization, but keratin is present in amphibians and is most pronounced in land animals: the reptiles, birds, and mammals. In the human embryo it occurs by the fourth month of pregnancy. As a result of keratinization, the cuboidal cells flatten, the nucleus degenerates, the cell loses its capacity to divide, and the fibrous keratin replaces the cytoplasm.

X-ray diffraction patterns that reflect macromolecular organization distinguish between two types of keratin, alpha or beta (Bell, 1965). For example, keratin that has the beta pattern composes avian feathers, but the cells of mammalian hair, stratum corneum, and nails are filled with keratin of the alpha type.

The fully keratinized cell consists of not much more than a tough cell membrane filled with an abundance of filaments. It acts as a barrier, keeping such materials as water inside the body and preventing other substances from entering. It is resistant to abrasive substances. As a result of keratinization, a layer of dried, horny cells known as the *stratum corneum* covers the surface of the skin. These cells are constantly lost (desquamated).

Replacement of the cells composing the epidermis, lost either through wear and tear or actual shedding, occurs continuously. Either the epidermis sloughs off in the form of small fragments, such as dandruff, or the loss may involve practically the entire outer covering of skin, scales, feathers, or hair. If the loss is extensive, it is usually referred to as a *molt*. The periodic shedding of integument allows the animal to

change from a heavier to a lighter coat or from dull to bright plumage, or merely to repair those cells that have worn away.

Sometimes the cells are shed periodically and are associated with seasonal and reproductive cycles. Genetic and neuroendocrine factors interact in the animal's response to environmental stimuli. In some animals, such as the amphibian, the thyroid gland plays an important role in molting. Also, the gonadal hormones may act in a synergistic fashion with other hormones to influence growth of the integument or its derivations. Progesterone, for example, stimulates molting in birds. The integument of the vertebrate represents one of the few areas of the body in which growth and cellular differentiation continue into adulthood.

The epidermis of the amphibian, unlike that of the fish, contains only one type of differentiated cell. It produces both mucus and keratin filaments (Flaxman, 1972). After cell division as the cells migrate from the basal layer to the surface of the skin, they secrete and release mucus into the intercellular spaces. Along the way to the surface of the animal, however, the mucus-secreting cells transform into horny cells filled with keratin.

Although bony scales covered the body of the earliest amphibians, the labyrinthodonts, most living forms lack scales. Only in the Apoda do remnants of these ancestral scales remain. Instead in modern amphibians, those that are primarily land dwellers, a dead outer *stratum corneum* appears, an adaptation to terrestrial life. The integument of the amphibians varies from the aquatic *Necturus,* in which a cuticle covers the skin, to the frog in which a few keratinized cells appear, to the more terrestrial toad in which the deposition of keratin forms a thick and horny skin. These strata cornea of salamanders, frogs, and toads contain alpha keratin in their cells. The secretion of mucus keeps the thin integument of the frog moist and helps it to retain some of its permeable characteristics. The dermis is very vascular and a large proportion of respiratory needs of the frog is carried out through this moist epidermis. Unlike most vertebrates, the epidermis of totally aquatic forms, *Cryptobranchus* for example, is supplied with blood vessels from the dermis and the skin actually becomes the primary organ for the exchange of gases.

Two well-defined layers compose the dermis of the frog. The outer layer consists of loosely arranged collagen fibers and contains blood vessels, nerves, pigment cells, lymph spaces, glands, but little fat. The inner layer is more compact and ties the skin to the underlying skeletal muscle.

The nature of the epidermis changed as the reptiles moved on to land. There was a loss of mucus-secreting cells and an increase in keratinization. According to some authors, the development of a flexible, lightweight keratinized skin is one of the factors that allowed aquatic animals to evolve into terrestrial forms and attain the large size of many species. The keratinized scales of the reptilian skin provide a flexible covering that protects the animal against abrasion and desiccation and aids in locomotion. The skin allows for growth, since it is periodically shed and replaced.

The main disadvantage of keratinized scales, however, is that they do not control the loss or gain of heat. This problem was not handled until the evolution of feathers and hair, both epidermal structures. The epidermis of reptiles and birds, in general, consist of a living germinative layer, an intermediate zone of cells and an outer covering of flat, dead cells, the *stratum corneum*. The dermis layer, upon which the epidermis rests, varies in thickness, depending on the species. The integument of reptiles and at least one bird, the ostrich, is thick enough that it can be prepared for leather.

The epidermis of mammals may contain as many as four different layers, depending on the location in the animal. In man, the skin of the soles of the feet and palms of the hands is much

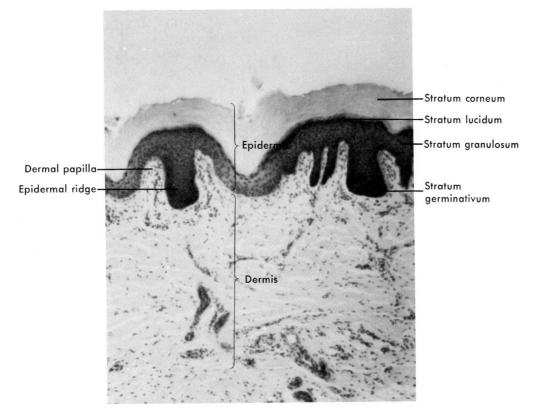

Fig. 10-2
Vertical section of skin showing thick epidermis. See text for description.

206 Organogenesis of vertebrate systems

thicker and exhibits all four layers, as compared to the thinner skin covering the eye lid. A vertical section through the thick part of the epidermis of man (Fig. 10-2) shows the first (or deepest) layer to consist of the cuboidal to columnar cells of the *stratum germinativum*. These are associated with another layer of cells that have short processes or spines that meet end to end and are attached by desmosomes, plate-like thickenings on apposing cell surfaces. As mitosis continues in the stratum germinativum, the cells move outward and form the next general layer, the *stratum granulosum*. This layer is three to five cells thick and may contain granules of keratohyalin, a substance whose function has not been agreed upon by authorities in the field (Bell, 1965).

As the cells continue to push outward, the *stratum lucidum* appears. It consists of several layers of flat cells that have lost their nuclei and contain droplets of material known as eleidin, believed by some biologists to be modified keratohyalin granules. This layer is present in the thicker regions of the skin but may be entirely lacking in the thinner portions. Several layers of flat cells that lack nuclei compose the surface layer or *stratum corneum*. The loss and replacement of these keratin-filled cells occur constantly. The outer surface of the epidermis is not smooth but contains grooves and ridges that create patterns; the most well known are responsible for the fingerprints. These patterns are so variable that they can be used to identify the individual.

The stratum germinativum rests on the dermal (mesoderm) component of the skin. The point of contact between dermis and epidermis is not a smooth one (Fig. 10-2), but rather the interface is wavy. The projections of the dermis into the epidermis are known as *dermal papillae* and contain many of the receptors described in the following chapter. The periodic downward invasions of epidermis into the dermis (as shown in vertical sections of skin) are referred to as *epidermal ridges*.

The mesodermal component of the mammalian integument is much thicker than the epidermis. It consists of a variety of different-sized collagen and elastic fibers that run in different directions and form networks of various degrees of denseness. The epidermis usually is avascular; the dermis, on the other hand, serves as a kind of packing tissue for blood vessels, muscle cells, fat, nerves, and nerve endings. Certain derivations of the epidermis such as hair follicles, sweat glands, and sebaceous glands extend down into the dermal layer to various levels.

The dermis, in turn, rests on a subcutaneous layer, the *hypodermis,* also derived from mesoderm. This layer contains a continuation of some of the dermal fibers along with different amounts of adipose tissue (fat) and muscle. The hypodermis anchors the integument in a loose fashion to the muscles, bones, and tendons of the body.

EPIDERMAL DERIVATIVES

Any discussion of the integument must include not only a consideration of the skin but of its derivatives as well. These structures can be roughly divided into three groups. Some form solely from epidermis although the mesoderm usually plays an inductive role in that some sort of papilla or core is present. Some of the more major epidermal structures are hair, feathers, horns, reptilian scales, scutes, beaks, claws, nails, chromatophores, and glands. A second group of structures involves the participation of both epidermal and dermal components. Examples of this type of cooperation may be seen in dermal denticles, vertebrate teeth, and some scales. The third group contains derivatives formed solely from the dermis (mesoderm) with no epidermal contribution. Such structures as antlers and the dermal bones of vertebrates may be classified in this manner.

The first group, those derived primarily from ectoderm, are considered in this chapter, and those structures derived from a combination of mesoderm and ectoderm or of mesoderm only are discussed later in the appropriate chapters.

Keratinized epidermal structures

The epidermis of the reptile folds upon itself about small dermal projections, the papillae, to form *horny scales* as illustrated in Fig. 10-3. The epidermis on both sides of a papilla becomes keratinized. The living mesodermal component then mostly withdraws leaving the two upper and lower epidermal layers in close apposition. These scales vary from the small projections of the chameleons to the overlapping, thin, keratinized scales of snakes.

Horny scales are a product of the stratum corneum layer of the epidermis and should not be confused with the bony scales of the fish that arise from the dermal layer. In the turtle the scales form flat scutes or plates and cover the bony plates of the carapace and plastron. Muscles attach to the transversely arranged bands of ventral scales in the snake and elevate and depress them. Reptilian scales, therefore, can be used in locomotion.

The remnants of the reptilian scales remain in the two higher groups of vertebrates. They persist on the legs of birds and the tails of certain rodents, insectivores, and marsupials and offer evidence of the reptilian ancestry of these forms.

The stratum corneum also gives rise to *claws* in the reptile and some mammals, which become modified to form *nails* and *hoofs* in most mammals. All three structures cover the digits and resemble epidermal scales as illustrated in Fig. 10-4. They possess a long hard nail plate (*unguis*) and a softer less cornified pad of tissue, the *subunguis*. They differ from one another, depending on the varieties of unguis and subunguis. Hoofs, for example, differ from nails in that they possess more than one shortened nail plate and the subunguis forms a pad within the curve of the hooftip.

The horny plate that makes up the nails covers the *nail bed* and is surrounded laterally and proximally by the *nail wall. A nail groove* separates the bed from the wall. The nailfold usually covers a whitish crescentic portion, the lunula (or "moon") located near the root of the nail. This fold has all the layers of the skin. Its underlying region, usually referred to as the *nail matrix*, forms new nail substances from the dead residues of the cornified epithelial cells. Thus the matrix forms the nail. Only the stratum germinativum covers the surface of the nail bed. Most authors agree that it does not contribute to the new nail substances but merely provides a surface for the nail to glide over.

The skin of the jaw in some amniotes becomes

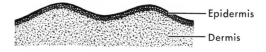
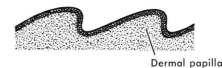
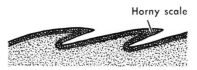

Fig. 10-3
Stages in development of the keratinized (epidermal) scales of reptiles.

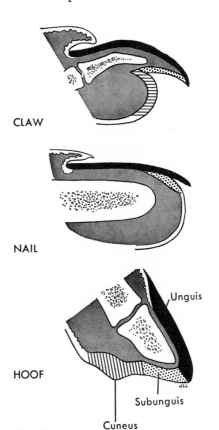

Fig. 10-4
Sagittal sections of mammalian terminal phalanges. Stratum corneum (*black area*) gives rise to the unguis of claws, nails, and hoofs. (From Kent, G. C., Jr.: Comparative anatomy of the vertebrates, ed. 3, St. Louis, 1973, The C. V. Mosby Co.)

modified. The stratum corneum that covers the upper and lower jaw gives rise to a *bill* or *beak* and takes the place of teeth in turtles, tortoises, and birds. The bill of the mammalian duckbill platypus is soft and pliable, unlike that of the birds.

Horns are found only among mammals. These are nonliving structures composed of keratin and have no nerves or blood supply. If horns are removed, they do not regenerate. The horns of sheep, goats, cattle, and antelopes have a core of bone, the *os cornu*, sheathed in keratin. They are not branched like the solid bony antlers of the deer and are never shed. Rhinoceroses have the simplest and most primitive horns composed of hardened, solid keratin. The pronghorn antelope *(Antilocapra americana)*, a native of North America has a horny covering over a bony projection. In this type of horn, the covering is periodically shed (Modell, 1969).

Feathers

Although the reptilian scales persist on the legs and feet of birds and become specialized to form beaks and claws, they are modified as feathers over the rest of the body. Feathers are composed of cornified epithelial cells. They represent the modification of the integument for flight and are the bird's most notable distinguishing feature. They occur in no other class of vertebrates. They are lightweight, have great strength, provide a water-repellent surface, and effectively insulate the body. Muscles at their bases control the feather's position, an important aid in a bird maintaining high (and relatively constant) body temperature.

There are three types of feathers. *Contour feathers* are the large complex feathers that cover the body, wing, and tail. *Down feathers* are the simple juvenile and adult feathers, and the very simple *filoplumes* are the "pinfeathers."

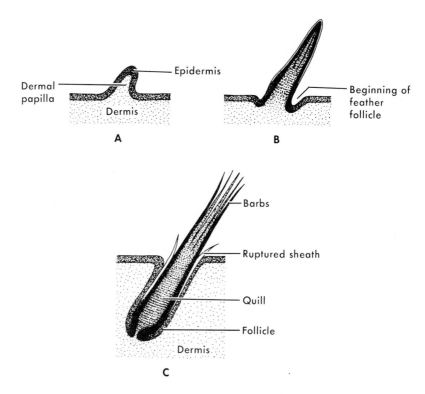

Fig. 10-5

Successive stages in the development of a down feather. Mesoderm cells induce the ectoderm to thicken and protrude as a cone-shaped structure, **A** and **B**. Feather germ is formed when a groove appears around the base of the papilla, **B**. Base of papilla becomes the quill, and ridges of ectoderm give rise to the barbs, **C**.

The contour feathers are not randomly distributed over the body of the bird, but occur in tracts with bare spaces in between. Down feathers and filoplumes, however, may be located in these spaces. They help to insulate the bird and aid in warming the eggs during incubation. Feathers are shed periodically. Molting, under the control of hormones, usually occurs in the fall or spring. All the feathers are not lost at one time; they are shed gradually. The feather follicle, which remains intact in the integument, replaces the feather.

Feathers arise in the embryo in much the same way as a reptilian scale. Mesodermal cells condense under the epidermal ectoderm and induce the ectoderm to thicken and protrude as a cone-shaped structure from the surface of the body, as diagrammed in Fig. 10-5. Although the early development of a feather resembles that of a scale, its further development differs greatly. A groove appears around the base of the papilla, indicating the beginning of the feather follicle. At this stage, the structure is known as the *feather germ.*

A collar of germinativum cells at the base of the papilla gives rise to ridges in the ectodermal covering of the elongated papilla. These ridges form the *barbs* of the down feather, which, in turn, give rise to the lateral outgrowths, the *barbules.* Blood vessels located in the mesodermal pulp (the papilla) nourish the developing structure. The base of the papilla becomes a short cylindrical *stalk* or *quill* and contains the radially arranged barbs. The dermal pulp and stratum germinativum gradually retract, leaving dried pithy remnants in the quill.

The down feathers appear externally as a small spray of branches. They cover the young bird and are known as "nestling down." Contour feathers replace these first feathers during the

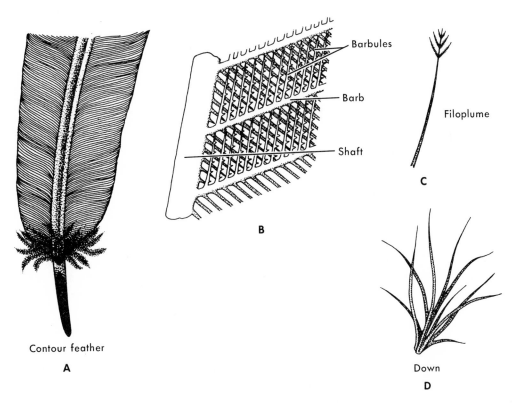

Contour feather

A

Barbules

Barb

Shaft

B

Filoplume

C

Down

D

Fig. 10-6
Diagram of three types of feathers. See text for structural details of a contour feather, **B.**

early life of most birds. Filoplumes are even more simple in structure. The quill gives rise to a short slender shaft from which arises a small tuft of barbs. These feathers are hidden by the contour feathers and become visible when feathers are plucked as in preparing a bird for cooking. They are usually singed off.

The contour feather develops in much the same way as the filoplume and down feathers. The feather germ forms, consisting of an epidermal cone filled with mesodermal pulp. An epidermal sheath covers the entire structure. As in the example of the down feathers, radially arranged barbs develop from the germinativum collar. Eventually one particularly strong process

grows out and gives rise to the shaft of the feather. The barbs migrate onto the shaft. These obliquely located branches (the barbs) form subbranches, the barbules, which interlock with one another, as shown in Fig. 10-6. As a result of the interlocking barbules, the feather appears as a continuous sheet.

Hair

Hair is a uniquely mammalian characteristic and in most forms covers nearly the entire integument. Like the feather, it is composed entirely of epidermal tissue but unlike the feather it is believed to have evolved from tactile sensory pits rather than from reptilian scales.

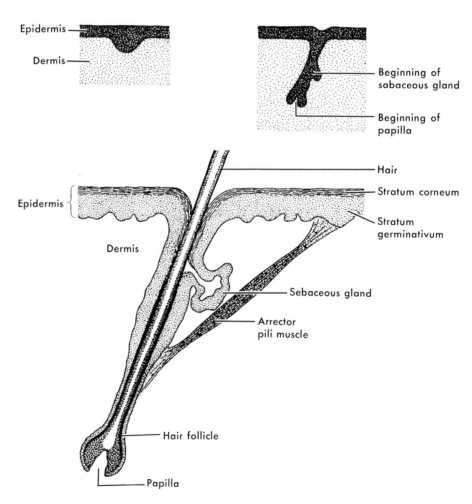

Fig. 10-7
Diagrams of longitudinal sections showing successive stages in the development of mammalian hair.

The bodies of all mammalian embryos at some time during development are covered with fine hair known as the *lanugo*. It is well developed in the human embryo by the seventh month but is usually shed by the time of birth.

The shedding and replacement of hair, like feathers, occur either periodically or constantly. If the stratum germinativum composing the hair follicle is lost through injury, no regeneration is possible. The density of hair varies in different mammals as well as over the body of the same animal. Manes, eyelashes, and eyebrows all differ from that covering the rest of the body.

The development of hair is initiated when the epidermal ectoderm grows obliquely down into the dermis (Fig. 10-7). The base of the column becomes bulb-shaped and the dermal mesenchyme pushes into the bulb to form a papilla. Blood vessels form in the papilla and supply nutritive material to bulb cells, the only living part of the hair. The papilla and its covering of epidermal cells make up a hair follicle. A hair consists of its *root* and, the main part, its *shaft*.

As the germinativum cells of the follicle undergo cell division, the new cells are pushed toward the surface through the original epidermal column where they form part of the root. As they continue to move outward, the cells gradually give rise to the shaft of the hair. Dead keratinized cells compose both the root and shaft of the hair.

Two thickenings occur on the side of the follicle. As shown in Fig. 10-7, one consists of a cluster of epidermal cells that give rise to a *sebaceous gland* opening into the hair follicle. The other group of cells provides an attachment for the *arrector pili muscle*, which forms from the mesenchyme of the dermal layer and is associated with each hair shaft. Since each hair shaft is at an angle, the contraction of the arrector pili muscle causes the hair to stand erect.

According to cross sections, two or three layers of cells form a hair. A thin cuticle of overlapping, transparent cells covers the hair. Hard keratin fibers with intervening air spaces compose the cells of the *cortex* located under the cuticle. The *medulla* makes up the central area of the fiber and consists of keratin, shrunken cells, and air spaces. The medulla may be absent in thin hair. If the section is made through the wall of the hair follicle, several layers of cells present can be divided into two main layers, the internal and outer root sheath.

Glands

A gland consists of a cell or a group of cells that not only carry on their own metabolic processes, but also manufacture and release certain specific materials. Such substances are either utilized (digestive enzymes) or eliminated from the body (sweat). A unicellular gland is located near the surface where it synthesizes and releases its specific secretion. Several cells (multicellular) formed from invaginations of the germinative layer compose most glands. These invaginations differentiate into a secretory portion and a nonsecretory portion, or duct, that carries the secretion to the surface. The term, *exocrine*, refers to this type of gland. *Endocrine glands,* on the other hand, lose their connection with the surface epithelium and are ductless.

Exocrine glands exist in a variety of shapes (Fig. 10-8). If the secretory cells are arranged in a simple tubelike form that opens into an unbranched duct, the gland is said to be *simple*. However, if the duct system is branched, the gland is *compound*. The secretory portions of either simple or compound glands may be arranged as tubules, in which case it is known as a *tubular gland*. If the secretory portion expands to form a sac-like structure, the gland is either a simple or compound *alveolar gland*.

Glands can be classified not only by their shape but also according to the type of material secreted. *Mucous glands* secrete a viscous, slimy material; the secretion of *serous glands* is more watery. Some *mixed* glands produce both types of secretion. The cells composing the glands release their secretory products in different ways. A *merocrine gland* releases its products through the cell membrane with the cell remaining intact. If some of the apical cytoplasm is lost along with the material secreted, the gland is referred to as *apocrine*. In a *holocrine gland*, the entire cell disintegrates, forming a part of the secretion.

Glands develop in the epidermis of all vertebrates. In general, the glands of fish are unicellular, although some multicellular glands exist.

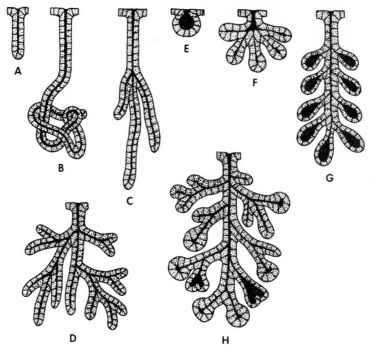

Fig. 10-8

Diagrammatic representations of various types of integumentary (exocrine) glands: **A,** simple tubular; **B,** coiled tubular; **C,** branched tubular; **D,** compound tubular; **E,** simple alveolar; **F** and **G,** branched alveolar; **H,** compound tubuloalveolar gland.

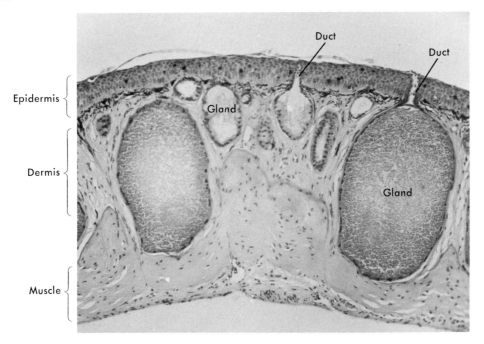

Fig. 10-9

Multicellular glands of frog skin are sac-like structures derived from epidermis but located in the dermis. They release their secretions to the surface by ducts.

They differentiate as small cells from the stratum germinativum and migrate toward the surface. Most are mucus-secreting glands; some are serous glands. The mucus forms a layer on the surface of the fish and makes it more impermeable to water. In some species, multicellular poison glands are associated with the base of the spine on the fins.

The aquatic amphibians continue to secrete mucus that aids in the maintenance of a moist skin and protects against loss of water. However, instead of the individual mucus cells of the fish, the cells of the amphibian are grouped together into simple glands. The mucous glands of the amphibian are small and composed of low cuboidal epithelium. The cells that compose the larger serous glands have a granular cytoplasm and are irregularly spaced. Thus, serous glands are often referred to as *granular glands*. They are usually poisonous, with their secretions ranging from mildly irritating to toxic. Both types of glands are sac-like structures derived from the epidermis but located in the loose dermal layers of the skin. They release their secretions to the surface by way of a duct, as shown in Fig. 10-9. Presumably the numerous and diversified mammalian glands evolved from ancestors possessing these two basic types of glands (mucous and serous).

A loss of mucus-secreting glands occurs in reptiles and birds, thereby water is conserved; the reptilian skin is dry and scaly. However, despite what is written in most textbooks, reptiles possess a variety of skin glands (Quay, 1972). They are very small and difficult to discern and easily confused with pores or horny outgrowths of the integument. Most of the reptilian glands are holocrine, that is, the secretion consists of the entire secretory cells sloughing off into the cavity of the gland and degenerating into an amorphous fluid. Most of the glands are specialized scent glands and reach a greater size and activity in the male during the breeding season.

The paired uropygial or preen glands at the base of the tail of birds secrete oil, which the bird dispenses with the help of its beak. This secretion is apparently necessary to maintain the structural integrity and water-repellent charac-

teristic of the feathers; these glands are especially well-developed in aquatic birds. There are also traces of sebaceous-like glands in the ear and trunk regions of some birds.

The mammalian skin contains many glands, but basically they are either modified *sebaceous glands* or *sweat glands*. The sebaceous glands are spherical or ovoid in shape and are simple or branched alveolar glands. They are believed to be homologous with the amphibian alveolar mucous glands. In the mammal the sebaceous gland secretes oil and is associated mainly with the hair follicles, as shown in Fig. 10-7. They develop first as thickenings of the outer sheath cells. Their ducts open into the neck of the follicle and their oily secretion appears to be the direct product of cellular disintegration. Several types of sebaceous glands are distributed over the body where hair is absent. They are located, for example, at the corners of the mouth and lips, and on the nipple, the eyelids, and glans penis.

Sweat glands may have evolved from the amphibian serous glands. They are found only in mammals. They appear in the embryo as solid, cylindrical ingrowths of the stratum germinativum. The deeper part of the ingrowth coils on itself and forms the body of the gland. The central cells eventually degenerate and produce a tubular structure that is simple coiled or branched. The coiled portion rests in the subcutis region of the skin and a long duct extends through the dermis, entering the epidermis between two papillae. The duct opens to the surface by way of a sweat pore. Some of the surrounding ectodermal cells give rise to myoepithelial cells and, presumably, are able to contract.

The sweat glands are apocrine glands since the distal ends of the cells are discharged as part of the secretion. The sweat glands are important excretory organs. Sweat is a watery secretion containing certain salts, urea, and other wastes; it is a significant method of eliminating metabolic wastes of various kinds. It also helps maintain the body temperature, since the evaporation of sweat on a hot day produces a cooling effect.

Mammary glands, ceruminous (wax) glands of the ear, and certain scent glands also have

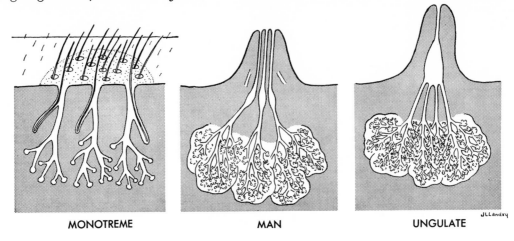

MONOTREME   MAN   UNGULATE

Fig. 10-10
Mammary glands, ducts, and nipples. The monotreme lacks nipples, and the glands resemble modified sweat glands. See text for further discussion of primate and ungulate glands. (From Kent, G. C.: Comparative anatomy of the vertebrates, ed. 3, St. Louis, 1973, The C. V. Mosby Co.)

an apocrine type of secretion and probably evolved from sweat glands. Mammary glands, present only in mammals, are responsible for the name of the class. Mammary glands assume various forms (Fig. 10-10). In the monotremes they consist of two glands in the abdominal wall that secrete a sticky material onto the surface; the secretion is licked off this mammary patch by the young. The glands are located in the pouch of the marsupial. At birth the young crawl into the pouch, and each attaches to a nipple. In ungulates, several ducts empty into a common collecting chamber and a single duct opens to the outside. The primate's mammary gland basically consists of several lobes (15 to 20), each of which is considered to be a compound gland with a duct opening into the tip of the nipple.

Mammary glands first form as linear ectodermal thickenings, known as the milk, or mammary, ridges, running down the ventrolateral region of the embryo of both sexes. Various areas of this region continue to develop; the precise number of glands usually corresponds with the number of offspring produced. The development of the mammary ridge normally occurs only in the pectoral region in man and the elephant and only in the inguinal region in the sheep, cow, and horse, but it is extensively developed down the middle of the ridge in such forms as the cat, dog, or pig.

Thickenings of the epidermis represent the beginnings of the nipples. The ectodermal cells undergo proliferation and become bulbous; they grow in toward the mesenchyme layer as shown in Fig. 10-11. Several buds (about 15 or 20 in the human embryo) push out into the dermis from the epidermal bulbous area. These buds are the primordia of the mammary gland ducts. Near the end of embryonic life, they undergo further branching, but then until puberty the mammary glands of both sexes remain in an infantile state. The secretion of estrogen by the female at sexual maturity stimulates duct growth; progesterone stimulates the growth of the alveolar secretory cells. During pregnancy when the estrogen and progesterone levels remain high because of production by both ovaries and placenta, the ducts and alveolae develop extensively, establishing a presecretory state. The lactogenic hormone (luteotrophic hormone, LTH) from the pituitary gland appears necessary in certain species for secretion to take place (see Fig. 3-18).

CHROMATOPHORES

The various color patterns of vertebrate animals function in various ways and are determined by heredity. They are involved in camouflage, protection, sexual attraction, and warning. Color has definite survival value. The pigment melanin, for example, may function in some

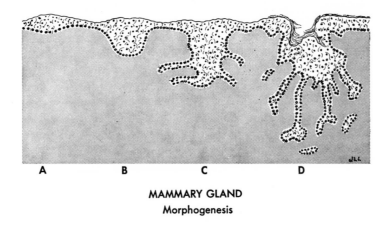

MAMMARY GLAND
Morphogenesis

Fig. 10-11
Successive stages of mammary gland development. **A**, Equivalent to a human embryo at 6 weeks. **B**, Equivalent to a human embryo at 9 weeks and to mouse embryo at 16 days. **C**, Intermediate stage. **D**, At birth. Gray area represents dermis. (From Kent, G. C.: Comparative anatomy of the vertebrates, ed. 3, St. Louis, 1973, The C. V. Mosby Co.)

cyclostomes as a screen, protecting the central nervous system against the sun. Since melanin is associated with both locomotion and spine response in the invertebrates (sea urchin), some authors suggest that pigment may play a role in regulating the vertebrate central nervous system. Integumental pigmentation has undoubtedly been important in evolution, but we do not understand its specific role. Pigment-containing cells also penetrate more deeply than the integument. They are often found along the blood vessels, along the walls of the coelom, and in the liver, all areas where it is difficult to determine a functional advantage for the pigment.

Neural crest cells invade the epidermis and dermis and differentiate into color-forming cells known by the general term *chromatophores*. Since they have been traced to the neural crest cells, they are considered ectodermal in origin. Soon after the completion of neurulation some of the neural crest cells (melanoblasts) migrate out to the various locations they will occupy in the postembryonic body. The specific color pattern of vertebrates depend on the distribution and activities of these cells. They allow the animal to respond to many environment stimuli by changing color.

Since the chromatophores are stellate and have long slender processes, they are sometimes referred to as *dendritic cells*. Pigment granules

may either be concentrated in the center of the cell in one mass, in which case little color appears, or else the pigment may be distributed throughout the cell including the long dendritic processes, as shown in Fig. 10-12. When dispersal of the pigment occurs, the color effect is maximum. The color-bearing cells are also able to shift their relative positions in the body of the animal by ameboid movement. The color changes displayed by such animals as the flounder and chameleon are attributable to both these mechanisms—the migration of the cells and the amount of dispersal of the granules within the individual cells.

Chromatophores are under hormonal control and are influenced by pituitary, thyroid, gonad, pineal, and adrenal gland secretions. For example, the central nervous system influences the intermediate lobe of the pituitary to release its melanotrophic hormone (intermedin) into the bloodstream of fish, amphibians, and some reptiles. Dermal capillaries carry the hormones to the pigment-synthesizing cells. Color changes controlled by intermedin take minutes or hours to occur.

In poikilotherms (cyclostomes, elasmobranchs, teleosts, amphibians, and reptiles), the chromatophores are also effector cells and respond to nervous stimuli. Consequently their response is rapid. Color pattern in the environment influ-

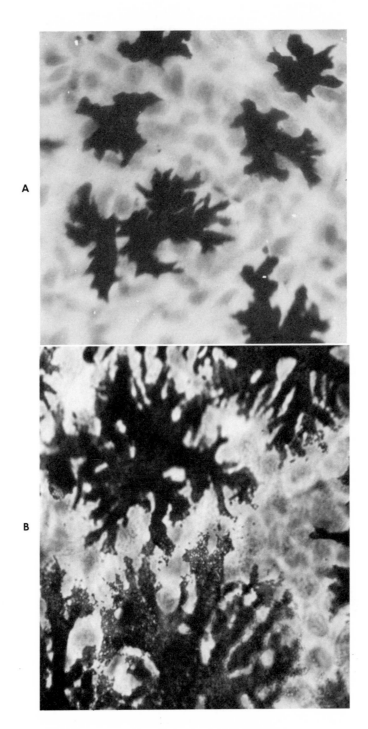

Fig. 10-12

Stages in the dispersion of pigment in chromatophores of frog skin. Pigment granules are concentrated in center of cells, **A**; pigment is dispersed throughout the cytoplasm of the chromatophores, producing the maximum of color effect, **B**. (× 450.)

ences color change in the animal by pathways leading from the eyes to the brain of the organism. If a single cutaneous nerve in a fish is destroyed, it is unable to change color in the area of the cut. Nerves produce their effect by liberating a chemical, a *neurohumor*, at their terminal ends that diffuses to the chromatophore and brings about the change. Epinephrine-like substances released by the nerve terminals cause the melanin to concentrate in the center of the cell and acetylcholine-like materials induce melanin granules to disperse into the dendritic arms.

Birds and mammals apparently lack a pigmentary effector system, since color changes associated with these classes of animals involve relatively slow alterations in the amount of pigment. The cells respond to seasonal changes, allowing the skin to tan in the summer or the coats of certain animals to change from brown to white. In some cases these color variations are caused by the amount of pigment present and in other cases to the type of pigment.

There are various kinds of pigments in the integument of all vertebrates. The specific type present depends on the synthetic process of the chromatophores. The chromatophore that synthesizes *melanin*, the predominant vertebrate pigment, is referred to as a *melanophore* and is located in both the epidermis and dermis of at least some member of each class of vertebrates. The skin color of man depends on the presence and amount of melanin deposited in the epidermal layers. Melanin granules vary in color from yellow through orange and reddish brown to dark brown, depending on their state of oxidation. Melanin also may be present as reduced leukoform, a bleached form. Thus it acts as an oxidation-reduction indicator; in its oxidized form melanin is dark, in the reduced state it is bleached.

Although the *epidermis* contains only melanophores, other types of chromatophores are present in the *dermis*. These cells may originate from a common cell type and differentiate into the various chromatophores according to the specific environmental stimuli they receive. *Iridophores* are described as reflecting cells that contain guanine, hypoxanthine, adenine, or a combination thereof. They are present in anamniotes and

the iris of some birds, but are usually absent from the integument of birds and mammals (Hadley, 1972). *Xanthophores* responsible for the secretion of yellow pigment, and *erythrophores*, containing red pigment, are usually found only in the dermis of elasmobranchs, teleosts, amphibians, and reptiles. Vertebrate color changes result when these different chromatophores interact.

The modern history of pigmentation shows that coloration in vertebrates is the result of interaction not only between pigment-containing cells, but also between these cells and other cells of the skin, such as the cells responsible for forming keratin. This interrelationship can be demonstrated in the human skin. The neural crest cells destined to form melanocytes take up a position at the interface between epidermis and dermis. They extend their branches between the basal cells of the germinativum layer and discharge their pigments into the keratinocytes. Pigmentation of the mammalian epidermis, therefore, is not caused by the melanocyte acting alone, but is the result of an interrelationship between the melanocyte and an associated group of keratinocytes, forming the *epidermal melanin unit*. These units, established during development, are the result of tissue interaction. According to Quevedo (1972) the melanocytes in man exist in a ratio of one to 36 keratinocytes. The maintenance of such a relationship suggests a precise control over mitotic activity.

The melanocytes contain tyrosinase, an enzyme that produces melanin by oxidation of the amino acid, tyrosine. Melanocytes are the only cells capable of synthesizing this material. The pigment is deposited in the cytoplasm within a membrane-bound organelle, the melanosome. Melanin is then transferred to the keratinocytes when these cells phagocytize pieces of the melanocyte dendrites containing the melanosomes. The pigment-containing organelle is transported, and ultimately shed, along with the cornified cells, or catabolized along the way by the keratinocytes.

There is significant variation in the number of melanocytes with regard to sex or race. Skin color, therefore, appears to depend upon the activity of the pigment cell rather than the number of cells present. This activity, in turn, is genetically determined.

Similar units located in the dermis, called *dermal chromatophore units,* are described for poikilothermic animals (Taylor and Bagnara, 1972). The basic types of chromatophores, previously described for poikilothermic vertebrates, are arranged in such a way in the amphibian that the xanthophores are situated in a top layer, the melanophores form a basal layer, and the iridophores are located in one or more rows in the middle. The dendritic arms of the melanocyte entwine about and between the layers above them. When the frog adapts to a dark background, melanosomes migrate to these dendrites of the melanophores, thus obscuring the other chromatophore types and causing the skin to darken. Migration of the melanosomes out of the dendrites to a more central location exposes the xanthophores and iridophores, causing the animal to lighten.

SUGGESTED READINGS

1. Bell, E.: The skin. In DeHaan, R. L., and Ursprung, H., (editors): Organogenesis, New York, 1965, Holt, Rinehart & Winston.
2. Flaxman, A. B.: Cell differentiation and its control in the vertebrate epidermis, Am. Zool. **12**:13-25, 1972.
3. Hadley, M. E.: Functional significance of vertebrate integumental pigmentaton, Am. Zool. **12**:63-76, 1972.
4. McLaoughlen, C. B.: Mesenchymal influences on epithelial differentiation, Symp. Soc. Exp. Biol. **17**: 359-388, 1963.
5. Modell, W.: Horns and antler, 1969, Readings from Scientific American, Vertebrate structures and functions, San Francisco, 1973, W. H. Freeman & Co.
6. Patt, D. I., and Patt, G. R.: Comparative vertebrate histology, New York, 1969, Harper & Row.
7. Quay, W. B.: Integument and the environment: Glandular composition, function, and evolution, Am. Zool. **12**:95-108, 1972.
8. Quevedo, W. C.: Epidermal melanin units: Melanocyte-keratinocyte interaction, Am. Zool. **12**:35-41, 1972.
9. Rawles, M. E.: Skin and its derivatives. In Willier, B. H., Weiss, P. A., and Hamburger, V. (editors): Analysis of Development, New York, 1955, W. B. Saunders & Co.
10. Taylor, J. D., and Batnara, J. T.: Dermal chromatophores, Am. Zool. **12**:95-108, 1972.

CHAPTER 11

SENSE ORGANS

If an animal is to survive successfully, it must be responsive to the condition of both its internal and external environments and to any changes that occur in them. In the primitive, one-celled animal, this information is easily made known to the active part of the organism, since all cells possess irritability. However, communication between various parts of the multicellular animal becomes more of a problem. As the result of neurulation, the central nervous system (the brain and spinal cord) moves from the surface of the animal to the interior, and the neural crest cells that form the ganglia of the sensory nerves end up in proximity to the brain and the cord. The epidermal ectoderm develops into an integument that covers, insulates, and protects the individual. The central nervous system, therefore, usually cannot be directly stimulated by any change that goes on in or around the organism.

A sensory receptor system evolved in the multicellular vertebrate that detects changes in the internal or external environment and transmits the information to the central coordinating areas. These areas, in turn, send appropriate instructions for action to muscles, glands, and organs. If a prompt reaction is necessary to remedy a temporary situation, the message to react is usually sent through the proper nerve to the muscles. On the other hand, if the body needs a slower more generalized adjustment to some situation, the endocrine system functions in producing the response. In general, sense organs are associated with the nervous system.

Sensory receptors are hypersensitive, intermediary structures, located between the environment and central nervous system, that receive and respond to stimuli. They are usually specialized cells that are sensitive to specific chemical or physical stimuli and are associated with nerves that relay the information to the central nervous system. Each receptor responds to one particular kind of stimulus, and depending on the nature of the stimulus, receptors are classified as *photoreceptors* (those that respond to visible radiation), *chemoreceptors* (those sensitive to dissolved chemical materials), *mechanoreceptors* (those stimulated by touch or pressure), *thermoreceptors* (those that react to temperature), *statoreceptors* (those stimulated by changes in body position), and *phonoreceptors* (those stimulated by vibrations).

The sensory receptors develop from ectoderm and their origin may be traced to epidermal ectoderm, neural ectoderm, or neural crest cells. In some instances, a combination of ectodermal types compose the sense organ; often mesoderm, in the form of connective tissue capsules, combines with the ectodermal cell. The receptors are associated with the somatic sensory and visceral sensory nerves. The somatic sensory nerves carry impulses from the cutaneous surface and muscles of the body wall to the central nervous system; visceral sensory nerves relay impulses from the viscera.

The higher centers of the brain interpret the impulses as *sensations* and the individual experiences cold, pain, warmth, sight, sound, etc. The receptors do not perceive anything; they merely refer information to the nervous system where it is sorted and integrated. Obviously most of our insight into sensation is based on man's *reaction* to stimuli, since there is no way of knowing whether the toad or the dog possesses similar sensations. There may be many sensations experienced by lower animals that man is unable to comprehend and, therefore, he has no way of knowing about them. The fact that similar structures (the eye, for example) originate in all vertebrate embryos in a similar manner and that they give rise to organs that are anatomically similar in the adult leads biologists to believe that some sensations, at least, are shared by both lower and higher animals.

Those receptors located over the general body are referred to as the *general sensory organs*, although in some cases bare fibers serve as the receptors and the term "organ" is applied from general use. Other receptors concentrate only in special areas of the body and react to very specific stimuli. They are known as the *organs of special senses:* the organs of olfaction, sight, hearing, and equilibrium.

We classify sense organs according to their morphology and usually recognize at least three levels of organization. These levels also reflect their evolutionary status, as shown in Fig. 11-1. At the simplest level, the epithelial cell, located

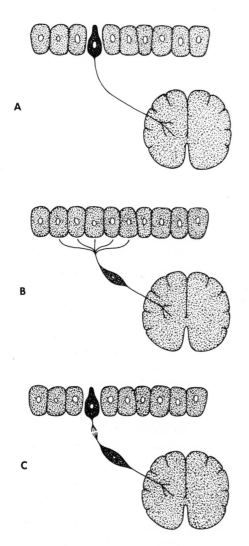

Fig. 11-1

Sense organs can be classified according to their morphological types and levels of organization. At the simplest level, **A,** the epithelial cell serves as both receptor of stimuli and conductor of impulse. At the second level, **B,** the body of the cell migrates inward and cell processes react to the stimuli and transmit information. A second cell is inserted at the surface in the third level, **C,** and reacts to stimuli, passing the impulse on to the nerve cell.

at the surface of the animal, serves as both receptor of stimuli and conductor of nerve impulses. At the second level, the cell body migrates inward and the modified cell processes react to the stimulus and transmit the information. In the third type of organization, a second cell, inserted in the pathway and located at the surface of the animal, reacts to the stimulus. The generated impulse passes to the nerve cell, which, in turn, transmits it to the brain.

Some organs are classified according to their functions. *Exteroreceptors* are those receptors that receive information about the external environment; *proprioceptors* are those located in the striated muscles and tendons. *Interoceptors* are associated with internal organs.

GENERAL SENSORY ORGANS

The receptors composing the general sense organs are less sensitive to stimuli than those of special senses. They react to touch, pressure, pain, temperature, position, movement, and the viscera. A variety of these stimuli apparently produce the sensation of pain. The most primitive type of sensory cell, found primarily in invertebrates, consists of a modified ectoderm cell located in the superficial layers with long pro-

cesses extending inward. The vertebrate's olfactory organs (which we shall discuss under the topic of special sense organs) consist of such a simple arrangement. In general, the cell bodies of the general sensory organs do not remain in the superficial ectoderm of the organism but move inward and become associated with the brain and spinal cord. They belong to the second level of organization mentioned above. These cells differentiate from neural crest cells that were brought in at the time the neural tube formed. The cell bodies collect in clusters (ganglia) outside the brain and cord and send processes into the central nervous system as well as to the integument of the organism. These distal processes, modified during evolution, provide a variety of nerve endings usually classified as *free (nonencapsulated)* or *encapsulated*.

The free type of nerve ending occurs when the peripheral process of the sensory nerve merely ends in a spray of terminal, nonmyelinated, slender twigs or knoblike swellings, as shown in Fig. 11-2. This type of sensory cell is distributed abundantly over the entire body, and its fibrils entwine or embed in epithelial cells, connective tissue, muscle, or serous membranes. The fibrils terminate in the epithelium of the

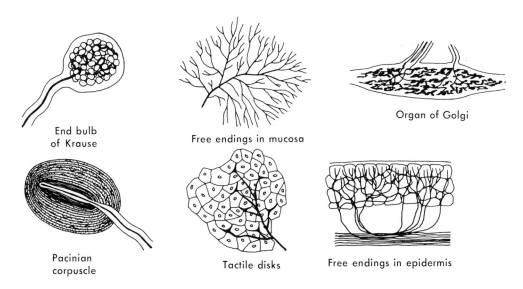

End bulb
of Krause

Free endings in mucosa

Organ of Golgi

Pacinian
corpuscle

Tactile disks

Free endings in epidermis

Fig. 11-2
Examples of encapsulated and (nonencapsulated) free nerve endings.

cornea, oral cavity, respiratory passages, and skin of all vertebrates. They also appear among the fibers of the connective tissue of the dermis, periosteum, blood vessels, and individual muscle fibers, to name a few examples. Properly stained histologic sections of the integument show this type of free ending to penetrate the skin as far as the stratum germinativum layer. Sections through the bronchial epithelium, on the other hand, reveal branches of the nerve wrapped around the cell, with the ends of the fiber actually pushing to the surface. Pain endings are of this type. The sense of touch appears to depend on stimulation of similar endings. For example, nerve endings in hair follicles are important tactile organs. The sensory fibers divide and form a meshlike ending around the hair shaft. Any pressure sufficient to move the hair shaft also stimulates the nerve and adds to the sensitivity of touch.

The epithelial cells associated with the nerve endings are generally similar to one another although they differ in some cases. The tactile cell is an example of an epithelial cell that varies in staining properties from its neighbor. This specialized epithelial cell, together with the arborization of its nerve endings, is known as a *tactile corpuscle of Merkel* and is located in the deeper epithelial layers of the skin. Other modified epithelial cells, the *neuroepithelial cells* or *neuromasts,* receive the termination of a special sensory nerve. The nerve fiber forms a net around one of these cells and receives the impulse transferred from it. The neuroepithelial cells of the taste buds, the hair cells of the organ of Corti, and the cristae and maculae of the inner ear are

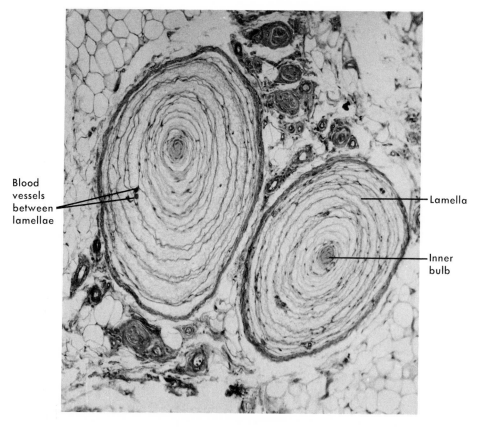

Blood vessels between lamellae

Lamella

Inner bulb

Fig. 11-3
Cross section through two pacinian corpuscles demonstrating the lamellar connective tissue wrapping. The corpuscles are examples of encapsulated nerve endings sensitive to mechanical pressure. (× 100.)

examples of this type of modified epithelial cell that is associated with free nerve endings.

When amniotes moved to land, the sensory endings became encapsulated, apparently so that there is a protective adaptation to terrestrial life. The encapsulated endings of the sensory nerve fibers are all similar in that each consists of a terminal nerve ending wrapped with connective tissue. Such structures as the tactile corpuscles of Meisner (touch), end bulbs (temperature), Pacinian corpuscle (tension and pressure), and neuromuscular and muscular-tendon bundles (tension and stretch) are examples of encapsulated nerve endings. They differ from one another in the degree of branching of the nerve, the number of supporting cells present (connective tissue), and the size and shape of the structure. The terminal nerve endings that pass to skeletal muscles and tendons, for example, entwine around a muscle fiber that is encased in a connective tissue capsule. When the muscle fiber stretches, it stimulates the nerve fiber, revealing the position of the body and its parts to the organism. In some instances the connective tissue wrapping around the ends of the nerve is so extensive that the structure can be seen with the naked eye (Pacinian corpuscle) Fig. 11-3.

ORGANS OF SPECIAL SENSES
Organs of taste

The *taste buds* develop from modified epithelial cells, the neuromasts, mentioned earlier in the chapter. In fish, these cells are distributed over the surface of the body and are innervated by extensions of the cranial nerves. Taste buds are also found buried in the epithelium of the gill rakers and gill arches as well as in the mouth and pharynx of fishes. Materials dissolved in the water stimulate the exposed ends of the cells; taste buds therefore are examples of chemoreceptors that are stimulated by substances at close range rather than at a distance. During their evolution, taste buds lost their generalized distribution over the body of the animal and became localized in special areas. In terrestrial animals they are usually restricted to the tongue, although they may also be present in the palate and pharynx.

The taste buds are usually associated with small elevations of the tongue epithelium, known as *papillae*. Trenchlike depressions separate one papilla from another, and the taste buds are located in the walls of these trenches (Fig. 13-2). The taste buds of man can discriminate between only four taste sensations: acid, bitter, salty, and sweet. All other "tastes" are actually olfactory sensations. Fish are believed to discriminate between these same four tastes, but amphibians show no response to substances classified as sweet or bitter. The horny tongues of birds lack taste buds.

Histologically, the epithelial cell differentiates into two types of cells, a *gustatory receptor* cell (neuromast) and a *sustentacular*, or supporting cell. A chemically sensitive hairlike process projects from the apical surface of the elongated neuromast. In mammals, clusters of neuromast cells group together with their supporting cells to form a taste bud, as shown in Fig. 11-4. The number of neuromast cells composing a taste bud varies. The supporting cells are interspersed among the neuromast cells and also surround them like staves of a barrel. The hairlike process of each neuromast is in contact with the surface of the epithelium by way of a taste pore.

Nerve fibers that break up into a basketlike arrangement of telodendria (nerve endings) surround the deep ends of the neuromast cells. The cell membrane of the nerve ending is in direct contact with the cell membrane of the neuromast cell. Consequently, when the neuromast cell responds to chemical stimulation, the physiologic changes activate the nerve endings. The nerve then relays the impulse to the central nervous system. Taste buds of all vertebrates are supplied with branches of the eighth, ninth, and tenth cranial nerves. Since these nerves contain visceral sensory fibers, the gustatory organs are considered special visceral receptors. Presumably as a result of the chemical stimulation, the primitive animal moved toward or away from such objects as food, enemies, or a mate.

Organs derived from placodes

Although most of the epidermal (ectoderm) covering of the embryo develops into the epidermis and epidermal derivatives, a number of

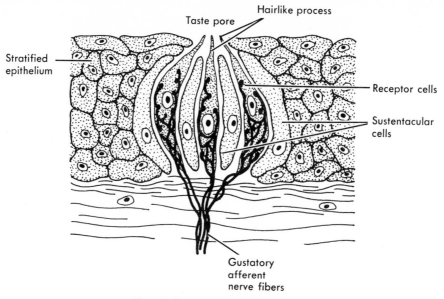

Fig. 11-4
Microscopic structure of taste bud.

other structures are derived from it. Many of these structures begin their development in the form of *placodes,* plate-shaped thickenings in the epidermal ectoderm. In the early neurula stage the placodes are arranged in an almost continuous horseshoe-shaped swelling around the open cranial neural folds. In most cases the initiation and further development of the placodes depends on induction by the tissues beneath it.

By the time the neural fold closes, the generalized swelling becomes identified as contributing to a specific sense organ. The thickened epidermal ectoderm located anterior to the neural plate (nasal placodes) is stimulated to form olfactory sacs. The optic vesicle contacts the epidermis and induces it to thicken *(lens placode)* and develop into the lens of the eye. An *auditory placode* located laterally to the hind brain gives rise to the ear. A *lateral-line placode* associated with the auditory placode becomes the lateral line sense organs of aquatic animals. Several placodes give rise to the cranial ganglia. These contribute to the fifth and seventh to tenth cranial nerves and are described in Chapter 12.

Olfactory organ

The olfactory or nasal placodes of all vertebrates first appear as oval thickenings on the ventrolateral surfaces of the head of the embryo, anterior to that part of the closed neural tube destined to become the brain (Fig. 11-5). With the exception of the cyclostome, which has a single nasal pouch, the olfactory placodes are bilaterally arranged. They appear in the human embryo as early as the fourth week of gestation. The cells composing the central part of the placode sink inward to form the *olfactory pit;* the walls of the pit soon thicken to become the *olfactory sac.* The opening of the sac to the outside is called the *external naris.*

Some of the cells in the wall of the olfactory sac differentiate into sensory cells. These take the form of rodlike projections ending in sensitive brushes extending to the surface. Processes develop on the proximal end of each cell (end closest to the brain) and grow into that part of the forebrain destined to become the *olfactory bulb.* In the bulb the processes (axons) synapse with the mitral cells, which carry the impulse via the olfactory tracts to the appropriate center in the brain. These processes of the nasal epithelial cells leading from the sac to the telencephalon make up the first cranial nerve, the *olfactory nerve.* Most nerves develop either from the brain itself or from ganglia that are associated with the brain or cord. The olfactory nerve

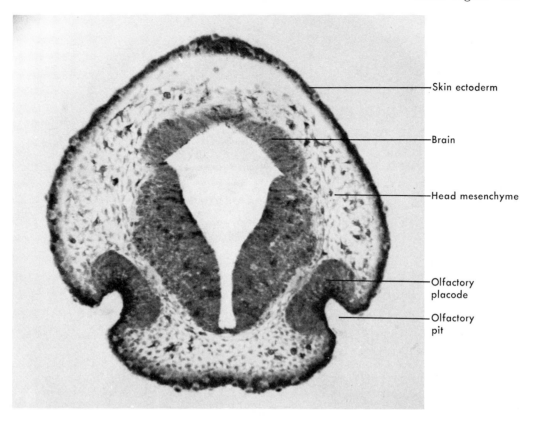

Skin ectoderm

Brain

Head mesenchyme

Olfactory placode

Olfactory pit

Fig. 11-5
Section through head of 5 mm. tadpole at level of olfactory placodes. (× 100.)

is an exception. It does not develop from nervous tissue at all but from the epithelium of the nasal sacs. It is, therefore, not considered a typical cranial nerve.

In most fishes the olfactory sacs of the embryo develop into similar adult structures. Their primary function is an important one since they act as distance receptors informing the organism of the presence of food some distance away. The olfactory receptors are good examples of exteroreceptors. The sacs remain as a pair of pockets in the fish without any communication with the mouth. Each pocket is usually divided into two openings. The water with its dissolved chemical substances flows in one side of the nasal pocket and out the other side. The mucosa of the sac consists of many folds of columnar epithelium thereby increasing its surface area. As the water passes over the sensory end brushes, the dis-

solved chemicals stimulate the nasal epithelial cells. The proximal processes of the cells conduct the generated impulse to the brain.

The olfactory organ increases in complexity in the Crossopterygii and in the tetrapods. The olfactory sacs in these animals are no longer blind pouches but communicate with the oral cavity by way of an opening, the *internal naris,* or *choana.* Fig. 11-6 is a cross section of a 10 mm. frog showing the internal naris opening into the mouth cavity. In these animals the nose is also involved in breathing. In the amphibians the nasal sac is a simple elongated structure that opens into the anterior region of the roof of the mouth and functions both on land and in the water. On land it becomes filled with air and special mucous glands keep the epithelial cells moist and capable of functioning. The sensory epithelium of the fish was thrown into folds. In

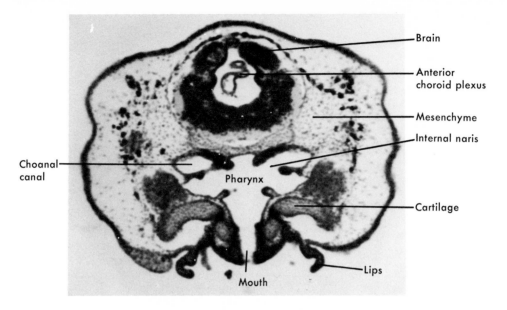

Fig. 11-6
Section through head of 10 mm. tadpole showing internal nares opening into mouth cavity. (× 100.)

contrast, the olfactory pouch of the amphibian is smooth, and only part of its surface contains the sensory cells.

The nasal organs of reptiles and birds are more complex. Although birds retain the reptilian plan of nasal structure, their olfactory organs are of modest size. Birds rely more on their eyes than on their sense of smell to learn about their environment. The olfactory sac divides into two main regions—a small anterior *vestibule* into which the air passes from the external naris, and a larger olfactory chamber opening into the oral cavity by an internal naris more posteriorly placed than in the amphibian. Only the dorsal area of the olfactory chamber contains sensory cells. This sensory epithelium covers the curved, lateral ridges known as the *conchae*, which increase the surface of this area. The walls of most of the chamber, however, function as an air passage and are free of sensory epithelium.

The nasal structures of most mammals increase in size and may occupy as much as half of the skull space (dog). As in the reptile, the olfactory area divides into a dorsal sensory area and a nonsensory air passage. The development of a secondary roof to the oral area, the secondary

and soft palates, moves the openings of the internal nares more posteriorly in the mouth. The chonchae, formed from coiled scrolls of the ethmoid, maxilla, and nasal bones, are highly developed and covered with sensory epithelium (see Fig. 15-15). The incoming air passes through the scrolls and is warmed and filtered in the process. The nasal cavities of eutherian mammals also communicate with cavities (sinuses) of adjacent bones, lightening the skull.

Except for some mammals, turtles, and crocodiles, a second sensory area appears in tetrapods, the *vomeronasal organ*, or *organ of Jacobson*. It forms from another part of the olfactory sac that retains its sensory function. It detects olfactory sensations from the food in the mouth. This "organ" is either a groove covered with olfactory epithelium, or else it exists as a separate pocket. In either case, it usually communicates with the oral cavity by way of the internal naris. Jacobson's organ is particularly well-developed in reptiles. It may consist of a medioventral, club-shaped pouch whose opening into the oral cavity is associated with the internal naris, or it may exist as a completely separated pouch with its own opening. In lizards and snakes, the cleft, flicking tongue also serves as an olfactory organ.

Sense organs **227**

When drawn into the mouth, the tips of the tongue are inserted into the vormeronasal pocket. Chemical particles adhering to their surface pass into solution and stimulate the sensory epithelium of the pocket. The pouch is absent in primates but is present in other mammals as a functional structure.

Acousticolateralis placodes

A lateral series of placodes, located on either side of the neural tissues of the head, develop into the lateral-line system in fishes and aquatic stages of amphibians. The cells composing this system in modern vertebrates are sensitive to mechnical stimulation. Apparently they evolved from the neuroepithelial cell (neuromast) considered common in ancestral types. A group of stereocilia and a long motile cilium extend from the apex of this nucleated, columnar cell as shown in Fig. 11-7. These processes are embedded in a knoblike mass of gelatinous material, the cupula, which adheres to the cell and is secreted by it. The terminal endings of the associated neurons wrap around the neuromast and receive

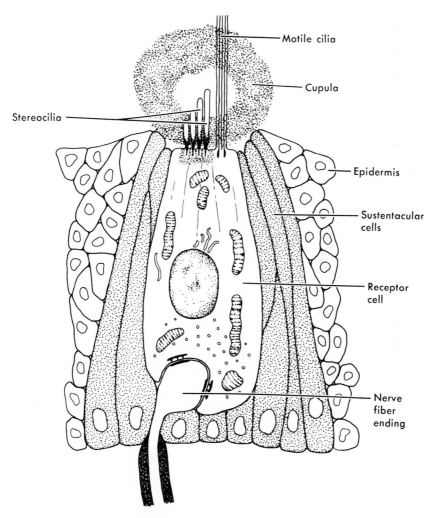

Fig. 11-7
Diagram of structure of neuromast.

the impulse of the stimulated receptor cell. Although some neuromast cells respond to chemical and thermal stimuli, they are considered primarily mechanical receptors in the acousticolateralis system, sensitive to the shearing forces that affect the stereocilia and cilia. Both the lateral-line organs and inner ear contain these mechanoreceptors. The inner ear, present in all vertebrates, presumably evolved from the acousticolateralis system of its ancestors.

LATERAL-LINE SYSTEM. The lateral-line system responds to pressure changes in the surrounding medium of fish and amphibians. Animals above them on the evolutionary scale, the amniotes, lack lateral lines. Even those reptiles and mammals that returned to the aquatic environment did not retain the system. The lateral-line receptors consist of clusters of neuromast cells located in pits or grooves that run in a definite line in the epidermis from head to tail. The pits open to the surface or communicate with one another under the surface through canals. The canals open to the outside by pores that pierce the scales. The cupula waves freely in the water of the pit or groove and stimulates the hairlike processes of the neuromast cells. The cilium is located on the apical end of the sensory cell at the periphery of a patch of stereocilia.

Apparently the lateral-line organs enable the organism to distinguish the direction of mechanical stimulation, that is, turbulence, vibration, or disturbances in the water. Lateral-line stimulation makes the fish aware of prey, enemies, or navigational obstructions.

The lateral-line placodes are associated with three of the cranial nerves: the seventh (facial), ninth (glossopharyngeal), and tenth (vagus). Specific nerves innervate different areas of the lateral line. The head canals become associated with the seventh cranial nerve and the temporal region with the ninth nerve. The vagus (tenth) sends fibers to the occipital region and forms a stout trunk that accompanies the lateral line down the length of the animal's body.

EAR. The mammalian ear is composed of three regions: *external ear, middle ear,* and *inner ear.* All vertebrates have inner ears, but the middle and external ears are relatively recent additions. The middle ear first appears in the amphibians and is an adaptation to aerial living. As the animal changed from an aquatic to a terrestrial existence, one of the gill pouches became the middle ear chamber and one of the bones of the gill apparatus became adapted to transmit vibrations from the outside to the receptors of the inner ear. The external ear merely collects and directs sounds to the middle ear where they are magnified. Some reptiles have an external ear, but it is most developed in the mammals.

Embryologic development of the inner ear suggests that it evolved from that part of the lateral line innervated by the eighth cranial nerve. The otic placodes located in the epidermis lateral to the hindbrain (rhombencephalon), on each side of the head, arise in much the same manner as other components of the lateral-line organs. The epidermis thickens to form a plate; it sinks more deeply into the loose mesenchyme cells of the head region than do the lateral-line placodes and becomes the otic sac. It may or may not retain its connection with the surface. The development of the inner ear of the bony fish is an exception. In these animals a solid plate of cells on the inner surface of the epidermis sinks downward and later becomes hollowed out.

Although the exact mechanism varies with the species, the otic sac is converted into the *otic vesicle,* or *otocyst.* This completely closed structure differentiates into the inner ear, composed of the organ of equilibrium and the organ of hearing. In the fish the organ of hearing is underdeveloped and the ear functions primarily in equilibrium. Since olfactory function was of primary importance in the primitive animal, auditory function in the ancestral vertebrates was perhaps of little value and may have been completely absent. However, the ability of the ear to function as an organ of equilibrium is more fundamental and remains relatively unchanged from fish to man. Hearing becomes an important part of the sensory system at the tetrapod level and increases in complexity as the evolutionary scale is ascended. The saccule of the fish, for example, is only a small structure, whereas in man the lagena, or organ of hearing, develops from its posterior end.

Neuroblast cells differentiate from the otic vesicle and form a club-shaped mass on the

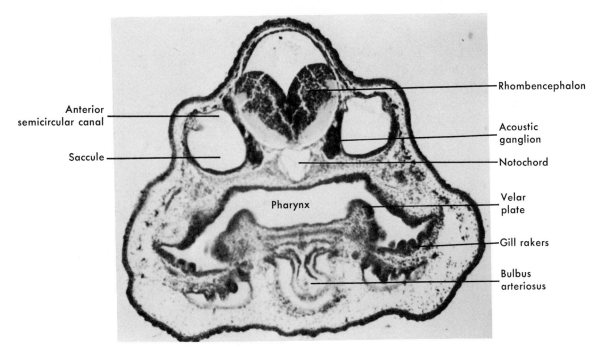

Fig. 11-8
Section through 10 mm. frog showing club-shaped acoustic ganglion. (× 100.)

medial wall (as shown in Fig. 11-8). These cells are destined to become the acoustic, or auditory, ganglion. Processes develop on the cells of the ganglion and penetrate the rhombencephalon, giving rise to the root of the eighth nerve. In adult animals this nerve divides into two main branches, the *vestibular nerve,* which passes to the anterior regions of the organ of equilibrium, and the *cochlear nerve,* which services the posterior part of the organ of equilibrium and the cochlea. The fact that neuromast cells provide the sensory receptors for both the lateral-line organs and inner ear offers additional evidence of their close phylogenetic relationship.

Ear as organ of equilibrium. The otic vesicle develops into a pear-shaped structure with the pointed end oriented toward the dorsal surface of the head. The pointed area becomes the *endolymphatic duct;* the expanded portion of the otic vesicle gives rise to the *membranous labyrinth* as demonstrated in Fig. 11-9. The labyrinth undergoes irregular growth and soon divides into two chambers, a dorsal *utricule* connected to a more ventral *saccule* by way of a narrow

sacculoutricular duct. The endolymphatic duct is attached either to this duct or to the saccule. Further expansion and constriction of the utricule give rise to the rudiments of the three *semicircular canals,* first present in the human embryo as early as the sixth week. In the adult of all vertebrates, these rudiments become three distinct canals, each of which is oriented in a different plane (two vertical and one horizontal) and is open at both ends into the utricule. They are referred to as the *anterior, posterior,* and *horizontal semicircular canals.* In lower vertebrates, the saccule forms a pocketlike structure, the *lagena,* at its posterior end. This elongates in reptiles and birds and expands in mammals into the *cochlear* duct. The utricule, saccule, semicircular canals, and lagena compose the inner ear (Fig. 11-10) and should be differentiated from the auxiliary middle- and outer-ear structures, which develop from different primordia.

The thin walls of the membranous labyrinth consist of flat epithelial cells. The medioventral area, however, thickens, and the cells develop

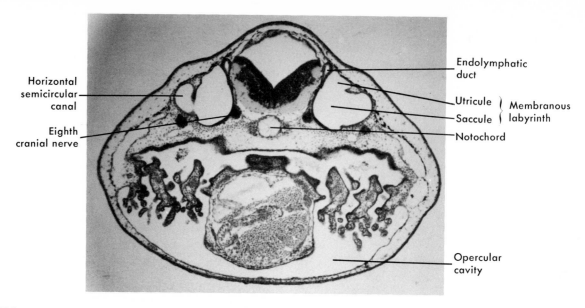

Fig. 11-9

Cross section through 10 mm. frog embryo showing the division of the membranous labyrinth into a dorsal utricle and ventral saccule. The horizontal semicircular canal is beginning to form. (× 4.)

into patches of supporting cells and sensory cells known as the *maculae*. In the adult organ they are distributed in a horizontal plane on the floor of the utricle and in a vertical plane on the inner wall of the saccule. These spots of sensory epithelium, known as the *utricular macula* and *saccular macula*, respectively, are associated with the branches of the auditory nerve. The fibers of this nerve grow between the epithelial cells early in development and arborize about the bases of the sensory cells. Stimulation of these sensory cells offers information about the tilt of the head, and the individual is made aware of static position. An expansion at the end of each semicircular canal, referred to as the *ampulla,* also contains sensory areas, termed *cristae.*

The hollow, irregularly shaped membranous labyrinth, consisting of the utricle, saccule, and semicirular canals, fills with fluid. The *endolymph,* which is more viscous than water, resembles the interstitial fluid. Supporting cells and hair cells with long processes compose the maculae and cristae (the actual receptors for the sense of equilibrium). The hair cells are histologically similar to neuromast cells and respond to pressure or movements of the liquid in which

they reside. The supporting cells are believed to secrete a jellylike substance, the *cupula,* in which the hairlike projections of the sensory cells of the cristae rest. Various concretions (otoliths) or grains of sand are associated with the gelatinous covering of the sensory cells of the macula. As the animal moves about, the weight of the otoliths, which rest on the sensory epithelium, stimulate different hair cells. This stimulation in turn causes an increase in the rate of impulses fired to the central nervous system by way of the vestibular branch of the eighth cranial nerve. The stimulation of these slightly elevated patches of cells furnishes the animal information about its turning movements. The endolymph also surges about in the tiny semicircular canals as the animal changes position, and the movement of the fluid stimulates the sensory hairs of the cristae, providing additional information about the activity of the animal.

As mentioned above, the original placode (induced to form by the rhombencephalon) sinks into the mesenchyme of the head area and gives rise to the otic vesicle. This vesicle develops into the labyrinth. Depending on the species, the mesenchyme (derived from sclerotomes) is in

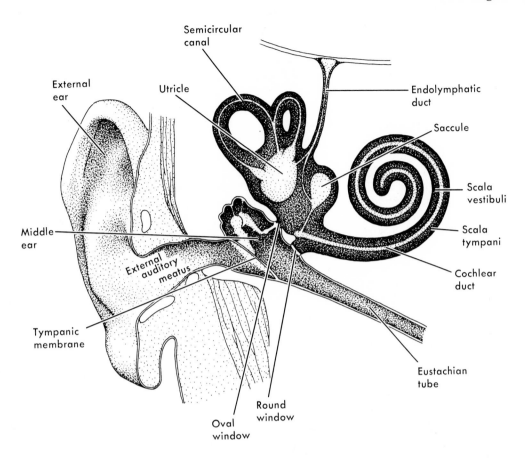

Fig. 11-10
Diagram showing the relationship of the structures of the external, middle, and inner ear.

turn induced by the otic vesicle to differentiate into skeletal tissue. It is of harder texture immediately surrounding the membranous labyrinth than elsewhere and forms a capsule about the ear known as the *cartilaginous* or *osseous labyrinth.* A space exists between the membranous labyrinth (derived from ectoderm) and the osseous labyrinth (composed of mesoderm). It fills with *perilymph,* a fluid very similar to the endolymph of the membranous labyrinth.

Ear as organ of hearing

MIDDLE AND OUTER EAR. The organ of equilibrium remains relatively unchanged in tetrapods, but hearing becomes an important additional sense. How well fishes hear remains a controversial topic, but, in general, investigators believe that the sensory maculae act as possible phonoreceptors. Skeletal structures of the head transmit sound waves from the water to the inner ear of fishes. The air bladder also may function as a transmitter of sound vibrations. However, since air waves are relatively faint, there is a need for some kind of device to amplify the vibrations in land animals. The development of the *middle ear* from the anterior gill pouch (the spiracular gill cleft) occurs in terrestrial animals. This first pharyngeal pouch does not break through to the outside to form a typical gill cleft; instead, it remains as an expanded lateral cavity, the primordium of the *middle ear,* or *tympanic cavity.* The addition of mesoderm to the thin membrane left between the pouch and the anterior ectoderm converts it to the *tympanic membrane,* or eardrum. Since the gill pouches are outpocketings of the pharynx, the internal lining of the tympanic membrane is endoderm. Its outer surface, however, is derived from superficial epidermal ectoderm. The resulting tympanic membrane thins and responds sensitively to air waves. The remnant of the attachment of the gill pouch to the pharynx becomes narrowed and remains as the *eustachian tube.*

Mesenchyme condensations give rise to the primordium of the transmitting apparatus of the middle ear. In amphibians and reptiles a piston-like bone, the columella (which evolved from the hyomandibular bone of fish, to be discussed later), crosses this pouch from the eardrum to a membrane-covered opening in the ear capsule, the *oval window (fenestra ovalis).* One end of the columella (stapes) rests against this membrane. It picks up vibrations received by the eardrum and transfers them internally to the fenestra ovalis. As a result, the liquid of the internal ear is set in motion on the other side of the membrane, stimulating the various sensory spots. A second membrane-covered opening, the *round window (fenestra rotunda),* is located at the other end of the perilymphatic duct (Fig. 11-10). It functions as a release valve. In mammals pressure waves, introduced to the perilymph by the action of the stapes, travel up the scala vestibuli and then across to the scala tympani (dorsal and ventral ducts of the original perilymphatic space) and back toward the middle ear. The membranous fenestra rotunda bulges into the middle ear cavity dissipating the pressure waves.

In mammals, three *auditory ossicles* (malleus, incus, and stapes) replace the columella and lead from the tympanic membrane to the fenestra ovalis (Fig. 11-10). The mammal also adds a cartilaginous *external ear (pinna)* to help collect and concentrate air waves. In many animals, muscles attach to the pinna and move the ear about and orient it in the direction of sound. A short canal, the *external auditory meatus,* leads from the outside to the tympanic membrane. Wax glands are usually present in the walls of this canal.

DEVELOPMENT OF COCHLEAR DUCT. The lagena, present in all vertebrates beginning with the fish, develops in higher animals into the basic structure of hearing, the *cochlear duct* with its *organ of Corti.* The evolution of the cochlea involves the *lagena,* the *perilymphatic duct,* and the *organ of Corti.* The lagena first appears as an endolymphatic papilla in the amphibian saccule. It expands into a long fingerlike extension in the crocodiles and birds, but in mammals it is so long that it must coil in order to fit within the ear capsule. In man, the cochlea makes 2¾ turns. Since the lagena is an extension of the saccule, endolymph also fills its cavity. This duct, formed by the extended lagena, is the *cochlear duct,* or *scala media.*

The *organ of Corti,* named after the Italian anatomist who first described it, is the true receptor organ for the sense of hearing. It extends down the length of the cochlear duct and its cells discriminate the sounds of different pitch. In the human embryo it develops as early as the third month as a local thickening of the floor of the cochlear duct. Between the third and fifth months the epithelial cells differentiate into the hair cells of the organ of Corti and establish the adult structure. The mature structure basically consists of a series of sensory hair cells (neuromast cells) intermingled with supporting cells. A gelatinous membrane, the *tectorial membrane,* extends over them and is in contact with the stereocilia of the hair cells, as shown in Fig. 11-11. This membrane may be compared to the cupula of the neuromast cells previously described as composing the lateral-line sense organs. A basilar membrane, capable of vibrating, forms the floor of the organ. The roof of the cochlear duct (scala media) is known as the *vestibular,* or *Reissner's membrane.*

The *perilymphatic duct* is the name given to the space between the cartilaginous capsule and lagena portions of the membranous labyrinth. It is present in amphibians, reptiles, birds, and mammals. It consists of a well-defined channel that follows one side of the cochlear duct from its origin at the membranous labyrinth to the end of the coil and then turns and follows the other side back. A portion of the perilymphatic duct, therefore, lies above and below the cochlear duct. This relationship of the cochlear duct to the perilymphatic canals can best be seen in a cross section of the duct (Fig. 11-11, *B*).

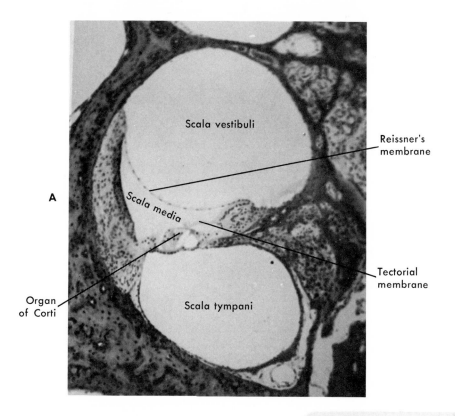

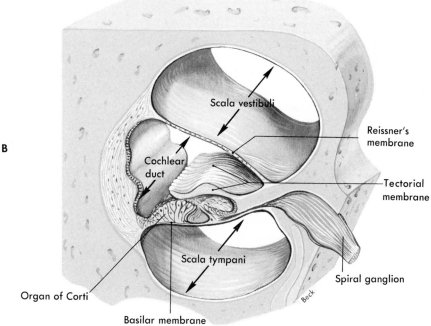

Fig. 11-11
A, Vertical section of the cochlear duct showing the scalae, tectorial membrane, and organ of Corti. (× 100.) **B,** Three-dimensional drawing of a section of one of the cochlear coils aids interpretation of the inner ear structure. (**B,** From Anthony, C. P., and Kolthoff, N. J.: Textbook of Anatomy and physiology, ed. 8, St. Louis, 1971, The C. V. Mosby Co.)

As a result of its relationship with the perilymphatic ducts, three main longitudinal chambers referred to as *scalae* compose the cochlea proper. The upper chamber is the *scala vestibuli* and the lower one is called *scala tympani;* both form from the perilymphatic ducts and fill with perilymph. In between the two chambers is the *scala media,* or cochlear duct, filled with endolymph and the only part derived from the membranous labyrinth. The scala media ends blindly at the apex of the coil, but the scala vestibuli and scala tympani communicate with one another at the apex, the *helicotrema,* through a small junction. They are, therefore, continuous with one another. The cochlear duct is attached to the sides of the bony labyrinth but is surrounded above and below by the perilymphatic ducts. Delicate strands of tissue cross these spaces and help anchor the fragile organ of Corti in place.

In the mammal the external ear directs the sound toward the tympanic membrane. Sound vibrations that impinge on this membrane cause it to vibrate. These vibrations are magnified and transmitted inward by the three auditory ossicles. The stapes vibrates against the fenestra ovalis at the same frequency as the original sound. The ascending scala vestibuli is on the other side of the fenestra ovalis, and a pressure change is produced in the perilymph when the stapes moves the window in and out. Since the perilymph is enclosed by a rigid bony casing and cannot be compressed, as stated above, the membranous fenestra rotunda bulges outward into the middle ear cavity dissipating the pressure.

Pressure changes initiated in the scala vestibuli (when the stapes vibrates against the fenestra ovalis) are believed to travel up the scala vestibuli to its junction with the scala tympani at the helicotrema and then move down this canal. However, many vibrations in the perilymph are transmitted across the membrane separating the scala vestibuli from the cochlear duct. This causes in the cochlear duct a disturbance of the endolymph, which displaces the basilar membrane toward the scala tympani. This displacement (caused by waves in the perilymph) alters the contact of the hair cells with the tectorial membrane. This change in relationship acts as a stimulus for the hair cells.

Terminal branches of the auditory nerve contact the hair cells. Presumably the stimulation of the hair cells is translated into a nerve impulse that passes to the medulla oblongata by way of the cochlear branch of the auditory nerve. Clinical and experimental evidence shows that the regionalization of response by the organ of Corti enables the individual to discern pitch. That part of the organ of Corti closest to the membranous labyrinth discriminates high tones; the receptors for low tones are located near the apex of the duct.

Eye

The eye is an exceedingly complex structure well developed in even the lowest vertebrate group. There are few clues as to how it evolved. It is a sensitive detector of light waves and differs from the other sense organs in that it develops from the wall of the brain. Its basic structure is the same from cyclostomes to mammals, although adaptive modifications allow it to function better in one ecologic niche than in another. It basically consists of a spherical *eyeball,* located in an *orbit,* protected by cartilage or bone, and connected to the brain by an *optic nerve.* The wall of the adult eyeball consists of three concentric coats: an outer *sclera,* a middle *uvea,* and an inner *sensory retina.* The eye also contains a crystalline lens and a transparent *cornea* (anterior portion of the sclera), which focus the light rays on the retina. Three cavities make up most of the eyeball: the *anterior* and *posterior chambers* and the *vitreal cavity,* which contain transparent viscous substances that allow the light rays to pass through to the retina. The eye results from a series of inductions, as pointed out in Chapter 8. It is derived from three main groups of tissues in the embryo. The retina forms from neural ectoderm, the lens develops from epidermal ectoderm, and the tunics of the eye develop from the surrounding mesenchyme.

Early development

Early in development, when the brain is still in the process of differentiation, lateral evaginations from the wall of the forebrain push toward the skin ectoderm. In the human embryo, the evaginations appear as early as the middle of the third week. These protrusions of the brain are the beginning of the *optic vesicles*. They become bulblike at their distal ends, where they are in contact with the surface of the head: each contains a cavity, the *opticoel*, continuous with the cavity of the brain *(prosocoel)*. A constriction soon separates the proximal end of the vesicle from the brain; the resulting connection between the two structures becomes the *optic stalk*, as shown in Fig. 11-12.

The underlying chorda-mesodermal roof induces the optic vesicles to form. As a result of this influence, the eye develops in a step-by-step manner, with specific tissue interactions necessary before the next stage of the development process can proceed. For example, mesenchyme cells must surround the evaginations of the brain for normal development to occur. Also, as the lateral evaginations from the diencephalon expand outward, they must contact the epidermal ectoderm for the retina to differentiate. If no contact is made, the presumptive neural retina becomes pigmented rather than sensory.

When the optic vesicle contacts the epidermal ectoderm, the vesicle flattens and the distal wall invaginates, with obliteration of the opticoel and formation of a double-layered *optic cup*. At first the wall of the optic vesicle is only one cell thick. However, the cells of the indented wall of the optic cup undergo mitosis and become the sensory *retina*, the photosensitive lining of the eye. Pigment granules invade the thin outer layer and form the *pigmented layer* of the retina. It absorbs any light that passes through the retina layer, thereby preventing scattering of the light and blurring of the image. The resulting structure is a double-layered cup attached to the diencephalon of the brain by a narrow, hollow, optic stalk. By the time the eye completes its differentiation, the retina and the pigmented layer fuse and form one layer.

The optic vesicle changes into the optic cup by an invagination that begins at the lower edge of the optic vesicle near the optic stalk and proceeds upward. As a result of the differential invagination, the ventral rim is not as well developed as the rest of the cup and a groove remains, the *choroid fissure*, shown in Fig. 11-13. The indentation that gave rise to the cup continues along the ventral surface of the optic stalk. As a result, during early development of the eye a troughlike structure extends from the ventral rim of the cup toward the brain. The central artery follows the trough of the choroid fissure and enters the optic cup where it is known as the *hyaloid artery*. A network of capillaries forms from the artery around the developing lens. This step appears necessary in the early stages for differentiation of the lens. By birth the hyaloid artery regresses, leaving the *hyaloid canal* in its place in the vitreous body. The edges of the choroid fissure eventually fuse and a small tube forms within the already tubular optic stalk. The central artery and vein remain in this canal and become the main blood vessels of the retina. When the optic nerve forms, the axons of the ganglionic cells converge to the walls of the optic stalk and follow its lumen into the brain. The walls of the optic stalk become the sheath of the optic nerve, enclosing the axons and the central artery and vein as well.

At first the opening of the optic cup is very large, but as development continues, the edges of the cup converge, resulting in a small opening, the pupil. The edges of the cup surrounding the pupil become the *iris*, and the cavity of the optic cup gives rise to the *vitreous body* of the eye, as illustrated in Fig. 11-14. The iris acts as a pigmented diaphragm that regulates the amount of light falling on the retina.

Formation of lens

The general pattern of lens induction is believed to be the same for all vertebrates. As stated in Chapter 8, first endoderm and then mesoderm induces the epidermal ectoderm to form a lens placode. When the lateral protrusions of the brain approach the surface of the embryo during the formation of the optic cup, the retina becomes the third inductor. The underlying nerve ectoderm induces the epidermal ectoderm to thicken into the lens placode and to form a lens. This inductive influence occurs even through porous sheets of material experimentally placed between the two layers

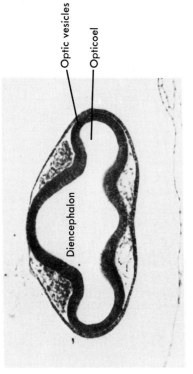

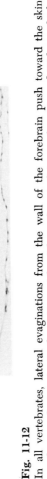

B

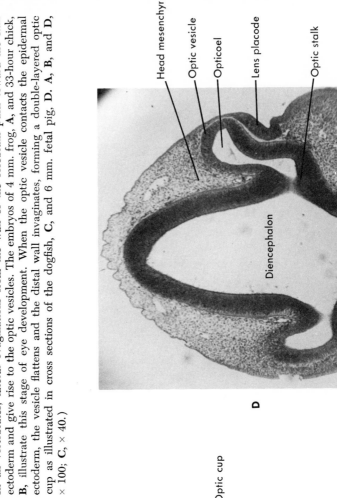

D

Fig. 11-12

In all vertebrates, lateral evaginations from the wall of the forebrain push toward the skin ectoderm and give rise to the optic vesicles. The embryos of 4 mm. frog, **A**, and 33-hour chick, **B**, illustrate this stage of eye development. When the optic vesicle contacts the epidermal ectoderm, the vesicle flattens and the distal wall invaginates, forming a double-layered optic cup as illustrated in cross sections of the dogfish, **C**, and 6 mm. fetal pig, **D**. **A**, **B**, and **D**, × 100; **C**, × 40.)

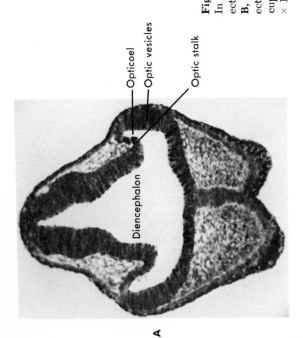

A

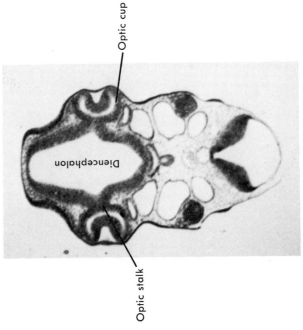

C

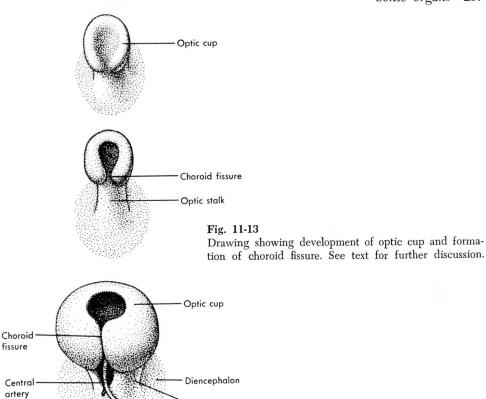

Fig. 11-13

Drawing showing development of optic cup and formation of choroid fissure. See text for further discussion.

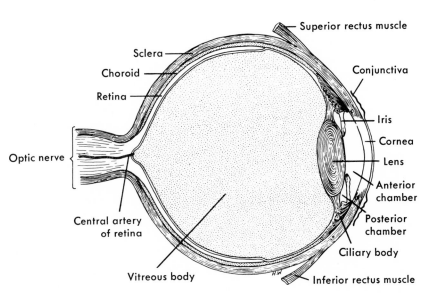

Fig. 11-14

Diagram of sagittal section of eyeball. (From Francis, C. C.: Introduction to human anatomy, ed. 6, St. Louis, 1968, The C. V. Mosby Co.)

of cells. The results of RNA-staining suggest that the optic vesicle changes chemically during the induction process. For example, its cytoplasm becomes less basophilic. At the same time, the presumptive lens ectoderm shows a gain in basophilia, as if "something" were transferred to it.

The influence of the optic vesicle on the epidermis can be further demonstrated by surgical removal of the lens placode. The surrounding epidermal cells move into the empty space and develop into a second lens placode when they come in contact with the optic vesicle. The optic vesicle, therefore, induces other areas of the epidermis to form a lens, and determines the exact position of the lens in relation to the eye cup. If the optic cup is removed, either no lens forms at all or it is defective. This ability of the epidermal ectoderm to respond to the optic cup is a clear example of an induction process and has been extensively studied.

The induced lens placode, under the continued influence of the retina, either bends inward or separates itself as a mass and reassembles to form a lens vesicle. In either case, the lens eventually occupies a position in the pupil of the iris almost filling the optic cup during early development. Once the presumptive lens separates from the overlying ectoderm, it differentiates further. The cells of the inner portion of the lens elongate, lose their nuclei, and transform into longer fibers, arranged in an orderly fashion. The outer layer of the lens becomes its epithelial capsule.

The lens takes its place at the mouth of the cup as a small crystalline structure, capable of either moving forward and backward (in anamniotes) or changing shape (amniotes). This difference in the mechanism of lenticular adjustments is correlated with the kind of adaptations the animal must make to its environment. For example, the ability to change the shape of the lens gives the animal a greater range of focus necessary for aerial vision. In cyclostomes the lens is not attached but the pressure of the vitreous humor and the cornea keeps it in its proper position. In other forms, a ring of fibers holds the periphery of the lens in place. The ability of the eyes to focus light on the retina is known as *accommodation*. It is accomplished, in general, in land animals by the curved surface of the cornea focusing the image on the retina and the lens bringing it into sharp focus. This is not the case in fish. The fish lens has a spherical shape and does most of the work of focusing the image.

Tunics of eye

While the basic structures of the eye differentiate, its accessory structures organize from mesenchyme. These structures are the fibrous and vascular tunics of the eye. The outer fibrous tunic (coat) gives rise to the *sclera* and *cornea*. The sclera is a whitish, tough, fibrous coat that forms a protective covering to the eye and is seen as the white of the eye. It varies in thickness from species to species but must be thick enough to withstand the intraoptic pressure. The adult sclera of some vertebrates is entirely cartilaginous. In several species of fish, birds, and reptiles, sclerotic bones, or ossicles, are embedded in the sclera near the cornea and give additional strength to the tunic. The tendons of the six optic muscles that move the eye attach to the surface of the sclera, and the fibers of the optic nerve perforate its posterior surface at the *lamina cribrosa*.

In the anterior portion of the eye the sclera combines with the epidermal ectoderm to form the transparent, circular cornea. The epidermis overlying the area of the lens and optic cup is induced to form the anterior epithelium of the cornea. Mesenchyme cells condense around the brain, optic stalk, and optic cup. These cells develop into the dura mater of the brain and optic stalk and the sclera of the eyeball. Those mesoderm cells that lie under the epidermal ectoderm (anterior epithelium of the future cornea) become transparent and contribute to the cornea. The cornea, therefore, is a composite structure, derived from both ectoderm and mesoderm.

It is at the corneal surface that much of the refraction of light occurs in terrestrial forms as pointed out above. Irregularities in its curvature bring about an impairment of vision in the human eye known as *astigmatism*. The cornea is an avascular structure, nourished by the secretions of the eye and able to repair itself rapidly if injured. It must be kept moist at all times. The location of many pain receptors in the cornea makes it an extremely sensitive structure.

The *uvea,* the inner tunic of the eye (the middle layer between retina and sclera), is derived from mesoderm and includes the *choroid coat,* the *ciliary body,* and the *iris.* The choroid coat is pigmented and extremely vascular, providing the nourishment for the eye. It contains arteries and veins of various sizes as well as capillaries. It also reflects light back through the retina in several species, a phenomenon that makes their eyes shine in the dark. The area of the choroid coat responsible for such eyeshine is known as *tapetum lucidum.*

The uvea differentiates into the connective tissue of the ciliary body, the fibers of the ciliary muscle, and the connective tissue of the iris. The iris (as well as the ciliary body) has a dual composition. This structure, present in all vertebrates, receives contributions from both the choroid coat and the nonnervous part of the retina. The presence of pigment in this layer is responsible for the color of the eyes. If no pigment is present at all, the blood vessels of the iris give the eye a pink color, characteristic of albino eyes. Blue eyes occur when the pigment is present only in the inner portion of the retinal layer. The colorless tissue covering the iris interferes with light rays in such a manner that the iris appears blue. The presence of dark pigment in both the choroid and retinal layers produces brown or black eyes. However, the eyes of newborn children, even those of the black races, do not reflect their true future color and are blue. The addition of pigment later to the layers of the iris gives rise to its true adult color.

Muscles are present in the iris, arranged in circular and radial patterns. Contraction of these muscles results in decreased pupil size. The iris, therefore, regulates the amount of light that passes to the lens and on to the retina. In dim light, the pupil opens wide, but in bright light it narrows. These muscles of the iris are derived from its retinal portion and are one of the very few examples of a muscle originating from neural ectoderm rather than the usual embryonic source of muscle, the mesoderm.

The ciliary body also receives contributions from the optic cup. It is a ring-shaped structure that encircles the equatorial zone of the lens and is located near the juncture of sclera and cornea. It functions in accommodation and may or may not actually contact the lens. When the muscles of the ciliary body contract in reptiles and birds, processes on the ciliary body push against the lens and cause it to thicken and shorten its focal length. The lens is a very elastic structure in mammals. It is anchored to the ciliary region by certain zonary fibers that hold the lens under tension and, therefore, flat. Contraction of the zonary muscles brings the ciliary body closer to the lens, the fibers relax, and the elastic lens becomes more rounded. This allows the mammal to accommodate for closer objects.

The eyeball consists of a series of cavities filled with transparent liquids of various consistencies. The *anterior chamber* of the eye is the space between the cornea and the iris; the *posterior chamber* is the small area between the iris and the lens. These two cavities are continuous with one another through the pupil. They are filled with a thin watery liquid known as the *aqueous humor* secreted by epithelial components of the ciliary body. This liquid is similar to the blood serum and nourishes the lens, iris, and cornea and produces the turgor of the eyeball. Drainage of the fluid into a series of sinuses that make up the canal of Schlemm, located in the angle of the iris, regulates the intraocular pressure. A thick gelatinous substance known as the *vitreous humor* fills the principal cavity of the eyeball, the space between the lens and the retina. The photosensitive cells of the retina secrete the material during the development of the eye.

Histogenesis of retina

As demonstrated by the manner in which it is formed, the retina is an extension of the brain. The origin of the rods and cones, the two types of cells sensitive to light, can be traced to the ependymal cells of the neural tube and to the presumptive neural ectoderm on the surface of the blastula. A knowledge of their development explains why light must pass through several layers of the adult retina before reaching the neurosensory photoreceptors. These receptors

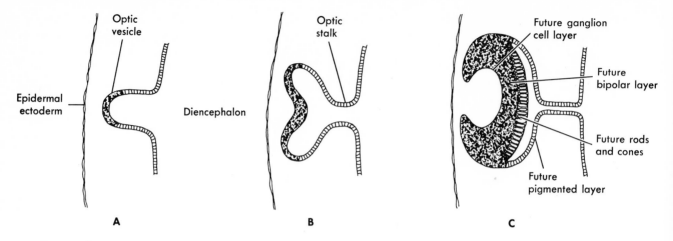

Fig. 11-15

A, Lateral extension of the brain, the optic vesicles, grow outward until they contact the epidermal ectoderm. **B,** Optic vesicles flatten and invaginate, forming the double-walled cuplike structure, the optic cup. **C,** Invaginated layer of optic cup, the future retinal layer, thickens and invaginates until it is adjacent to future pigmented layer. Light must pass through the depth of the retina before it reaches the receptor cells, the rods and cones.

are located in the outermost part of the retina, that layer closest to the choroid coat and farthest from the pupil. In the early embryo the ependymal layer lines the neural cavity. As the optic cup forms, this layer becomes adjacent to the pigmented layer of the cup as shown in Fig. 11-15. As a result, the rods and cones are located away from the surface exposed to the vitreous body and away from the source of light.

Three layers of cells make up the retina of vertebrates as illustrated in Fig. 11-16. Listed in order, the processes of the rod and cone cells are located next to the pigmented cells; the cell bodies of these photoreceptor cells make up the outer nuclear layer. This is followed by the *bipolar neurons,* with the layer of *ganglion cells* situated nearest the vitreous humor. The plexiform layers separate one cell layer from another and consist of cell processes synapsing with one another. The *outer plexiform layer* is the area of synapse between the rods and cones and the bipolar cells; the *inner plexiform layer* consists of the synapses between the bipolar cells and the ganglion cells. The distribution of rods and cones in the vertebrate retina differs among the various species. Nocturnal vertebrates, for example, usually have more rods than cones, and the retina of diurnal vertebrates contains more cones. A depression, known as the *fovea,* often

marks the site of sharpest vision in certain teleosts, birds, and primates.

The rods and cones differ from one another in shape, number, sensitivity to light, and specific visual pigment contained in the receptor. Vertebrate rods are slender, filamentous cells, sensitive to degrees of darkness, are more numerous than cones (at least in the human eye), and contain in their outer segments a specific reddish purple pigment called *rhodopsin.* The cones, on the other hand, are shorter and thicker, are sensitive to color, and contain the visual pigment called *iodopsin.* The visual pigment consists of the protein opsin and a particular configuration of an aldehyde of vitamin A. When stimulated by light, the retinaldehyde is converted to an unstable form.

The impulse generated as a result of this chemical transformation passes on to the processes of the bipolar cell that connect with the rods and cones on one hand and with the associated processes of the ganglion on the other. It appears that several rods can synapse with one bipolar cell. The long processes of the ganglion cell pass to the brain and relay the impulse generated by the light. These long processes (axons), originating on the inner surface of the retina, converge at a common point, penetrate the retina, and continue on to the

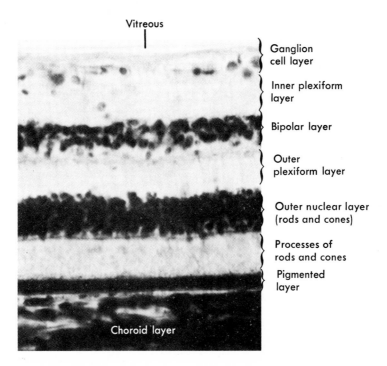

Vitreous

Ganglion cell layer

Inner plexiform layer

Bipolar layer

Outer plexiform layer

Outer nuclear layer (rods and cones)

Processes of rods and cones

Pigmented layer

Choroid layer

Fig. 11-16
Three layers of cells make up the retina of vertebrates (rabbit). (× 450.)

brain in the walls of the optic stalk. They form the optic nerve. As we stated earlier, the eye is an extension of the brain itself; the optic nerve is actually a brain tract that links one part of the brain (the eye) with another. Rods and cones are absent at the point in the retina where the fibers of the ganglion cells leave. Consequently, this point is known as the *blind* spot of the eye.

The optic nerve fibers pass to the floor of the diencephalon and cross to the opposite side of the brain at the X-shaped *optic chiasma*. There is complete *decussation* (crossing of fibers) in all classes except mammals. In these animals, decussation is incomplete and only the fibers from the medial half of the retina cross to the other side. This leaves about one third to one half of the fibers uncrossed in man (Fig. 11-17). This incomplete decussation is associated with the development of *stereoscopic vision*. Physiologists believe that two duplicate mental pictures form in most animals. In mammals, however, the development of stereoscopic vision

enables each brain hemisphere to build up a half-picture of the total image. Interconnections between the two cerebral hemispheres allows the individual to "see" the total picture.

In all nonmammalian vertebrates the optic fibers continue in the walls of the thalamus to the roof of the midbrain (mesencephalon). Here they terminate in the optic lobes of the mesencephalon where the primary visual center is located. When the cerebral hemispheres assume their prominence as a coordinating and association center in mammals, the mesencephalon loses its importance and no longer acts as a visual center. As a result, most of the optic fibers in mammals are no longer sent to the mesencephalon. Instead, the optic impulses in man are shunted from the thalamus to the new visual centers of the cerebral cortex. It is in the cerebrum that the sensation of sight occurs.

Accessory structures of eye

Certain accessory structures protect the eye or aid it in its function. Folds of developing skin,

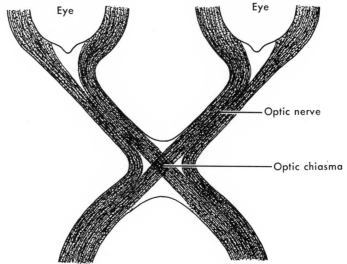

Eye   Eye

Optic nerve

Optic chiasma

Fig. 11-17
Nerve fibers of optic nerve cross to the other side of the brain at the X-shaped optic chiasma. In mammals there is incomplete decussation and about one third to one half of the fibers remain uncrossed. Duplicate images are created on each side of the brain and stereoscopic vision is especially well developed.

consisting of ectoderm and mesoderm, arise above and below the cornea and give rise to the eyelids of tetrapods. Most fish lack a movable eyelid. The blinking of the eyelids of tetrapods keeps the cornea moist and clean and prevents it from becoming dry and opaque. A transparent third eyelid, the *nictitating membrane,* is present in birds and some reptiles and mammals. It passes from the inner angle of the eye to the outer surface. Rows of hairs, the eyelashes and eyebrows, furnish additional protection to the eye.

In land animals, lacrimal glands (tear glands) secrete a watery fluid that keeps the cornea moist and clean and provide nourishment to this avascular structure. Epithelial buds form on the undersurface of the eyelid and during development converge as a group to one area of the eyeball. In most animals, they become branched and form an acinous gland that secretes constantly. A lacrimal duct drains the secretions into the nasal passageway.

SUGGESTED READINGS

1. Coulombre, A. J.: The eye. In DeHaan, R. L., and Ursprung, H. (editors): Organogenesis, New York, 1965, Holt, Rinehart and Winston.
2. Cordier, R.: Sensory cells. In Brachet, J., and Mirsky, A. (editors): The cell, vol. VI, New York, 1964, Academic Press Inc.
3. Patt, D. I., and Patt, G. R.: Comparative vertebrate histology, New York, 1969, Harper & Row, Publishers.
4. Twitty, V.: Eye. In Willier, B. H., Weiss, P. A., and Hamburger, V. (editors): Analysis of development, Philadelphia, 1955, W. B. Saunders Co.
5. Yntema, C. L.: Ear and nose. In Willier, B. H., Weiss, P. A., and Hamburger, V. (editors): Analysis of development, Philadelphia, 1955, W. B. Saunders Co.

CHAPTER 12

NERVOUS SYSTEM

The nervous system is one of the first systems to undergo morphogenetic development. In the adult, along with the endocrine system, the nervous system coordinates the functions of the various organs. It is divided into the *central nervous system* (CNS), composed of the *brain* and *spinal* cord, and the *peripheral nervous system,* consisting of sensory and motor nerves. This division is mainly one of convenience, since both act together as one unit. The central nervous system develops from the neural plate of the late gastrula stage. The peripheral nervous system derives partly from the neural plate, partly from neural crest cells, and partly from the thickened ectodermal areas we have identified as placodes.

The basic structural unit of the nervous system is the nerve cell, or *neuron,* consisting of a *cell body* and its processes, the *dendrites* and *axons.* An intricate network of neuron communications carries out coordinating functions. Individual nerve cells (neurons) generate messages, which they conduct from one part of the body to another by way of their cell processes. These messages are then chemically transmitted to other nerve cells or to other cells of the body.

The analysis and interpretation of these communications and the attempts at describing them in terms of neural mechanisms mark the frontiers of biological investigation in this decade. Many physiologists believe that the complexities of the nervous system will never be comprehended. They believe that man is at the limits of his understanding and that the inadequacies of his brain will prevent him from completely analyzing and explaining its physiology.

Only fragments of behavior have been correlated with their neural mechanisms. Perhaps the simplest reflex, present in all vertebrate animals, is most readily understood. A stimulus produces a quick withdrawal movement and involves what is described as a *reflex arc.* This simplest of reflexes, considered to be a monosynaptic (one neuron in contact with one neuron) reflex action, may actually produce many more side effects in the central nervous system than we previously believed. Some of these effects are only beginning to be identified and described.

Although such a simple reflex arc is possible,

nervous reactions seldom involve only two neuron chains but are considerably more complex than this. Literally, billions of nerve cells make contact with one another, forming a maze of interacting fibers. In an attempt to understand basic nerve circuits, the investigator must seek common properties of neural structure and function. To accomplish these ends, the crayfish, the frog, and the cat have been used extensively in the past as investigative animals. However, at the present time, the research carried out on mammals, including man, exceeds that for all other animals.

DEVELOPMENT OF CENTRAL NERVOUS SYSTEM
Development of neural tube

By the end of neurulation (as discussed in Chapter 7) the neural ectoderm is in the form of a dorsal, hollow neural tube that extends under the surface epithelium of the embryo from its anterior to its posterior end. From the beginning, the neural tube expands in the anterior regions of the body. During gastrulation the notochord assumes a position under the neural plate. As a result of this migration the prechordal plate region lies immediately beneath the presumptive brain areas and the notochordal and somitic mesoderm under the middle and posterior regions. The brain of the organism develops from the expanded anterior region of the neural tube, and the spinal cord develops from the more posterior parts. As a result of further differentiation, induced by the prechordal plate and notochordal and somitic mesoderm, the primary rudiment (the neural tube) gives rise to the central nervous system of the adult.

After the neural tube is established, it undergoes a general organization. At early stages one can distinguish certain concentric layers and longitudinal bands in the walls of both the presumptive brain and neural tube regions. The three concentric layers are (1) an inner layer lining the central canal of the tube, (2) a middle cellular region, the *mantle layer*, and (3) an outer *marginal layer* consisting of fibers from the cells located in the first two layers.

As development continues, the cell bodies located in the mantle layer give a characteristic

configuration to the tube. In transverse section, the cellular (mantle) region appears darker because of the closely packed nuclei and is now referred to as the *gray matter* of the tube. The marginal layer lacks cell bodies and contains fibers wrapped with a white, fatlike material, myelin. This layer becomes the *white matter* of the neural tube. The tube grows in diameter by the proliferation of cells from the inner layer and their migration into the mantle layer, and also by the further deposition of myelin around the fibers.

The primitive neural tube can also be divided into six longitudinal bands. A relatively thin *roof* (roof plate) and *floor* (floor plate) form the dorsal and ventral areas of the tube. Each lateral wall consists of a dorsal *alar plate* and a more ventral and thicker *basal plate*, as shown in Fig. 12-1. Once this basic organization is established, the brain and spinal areas of the cord organize further, both internally and externally, and give rise to the central nervous system unique to the specific organism.

Evidently the neural epithelium at the time of cellular proliferation becomes determined, forming a rather rigid mosaic. Each region of the early neural tube is destined to give rise to a particular functional part of the future cord. For example, removal of the right dorsal half of the neural tube from the chick embryo at 44 hours of incubation results in a normal left side of the spinal cord but the right half is missing (Wenger, 1950).

Regionalization of neural cord

The anterior region of the neural tube soon divides into three major regions usually referred to as the *primary brain vesicles*: the forebrain, midbrain, and hindbrain, better known by their more technical terms as the *prosencephalon, mesencephalon,* and *rhombencephalon,* respectively. These primary vesicles are associated with the three major sense organs. The prosencephalon receives impulses from the olfactory organs, the mesencephalon from the eye, and the rhombencephalon from the ear and lateral-line organs.

The walls of the brain undergo further differentiation (Fig. 12-2) and the prosencephalon soon divides into an anterior *telencephalon* from

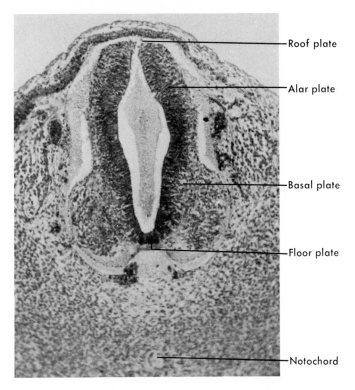

Roof plate
Alar plate
Basal plate
Floor plate
Notochord

Fig. 12-1
Primitive neural tube differentiates into roof, floor, dorsal alar plate, and ventral (thicker) basal plate as shown in this section through 9 mm. human embryo. (× 4.)

which the olfactory lobe and cerebral cortex form, followed by a *diencephalon*, from which the eyes and thalamus develop (Table 12-1). The mesencephalon does not divide further. The rhombencephalon differentiates into the *metencephalon*, which gives rise to the cerebellum and the pons, and the *myelencephalon*, from which the brainstem and upper part of the spinal cord develop. The rest of the tube remains of uniform diameter along its length and is destined to become the spinal cord. As the neural tube develops, it bends and gives rise to the *cephalic* and *cervical flexures* described in Chapter 7. Fig. 12-3 is a sagittal view through the five brain divisions and spinal cord of the chick.

Cavities of brain and spinal cord

The cavity of the neural tube, the *neurocoel*, remains in the adult animal and fills with cerebrospinal fluid. As the brain develops, the original small neurocoel in the telencephalon expands to form the *lateral ventricles* of the future cerebral cortex, *first and second ventricles*. The *third ventricle* is a median cavity located in the diencephalon and is connected to the first two ventricles by the *interventricular foramen,* or *foramen of Monro*. In amniotes a thin passageway (the cerebral aqueduct) in the midbrain connects the third ventricle with the fourth, located in the medulla oblongata. In lower animals the cavity of the mesencephalon remains large, forming the mesocoel. The ventricles of the brain continue into the spinal cord as the small central canal.

Meninges

The skull and neural arches of the vertebrae are laid down around the brain and spinal cord in the embryo. Connective tissue membranes, the *meninges,* wrap intimately around the nervous tissue and offer additional mechanical protection and support for the blood vessels of the central nervous system. The outer membrane is derived from the surrounding mesenchyme; the

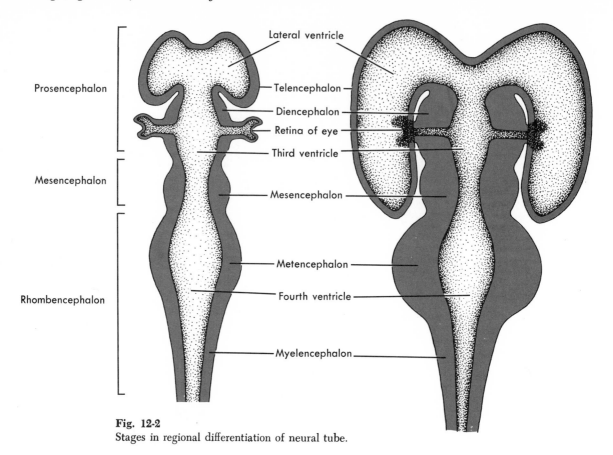

Fig. 12-2
Stages in regional differentiation of neural tube.

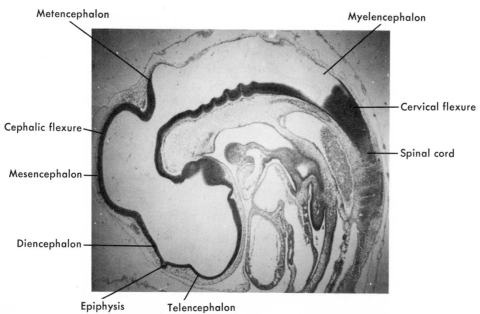

Fig. 12-3
Sagittal section through 72-hour chick embryo showing the 5 brain divisions, spinal cord, and flexures. (× 2).

TABLE 12-1. Development of the neural tube

Primary brain vesicles	Subdivisions	Parts of adult brain	Associated nerves	Summary of evolutionary changes
Prosencephalon	Telencephalon	Rhinencephalon (paleopallium and archipallium) Corpus striata Cerebral cortex	Olfactory (I)	More independent action Shift in gray and white matter Increase in bulk Association centers increase
	Diencephalon	Epithalamus Thalamus Hypothalamus Optic chiasma Tuber cinereum Mammillary bodies Infundibulum		Increase in size because of centers of correlation
Mesencephalon		Tectum (corpora quadrigemina) Tegmentum	Optic (II) Oculomotor (III) Trochlear (IV)	Changes from dominant visual area to tracts leading to cerebrum
Rhombencephalon	Metencephalon	Cerebellum Pons		Development of sensory and motor tracts
	Myelencephalon	Medulla oblongata	Trigeminal (V) Abducens (VI) Facial (VII) Acoustic (VIII) Glossopharyngeal (IX) Vagal (X) Spinal accessory (XI) Hypoglossal (XII)	
Spinal cord		Spinal cord	Peripheral	

inner membrane appears to be composed, at least in part, of neural crest cells.

In fish, only one membrane, the *meninx primitiva*, covers the brain and spinal cord. Fine collagen fibers pass through the meninx to the lining of the brain case. Two membranes are present in amphibians, reptiles, and birds: an outer, tough, connective tissue membrane, the *dura mater*, and an inner, more fragile, vascular, *pia-arachnoid layer*. The *subdural space* separates the two membranes; a second space exists between the dura mater and lining of the braincase, or neural arch.

In mammals, the pia-arachnoid layer divides, and as a result three membranes are present. There is the outer, tough dura mater, a middle *arachnoid layer*, and an *inner pia mater*. The pia mater is intimately applied to the brain and follows its contours (Fig. 12-4). A space, the *subarachnoid* space, separates the pia mater

from the arachnoid and is traversed by delicate fibers that tie the two membranes together. The middle layer, unlike the pia mater, does not dip down into the sulci and fissures of the brain. The outer layer, the dura mater of mammals is closely applied to the lining of the skull, obliterating any space, although in the spinal cord a space continues to exist between this membrane and the lining of the vertebral canal. The dura mater involutes and forms a septum (falx cerebri) that helps to divide the right and left cerebral hemispheres longitudinally. It also contributes to a transverse septum (the tentorium) separating the cerebrum from the cerebellum.

Cerebrospinal fluid fills the ventricles of the brain and central canal of the cord, as well as the spaces traversed by the connective tissue fibers. The fluid has two functions. It carries the nutrients derived from the blood vessels to the tissue of the central nervous system, and it acts

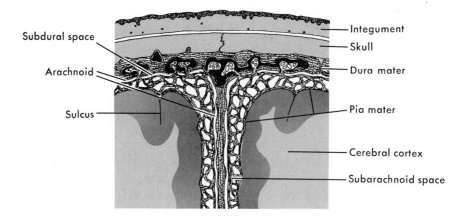

Fig. 12-4
Diagram showing relationship of mammalian meninges to skull and brain.

as a cushion to the brain and spinal cord. The *choroid plexuses,* vascular networks located in the roof of the diencephalon and medulla oblongata, secrete the fluid into the third and fourth ventricles. It flows from the ventricles into the subarachnoid space. Here it makes its way into the lymphoid vessels, or arachnoid villi, that connect with certain large venous sinuses under the dura mater. Since secretion of the cerebral fluid occurs continuously, its removal must also go on constantly in order to maintain a stable intracranial pressure.

Basic embryonic plan

This basic plan of five cranial divisions plus the spinal cord, along with their cavities and connective tissue membranes, make up the primordium of the central nervous system. It forms early in the development of the organism and is similar in all vertebrate embryos at this early stage. It is far more advanced in the simplest vertebrate, the cyclostome, than in any member of the invertebrate phylum.

Although the nervous system is basically the same in the embryo of all vertebrates and it functions in a similar manner in the adult, the increase in complexity from the lowly cyclostome to the mammal is truly outstanding. The growth of the cerebral cortex brings about an increase in coordination and association centers. It is this growth in the cerebral cortex that offers man his great potentialities. According to Romer,

"The evolution of the cerebral hemispheres is the most spectacular story in comparative anatomy."

HISTOGENESIS OF NERVOUS TISSUE

Although the presumptive neural tissue at the blastula and gastrula stages is only one cell thick, by the time the neural tube is established its walls consist of a pseudostratified epithelium composed of columnar cells and rounded cells. These cells attach not only to one another, but also at the lumen of the neural tube by special devices known as terminal bars. Watterson (1965) suggests that this attachment at their terminal ends imposes a radial orientation on the neuroblasts and helps to collect similar cells together. All the cells composing the early neural tube are capable of division. They appear similar to one another, but differentiate along two lines. They give rise to the *neuroblasts* that are destined to form the neurons, or else they form the supporting tissue, the *neuroglia.*

Formation of neuroblasts

When a neuroepithelial cell divides, its nucleus moves (in the cytoplasm of the cell) toward the neural lumen; the cell rounds up and undergoes mitosis. The daughter cells produced at the end of the telophase retain their attachment at the lumen, but they elongate and stretch out away from their point of attachment. Their nuclei then migrate laterally in the cells. This migration of the nuclei within the cells gives the impression that mitosis occurs only at the region of the lumen.

Eventually the embryonic nerve cells (neuroblasts) lose their attachment to the lumen of the neural tube and migrate laterally into a cell-free zone. Eventually, this zone becomes packed with cells, forming the *mantle layer*. Most of the cells that migrate peripherally are in the undifferentiated state, and as they move outward, they differentiate into neurons. However, some of the motor neuroblasts undergo histologic differentiation while still attached to the neuroepithelium; when they migrate, they can be followed with the aid of certain staining techniques. These cells have one process attached to the lumen of the tube and a slender process extending from the other end of the cell. They are known as *bipolar cells*. As differentiation continues, the cells lose their attachment to the lumen and become pear shaped, retaining the more distal process believed to be the *axon* of the future neuron. The cells are now considered to be temporarily *unipolar*. Later, as other branched processes appear on the neuroblasts, they are converted to *multipolar cells* as shown in Fig. 12-5. The axon is destined to conduct impulses to some effector organ. The branched secondary processes responsible for the multipolar state make up the dendritic zone.

As the cells migrate into the mantle layer, they do so at the level of their attachment to the lumen. Consequently groups of like cells gather at certain areas of the neural tube rather than scatter at random throughout its length. Some of these cells in the gray matter become intermediate or *association neurons*. Others, as a result of this grouping tendency, give rise to the motor neurons and end up in close association with one another in the ventrolateral portion of the mantle region. Such an aggregation of cell bodies within the gray matter is defined as a *nucleus*. Therefore, those cell bodies located in the ventrolateral portion of the neural tube compose the *motor nuclei* of the cord. Similar aggregations of cell bodies outside the spinal cord or brain are referred to as *ganglia*.

In the 1800s neural anatomists did not know

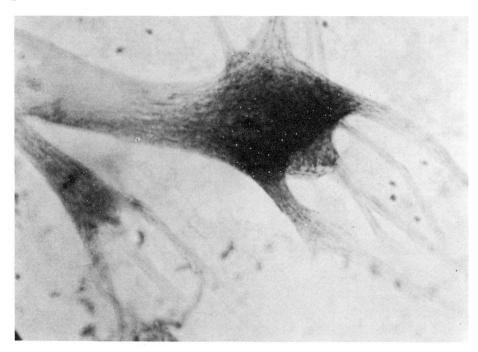

Fig. 12-5
Most numerous type of neuron is the multipolar neuron, characterized by a single axon and several receptor processes. (× 450.)

that the fibers present in nervous tissue, now recognized as dendrites and axons, were a part of the neuron. Most of the information about a neuron came from histologic preparations. Sectioned nervous tissue showed only bits and pieces of the long fibers, often not associated with the nerve cell body. Several theories arose to explain the origin of these fibers. One, acceptable today, suggested that the fiber formed as an outgrowth from a single cell, the neuroblast.

Ross G. Harrison is credited with first demonstrating conclusively that the neuroblast is responsible for forming the nerve fiber. In 1907 he removed fragments of neural tube from frog embryos shortly after the neural tube had formed and cultivated them in an artificial medium containing frog lymph. This was the beginning of tissue culture. He found that the nerve fiber was not something laid down by another cell along preformed pathways because he watched it grow out from the neuroblast as a *cone of growth.* This cytoplasmic projection extended out into a long thread, the axis cylinder, which retained ameboid movement at its cytoplasmic tips.

Differentiation of neuroglia

All the neural epithelial cells in the early neural tube do not form neuroblasts capable of responding irritably to stimuli and conducting impulses. Some of these primitive cells differentiate into the nonnervous supporting, or protective cells, the *neuroglia.* They give rise to the *ependymal cells.* These cells remain located at the neural canal but extend their processes outward for varying distances beyond their cell bodies. Other primitive cells, the *spongioblasts,* develop further and give rise to migrating glial cells that take up a position in the mantle and marginal layers of the neural tube and give stability to the differentiated nervous tissue.

Contributions of neural crest cells

When the neural tube forms, some of the cells are neither included in the walls of the tube nor remain with the epidermal ectoderm. These *neural crest cells* leave their original position dorsal to the newly formed neural tube and migrate laterally on either side between the tube and myotomes. Some of them line up in clusters on either side of the neural tube and give rise to the segmentally arranged *cerebrospinal ganglia,* which are sensory in function, and to the *autonomic ganglia,* which are motor. The segmental presence of myotomes determines the segmental arrangement of the neural crest cells, since the removal of a myotome affects this arrangement. Within the ganglia, the neural crest cells differentiate along two pathways; they either develop into neuroblasts destined to become neurons, or they become interstitial cells surrounding the nerve cells. Fig. 12-6 shows a histologic section through a cerebrospinal ganglion with the small interstitial cells surrounding the larger ganglion cells.

Neurogenesis

Neurogenesis is the process by which neuroblasts differentiate into *neurons,* the definitive nerve cell. It has been estimated that approximately 14 billion of these cells compose the nervous system of man (Bloom and Fawcett, 1968). They are usually classified according to the number of processes they have (that is, unipolar, bipolar, or multipolar) or to the direction in which they conduct impulses. If they conduct impulses toward the cord, they are *sensory,* or *afferent, neurons. Motor,* or *efferent,* neurons conduct impulses away from the cord toward the muscle or gland (effector organ). *Intermediate neurons,* located within the gray matter of the cord, connect the sensory and motor neurons.

The neuron is considered a highly specialized cell. Once the neuroblast becomes specialized, it can no longer divide and give rise to new cells. Since there are no nerve stem cells in the adult animal, apparently an individual possesses at birth most of the nerve cells he will ever have. If the nerve cell body is destroyed, the nerve processes degenerate and are not replaced. However, if the processes are cut and the cell body remains intact, the part distal to the cut degenerates and the part attached to the cell body may regenerate.

Typical neurons

The cell body, or *perikaryon,* of a typical neuron is usually round or oval, but it may take various shapes. Its large, lightly basophilic nu-

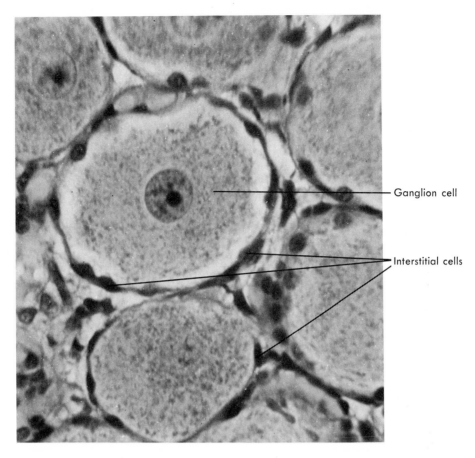

Ganglion cell

Interstitial cells

Fig. 12-6
Section through spinal ganglion showing several neurons surrounded by nuclei of interstitial cells. (× 450.)

cleus contains a single prominent nucleolus. Basal condensations, *Nissl substances,* are present in the cytoplasm of the cell body and dendrites. The electron microscope reveals these substances to be composed of a dense network of endoplasmic reticulum and RNA granules. As we indicated earlier in the text, RNA is usually associated with protein synthesis and its presence in the nerve cell is believed to be related to the turnover of cytoplasmic material in the axon. The mature neuron is in perpetual growth, since the macromolecules of the neuron undergo continuous degradation and must be replaced. Axoplasm is constantly synthesized in the cell body, replenishing the enzyme and structural protein composition of the axon. *Neurofibrils,* cytoplasmic inclusions, are now believed to be artifacts produced in preparing the tissue for histologic

sectioning. However, the *neurofilaments* and *microtubules,* seen in the electron micrographs, are considered part of the cytoplasm, although we do not completely understand their function.

Two types of processes extend from the cell body, the *dendritic* and *axonal* processes. In the past, their identification was based on what was traditionally considered a typical nerve cell, the motor neuron. However, anatomists named the processes one way, neurophysiologists, another way. Today, we realize that no cells in the body differ from one another more than the cells of nervous tissue and that there is no such thing as a typical nerve cell. In an attempt to take into account current functional-anatomical concepts, the conventional terminology was reexamined and a modified nomenclature of vertebrate neuron structure was proposed (Bodian, 1962).

Since the perikaryon (cell body) is considered primarily a growth center, its position on the fiber has little to do with electrochemical functions. Therefore, terminology based on the direction of travel of the nerve impulse, that is, toward or away from the cell body, is meaningless. The new nomenclature refers to a *dendritic zone* of a neuron (Fig. 12-7). In this zone the receptor membrane consists of cytoplasmic branches modified either to receive synaptic endings of other neurons (such as an association neuron), or to respond to stimuli by generating a nerve impulse (as in a sensory neuron). The many dendrites (*dendron*, 'tree') branch in the motor neuron and end in knoblike structures called *gemmules*. One Purkinje cell of the cerebellum, for example, may have as many as 200,000 terminals.

The *axon* is a long extension of cytoplasmic material differentiated to carry nerve impulses away from the dendritic zone. It is synonymous with the general terms "long peripheral fiber" or "axis cylinder." It may be branched and is of uniform diameter. A *neurolemma* (specialized sheath cells) usually wraps around the axon.

Axon telodendria are the endings of axons, functioning in synaptic transmission and neurosecretory activity. They may terminate in buttonlike enlargements, *boutons*. These are in contact with the processes or cell membrane of another neuron, or they terminate at a gland, a special unfolded area of a muscle (Fig. 12-8), or at a blood vessel. According to electron micrographs, many small *presynaptic vesicles* are present in the axonal endings or boutons. Anatomists believe that these vesicles are associated with the storage, release, and uptake of transmitter substances and are the only organelles unique to the

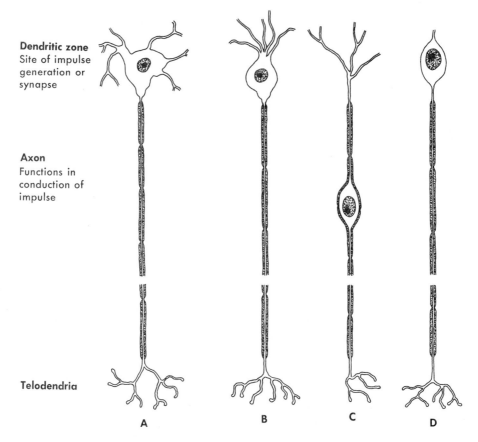

Dendritic zone
Site of impulse generation or synapse

Axon
Functions in conduction of impulse

Telodendria

A   B   C   D

Fig. 12-7
Diagrams of a typical motor neuron, **A,** and three different types of receptor neurons, **B** to **D.**

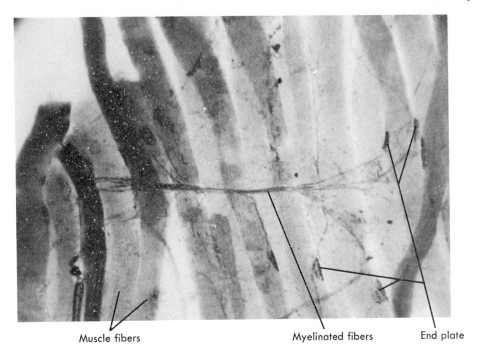

Muscle fibers   Myelinated fibers   End plate

Fig. 12-8
Axon telodendria terminate in a one-to-one relationship with individual muscle fibers at sites of contact known as motor end plates. A single motor neuron usually innervates several thousand muscle fibers. (× 450.)

neuron. The vesicles are morphologically diverse, possibly indicating a variety of chemical transmitters, the most common of which are *acetylcholine* and *norepinephrine.*

Impulses are usually received either by the ends of the dendritic branches or by the membrane of the cell body and transmitted in the direction of the axon. The receptor processes of the sensory nerves are either free or encapsulated, as discussed in Chapter 11. They are either directly in contact with the environment (pain endings) or with another specialized cell that, in turn, is capable of responding to environmental stimuli (rods or cones of the eye, for example). A stimulus generates an impulse in the sensory nerve which carries it to the cord or brain; here the neuron makes contact with association or motor neurons. A nerve fiber itself can conduct an impulse in either direction, but depending on its terminal arborizations it can either receive impulses (gemmules) or transmit them (boutons). The synapse, therefore, can conduct the nerve impulse in only one direction.

Except at their point of origin from the cell body and at their terminal fibers, specialized sheath cells, arranged end to end, cover the axons of the peripheral nervous system and most of the axons of the central nervous system. In the peripheral nervous system these cells are derived from the neural crest cells and are known as the *neurolemma,* or *Schwann cells.* Most of the axons also have a sheath of fatty material, *myelin,* inserted between the outer membrane of the Schwann cells and the membrane of the axonal fiber. Those nerve fibers that contain this fatty sheath are referred to as *myelinated fibers;* those fibers that lack the sheath are *nonmyelinated.*

The myelinated fibers are usually larger than the nonmyelinated and conduct impulses at a faster rate. The postganglionic fibers of the autonomic system, those that pass from the autonomic ganglion to a muscle or gland, are examples of fibers that lack myelin sheaths. The axons of these fibers are usually grouped together with as many as 20 axons in a bundle. Each axon sinks into an invagination of the cell membrane

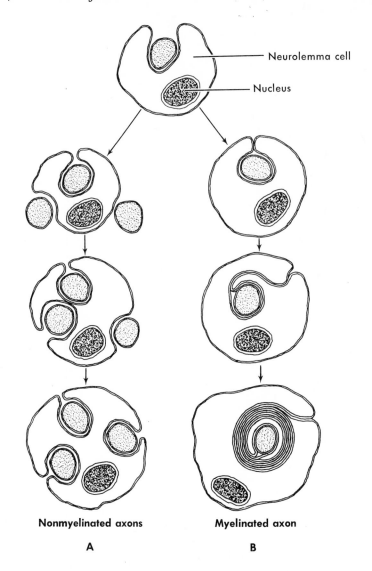

Neurolemma cell

Nucleus

Nonmyelinated axons

A

Myelinated axon

B

Fig. 12-9
A, Several axons sink into evaginations of the cell membrane (mesaxons) of a neurolemma cell and become enclosed by it. The numerous axons are nonmyelinated. **B,** One axon sinks into the mesaxon. The rotation of the neurolemma cell results in wrapping the axon, "jelly-roll fashion," with double layers of neurolemma cell cytoplasm. The fibers wrapped with such a sheath are said to be myelinated.

of a neurolemma cell, the so-called *mesaxon,* as shown in Fig. 12-9, *A.* As a result, one sheath cell encloses a bundle of axon fibers.

On the other hand, as shown by electron microscopy, a single Schwann cell wraps a myelinated fiber, often as many as 50 times or more, as illustrated in Fig. 12-9, *B.* This is sometimes referred to as the "jelly roll" formation of myelin. A cross section of a myelinated nerve fiber re-

veals a sheath composed of several concentric layers of the Schwann cell's plasma membrane. As the Schwann cell wraps itself around the axonal fiber, the cytoplasm is squeezed out in some manner and the plasma membranes of the Schwann cells are left. These membranes consist of a lipid layer of molecules sandwiched between two protein layers. The protein layers of two adjacent membranes fuse, freeing the lipid layer. It is this lipid component of the Schwann cell membrane that constitutes the myelin. Myelination begins to develop in the human fetus about the fourth month and may continue until the second or third year after birth (Hamilton, Boyd, and Mossman, 1962).

A constriction, the *node of Ranvier,* marks the point where one Schwann cell ends and another begins. Although the myelin sheath is absent at these nodes, the axonal fiber is not naked at this point. The ends of one Schwann cell overlap another at the nodes and form a protective membrane. Since the cytoplasm is squeezed out from between the layers of the membrane as the Schwann cells rotate around the fiber, most of the cytoplasm accumulates along with its nucleus in the outermost membrane. It is this outer portion of the Schwann cell that is customarily referred to as the neurolemma.

The cells of the central nervous system lack Schwann cells (neurolemma). Instead, one type of glial cell (oligodendroglia cells) provides the myelin around the fibers. The myelinated fibers of the central nervous system, therefore, structurally resemble the myelinated fibers of the peripheral nervous system.

We do not understand the exact function of the myelin sheath, but assume it acts as an insulating material that prevents nerve impulses from jumping from one axon to another. The thickness of the myelin sheath apparently influences the speed of conduction, since the thickest fiber is the fastest conductor. The myelin may also function in a nutritive role for the enclosed axon.

Neurosecretory cells

Although the neuron functions conventionally as the conductor of nerve impulses, some neurons are modified to secrete. These neurons, referred to as *neurosecretory cells,* are found in the hypothalamus and other parts of the nervous systems of both vertebrates and invertebrates.

Sensory neurons, relaying all possible types of information from other parts of the body, synapse with the dendrites of the neurosecretory cells. Unlike ordinary neurons, the axons of these cells end near a capillary bed. They do not synapse with other neurons nor innervate effector organs. A stimulated neurosecretory cell synthesizes its product and transports it in the form of visible droplets down the axon toward the blood vessel. Here it is either temporarily stored or discharged into the bloodstream, as suggested in Fig. 12-10. The circulatory system carries the product of the neurosecretory cell to some distal site in the body where it produces prolonged effects.

The neurosecretory cells link the nervous system with the endocrine system, the two coordinating systems of the body. Transmission of information to these cells enables them to convert sensory information into a hormonal message that can produce a physiologic response in the organism. Such a circuit is referred to as a *neuroendocrine reflex.*

Synapse

New information resulting from electron microscopic studies and microelectrode and pharmacologic analysis forced the neuroanatomists to change some of their concepts of the organization and structure of nervous tissue. The nature of the *synapse* morphology is one of these areas. Anatomists no longer talk of THE SYNAPSE but realize that there is a variety of mechanisms involved in cell-to-cell communication. A synapse is traditionally described as the end-to-end coupling of the axon telodendria of one neuron with the dendritic receptor sites of another neuron. New data reveal, however, that this conventional picture is only one of several relationships that exist between neurons. Fig. 12-11 demonstrates some of the diversity of neural linkages that have been described and that do not fall readily into the suggested nomenclature system proposed earlier. The coupling of one cell body with another, dendrite to dendrite, and axon to axon occur frequently. However, cell body to dendrites and cell body to axons have also been described (Bodian, 1972).

Impulses travel down nerve processes until they come to the point where one cell process contacts the cell process or membrane of the cell body of another. This physical junction between the transmitter site of one neuron and the receptor site of another is known as the

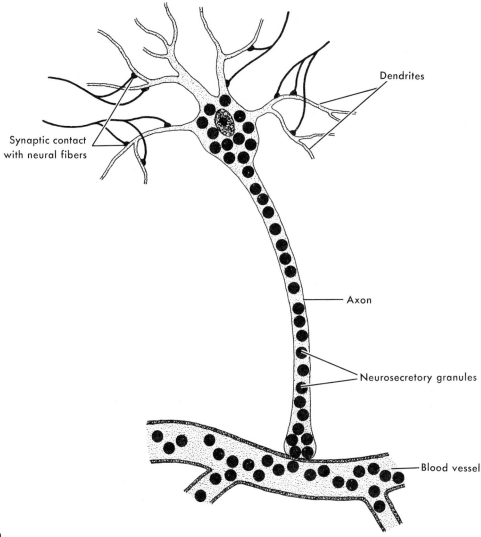

Fig. 12-10

Sensory neural fibers synapse with the dendrites of a neurosecretory cell, stimulating it to synthesize its product. These neurosecretory materials are then transported in the form of visible droplets down the axon toward the blood vessel.

synapse. The two membranes, closely apposed to one another, have only a small but variably sized *synaptic cleft* between them. The impulse passes from one neuron to another by the aid of the transmitted substance believed stored in the vesicles of the many terminal boutons. For example, norepinephrine, one kind of synaptic substance, is associated with a specific type of vesicle with a dense core. Stimulation of nerves known to release norepinephrine causes these vesicles to disappear. The transmitter substance alters the ion permeability of the receptor site by

depolarizing its membrane and initiating a new nervous impulse in the second neuron.

Reflex arc

The quick, automatic withdrawal of a finger when it touches a hot object is the result of a reflex action. The knee jerk is another common illustration. In these examples, a chain of neurons carries the impulse from the point of stimulus, at the finger or patellar ligament, to the responding muscle. Such a chain of neurons composes a *reflex arc,* considered the *functional unit* of the nervous system. It first makes its appearance in the human fetus about the fourteenth week of gestation.

Although it is possible for the sensory neurons to contact the motor neurons directly, thereby involving a two-neuron chain (monosynaptic reaction), most reflexes are more complicated than this. In general, the simplest reflexes involve at least three neurons. For example, a receptor (dendrite) responds to a heat stimulus and a nerve impulse is generated in the sensory neuron. It passes through the cerebrospinal ganglia outside the cord and, by way of axonal fibers, enters the spinal cord where it makes contact with many connecting and integrating circuits in the central nervous system. Here analysis and integration of the message occur. The association neurons relay the commands back to the motor neurons. The motor neurons carry the impulse to the effector organ and complete the reflex arc (Fig. 12-12, *A*).

In a three-neuron chain reflex, the axonal telodendria of the sensory neurons synapse with several intermediate or association neurons located in the gray matter of the spinal cord. These synaptic connections increase considerably the number of possible pathways. Each association neuron, in turn, receives impulses from several different sensory neurons. The spray of branches at the end of the axonal fiber then

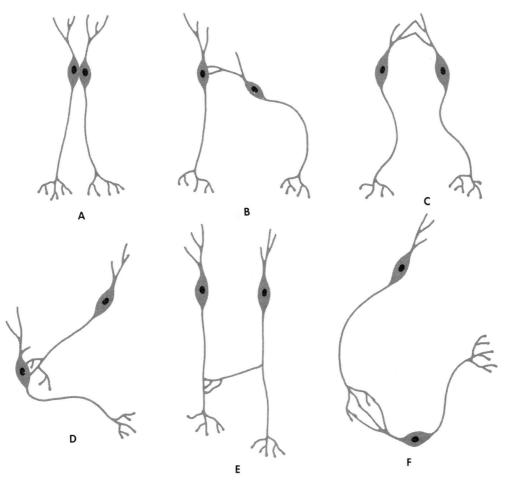

Fig. 12-11

Diagram of various types of synaptic relations between neurons. A cell body of one neuron may contact that of a second neuron, **A**, or its dendrites, **B**, or axons, **D**. There can also be dendrite-to-dendrite, **C**, or axon-to-axon, **E**, coupling. **F**, Conventional axon-to-dendrite junction.

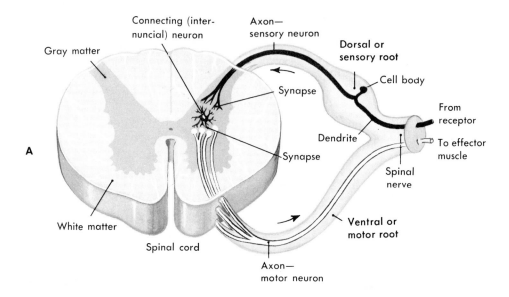

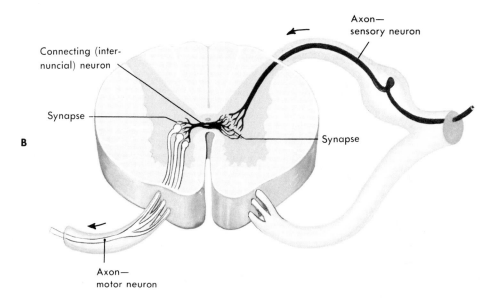

Fig. 12-12

Diagram of a reflex arc involving three neurons: a sensory, an association (intermediate), and a motor neuron, **A.** Such an arc involves two synapses in the gray matter of the cord. In many instances the intermediate neuron passes to the other side of the cord and relays the impulses to motor neurons on this side. Such neurons are considered commissural neurons, **B.** (Modified from Anthony, C. P., and Kolthoff, N. J.: Textbook of anatomy and physiology, ed. 8, St. Louis, 1971, The C. V. Mosby Co.)

allows the association neurons to relay the impulses to several motor neurons. Obviously such interrelationships result in a kind of nerve net.

Sometimes the response is visible, such as an overt behavior reaction (running away) or the knee jerk mentioned above; sometimes the response is invisible and involves regulative changes in internal organs (for example, secretion by glands or changes in circulation). It is those *automatic reactions,* visible or invisible, that are defined as *reflex actions.*

A reflex may go on at one level of the central nervous system or it may involve other parts of the nervous system as well. For example, in the withdrawal of the toe from the stimulus of a sharp object, the individual may move his arms and utter an exclamation of pain as he removes his foot. If both arms are raised, fibers of the intermediate neurons must have crossed to the other side of the cord and relayed the impulse to motor neurons on this side, the opposite side to that in which the stimulus had occurred. Intermediate neurons that cross to the other side of the cord are referred to as *commissural neurons* (Fig. 12-12, *B*).

There is evidence that reflex circuitry is laid down early in the embryo and that the nervous system develops orderly patterns of behavior long before they are actually used. One can demonstrate this by anesthetizing a young embryo at its learning stage. A young amphibian embryo anesthetized before its muscles have functioned remains quiescent during the completion of their development. If the anesthetic is then washed away when the untreated controls demonstrate their ability to swim, the experimental embryos soon recover and join in the vigorous swimming movements. Apparently, the swimming pattern was not learned. Instead, all the neural pathways for reflex swimming movements developed during the anesthetized state. Evidently much of behavioral circuitry is built into the nervous system and is not something imposed upon an established order. The recognition of this fact has caused many researchers to turn from a study of psychology to that of neuroembryology in their attempts to understand behavior (Sperry, 1965).

DEVELOPMENT OF PERIPHERAL NERVOUS SYSTEM

The peripheral nervous system consists of paired spinal and cranial nerves that innervate the surface of the body or penetrate to the deeper organs. In the regions of the forelimbs and hindlimbs, several spinal nerves enter the limb buds, establish interconnections, and form a *nerve plexus.* The group of nerves entering the forelimb bud make up the *brachial plexus;* those that innervate the hindlimb bud compose the *lumbosacral plexus.*

Formation of spinal nerves

The location of the somites on either side of the neural tube in the young neurula determines the position that some of the neural crest cells (future sensory nerve cells) take as they migrate away from the newly closed neural tube. One can demonstrate the importance of the somites by surgically removing them or transplanting additional somites along one side of the body. The opposite unoperated side remains as a control. A corresponding decrease in neural crest cell clusters occurs when somites are removed. Conversely, additional somites induce an increase in numbers of cell clusters when compared with the unoperated side.

There are 31 pairs of spinal nerves in the human embryo, but only 10 pairs in the frog. Each spinal nerve is connected to the spinal cord by way of two roots, *dorsal* and *ventral,* that have different embryonic origins. In amphioxus and some cyclostomes the two roots remain separated, but in all gnathostomes they unite to form a *spinal nerve.* Both sensory and motor elements must be present in the nerves if reflex arcs, the functional units of the nervous system, develop.

The axons of the neuroblasts located in the motor nuclei grow laterally and penetrate the outer wall of the neural tube, the *marginal zone.* Here they emerge as the *ventral,* or *motor,* root of a spinal nerve, as shown in Fig. 12-12, *A.* These motor fibers are classified as either *somatic* or *visceral fibers.* Somatic motor fibers carry impulses to the voluntary muscles of the body, those usually derived from myotomes. Visceral motor fibers, on the other hand, pass deeply into the body of the organism and innervate such internal organs as the heart, stomach, and intestine. They maintain those routine functions of the body that are under more or less automatic control. The motor fibers of this visceral system are involuntary in nature and are usually referred to as the *autonomic nervous system,* as compared to the conscious, or willful, nature of the somatic system.

The neuroblasts located in the cerebrospinal ganglia develop into *sensory* neurons, either *somatic* or *visceral,* depending on the organs they innervate. In either case, processes extend from the neuroblast (formerly the neural crest cell) in both directions, out to the receptor and in toward the spinal cord. In the gray matter of the spinal cord they synapse with association neurons. The fibers of the nerve cells collect into bundles outside the spinal cord and give rise to the *dorsal,* or *sensory, root* of the spinal nerve.

The dorsal root unites with the ventral root to form a *spinal nerve,* as can be seen in the section of a 10 mm. pig (Fig. 12-13). A spinal nerve is usually a *mixed nerve;* it can be composed of four different types of nerve processes. It may contain somatic sensory (afferent) and visceral sensory (afferent) fibers, as well as somatic motor (efferent) and visceral motor (efferent) processes.

Growth of nerves

The factors responsible for directing or guiding certain neurons to specific structures or other neurons have been the subject of much investigation. According to Weiss (1955), there are three phases in the development of nerves: the pioneering phase, the application phase, and the towing phase. In the pioneering phase the cytoplasm protrudes from the side of the nerve as a short thread. The thread lengthens because of the synthesis of protoplasm by the cell body and its flow to the tip of the sprout where ameboid processes develop. During the application phase the free pioneering tip of the fiber attaches itself to a receptor or to an effector cell, located nearby at this early stage. As the embryo grows,

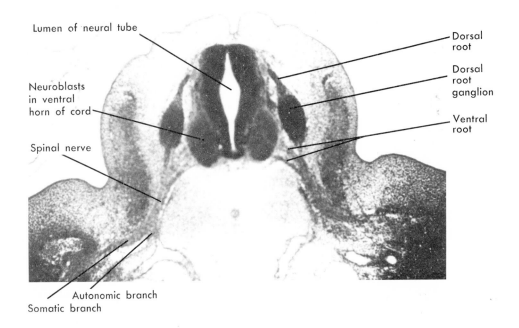

Fig. 12-13
Cross section through 10 mm. pig embryo showing dorsal and ventral roots of a spinal nerve. (× 100.)

the peripheral cell shifts and during this migration "tows" (third phase) the nerve fiber with it. If these peripheral cells migrate outward and become, for example, the big toe of a hindlimb, the distance the axonal fiber is towed can be considerable.

We do not understand why the pioneering fiber attaches to a particular cell. The problem of innervation obviously concerns the orientation of the pioneering fibers. Once the application phase is established, additional new fibers from other cells follow the course set by the pioneers, obviously using it as a solid substrate. There is general agreement that nerve fibers follow oriented structural or ultrastructural elements. One hypothesis suggests that the tips of nerves grow into actively growing limb buds by following the stress lines set up as the rapidly dividing mesenchyme cells absorb water. The tendency of nerve fibers to grow along solid objects is referred to as *stereotropism*. The growth of the optic nerve offers a more obvious illustration. The fibers from the inner layer of ganglion cells in the retina converge, pierce the choroid and sclera, and follow the optic stalk as a pathway into the brain. As the fibers grow back into the brain substance, they group together and give rise to the optic nerve.

There is general agreement that growing nerves are subject to contact guidance. Whether additional factors (chemical or electrical) are involved remains a controversial issue. Some investigators explain the migration of nerve fibers toward the source of their stimuli by postulating a difference in electric potential. However, the application of actual electrical currents does not affect either the rate or direction of growth of the fibers. There is little evidence that a fiber can electrically select a particular pathway.

According to Sperry (1965), the modern concept of inherent chemical affinities of the neurons can best explain the selectivity of a growing nerve fiber for a particular pathway. Each of the billions of cells within the nervous system has a specific chemical identification tag dictated by the genetic code. According to this thesis, as the neurons mature and begin to form associations with other neurons, they are attracted to chemically compatible cells or fibers from the millions, or billions, of nerve cells with different chemical identities. As a result, numerous neurons having similar chemical identities establish brain pathways. However, chemical affinity must not be the total answer. There are too many different connections that must be made in the total organism for such a simple explanation to apply.

Like most embryonic cells, the developing peripheral nerves appear to be unspecialized as they grow out toward an end organ. There is evidence that a motor nerve makes connection with any muscle cell in its path and becomes specialized after it makes this contact. Motor fibers connect to muscles and glands, and sensory fibers connect to receptors. Evidently these end organs bring about specific chemical changes in the nerves they contact.

Once attained, the specificity of a neuron is irreversible. Sperry (1951) obtained evidence for this specificity when he crossed the cutaneous nerves of the left hind foot to the right hind foot in rats 14 to 26 days old. After the rats recovered from the operation, he found that stimulation of the right foot caused the animal to lick its left foot. No response occurred on the stimulated right side and the proper reactions to the stimuli could not be induced by training. These reactions suggested that during development the nerves reacted with the end organs of their receptors and this reaction determined the specificity of these nerves. This information was recorded in the brain.

As development proceeds, the brain irreversibly registers a copy of the nonneural portion of the body. A condensed, point-by-point map of all the body's surfaces, both internal and external organs and muscles, is imprinted on the nervous system. By the time the operation was carried out in the above experiment, the nerves passing to the left side of the animal had contacted the end organs, become specialized as the left sensory or motor leg nerves, and been registered as such in the central nervous system. Therefore, when the left nerve was transplanted to the right side in the postnatal animal and the right side was stimulated, the animal lifted its left foot. This lack of plasticity offers a possible explanation as to why an amputee continues to feel pain in his leg when the stump is stimulated.

Formation of cranial nerves

The origin of the cranial nerves is much the same as spinal nerves, in that motor fibers arise from nuclei located in the gray matter and sensory neurons form from neuroblasts derived either from neural crest cells or ectodermal placodes. There is one difference, however. Although cranial nerves may be mixed nerves, in many cases they are one or the other, either sensory or motor in function. Some biologists believe that cranial nerves at one time contained two roots that did not unite, like the spinal nerves in amphioxus and the cyclostomes. In some cases, the dorsal root became the predominant component and the ventral root degenerated leaving a purely sensory nerve. In other instances, the dorsal root was lost and the ventral root remained as the motor nerve.

Segmentation is also lost in the cranial region since some of the cranial nerves represent roots from more than one segment. As an illustration, the hypoglossal nerve (twelfth nerve) forms from the union of ventral roots from several occipital nerves.

Structure of a nerve

A spinal nerve consists of axons from the somatic as well as the visceral nervous systems. A cross section of the nerve as seen in Fig. 12-14 best reveals its structure. Each nerve axon is surrounded by a sheath of Schwann cells (neurolemma), but may or may not be myelinated. The axons, therefore, are of various sizes ranging from large axons with a thick myelin sheath, fibers of smaller diameter and thinner sheath, and thin fibers with no sheath. The large myelinated fibers have a more rapid rate of conduction than do the smaller myelinated fibers. The fibers are arranged in parellel groups and collected into bundles, or *fascicles*, by a connective tissue sheath, the *endoneurium*.

When we refer to a nerve, we are speaking of a group of fascicles bound together by the *perineurium*. This connective tissue sheath not only protects the nerve bundles, but also functions as a diffusion barrier. Several nerves make up a *nerve trunk*. A connective tissue membrane, the *epineurium*, ensheathes a nerve trunk. This

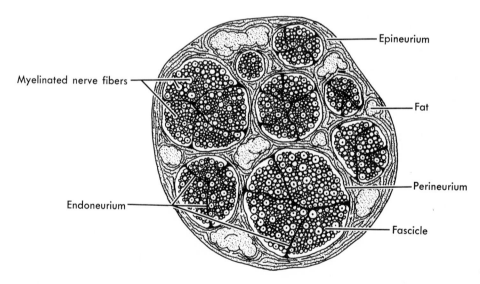

Fig. 12-14

Cross section through a nerve trunk showing myelinated nerve fibers divided into fascicles by the endoneurium. Several fascicles, wrapped by the perineurium, compose a nerve, and several nerves make up a nerve trunk. The nerve trunk is ensheathed by the epineurium.

membrane may extend into the nerve trunk as a septum helping to further separate the groups of nerves.

SPINAL CORD
General description

At first the spinal cord is a thick-walled tube with a central canal. This canal gradually diminishes in size as development continues; in the human adult it is usually obliterated. The spinal cord extends down most of the length of the body and undergoes considerably less modification than that of the brain. The adult cord is usually oval in shape and flattened more on its ventral side than on its dorsal side. There is no special boundary between it and the brain at the anterior end, other than the cervical flexure present in amniotes. At the posterior end, the spinal cord tapers to an end, the *filum terminale*. In tetrapods, two prominent bulges appear, a cervical enlargement at the level of the forelimbs and a lumbar enlargement opposite the hindlimbs. They are most pronounced in amniotes and reached their greatest size in dinosaurs, where they are believed to have been much larger than the brain itself. The enlarge-

ments are the result of an increase in numbers of cell bodies at the level of the limbs and mark the point of departure from the cord of neurons that pass laterally into these structures.

Early in their development, the neural tube and vertebral column are approximately the same length. However, the vertebral column (cartilage or bone) develops at a faster rate than does the cord. The coccygeal end (posterior) of the cord terminates at the lumbar region in most vertebrates, and the cord, except for the filum terminale, is absent from the posterior regions of the vertebral column. In man the spinal cord terminates at the level of the third lumbar vertebra; in other animals it may be longer but does not usually reach the full length of the vertebral column. As a result of this unequal growth, the spinal nerves in the cervical regions pass laterally into the organs they innervate, but in the posterior part of the cord they are arranged in a more craniocaudad direction.

A *ventral fissure* is present on the undersurface of the cord of higher vertebrates. A longitudinal *dorsal septum* extends inward from a *dorsal sulcus* (depression). This septum, to-

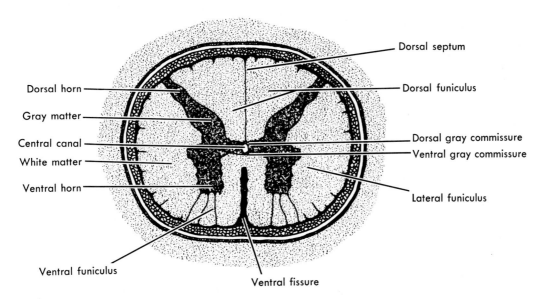

Fig. 12-15
Diagram of cross section through mammalian spinal cord showing relation of gray and white matter.

gether with the dorsal sulcus and ventral fissure, partially divides the cord into two symmetrical halves as may be seen in Fig. 12-15. The two halves are connected with one another by nerve fibers *(commissures)*.

Gray matter of cord

A cross section of the adult cord of amniotes shows that the mantle area of the orginal neural tube has undergone considerable expansion during development. It forms a "butterfly," or "H-shaped," structure that fills the central part of the section. Anatomists speak of the *dorsal* and *ventral horns* of the gray matter. These are actually cross sections of *columns,* areas of common function, that run up and down the cord. In all vertebrates *dorsal* and *ventral gray commissures* located on either side of the central canal connect the two sides of the cord. The presence of sulci and fissures, as well as dorsal and ventral columns, is much more pronounced in higher vertebrates than in lower forms. For example, the spinal cord of cyclostomes lacks sulci and fissures, and there is no definite demarcation between gray and white matter.

The cell bodies of the *association neurons* are located in the dorsal columns of the gray matter. These multipolar neurons receive the impulses from the axons of the afferent (sensory) neurons. They coordinate the impulses brought in by the sensory neurons to those sent out by the motor neurons. The fibers of the association neurons may remain on the same side of the cord or cross to the other side. They may make contact ventrally (synapse) with the dendrites of the motor neurons, or they may send their axons into the white matter where they ascend to the brain.

The cell bodies of the motor neurons, located in the ventral columns, are distinguishable by their large size and large amount of Nissl material. Their axons pass out laterally, forming the ventral root fibers of the spinal nerves. The gray matter, therefore, consists of interstitial cells, association neurons, cell bodies and dendrites of motor neurons, portions of myelinated and nonmyelinated fibers, and synapses.

Neural anatomists distinguish functional areas (somatic or visceral) within the dorsal and ventral columns of the gray matter. They identify four such areas on each side of the cord: two areas in the dorsal column where somatic and visceral sensory neurons synapse with association neurons, and two in the ventral area where the cell bodies of the visceral and somatic motor neurons are located. From dorsal to ventral, the areas may be listed sequentially as the somatic afferent and visceral afferent, located in the dorsal column of the gray matter, and visceral efferent and somatic efferent, in the ventral column, as shown in Fig. 12-16, *A*. The somatic areas are usually larger than the visceral ones. These general regions persist and can be identified as far forward as the medulla oblongata in higher animals. Anterior to the medulla, this structural plan changes. However, in the amphibian, for example, the entire central nervous system (brain and cord) resembles the cord of higher animals.

White matter of cord

Longitudial tracts, referred to as *funiculi* (to differentiate them from the columns of the gray matter) compose the white matter of the cord. Myelinated and some nonmyelinated fibers of sensory, motor, and association neurons make up the funiculi. Some transverse fibers are also present running to and from the gray matter. In general, there are no cell bodies and no dendrites in the white matter. The shape of the gray matter divides the surrounding white matter into three general areas on each side of the cord (Fig. 12-15). They are the *dorsal funiculi* located between the dorsal sulcus and dorsal column, the *lateral funiculi* situated between the dorsal and ventral columns, and the *ventral funiculi* between the ventral column and ventral fissure. A white commissure connects the two halves of the cord.

The three funiculi can be further divided into specific *fiber tracts* (fasciculi). A detailed discussion of the fiber tracts of the cord is beyond the scope of this book. One should realize, however, that these tracts connect one part of the cord with another and join the brain with the peripheral system. Their importance increased as the brain evolved and assumed more of the coordinating and association

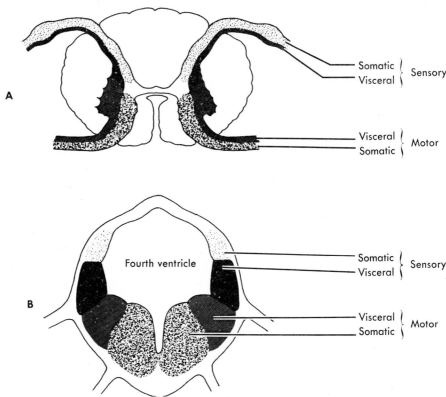

Fig. 12-16
Diagram showing similarity in distribution of sensory and motor columns in spinal cord, **A,** and embryonic medulla oblongata, **B.**

functions of the body. The fiber tracts developed to a greater degree in higher animals than in the fish where the trunk is more or less semi-autonomous. They are two-way conduction paths, consisting of ascending axons carrying impulses up the cord and to the brain and descending axons relaying messages back to the cord and to the peripheral neurons. Bundles of axons compose the tracts and many tracts make up the funiculi.

In general, ascending fibers from some of the sensory neurons compose each dorsal funiculus. The fibers enter the cord through the dorsal root and then ascend to a higher level instead of synapsing with an association neuron. Ascending axons from association neurons are also present in this region of the cord. The ventral funiculi carry impulses down the cord and from the brain centers. The cell bodies of these neurons are located in the higher centers in the brain, and the descending fibers synapse either directly with a motor neuron in the ventral column of the cord or with an association neuron, which then contacts the motor neuron. The lateral funiculi consists of both ascending and descending fibers that appear to connect one area of the cord with another.

BRAIN
Myelencephalon

The myelencephalon is the anterior continuation of the spinal cord and is well-developed in all vertebrates. In the adult, it is recognized as the *medulla oblongata* and along with the pons and midbrain composes the *brainstem*. The central canal expands into a triangular structure, the *fourth ventricle*, covered by a thin, highly vascular roof, the *tela choroidea*. Anteriorly, the cerebellum overlaps the medulla. The *posterior choroid plexus* (the mass of capillaries located in the tela choroidea) secretes the cerebrospinal fluid. The white funiculi and gray columns of the cord continue as the walls of the medulla oblongata. The gray matter retains its dorsoventral arrangement of sensory and motor components, as shown in Fig. 12-16, *B.* Some of the fibers of the medulla cross over to the other side (decussate), thereby integrating the two sides. Consequently, one side of the brain controls the opposite side of the body. Other fiber tracts continue either anteriorly or posteriorly from the medulla. Obviously all tracts between the cord and higher brain areas must pass through the medulla.

Afferent fibers from the posterior regions synapse at two prominent nuclei in the walls of the medulla oblongata. The axons of these cells carry impulses upward to the thalamus and cerebellum. The medulla is the seat of reflex control for such important functions as respiration, heartbeat, and blood pressure. These functions are so necessary for survival that the nuclei of the medulla are referred to as *vital centers.* An injury to this area of the brain often results in death. The reflex centers for certain nonvital functions are also located here, including centers for vomiting, coughing, sneezing, swallowing, hiccuping, and salivation. The majority of the cranial nerves are associated with the medulla oblongata. The fifth to twelfth cranial nerves leave or enter the medulla.

Metencephalon

The metencephalon gives rise to the anterior regions of the medulla oblongata, the cerebellum, and the pons. The dorsal part of the metencephalon becomes the elevated and thickened *cerebellum,* which seems to be directly related to the locomotor activity of the organism. The cerebellum does not itself direct activities, but it moderates and coordinates those of higher brain centers. It is poorly developed in sedentary forms of vertebrates and most highly developed in birds and mammals. It is a receiving center for sensory and motor information and functions by controlling skeletal muscles. The cerebellum is poorly developed in the cyclostomes, some fishes, amphibian, and reptiles. In these sluggish and poikilothermic forms, it consists of little more

than a shelf of tissue anterior to the fourth ventricle.

The posterior dorsal area of the metencephalon receives information from the vestibular portion of the eighth cranial nerve carrying impulses from the semicircular canals. Also nerves returning from the lateral-line organs give information about vibrations, water currents, and movement of nearby objects. After receiving these sensory data, the cerebellum sorts, correlates, and regulates the body movements. In more active animals (Elasmobranchii, Dipneusti, etc.), irregular-shaped lobes called *auricular lobes,* or *restiform bodies,* project laterally from each side. Their cavities are continuous with the fourth ventricle and they represent the most ancient part of the cerebellum. These lobes are intimately connected with the inner ear and function primarily as organs of equilibrium.

In amniotes, the lateral line components drop out, and as the muscles associated with terrestrial living develop, the proprioceptors increase in importance. The cerebellum of birds is more advanced than in most of the lower animals. It is divided into a middle "worm-shaped" portion, called the vermis (consisting of many horizontal ridges), between two lateral lobes or hemispheres. Its development is associated with the coordination of the intricate flight muscles. In the mammal the cerebellum reaches its greatest degree of development. It also receives information about the position of body parts from the organ of equilibrium and on the state of muscle tension from muscle and tendon spindles, types of receptors described in Chapter 11.

The cerebellum sends and receives fibers to and from the higher brain centers. In the mammal the highly developed cerebral cortex takes over much of the control from the cerebellum. Conspicuous fiber tracts connect the spinal cord and medulla with the cerebellum, and the cerebellum with the cortex. These tracts are located on the ventral part of the myelencephalon and metencephalon and externally appear as a bulge, the *pons* (Latin word meaning 'bridge'). The cerebral cortex increases in importance and establishes sensation centers for touch, vision, hearing, and muscle tone. Impulses from the

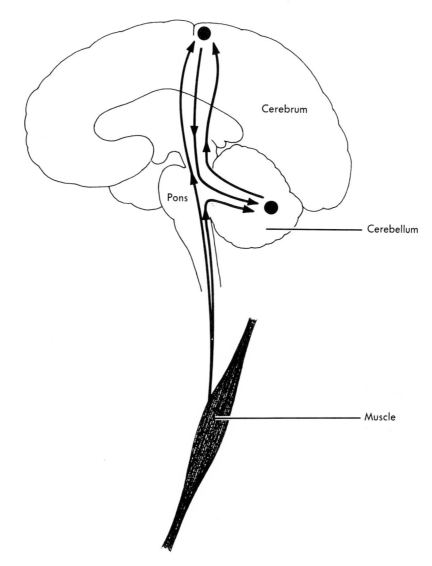

Fig. 12-17
"Wiring diagram" indicating that impulses from spinal cord may pass either directly to cerebrum or first to cerebellum and then to the higher center. The cerebrum sorts the information it receives and then sends instructions back to the cerebellum as to what should be done.

cord may now pass directly to the cortex, where the information is sorted and sent back to the cerebellum by way of the pons for final adjustment as to what should be done. "Commands" are then relayed back to the effector organs. On the other hand, impulses may pass first to the cerebellum and then to the cortex and back to the cerebellum (Snider, 1958). The

"wiring" diagram of Fig. 12-17 indicates these possibilities.

The distribution of gray and white matter in the cerebellum is the opposite of that of the cord. The white matter is concentrated in the center of the cerebellum, and the gray matter, which has increased in amount, forms a convoluted covering over the white matter. The sur-

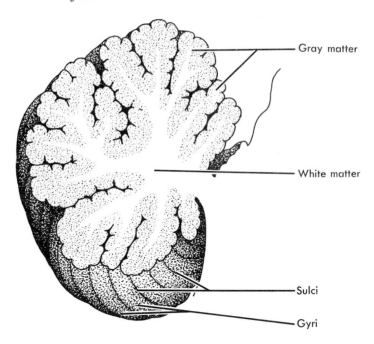

Gray matter

White matter

Sulci

Gyri

Fig. 12-18
Diagram of cross section through cerebellum showing distribution of white and gray matter to be the reverse of that of the cord.

face of the gray matter has numerous grooves (sulci) and convolutions (gyri). A sagittal section through the cerebellum shows that the white fiber tracts spray out into the gray matter of the cerebellar cortex (Fig. 12-18).

Mesencephalon

Unlike the other parts of the embryonic brain, the midbrain does not divide further. In lower animals it is linked to the visual sense and is an important association center. In higher forms many of its activities are taken over by the cortex, and it remains primarily a tract to and from these higher centers.

In cross section, the mesencephalon consists of the thickened dorsal region of gray matter, the *tectum,* and the thinner walls and floor of gray matter referred to as the *tegmentum.* The cavity of the mesencephalon decreases during development, forming the narrow *aqueduct.* It communicates posteriorly with the fourth ventricle and anteriorly with the third ventricle. In lower animals the tectum, or roof, an important visual center, appears as a pair of

dorsolateral *optic lobes (corpora bigemina).* The fibers of the optic nerve enter the diencephalon and then pass into the roof of the mesencephalon. Fibers from the spinal cord and medulla also terminate in these lobes. The optic lobes are thus important correlating centers for optic and exteroceptive impulses. The tectum is most important in fishes and amphibians, a little less important in reptiles and birds, and least important as a visual center in the mammal. If the cerebral hemispheres are removed from a higher animal, it can no longer function. A frog, on the other hand, after recovering from such an operation, can continue functioning in an apparently normal fashion as long as the brainstem remains intact.

The tectum of mammals is reduced to four prominent swellings known as the *corpora quadrigemina.* The larger anterior pairs are the *superior colliculi* (containing visual receptive centers); the posterior pairs are the *inferior colliculi* (integrating centers for auditory sense). Although optic and auditory fibers are still sent to the superior and inferior colliculi, the ascending spinal tracts, in general, bypass the mesencephalon of mammals and continue anteriorly to the diencephalon, or higher centers. The highly evolved cerebral cortex of mammals takes over the major visual and auditory control, leaving the tectum as essentially a reflex center for light and sound.

Nuclei of the third and fourth cranial nerves are located in the gray matter of the midbrain. Ascending and descending fiber tracts from the rear and from the anterior cerebral cortex form the tegmentum. These are more prominent in mammals than in some of the lower animals, as might be expected, and constitute the major bulk of the mesencephalon. The majority of these fibers originate in the cerebrum and pass by way of the midbrain to the pons, medulla, or spinal cord.

Diencephalon

The diencephalon, or the tween-brain represents an ancient reflex center. It can be divided into a thin roof, the *epithalamus;* the thickened sides, the *thalamus;* and the floor, the *hypothalamus,* each part carrying out specialized functions. The third ventricle forms the cavity of the diencephalon. Several dorsal and ventral outgrowths arise from the diencephalon.

Epithalamus

The anterior portion of the roof of the diencephalon resembles the covering of the fourth ventricle in the medulla. It is a thin, nonnervous, vascular membrane that extends into the third ventricle and contains the *anterior choroid plexus.* Along with the posterior choroid plexus, it forms the cerebrospinal fluid, which fills the cavities of the nervous system. In some forms, a fold of the membrane gives rise to the paraphysis, a structure of unknown function.

The posterior portion of the roof of the diencephalon evaginates to form a pair of median stalklike structures, the *anterior parapineal body* and a *posterior epiphysis,* or *pineal* structure. The function of the pineal has long intrigued the biological investigator, but Turner and Bagnara (1971) state that the "time has probably arrived when it is justifiable to consider the pineal as an endocrine gland." There

appears to be a decided seasonal interaction between the pineal and the reproductive organs, but other functions are not consistently present among the classes of vertebrates. According to a symposium presented by comparative endocrinologists of the American Society of Zoologists (1970), the pineal may control some basic homoiokinetic mechanism that allows the organism to adjust seasonally to its environment.

Thalamus

The thalamus is an integrating center for fibers that pass to and from the cortex, and it contains several important areas (nuclei). The walls of the diencephalon can be divided into a dorsal and a ventral half. In general, the cells located in the dorsal half are involved with sensory impulses and, next to the cerebrum, reflect the greatest evolutionary change. All sensory pathways, with the exception of the olfactory one, pass to the cerebral cortex of amniotes by way of these tracts. In lower animals the dorsal thalamus is of less importance. The ventral half of the thalamus is concerned with motor impulses.

Hypothalamus

The hypothalamus is of great importance, since it controls involuntary actions relating to sleep, temperature regulation, rate of breathing, genital impulses, and metabolism. In the human being it weighs a little more than 7 grams. It is possible to identify four areas.

The *optic chiasma* is located in the anterior parts of the hypothalamus. It is here that the optic nerve fibers cross to opposite sides of the brain before they proceed to terminate in the tectum of the midbrain of the lower animal. In higher animals, they pass to special areas in the gray matter of the cortex (Fig. 11-17). The *tuber cinereum,* believed to be the center of the parasympathetic system, is located behind the optic chiasma. Posterior to this center are the *mammillary bodies,* centers of olfactory function.

The fourth area, the *infundibulum,* grows ventrally between the optic chiasma and mammillary body to meet the ectodermal material from the stomodeal region, as shown in Fig. 12-19. Together they give rise to the pituitary gland of the individual. The infundibulum contributes to

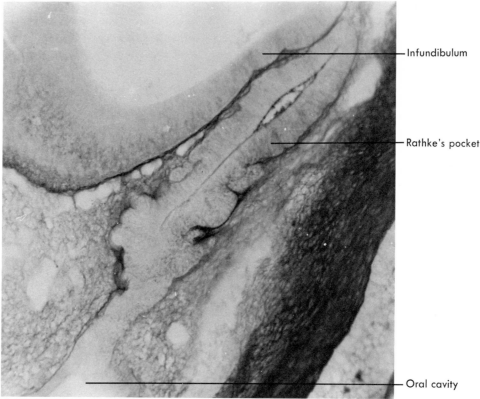

— Infundibulum

— Rathke's pocket

— Oral cavity

Fig. 12-19
Sagittal section through hypothalamus of 5-day-old chick embryo showing the relationship of infundibulum (nerve ectoderm) to Rathke's pocket (epidermal ectoderm). (× 100.)

the neurohypophysis (posterior pituitary and median eminence), and the stomodeal ectoderm contributes to the adenohypophysis, consisting of the anterior and intermediate lobes of the pituitary. In the hypothalamus are located the neurosecretory cells described in Chapter 11.

The hypothalamus regulates the function of the anterior pituitary gland, not by way of nerve fibers but by releasing into the portal blood vessels chemicals that stimulate or inhibit its activity. According to present information, the hypothalamus secretes nine regulating or releasing hormones (RH) that affect the pituitary gland (Schally, Arimura, and Kastin, 1973). Most of them stimulate the pituitary to both synthesize and release particular hormones. Some, however, inhibit the production of pituitary hormones.

A dual system of hypothalamic control regulates three of the pituitary hormones: the growth hormone, prolactin, and melanocyte-stimulating hormone. One factor stimulates the synthesis and release of the hormone and one inhibits its production. These hormones need a dual regulatory system since their target organs release no negative-feedback products. On the other hand, the thyroid, gonads, and adrenals all produce hormones. As indicated in Chapter 3, the circulating levels of these hormones inhibit the pituitary and hypothalamus secretions by a negative-feedback mechanism. Therefore, only a hypothalamic-releasing factor controls each of these glands.

The hypothalamus also synthesizes oxytocin and vasopressin. The long axonal fibers transport these hormones to the posterior lobe of the pituitary where they are stored until needed.

Telencephalon

Of all the parts of the brain, the telencephalon, or forebrain, evolved the most. Originally a single anterior expansion of the neural tube, it divides into the olfactory lobe and the cerebral hemisphere. In tetrapods, the hemisphere increases in size and separates into two definite lateral swellings, the *cerebral hemispheres.* The olfactory sense is the most important sense influencing behavior in fish, amphibians, and most reptiles. In primates, on the other hand, the sense of smell is of less importance. The story of the evolution of the telencephalon involves the structural and functional expansion of its cerebral part. This progressive enlargement of the cerebrum in higher groups is diagrammed in Fig. 12-20. The function of the telencephalon shifts from a primarily olfactory one in primitive forms to that of the dominate association and coordinating center for all the senses in the mammals. The cerebral hemispheres are responsible for the complex thought, intelligence, and acute sensation associated with man.

The evolutionary history of the telencephalon involves a shift in the location of gray and white matter as compared with that of the spinal cord. The cells of the gray matter move progressively outward as the phylogenetic scale is ascended. The migration of the gray matter outside the white matter occurs slowly and is associated with the growth of a new area, the neopallium. As a result of this reversal of position, the cells of the gray matter occupy a peripheral position in the telencephalon of mammals where there is room for greater surface expansion. The white fiber tracts occupy the central position.

When viewed in cross section, the forebrain of vertebrate embryos consists of two general areas surrounding the *telocoel,* or ventricle; the dorsal roof, or *pallium;* and a thickened floor, the *basal area.* The pallium becomes greatly modified during evolution; it is the primordium of the cerebral cortex. The basal area develops into the *basal nuclei,* essentially equal to the *corpus striatum* of mammals. It forms a part of the brain most concerned with basic instinctive behavior patterns. Certain cells representing additional sense centers appear in the basal nuclei of the more active fish.

The pallium is thin in the lower vertebrates. Only a small amount of gray matter lines the ventricle; the rest of the pallium consists of an outside covering of white fibers. In the primitive vertebrate and in the early embryo of all types, the telencephalon consists of a single cavity. Bilaterally located olfactory bulbs project forward from the forebrain toward the nasal sac. In the cyclostomes the pallium is related entirely to the sense of smell and the basal nuclei is poorly developed.

Even in the cyclostomes, the olfactory bulb of fishes separates from the forebrain and extends toward the olfactory sacs. In the elasmobranchs, for example, a slight longitudinal depression indistinctly divides the single telencephalon into two anteroventral *olfactory lobes* and two posterodorsal *cerebral hemispheres.* The olfactory lobes have only an olfactory function; the hemispheres are probably mostly olfactory, but they may contain a few other centers. Attached to the olfactory lobes are two stalklike anterior *olfactory tracts,* which pass into the rostrum of the fish, terminating in the *olfactory bulbs,* as shown in Fig. 12-21. The bulbs are the true anterior ends of the brain. The receptor cells located in the epithelium of the adjacent olfactory sac send their fibers into the olfactory bulb. These fibers form the olfactory, or *first cranial nerve.*

The paired amphibian hemispheres are larger than those of the fish, but it is difficult to differentiate between olfactory lobes and cerebral hemispheres. In these forms the pallium divides into two general regions, a dorsomedial *archipallium* and a lateral *paleopallium* (Fig. 12-22). Although the archipallium continues to be predominantly an olfactory center, the new association centers of other sensory impulses first appear here in the amphibians; the paleopallium and the basal nuclei remain olfactory centers. The changes that occur in the amphibians correlate with the transition to a terrestrial life. Dependence on the sense of smell begins to diminish, the sensitivity to light, sound, and cutaneous stimulation increases. The shift of additional sense centers from a more posterior area into the cerebral hemispheres represents another trend in the evolution of the mammalian brain. It is also in the amphibians that a few cells from the gray matter begin to move away from the ventricle and into the walls of the pallium. Most of

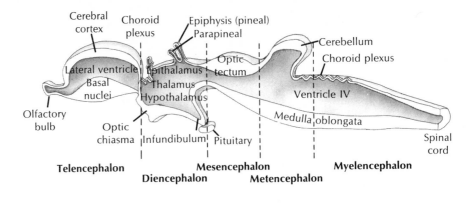

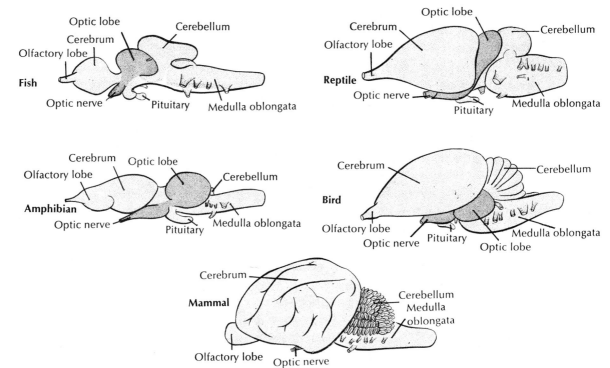

Fig. 12-20
Story of the evolution of the telencephalon involves the structural and functional expansion of the cerebral part of the telencephalon and the restriction of the olfactory center. (From Hickman, C. P., Sr., Hickman, C. P., Jr., Hickman, F. M.: Integrated principles of zoology, ed. 5, St. Louis, 1974, The C. V. Mosby Co.)

the gray matter of amphibians, however, is internal. All of the areas receive fibers from the olfactory center and the thalamus. Fibers that connect the archipallium with the paleopallium and with the basal nuclei also develop, and so these regions are able to correlate olfactory function with a few other simple impulses, possibly gustation. The basal nuclei relays impulses back

to the thalamus and to the midbrain. It begins to form an important correlation center that increases in complexity in more advanced groups.

A fourth region, the *neopallium*, differentiates laterally to the archipallium in some reptiles and all mammals. According to Romer, "the evolutionary history of the mammalian brain is essentially a story of neopallial expansion and elab-

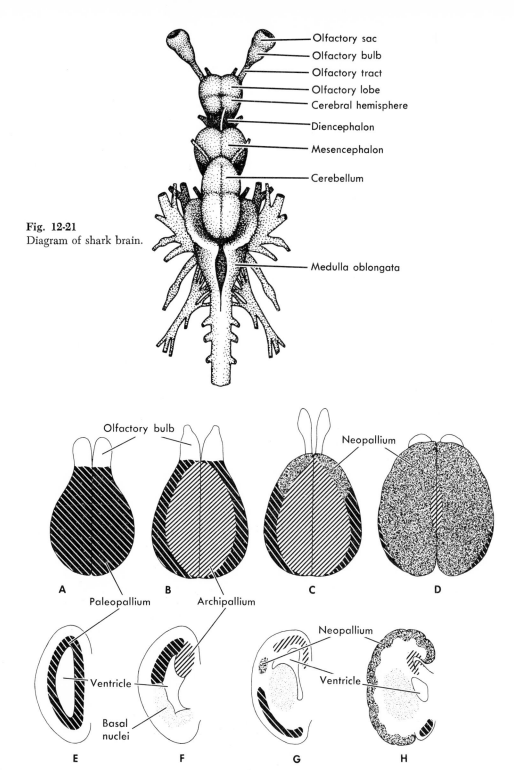

Olfactory sac
Olfactory bulb
Olfactory tract
Olfactory lobe
Cerebral hemisphere
Diencephalon
Mesencephalon
Cerebellum

Medulla oblongata

Fig. 12-21
Diagram of shark brain.

Olfactory bulb

Neopallium

A   B   C   D

Paleopallium   Archipallium   Neopallium

Ventricle   Ventricle

Basal nuclei

E   F   G   H

Fig. 12-22
Evolution of cerebral hemispheres as seen in diagrammatic dorsal view (*top row*) and cross section of left lobe (*bottom row*). Amphibian stage, **B** and **F**, adds archipallium and basal nuclei to primitive stage, **A** and **E**. The neopallium appears for the first time in reptiles, **C** and **G**, and continues to expand in mammals, **D** and **H**, where it becomes the cerebral cortex. The corpus striatum and archipallium are pushed to the interior, and the olfactory lobe diminishes in significance.

oration." It represents a complex association center that provides unlimited intellectual capacity. From the beginning it received sensory impulses from the brainstem, correlated them with other information, and relayed commands back to the brainstem. The neopallium consists of only a small area of superficial gray matter in reptiles and a somewhat larger region in the primitive mammals; in advanced mammals its surface area is considerable. It reaches its greatest development in man and is mainly responsible for the large size of the cerebral hemispheres.

The neopallium assumes more and more of the functions that in the lower vertebrates were centered in the brainstem and in the basal nuclei. As it increases in size, it covers the other areas, pushing them to the inner part of each hemisphere as shown in Fig. 12-22. In the majority of mammals it overlaps the midbrain and part of the cerebellum. The paleopallium is restricted to a small ventral area, the *piriform lobe*. The well-developed corpus striatum or basal nuclei moves toward the interior of the hemispheres, and the archipallium is forced medially, where it is

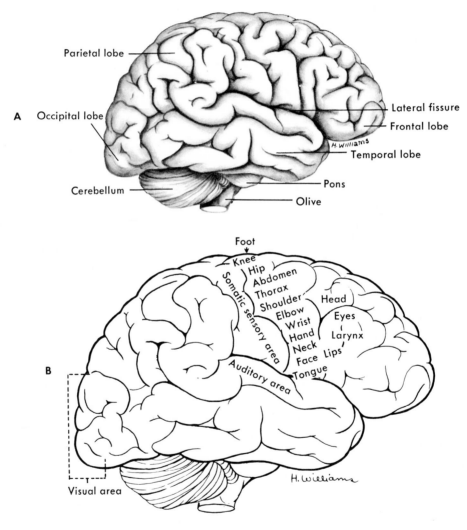

Fig. 12-23
Convolutions of mammalian cerebral cortex divide it into temporal, occipital, frontal, and parietal lobes, **A.** Except for the frontal area, specific functions have been ascribed to specific areas as indicated in **B.** (From Francis, C. C.: Introduction to human anatomy, ed. 6, St. Louis, 1973, The C. V. Mosby Co.)

known as the *hippocampus*. Automatic reactions remain centered in the corpus striatum. Beginning with the marsupials, a band of white myelinated fibers, the *corpus callosum* connects the two hemispheres.

As expansion continues, the cells of the gray matter composing the neopallium migrate nearer the surface. Here they become concentrated and are known in mammals as the *cerebral cortex*. Billions of neurons comprise the cerebral cortex. The walls of the cortex (neopallium) measure in man about 1/2 to 1/12 inch in thickness. As many as six different layers of neurons, with millions of neurons in each layer, make up the gray matter of the placental animal's cortex. The cells of the various layers of this continuous blanket enter into complex connections with one another by means of their axons and dendrites. It is impossible to comprehend the exact number of correlations that can be made.

The roof of the cerebral hemispheres is smooth in many of the lower vertebrates. In mammals, however, the more rapid increase in number of neurons at the surface of the neopallium as compared to the deeper lying parts, as well as the increase in underlying fiber volume causes the surface to be thrown into convolutions. The folds are referred to as *gyri;* the indentations are *sulci*. The convolutions divide the brain into various general areas. They are identified according to the skull bones surrounding them and are referred to as the temporal, occipital, frontal, and parietal lobes of the cerebral cortex (Fig. 12-23, *A*). With the exception of the frontal lobe, specific functions are ascribed to specific areas. For example, the occipital lobe is the center for vision; the rest of the centers are identified in Fig. 12-23, *B*.

As a result of the progressive development of the neopallium, the tectum of the mesencephalon loses its coordinating function. It now consists primarily of a center that relays information to the new association centers in the cortex. The somatic impulses relayed by the thalamus to the corpus striatum of lower animals are carried through and beyond the corpus striatum by fibers that now terminate in the neopallial surface. The cortex receives all data, integrates and coordinates the information, and then relays the commands back to either the cerebellum, the corpus striatum, or the hypothalamus, or by way of the pyramidal tracts to the brainstem and spinal cord.

PERIPHERAL NERVOUS SYSTEM
Autonomic nervous system

The *autonomic nervous system* is part of the peripheral nervous system and includes both sensory and motor neurons, since it functions reflexively. It is usually further divided into *sympathetic* and *parasympathetic* systems, which have antagonistic functions. In general, the term "autonomic nervous system" refers to the visceral motor fibers that innervate the smooth muscles of the internal organs, that is, those involuntary muscles of the heart, blood vessels, and digestive, urinary, and reproductive organs. The visceral sensory system differs from the somatic sensory system only in that it carries impulses to the cord from the viscera rather than from the body wall. However, the input of any somatic sensory nerve can also produce an automatic motor response. For example, something that an individual sees and finds disturbing can cause his heartbeat rate to increase. The visceral motor system differs distinctly from the somatic motor system; in fact, most authors define the antonomic system as consisting of only these visceral efferent fibers. Sometimes the student has the impression that the autonomic system is an independent system, but it should be considered as a functional division of the whole. Its control is located in the central nervous system and it is intimately bound together with the rest of the nervous system.

Comparison of somatic and autonomic nervous systems

Earlier in the chapter we described a typical spinal nerve as being composed of somatic and visceral fibers. Certain functional and structural characteristics help to differentiate the autonomic (visceral) system from the somatic.

When an impulse leaves the somatic motor nuclei in the cord, it passes down an axon to a muscle or gland. Should that muscle be located in the big toe, the axon extends from its cell body in the posterior regions of the cord to the big toe, a distance of perhaps 3 feet. Only *one* neuron is involved between the cord and the muscle. In the autonomic system, however, the impulse is conveyed from the cord to the effector organ via *two* neurons. The cell body of the first neuron is typically located in the visceral motor area of the gray matter, previously described. Its axon may extend to the *lateral ganglia*, lined up in a chain outside the central nervous system on either side of the vertebral column, or it may extend to the *collateral ganglia* located farther away, or even to the organ itself. The ganglia are those described as originating from the neural crest cells. In the ganglion the first neuron may synapse with a second neuron, the axon of which passes to the organ it innervates. In some cases, as will soon be described for the parasympathetic system, this ganglion is actually embedded in the tissues of the organ.

Preganglionic fibers, as their name implies, are axons that transfer the impulse from the cord to the lateral ganglion. The second neuron,

whose axons terminate in the muscle or gland, is referred to as the *postganglionic* neuron. Unlike the preganglionic fibers, they lack myelin sheaths.

When the ventral and dorsal roots of a spinal nerve unite outside the cord, they form a nerve trunk consisting of many fibers. This trunk soon divides into three branches, or *rami*. A *dorsal ramus*, composed primarily of somatic afferent and efferent fibers, passes to the dorsal epaxial region of the organism; a *ventral ramus* extends to the somatic hypaxial region of the organism; and a *visceral ramus* sends branches to the internal organs. The visceral rami can be further divided into two components, the *white* and *gray rami*, best understood by referring to Fig. 12-24. The preganglionic fibers of the sympathetic system leave the cord in the ventral root along with somatic motor fibers, but then pass to the lateral ganglia by way of the visceral rami. The myelinated preganglionic fibers make up

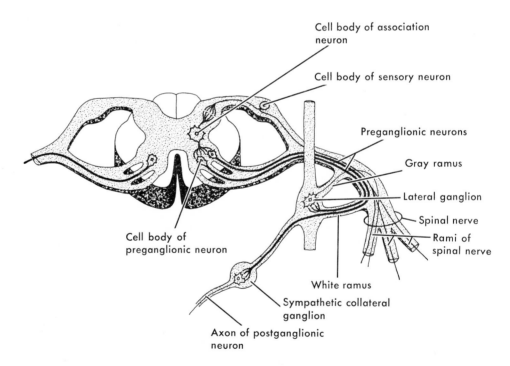

Fig. 12-24
Diagram showing visceral motor pathway from spinal cord to viscera. Two neurons are involved. The cell body of first neuron is located in spinal cord; its axons synapse at lateral ganglion or at sympathetic ganglion. A postganglionic fiber carries impulse to viscera. The myelinated fibers of the preganglionic fiber form the white ramus. The nonmyelinated fibers of the postganglionic fiber compose the gray ramus.

the white ramus. In the ganglion some of the preganglionic fibers synapse with postganglionic neurons, and these nonmedullated (nonmyelinated) postganglionic fibers give rise to the gray ramus.

As stated above, all sympathetic fibers do not synapse at the lateral ganglion; some may pass through the ganglia and extend anteriorly or posteriorly in the sympathetic chain before synapsing at levels other than where they originated. A third possibility exists for the preganglionic fiber to pass through the lateral chain ganglia to certain large ganglia located some distance away known as the *collateral ganglia*. The celiac, anterior mesenteric, and posterior mesenteric ganglia compose these collateral ganglia. Regardless of the location of the synapse, any one preganglionic neuron synapses with several postganglionic neurons. The latter, in turn, may then carry the impulse to several different organs. As a result sympathetic responses are widespread and involve many different structures.

Sympathetic and parasympathetic divisions

On the basis of function, structure, and location, the autonomic system of higher animals is further divided into two main divisions, the *sympathetic system* and the *parasympathetic system*. Both types of fibers innervate most internal organs. The two systems can be differentiated in several ways.

They differ in their physical relationship to the central nervous system. The preganglionic fibers of the sympathetic system leave the cord in the thoracolumbar regions. For this reason they are sometimes referred to as the *thoracolumbar autonomic system*. However, the preganglionic neurons of the parasympathetic fibers are mostly located in the medulla oblongata. Included are a few fibers to the iris and ciliary body that travel with the third cranial nerve, as well as a part of the facial (seventh), the glossopharyngeal (ninth), and the vagus (tenth) nerves. Also, nerves from the posterior parts of the cord belong to this system and send fibers to the large intestine, bladder, and reproductive tract. As a result, the parasympathetic portion of the autonomic system is referred to as the *craniosacral system*.

The locations of the synapses between preganglionic and postganglionic fibers is a second difference between the sympathetic and parasympathetic systems. The preganglionic fibers of the parasympathetic system do not synapse with the postganglionic fibers in the lateral or collateral ganglia as described above for the sympathetic system. Instead, they pass directly to the organs they innervate. Here, either in or near the organ itself, synapses occur with the second neuron. Since synapsis occurs some distance from the cord, the axons of the preganglionic neurons of the parasympathetic system are long compared to those of the sympathetic system that synapse just outside the cord. Of course, the postganglionic fibers are short in the parasympathetic system and long in the sympathetic system.

The two systems have opposite effects on the organs that they innervate. On the whole, the sympathetic system alerts the body for activity. It prepares it to meet an environmental challenge by speeding up its heartbeat and respiration rate and stimulating the integumentary glands, hair muscles, and skin capillaries. It depresses those activities not conducive to body activity, such as digestion, excretion, etc. The parasympathetic system, on the other hand, is sometimes referred to as the vegetative system, since it produces a reverse effect. Neither system is entirely stimulative or repressive, but can produce both excitatory or depressant effects depending on the structure under consideration. Under normal circumstances, the organism coordinates their effects and maintains a homeostatic state, with either system being able to take over temporarily if the occasion demands it.

The systems produce their effect by liberating certain chemicals, acetylcholine or norepinephrine, at their end organs. These were referred to as transmitter substances earlier in the chapter and are given the general term of *neurohumors*. The ends of all somatic neurons liberate acetylcholine. It is also released by the preganglionic fibers of both sympathetic and parasympathetic axons and by the axons of the parasympathetic postganglionic neurons. Such neurons are referred to as *cholinergic nerves*. Epinephrine-like (adrenaline-like) compounds are libered by the postganglionic endings of the sympathetic system and consequently this system is referred to as *adrenergic.*

Cranial nerves
General characteristics

The nerves that arise from the ventral surface of the brain and emerge through special openings (foramina) of the skull are referred to as *cranial nerves.* Together with the spinal nerves, they complete the peripheral nervous system. There are 10 pairs present in most anamniotes and 12 pairs in reptiles, birds, and mammals. The nerves are numbered starting at the anterior end. Roman numerals are often used. The name, number, origin, and distribution of the nerves from fish to man are similar, although, of course, where structures have been added or deleted through evolution, modifications occur. For example, nerves pass to the gills of aquatic animals. When amniotes undergo development, these nerves are either lost or they innervate the structures that evolved in the gill region. Although absent in man, a terminal nerve is present in most vertebrates, anterior to the first cranial nerve. Since it was discovered after the other nerves were numbered, it is usually labeled 0.

Earlier in the chapter, we described four functional components of the spinal nerves. These same general components are present in the cranial nerves. The cell bodies of the cranial motor nerves are located in nuclei in the brainstem. The cell bodies of the sensory neurons collect in ganglia near the brain. Somatic sensory fibers send twigs to the skin of the head and other somatic structures. Visceral sensory fibers relay information from the membranes of the pharynx, the anterior part of the gut. Somatic motor fibers terminate in structures derived from myotomes, for example, the eye muscles, and visceral motor fibers pass to the muscles of the gut. However, a special group of nerves, distinguished from the general nerves described above form an additional category of cranial nerves. They are the *special somatic sensory, special visceral sensory,* and *special visceral motor nerves.*

The terms "special" and "special visceral" need further clarification. As indicated in Chapter 11, the nose, eye, and acoustolateralis organs are defined as special sense organs, distinguished from the simpler receptors. The sensory nerves that pass from these organs to the brain retain this term and are known as the special somatic sensory nerves. A special visceral sensory nerve consists of fibers from the taste organ. The muscles that work the gill bars of fish are a special kind of muscle. They are not derived from myotomes and, although they are formed from lateral plate mesoderm, they differ from the smooth muscle of the gut (of splanchnic mesodermal origin). These gill muscles, referred to as visceral muscles, are striated, and in this respect are similar to skeletal muscles. They are innervated by cranial nerves known as special visceral motor nerves.

Classification of cranial nerves

In order to minimize rote memorization of names and functions of the cranial nerves, we advise grouping them in different ways. For example, two of the nerves, cranial nerve I (olfactory) and cranial nerve II (optic), are considered atypical nerves, since their embryonic origins do not conform to the usual pattern. These sensory nerves do not possess ganglia. The cell bodies of most sensory nerves are located near the spinal cord or brain, but cranial nerve I does not actually develop from neural tissue. Instead, the olfactory receptor cells, derived from the olfactory placode, send their projections into the olfactory lobe of the brain. These fibers combine to form the olfactory nerve. Cranial nerve II is actually a brain tract, since the retina is an evagination of the diencephalon and is considered a part of the brain. The optic nerve forms by a combination of fibers from the ganglionic cells located in the wall of the retina. These cells send their fibers back into other regions of the brain.

It is also helpful to remember that the forebrain arose in relation to the olfactory sense, the midbrain with the visual sense, and the hindbrain with the acousticolateralis sense. Cranial nerves can be grouped therefore, as in Table 12-1, according to the region of the brain with which they are associated. The fibers of the olfactory nerve extend to the telencephalon and the optic fibers extend to the diencephalon and then on to the tectum of the mesencephalon; cranial nerves III and IV arise from the mesencephalon, and nerves V to XII from the medulla oblongata.

The cranial nerves can also be divided into three general groups. Cranial nerves 0 (terminal nerve), I (olfactory), II (optic), and VIII (auditory) are all sensory nerves. Motor nerves consist of cranial nerves III (oculomotor), IV (trochlear), VI (abducens), and XII (hypoglossal). The remaining nerves, cranial nerves V (trigeminal), VI (fascial), IX (glossopharyngeal), X (vagus), and XI (spinal accessory), are all mixed nerves.

Specific cranial nerves

The following cranial nerves are grouped according to their functional components:

SOMATIC SENSORY

0, Terminal nerve. This is a small nerve of unknown function that runs parallel to the olfactory nerve but enters the diencephalon. It is apparently sensory in function, since it bears one or more ganglia. It may represent the remnants of an anterior nerve existing in ancestral vertebrates.

SPECIAL SENSORY. These nerves transmit impulses from the special sense organs.

I, Olfactory nerve. This is a sensory nerve that carries impulses from the olfactory sac to the telencephalon. It has no ganglion, but develops from the cells of the epithelial lining of the olfactory sac.

II, Optic nerve. This is a sensory nerve that carries impulses from the eye to the higher regions of the brain. The fibers from each side of the head unite in the floor of the diencephalon where some of them cross to the other side and give rise to the optic chiasma. The fibers then continue in the brain as optic tracts passing to the mesencephalon (in lower animals) or to the cerebral cortex (in higher forms).

VIII, Acoustic nerve. The ganglion giving rise to this nerve divides into two parts in higher animals: the spiral ganglion with fibers passing to the cochlear duct, and the vestibular ganglion that sends fibers to the semi-circular canals and the sacs of the inner ear. The lateral line nerve is closely related to the acoustic nerve. It enters the medulla of fish with nerve VIII, but is usually considered to be more closely combined with nerve VII.

SOMATIC MOTOR. These nerves carry impulses to the muscles that move the eyes and to the tongue muscles. Apparently they lost their dorsal roots; the remaining ventral roots compose the nerve.

III, Oculomotor nerve. This nerve arises from the mesencephalon and supplies the eye muscles that are derived from the first cranial myotome: the inferior oblique and the superior, inferior, and medial rectus muscles. A few fibers from nerve V usually accompany nerve III as they pass to the smooth muscles of the iris and ciliary body. However, these fibers are usually not considered a part of nerve III.

IV, Trochlear nerve. This nerve arises from neuroblasts in the floor of the mesencephalon just posterior to nerve III; it innervates the eye muscle derived from the second myotome. Its fibers pass upward in the wall of the brain where they then pass dorsally and cross to the opposite side. They emerge dorsally from the brain and pass to the superior oblique muscle of the eye.

VI, Abducens nerve. The abducens nerve originates from the motor nucleus located in the pontine region of the mesencephalon. It innervates the external rectus muscle of the eye, derived from the third myotome.

XII, Hypoglossal nerve. The hypoglossal nerve has several origins. The ventral roots of three or four nerves from the occipital region (back of head and neck) leave the medulla oblongata and merge into one nerve. This nerve innervates the occipital myotomes, which in the fish embryo migrate beneath the gill region to form the hypobranchial muscles. In higher forms, when the gills are lost, this region is remodeled. These muscles are lost in amphibians but contribute to the tongue musculature of amniotes. The hypoglossal nerve therefore innervates the tongue.

Mixed nerves

Mixed nerves all arise from the medulla oblongata and each is related to a gill arch of the fish. As a result, they are sometimes referred to as the *branchial nerves.* When amniotes lose their gills, the nerves innervate the structures derived from the gill area. Each nerve usually includes somatic sensory as well as special visceral sensory fibers and special visceral motor fibers. Cranial nerves V, VII, IX, and X are all considered mixed nerves. Originally, each nerve consisted of three main branches, a pharyngeal branch passing inward to the pharynx, a pretrematic branch running in front of the gill slit, and a posttrematic branch running in back of the gill slit.

V, Trigeminal nerve. This is a stout nerve that has a large semilunar (or gasserian) ganglion located outside the hindbrain. It is usually divided into three main branches: the ophthalmic, maxillary, and mandibular nerves. The fibers are primarily sensory from the face, nose, and mouth; they enter the brain at the somatic sensory column of the gray matter of the medulla. Motor fibers pass to the muscles of mastication. Since these muscles are derived from the muscles of the original first branchial arch, the nerves are considered special visceral motor nerves.

VII, Facial nerve. In fish, the facial nerve passes to the second arch and the spiracular gill slit (considered the second gill slit). It contains both somatic and visceral sensory, as well as visceral and special visceral motor fibers. Some of the fibers become intimately associated with fibers from nerve V and pass along with them to the anterior regions of the head. This nerve is called the facial nerve because in mammals the muscles of the second arch become the muscles of expression and retain the same innervation. There is a sensory ganglion, the geniculate ganglion, housing the cell bodies of the sensory portion of

the nerve. The visceral sensory fibers pass to the taste buds and to the lining of the pharynx. The large somatic sensory portion of the nerve passes to a lateral line system.

IX, Glossopharyngeal nerve. In fishes this nerve passes to the first functional gill and therefore contains both special visceral sensory and special visceral motor fibers. Its sensory cell bodies are located in two ganglia, one near the myelencephalon, the superior ganglion, and the other more laterally located, the petrosal ganglion. In fishes it contains both a pretrematic and a posttrematic branch; in mammals this nerve is lost to a great extent. Its visceral motor fibers innervate some of the muscles of the pharyngeal areas and parotid salivary gland; its visceral sensory fibers pass to the taste buds.

X, Vagus, and XI, spinal accessory nerves. The vagus is one of the most important nerves. It is a composite nerve formed by the union of several branches that pass to the posterior gill arches, those numbered four to six. When the amniotes lose their gill arches, some of these branchial fibers degenerate, but a few remain and innervate those structures derived from this region, such as the pharyngeal musculature. The main branch of the vagus is visceral and extends backward into the body along the gut where it gives off branches to the stomach, heart, lungs, and anterior intestine. It carries the visceral impulses to the medulla oblongata. It also relays visceral motor impulses back to these organs by way of the preganglionic branch of the parasympathetic system. Since the vagus represents a union of several nerves, it has several sensory ganglia as might be expected. A motor portion of the vagus of lower animals divides into a separate nerve. In mammals, it is known as nerve XI, or the spinal accessory nerve.

SUGGESTED READINGS

1. Bodian, D.: The generalized vertebrate neuron, Science **137**:323-326, 1962.
2. Bodian, D.: Neuron junctions: A revolutionary decade. President's address. Proceedings of the AAA Eighty-fifth meeting, Anat. Rec. **174**:73-82, 1972.

3. Hamburger, V.: Origins of integrated behavior. In Locke, M. (editor): Emergence of order in developing systems, New York, 1968, Academic Press Inc.

4. Jacobson, M., and Hunt, R. K.: The origins of nerve cell specificity, Sci. Am. **228**:26-35, 1973.

5. Kallen, B.: Early morphogenesis and pattern formation in the central nervous system. In DeHaan, R. L., and Ursprung, H. (editors): Organogenesis, New York, 1965, Holt, Rinehart & Winston.

6. Hamilton, W. J., Boyd, J. D., and Mossman, H. W.: Human embryology, Baltimore, 1962, The Williams & Wilkins Co.

7. Nawar, G.: Experimental analysis of the origin of the autonomic ganglia in chick embryo, Am. J. Anat. **99**:473-505, 1956.

8. Romer, A. S.: The vertebrate body, Philadelphia, 1962, W. B. Saunders Co.

9. Schally, A. V., Arimura, A., and Kastin, A. J.: Hypothalamic regulatory hormones, Science **179**:341-350, 1973.

10. Snider, R. S.: The cerebellum, Sci. Am. **199**:2-7, 1958.

11. Sperry, R. W.: Embryogenesis of behavioral nerve nets. In DeHaan, R. L., and Ursprung, H. (editors): Organogenesis, New York, 1965, Holt, Rinehart & Winston.

12. Watterson, R. L.: Structure and mitotic behavior of the early neural tube. In DeHaan, R. L., and Ursprung, H. (editors): Organogenesis, New York, 1965, Holt, Rinehart & Winston.

13. Weiss, P.: Neurogenesis. In Willier, B. H., Weiss, P., and Hamburger, V. (editors): Analysis of development, Philadelphia, 1955, W. B. Saunders Co.

14. Wenger, E. L.: An experimental analysis of relations between parts of the brachial spinal cord of the embryonic chick, J. Exp. Zool. **114**:51-86, 1950.

CHAPTER 13

DIGESTIVE AND RESPIRATORY SYSTEMS

The primitive gut tube extends from the anterior to the posterior end of the early embryo and contributes to both the digestive and respiratory systems of vertebrates. Most of the gut develops into the digestive tract. However, gills form in the walls of the pharynx of aquatic animals and a ventral diverticulum develops into the lungs of terrestrial animals, giving rise to the respiratory system. The allantois, a diverticulum from the gut in such animals as the chick (discussed in Chapter 9), acts as a respiratory membrane in the embryo. Thus, the digestive and respiratory systems have a common embryonic origin although they function in entirely different ways.

Other organs of the body also originate from the primitive gut. Digestive glands, such as the liver and pancreas, form as outgrowths of the original endodermal tube. Endodermal cells compose the endocrine glands, thyroid and parathyroid, as well as the two important lymphoid structures, the thymus and bursa of Fabricius.

The tube-within-a-tube arrangement, characteristic of vertebrate body plans, refers to the long tube of the digestive system that lies within the body tube. Ectoderm contributes to the outer epithelial surface of the body tube. However, epithelium derived from endoderm lines the inner surface of the digestive tract. The two surfaces are continuous at the oral cavity and anus (described in Chapter 7) where the epithelial lining of the digestive tract merges with the epidermis of the skin. Mesoderm contributes to the bulk of the body located between the two surfaces. The endoderm gives rise only to the lining of the gut and its associated structures; the rest of the tract, that is, the submucosa, muscularis, and serosa, form from the splanchnic mesoderm surrounding the endoderm.

The lumen (cavity) of the gut is considered a part of the external environment. Anything in the lumen is outside the body. Nothing gains entrance to the body unless it leaves the cavity of the gut and penetrates the cells, passing to the other side of the epithelial barrier. Digestive glands derived from endoderm line the stomach and intestine, and secrete their products into the lumen. The pancreas adds enzymes and the liver, bile, to the contents of the gut by way of their ducts, and digestion occurs in the lumen (outside the body proper). After these various chemicals break the food materials down into smaller absorbable molecules, they pass into the body. The remaining undigested substances are eliminated by way of the anus.

The digestive enzymes are secreted as inactive molecules that become active when they reach the acid contents of the stomach or the alkaline intestine. For this reason, the walls of the digestive tract are not digested by the enzymes they produce. A layer of mucus, secreted by the numerous goblet cells located along the length of the digestive tract, provides further protection to the lining.

As the respiratory system develops, the gut epithelium changes and adapts to one of two different respiratory media, water or air. In aquatic animals, gill filaments develop on the sides of the gill slits formed by the outpocketing of the walls of the pharynx. In terrestrial animals, a diverticulum from the gut either gives rise to the simple pouchlike lungs of amphibians and reptiles or to the highly branched respiratory tract of mammals.

A vascular system intimately associated with the gill and lung membranes transports the needed oxygen to the cells and the carbon dioxide away. Blood vessels are also closely associated with the rest of the gut lining. Food materials pass through the gut epithelium into the blood stream and the hepatic portal system carries them to the liver. The lymphatic system adds its products to the general circulatory system.

Since the surface of the gut and its diverticula is exposed to the external environment, it represents a vulnerable barrier to microorganisms and toxic agents. Consequently many patches of lymphoid tissue cluster along the length of the gut and the structures that form from it. Aggregations of lymphoid tissue, located along the adult respiratory, gastrointestinal, and urogenital tracts act as a line of defense for these surfaces.

DEVELOPMENT OF PRIMITIVE GUT TUBE
Formation of gut in lower animals

In all vertebrates the endoderm of the gastrula stage changes into a primitive endodermal tube that stretches from the mouth to the anus. Early in development it divides into three main divisions: (1) the foregut, (2) the midgut, and (3) the hindgut. The relationship of the archenteron to the primitive gut tube varies between those animals with total cleavage (cyclostomes, certain fish, and amphibians) and those with incomplete cleavage (reptiles, birds, and mammals).

In amphioxus and holoblastic animals, the archenteron consists of a tube; endoderm composes the floor and sides, but presumptive notochord and mesoderm completes the roof of the tube. In amphioxus the notochord separates from the mesoderm and the ends of the mesodermal pouches pinch off from the endoderm and fuse. The endoderm cells then migrate into the gap left by the mesoderm and notochord, forming a roof to the archenteron. In holoblastic-cleaved eggs, such as those of the frog, the endoderm separates from the roof of notochord and mesoderm, and the edges of the endoderm grow inward from each side under the notochord. In either case, a complete endodermal tube forms and its cavity becomes that of the alimentary canal. This process has been previously illustrated (Fig. 7-1) and described in Chapter 7.

During tubulation and elongation of the neural tube, the gut tube also extends in an anteroposterior direction. Underneath the notochord the cephalic portion of the gut projects forward into the developing head as the foregut. Two diverticula are associated with the early foregut and are more pronounced in some forms than in others. A dorsal portion, the *head gut,* projects toward the brain, and an anteroventral evagination pushes below the brain toward the epidermal ectoderm. This area gives rise to the *pharyngeal* region of the embryo, including the mouth. Unlike the foregut, the cavity of the midgut is small, since the floor of the primitive tube fills with yolk-laden cells. The young embryo lives off this stored intracellular food material until it can forage for itself. The posterior extension of the gut into the tail region gives rise to the hindgut. Evaginations similar to those of the foregut arise to form the dorsal *tail gut* and a more ventral *cloacal chamber*. The anus will form in this region. These areas can best be identified in the sagittal section of a young 3.5 mm. tadpole shown in Fig. 13-1.

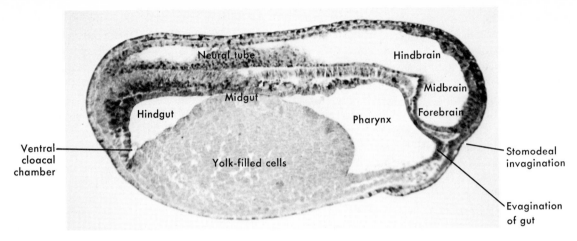

Fig. 13-1
Sagittal section of 3.5 mm. frog tadpole showing the early regions of the gut. ($\times$ 40.)

Formation of gut in meroblastic animals

The formation of the gut in animals with mero-blastic cleavage is more complicated than in those with holoblastic cleavage, since the flat sheet of endoderm must give rise to a tubular structure. In these embryos, the ectodermal and mesodermal parts of the blastodisk are spread out above the endodermal sheet, and it, in turn, grows around the yolk as the inner layer of the yolk sac. Early in development, head folds and tail folds project upward, undercut by the ectoderm. As a result, these areas of the embryo are lifted off the yolk, thus defining the head and tail ends. Since the anterior portion of the endoderm is closely applied to the ectoderm, it also is carried forward into these folds. The endodermal material, along with the ectodermal layer, rolls back under the head fold in such a manner that this area of the gut, the foregut, gains a floor as well as a roof and sides. The *anterior intestinal portal* marks the opening into the foregut region.

A similar posterior undercutting occurs simul-taneously in mammals, or later in such forms as the chick, and gives rise to a posterior endo-dermal tube, or hindgut. The opening into this area is the *posterior intestinal portal*. In between these two areas the midgut has only a roof and sides and is open ventrally to the yolk sac. Lat-eral folds move inward toward the median line and, accompanied by a dorsal arching of the

embryo, help lift the body from the extraembry-onic membranes. As the embryo continues to develop, anterior, posterior, and lateral under-cuttings continue until only a small area in the midgut is left attached to the yolk sac. In the chick this point of atttachment is known as the yolk stalk (see Fig. 9-2).

Once the foregut and hindgut are established in the meroblastic animal, development con-tinues in a manner similar to that described for the holoblastic animals.

FATE OF EARLY GUT TUBE

The foregut is a wider and more flattened area than is the hindgut. It is usually divided into several basic embryonic regions: (1) headgut, (2) stomodeal area, (3) pharyngeal region, (4) esophagus, and (5) stomach. The hepatopyloric segment located at the junction of the foregut and midgut is associated with the liver and pan-creas. The midgut gives rise primarily to the in-testine. From the hindgut the transitory tail gut projects dorsally into the tail region. The endo-derm evaginates ventrally where it meets the ectoderm and forms the proctodeal plate.

Foregut
Headgut

The headgut is the most anterior region of the foregut and projects forward toward the end of the notochord and the brain. A transitory structure not found in the adult animal, it acts as part of the head organizer in the early stages of development.

Stomodeal area

The stomodeum gives rise to the oral cavity that appears rather late in embryonic life. The mouth forms by the anterior endoderm pushing outward (evagination) and the ectoderm (stomodeal ectoderm) invaginating to form an *oral plate* or *membrane*. Later this membrane thins and eventually ruptures, forming a *mouth* and an *oral cavity*. Experiments indicate that the contact of the endoderm with the ectoderm near the end of the gastrulation stage initiates the stomodeal invagination. If the anterior endoderm is experimentally removed before it comes in contact with the ectoderm, the ectoderm does not invaginate and no mouth forms. However, if the endoderm is removed later, in the neurula stage after the two germ layers have contacted one another, the ectoderm continues to invaginate. The neural tube located immediately dorsal to this area of gut also helps to induce the formation of the mouth. Fig. 13-1 shows the relationship of brain to gut in a saggital view of a young tadpole.

Structures of oral cavity

In general, the same thin stratified epithelium described in Chapter 10 as composing the integument, covers the surface of the oral cavity. Some anatomists believe that ectoderm from the stomodeal invagination lines most of the cavity, but certainly endoderm also contributes to it.

TONGUE. In lower animals, a fold projecting from the floor of the oral cavity is considered a tongue. It lacks muscles. Movements of the gills produce some movement in the fold of tissue, since cartilage associated with the gill system contributes to its support. It probably functions to hold the prey of the animal; in fact, in the bony fishes this elevated ridge in the floor of the mouth contains teeth. It is not until land animals evolved that the tongue became flexible and protrusible and was used in the acquisition of food.

The "true" tongue of higher animals forms from a fusion of three primordia. In the bird, the *tuberculum impar* develops as a median swelling on the floor in front of the *copula*, the most posterior median elevation. The tuberculum impar make up the middle part of the tongue. Extensions of the tuberculum impar give rise to the most anterior part of the tongue in the bird. In mammals, the fusion of two anterior *lateral swellings* contribute further to its formation. As a result, the mammalian tongue is a heavy structure containing both intrinsic and extrinsic muscles.

If you recall, only the covering of the tongue forms from either stomodeal ectoderm or endoderm. Mesoderm gives rise to the main bulk of the tongue, that is, the muscles and its supporting skeletal structures. Nerves invade its tissue. The surface of the tongue of vertebrate animals and in some cases the oral cavity itself contain numerous projections, or papillae, classified into two or three different types according to their shape. The oral cavity contains taste buds that in mammals are concentrated in the papillae, as shown in Fig. 13-2. Mucus-secreting goblet cells also are present. Adaptations of the tongue help the animal secure various types of food materials. For example, the tongue of insectivores is tubular and that of the woodpecker is extremely long. The amphibian tongue is attached anteriorly; its free end is folded back on the floor of the mouth and is flipped out to catch insects.

ORAL GLANDS. The evolution of the mouth glands is correlated with the movement toward land and the adaptation of the animal toward specific foods. Glands are not so important in aquatic animals, since the water aids in swallowing the food. The oral cavity of fishes contain simple mucous glands, described in Chapter 10; multicellular glands are rarely present. An exception is the lampreys, which secrete a special material preventing the blood of their prey from coagulating.

The membrane lining the oral cavity of the amphibians is similar to that of the fishes, except it is thinner and more vascular. Amphibians depend on their integuments for much of their oxygen exchange, since their sac-like lungs are inadequate. Branched multicellular glands appear

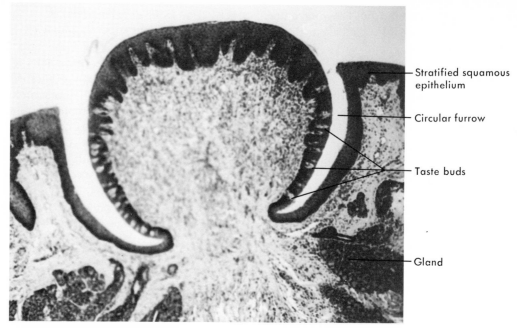

Fig. 13-2
Anterior dorsal surface of tongue is covered by three types of small excrescences or papillae. Section through a circumvallate papilla of rhesus monkey (*Macaca*) shows many taste buds located on the lateral surface of the papilla. (× 4.)

for the first time in the amphibia and are comparable to the salivary glands of mammals.

The reptiles retain the goblet cells and the branched tubular glands of the amphibians. Keratinization of the oral epithelium represents the major change as the reptiles moved to land, and water loss from moist surfaces became an important problem. Modified salivary glands form the poison glands of snakes and Gila monsters. As many as seven types of salivary glands are present in birds, depending on the type of food eaten. Aquatic birds, which eat the slippery food of the seas, have less developed glands. Grain eaters, on the other hand, need to mix their food with mucous secretions to make swallowing easier. In addition, some of the secretions are used to glue the components of the nest together. In general these glands lack enzymes, although amylase is reported in the salivary secretion of turkeys and pigeons.

One of the functions of the digestive system is to break down the large food particles into smaller absorbable units. Most of this process takes place in the more posterior regions of the digestive tract, but it begins in the oral cavity with the development of teeth that physically break up the food. Glands containing *ptyalin,* an amylase, initiates starch digestion in the mouth. The glands release both mucus and a more watery type of secretion. Among the several oral glands are three prominent salivary glands that arise in the embryo as three pairs of epithelial buds. These buds invaginate but remain connected to the surface by ducts. They are the *parotid, submaxillary,* and *sublingual glands,* most developed in the mammals.

TEETH. There are two types of teeth in the oral cavity of vertebrates: horny teeth and "true bony teeth." The horny type is limited to the cyclostomes, frog and toad larvae, and prototherian mammals. The horny teeth of the jawless lamprey are situated in its sucker, with the sharpest ones located on its rasping tongue. In the frog larva these teeth are nothing more than a horny covering of the jaws and are lost at the time of metamorphosis, being replaced by the bony type. The adult platypus shows the reverse; the young have true vertebrate teeth that are replaced by horny structures that grow over them. They are used for breaking the shells of mollusks.

Although teeth are lacking in some fishes, reptiles, and birds, most jawed vertebrates have teeth basically similar to the one diagrammed in Fig. 13-3. The typical vertebrate tooth, formed from a combination of epithelium and mesoderm, consists of the exposed *crown*, a *neck*, and one or many *roots*. Vertebrate teeth are composed essentially of dentine, with a covering of enamel or enamel-like material, and a core, or pulp cavity.

Early in development a thickened *dental lamina*, a ridge of oral epithelium, differentiates and at intervals sends epithelial buds, tooth germs, down into the underlying mesoderm. This process is depicted in Fig. 13-4. The cells of these buds give rise to the enamel organ of the tooth. Each bud develops into a cup-shaped organ enclosing mesenchyme. The cells on the surface of the cup surrounding the mesenchyme are arranged in a row and differentiate into *ameloblasts* capable of secreting enamel. The cluster of enclosed mesenchyme cells (dental papilla) form the tooth pulp and give rise to the *odontoblasts*. These cells are responsible for depositing the dentine of the tooth.

The odontoblasts initiate tooth formation when they start depositing the matrix for the dentine. This is later impregnated with inorganic calcareous materials and converted to a hard

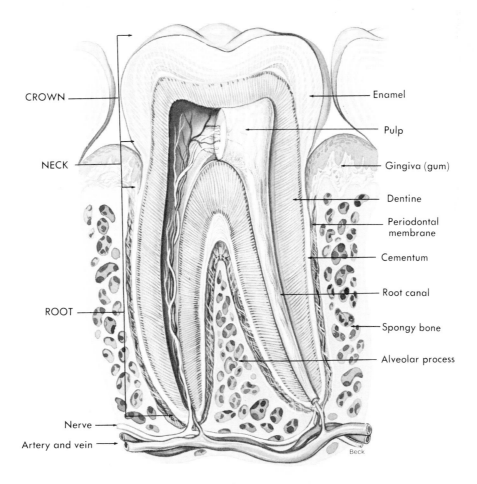

Fig. 13-3
Diagram of typical vertebrate tooth showing crown, neck, and root. It is composed of dentine covered with enamel or enamel-like material and contains a pulp cavity with nerves and blood vessels. (From Anthony, C. P., and Kolthoff, N. J.: Textbook of anatomy and physiology, ed. 8, St. Louis, 1971, The C. V. Mosby Co.)

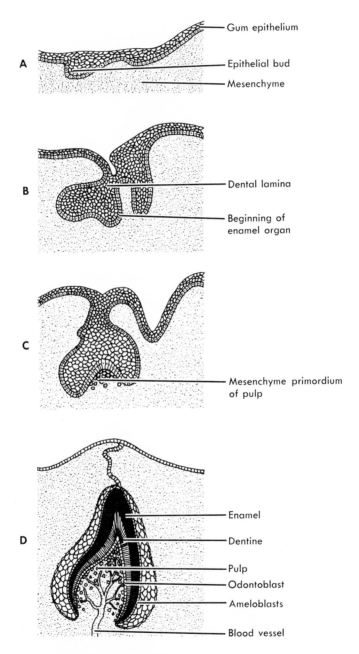

Fig. 13-4

Development of tooth. Epithelial bud, **A**, develops into a cup-shaped structure, the enamel organ, **B** and **C**, which gives rise to the crown of the tooth. Blood vessels in the pulp supply materials to the odontoblasts, **D**, and dentine is deposited on the inner surface of the enamel organ.

bonelike substance, the dentine. As deposition of the dentine continues, the odontoblasts are pushed toward the mesodermal pulp.

The ameloblasts on the inner layer of the enamel organ deposit a cap of enamel around the dentine of a reptilian or mammalian tooth. Once the tooth erupts through the gums, the ameloblasts degenerate. Consequently, after the enamel forms, it cannot grow or be replaced. In lower animals, other hard materials (vitrodentine) may be substituted for the enamel. Blood vessels and nerves grow into the pulp located in the center of the tooth. The formation of the tooth occurs beneath the gums, but the process continues downward from the crown toward the developing root. As this occurs, the whole tooth pushes upward.

Anchorage of the tooth in the mouth occurs in various ways and its type of attachment forms the basis for classifying the tooth. About the time the crown erupts through the gums in most vertebrate forms, it is cemented into the socket of the jaw. This type of socket relationship is referred to as a *thecodont* tooth. Some teeth, however, fuse to the jaw, either on its upper edge or on its inner surfaces. In some cases teeth are not limited to the jaw region, but appear in the roof of the mouth or on any surface where the dental lamina appears.

Vertebrate teeth are basically conical structures, modified in various forms and adapted to feeding habits of the individual species. Conical teeth tear the food; the surfaces of other teeth bite, cut, grind, or crush. All the teeth of a shark are conical; in mammals, although some of the anterior teeth are conical, some of the back ones are modified for grinding (premolars) or for chewing (molars). The elephant's tusk is an incisor tooth that grows constantly. The fangs of some snakes are basically tubular teeth, others have a deep groove in them. These teeth open by a duct to a salivary gland that synthesizes venom.

In some vertebrates (such as sharks), teeth are constantly lost and replaced (polyphyodont). New teeth form from buds located deep in the oral tissue. The mouths of fishes are often found to contain old teeth, mature teeth, as well as teeth that are just beginning to erupt through

the gums. Some fishes, however, have only one set (monophyodont). Mammals have two sets of teeth (diphyodont), the so-called "milk teeth" and the permanent set.

Pharynx

The pharynx is defined as that portion of the foregut between the oral cavity and esophagus. In the early embryo it is a large structure, but it becomes modified in the adult of higher animals where it forms a passageway to the digestive and respiratory systems.

FORMATION OF GILL SLITS. The presence of gill slits in the pharynx is one of the three characteristics that link all chordates together. Along with the hollow dorsal nerve cord and notochord, gill slits are present in the embryo of all animals that belong to the phylum Chordata. They are also present in such seemingly unrelated animals as the filter-feeding, tiny acorn worm, *Balanoglossus,* which belongs to the Hemichordata. It is because of the presence of these three chordate characteristics that some investigators trace the ancestry of the vertebrates to the protochordates and from there to ancestors common to the echinoderms. See Fig. 2-9.

The gill slits of the primitive chordates function in filter-feeding. Water with debris and food particles pass into the pharynx by way of a mouth or incurrent syphon, often aided by cilia. The food is trapped in layers of mucus and carried to the bottom of the pharynx by ciliary action; the water then continues to the outside by way of the many gill clefts that open in the pharyngeal region. It appears that originally the pharynx was a highly specialized structure that functioned for food collecting. The animal was sessile. It waited for the food to come to it and then merely strained the food out as the liquid flowed through the pharynx.

Gill slits form when the endoderm lining of the pharynx pushes outward (laterally), forming *pharyngeal pouches.* These outpocketings of endoderm are also referred to as *visceral,* or *branchial, pouches.* The pouches induce the skin ectoderm to invaginate and form *visceral,* or *branchial, furrows.* The invaginating ectodermal furrows and evaginating endodermal pouches approach one another, separated by a *branchial*

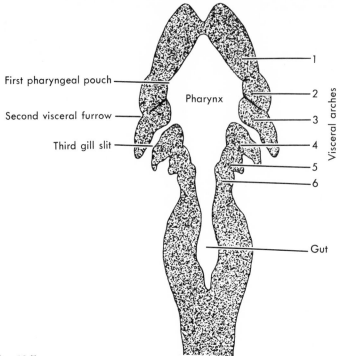

Fig. 13-5
Horizontal section of frog larva showing relation of arches, pouches, furrows, and clefts.

membrane. If the membrane ruptures, a continuous *gill slit,* or *gill cleft,* forms, connecting the interior of the pharynx with the outside of the animal. This relationship is diagrammed in Fig. 13-5.

The formation of clefts divides the hypomere of this region into blocks of mesodermal tissue. These blocks of mesoderm (sandwiched between two clefts) are referred to as *arches.* As was true for the pouches and furrows, they are given a variety of names. Branchial, visceral, or pharyngeal arches are all synonymous terms. (Do not confuse the term branchial with *brachial;* the latter term refers to the anterior limb.) Since these arches have filamentous gills attached to them in the fishes, they are also called gill arches. The term "pharyngeal arch" is usually reserved for the arches of amniotes on which gills never develop.

Gill pouches form in the pharynx of all vertebrate embryos, but under no circumstances should these be confused with gills. Gills are filamentous structures that develop on the walls of the gill slits and function in respiration. Amniote embryos have pharyngeal pouches but never develop gills. Gill slits are transitory structures in reptiles and birds and may never open at all in the mammals. Their formation is another example of the conservative manner in which the amniote repeats the developmental processes of many ancestral generations.

The visceral slits and the visceral arches are numbered and given names, starting at the anterior end of the animal. Probably the first visceral pouch, or perhaps several anterior visceral pouches, of some ancestral vertebrate were incorporated into the formation of the mouth. The first pouch in modern forms is usually considered the one that gives rise to the spiracle or middle ear. The *first arch* is anterior to the first cleft and contributes to the jaws; this arch is also known as the *mandibular arch.* The *second arch* is the *hyoid arch,* but the remaining arches are known merely by their number. Later on when we discuss the circulatory system, we shall learn that an aortic arch, an arterial branch of the vascular system, grows into each visceral arch. The names of these aortic arches correspond to their location; that is, aortic arch number three is located in the third visceral arch. Since a meaningful discussion of the aortic arches depends on an understanding of the visceral arches, it is a good idea to get the names and numbers of these arches straight in your mind at this time.

The number of gill clefts that form in the pharynx varies with the organism. There may be as many as 50 gill slits present in amphioxus, but this number is much reduced in the vertebrates. Probably the primitive vertebrate had as many as 10 to 14 gill slits. Most of the present-day cyclostomes (*Petromyzon*) retain seven, but in a few of the cyclostomes the number may vary from six to 14, depending on the species. The sharks usually have only six, with the first one modified to form the spiracle. The amphibians develop five clefts and amniotes have only four. A 4-week-old human embryo has five arches separated by four clefts. Gills develop on the sides of the clefts in adult fishes and some amphibians and become part of the respiratory system. Adult amniotes lose their gill clefts, but their development in the embryo represents the imprint of ancestral patterns.

DERIVATIVES OF PHARYNGEAL POUCHES. The first gill cleft of the elasmobranchs gives rise to the spiracle, but in amphibians and all amniotes this pouch never breaks through. Masses of epithelial cells from the walls and floor of the second, third, and fourth pouches give rise to the tonsils, thyroid, parathyroid, and thymus glands and ultimobranchial bodies.

Middle ear. The first pouch in the tetrapods never breaks through but remains drawn out from the pharynx and develops into the middle ear as described in Chapter 11. As the cavity expands, its walls wrap themselves like a mesentery, around the cartilage precursors of the auditory ossicles. These ossicles organize from the adjacent mesenchyme. Even in the adult they do not lie free in the cavity of the middle ear but are covered by an epithelium continuous with the lining of the cavity (as suggested in Fig. 13-6). As the wall of the pouch approaches the surface, the epidermal ectoderm invaginates and a membrane, the *tympanic membrane,* forms of

endoderm and ectoderm. The first ectodermal furrow gives rise to the external auditory meatus in those animals with an external ear. That part of the original pouch remaining connected to the pharynx becomes the constricted *eustachian tube* (see Fig. 11-10).

Thyroid gland. All vertebrates have a thyroid gland. It develops as a median diverticulum from the floor of the pharynx between the first and second pouches. The distal end of this median cluster of cells migrates ventrally into the underlying mesenchyme and takes up a position on the anterior surface of the trachea. It remains temporarily attached by the remnants of the original duct, now referred to as the *thyroglossal duct.* It eventually loses its connection to the floor of the pharynx and takes a variety of forms. The thyroid tissue may be dispersed, as in the fishes, and scattered along the ventral aorta. In other forms, a capsule surrounds the thyroid and its tissue is concentrated in one or two lobes. The human thyroid is bilobed, connected by a thin isthmus, and located on either side of the trachea just below the larynx.

The structural unit of the thyroid is the *follicle,* a hollow ball of cells, one layer thick. A section through the gland (Fig. 13-7) shows the arrangement of the thyroid cells into follicles. A gelatinous, amber-colored secretion, the *colloid,* fills the center of the follicle and makes its first appearance in the human embryo by the third month. The colloid serves as a storage area for the thyroid hormone. In storage form, the thyroid hormone combines with a protein to form a large molecule of *thyroglobulin.*

The thyroid hormone is a general term referring to thyroxine, 3,5,3'-triiodothyronine, and other active products synthesized by the gland. It regulates the metabolic rate in homoiothermic animals and controls metamorphosis in amphibians (poikilothermic). One of the pituitary hormones, the thyroid-stimulating hormone (TSH) regulates the synthesis, storage, and release of thyroid hormone. The hypothalamus, which is sensitive to the levels of the circulating thyroid hormone, controls the entire process. When the level of this hormone in the blood is low, the neurosecretory cells, described in Chapter 12, manufacture a "releasing factor" that stimulates

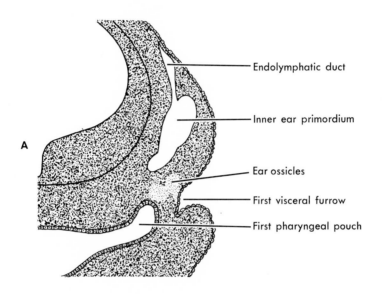

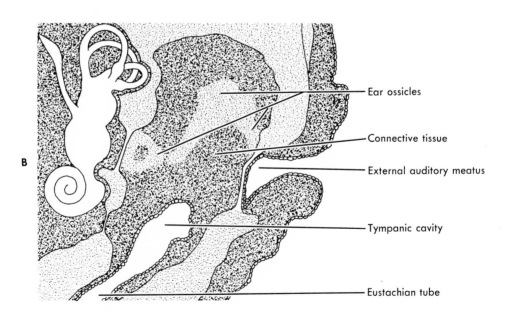

Fig. 13-6
Diagram showing development of middle ear. The first pharyngeal pouch, **A**, differentiates into the tympanic cavity and eustachian tube. The first visceral furrow becomes the external auditory meatus in those animals possessing an outer ear, **B**.

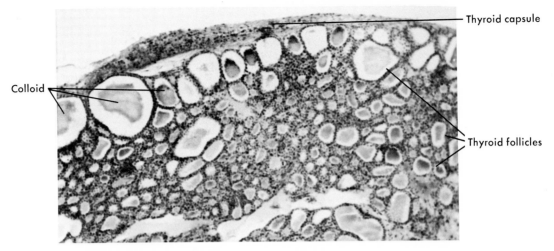

Colloid

Thyroid capsule

Thyroid follicles

Fig. 13-7
Section through rabbit's thyroid gland showing different-sized follicles typically filled with a gelatinous secretion, the colloid. (× 10.)

the pituitary to release TSH (Chapter 12). This, in turn, stimulates the thyroid to synthesize and/ or secrete more of its hormone. The relationship between the hypothalamus, pituitary, and thyroid is another example of a feedback mechanism controlling vital functions in the body. The concept of this negative feedback mechanism was first discussed in Chapter 3 when we considered the control of the reproductive system.

The thyroid gland also synthesizes a hypocalcemic factor, *thyrocalcitonin,* a hormone antagonistic to parathormone (parathyroid hormone). It is present in mammals and has been reported in birds, but its role in the lower animals is unknown. The thyroid cells responsible for the synthesis of this principle are believed to derive from the last pair of pharyngeal pouches. In fishes, amphibians, reptiles, and birds these cells form the ultimobranchial bodies.

Tonsils. The dorsal half of the second pouch gives rise to the *palatine tonsil,* one of the several varieties of tonsils found in man. Phagocytic lymphocytes infiltrate these clusters of cells. Situated at the anterior opening into the digestive tract, they represent one of the body's defense mechanisms.

Parathyroid glands. Parathyroid glands are present in all tetrapods—amphibians, reptiles, birds, and mammals—but they have not been identified in fishes. They vary in number from one to four pairs, depending on the species, and arise in the embryo from the corners of the third and fourth pouches. If only one pair remains in the adult, it is usually derived from pouch three. In man and certain other animals, the cells break away from the pouches and migrate into the neck region where they lie near or are embedded in thyroid tissue (Fig. 13-8). The gland contains no follicles but consists of secreting cells known as *chief cells.* In man, a second type of cell is also present, the *oxyphils,* believed to be nonsecretory in nature. Since the parathyroid glands control mineral (calcium) metabolism, they are essential for life, at least in the amniotes. Their removal causes the animal to go into tetany, a neuromuscular dearrangement that results in death.

Dogs are particularly sensitive to any change in their mineral metabolism. In the early days of endocrine research, the removal of the thyroid usually brought on the convulsions of tetany. The investigators of this period did not realize that the parathyroid was embedded in the tissue and, therefore, removal of the thyroid also eliminated the parathyroid gland. The resulting syndrome was erroneously attributed to the loss of the thyroid hormone. In the rabbit, accessory parathyroids, distinct from the thyroid tissue, are unusually prevalent; therefore, thyroidectomy (surgical removal of the thyroid

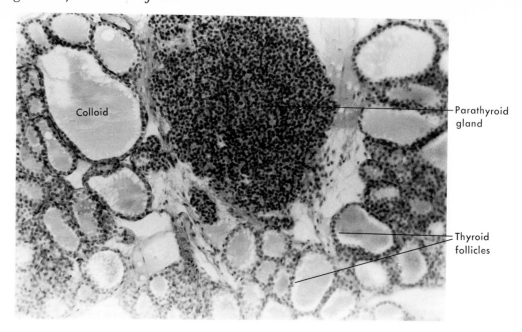

Colloid

Parathyroid gland

Thyroid follicles

Fig. 13-8
Section showing parathyroid gland embedded in thyroid tissue of rabbit. (× 100.)

glands) does not induce tetany. It was not until this animal was studied that the functions of the two glands were established and the true effect of removal of the parathyroid described. The parathyroid gland produces the hormone, *parathormone*. It acts on the cells of bone and kidney tubules and regulates the metabolism of such ions as calcium, phosphate, pyrophosphate, citrate, and magnesium.

Ultimobranchial bodies. The ultimobranchial bodies originate from the posterior margins of one of the posterior branchial pouches. As the thyroid gland enlarges, it incorporates these structures. Their fate is somewhat controversial; some believe they degenerate and are resorbed, but others report a conversion to thyroid tissue. Their embryology and histology suggest that in fishes, which lack parathyroid glands, the ultimobranchial bodies with the aid of high levels of vitamin D may take over the function of regulating calcium levels. The problem, however, remains to be resolved, since there are no conclusive data at this time demonstrating this function in fish.

Thymus gland. The thymus arises from the third and fourth pouches as sacs that rapidly form bars and become attached to the pericardium. A spongework of fibers furnishes a foundation for the organ; thymic corpuscles develop from the endodermal cells and invade the gland. The gland is large during infancy and prepuberty, but around the time of puberty it starts to regress. Over the years, attempts were made to identify a hormone produced by the thymus, but to this date none has been isolated. Histologically, it is part of the lymphoid system and is present in all vertebrates (Fig. 13-9).

The results of recent investigations show that the thymus plays a role in establishing the body's immune response. Removal of the thymus from a mature animal produces no demonstrable effects. However, if it is removed from a newborn, the production of lymphocytes decreases. During the past decade, evidence accumulated on mammals, at least, shows the body's immune mechanism to involve two types of lymphocytes, the thymic-independent, or B, cell and the thymic-dependent, or T, cell. Immunoglobulins and the antibodies they produce are part of the B-lymphocyte system. The other type of lymphocytes, the T cells, are specialized against cancer and organ transplants. The introduction of

Capsule

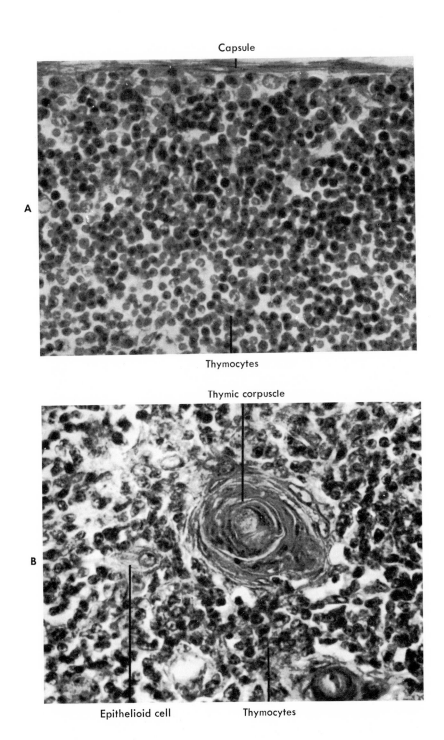

A

Thymocytes

Thymic corpuscle

B

Epithelioid cell   Thymocytes

Fig. 13-9
A, Section through cortex of thymus showing densely packed small lymphocytes. **B,** Number of lymphocytes decreases in medulla of thymus. Thymic corpuscles, characteristic of the thymus, are present. (× 640.) (With permission of Bevelander, G.: Essentials of histology, ed. 7, St. Louis, 1974, The C. V. Mosby Co.)

foreign antigens into the adult animal, either in the form of macromolecules or tissue grafts, stimulates the formation of antibodies against the antigen and results in rejection of the grafts. This reaction is described as a *cell-mediated immune response.* The lymphocytes involved are called T cells, because they are dependent on the thymus gland for their differentiation.

Evidence for the binary nature of the immune system is based on work carried out in chickens. A lymphoid organ, known as the bursa of Fabricius, arises from the posterior gastrointestinal tract. The fact was discovered accidentally that removal of the bursa interfered with B cell production, and removal of the thymus reduced the number of T cells. Thus, in the immune system of the chick, each organ is responsible for a distinct cell line of lymphocytes.

Man has no bursa, but it has been suggested that bone marrow and /or Peyer's patches, clusters of lymphoid tissue along the gut, may be the source of his B cells. Apparently, the bone marrow is also the source of T cells, which journey to the thymus where they proliferate and acquire a specific thymic factor. Interactions between these two systems are believed to occur. In some cases, for example, the B cells appear to need the help of T cells to produce their antibody against a given antigen.

There is evidence that the thymus is also involved in the immune response in lower animals. As shown in studies of immunity in amphibians *(Xenopus),* the larva's lymphocytes develop the capacity to invade a foreign tissue graft soon after the lymphoid maturation of its thymus. This can occur as early as 17 days after fertilization.

ORGANS OF RESPIRATION. As the chordates evolved, the function of the gill clefts changed from food gathering (filter feeding) to respiration. In aquatic animals, gill filaments develop on the sides of the pouches. Some posterior pouches are modified to form air bladders, functioning either in respiration or as a hydrostatic organ.

Most of the body cells of terrestrial animals are too far removed to exchange their gases directly with air. In these animals a ventral diverticulum from the gut, possibly representing posterior gill pouches, gives rise to special structures: a set of conducting tubes and lungs. The development of the respiratory system, that is, the system of anatomical structures that allows the exchange of oxygen and carbon dioxide between the organism and the environment, is closely associated with the development of the gut, specifically, the anterior portion, the pharynx.

For this exchange of gases to occur, the respiratory system must be in intimate association with the circulatory system. Oxygen from the outside environment passes into the blood, and carbon dioxide moves from the bloodstream to the outside. The circulatory system acts as a transport system between the external environment and the internal environment of the cells. To handle the respiratory needs of the animal, the respiratory structure must have a thin, moist, vascular membrane through which necessary gases diffuse. Simple squamous or low cuboidal cells in close contact with blood vessels usually compose this membrane. Actually, any membrane in contact with an oxygen supply can function in gaseous exchange. Amphioxus uses its thin skin as a respiratory organ. In most cases gills or lungs furnish the respiratory membrane, but it is possible to take advantage of other vascular surfaces. Many amphibians utilize the integument as an accessory respiratory organ, as described in Chapter 10, but the roof of the mouth, the cloaca, or hairlike projections from the pelvic fins or limbs also act as respiratory surfaces.

The exchange of oxygen and carbon dioxide between the animal and the outside environment is only one aspect of respiration. The term "respiration" also includes the mechanical operation of the system (external respiration) and those processes that go on at the cellular level (internal respiration). These functional aspects of respiration are usually considered within the realm of physiology. We are primarily interested in the morphogenesis of this system, that is, the development and anatomy of the organs that expedite this gaseous exchange.

Internal gills. Gills may be of two types: *internal gills* and *external gills.* Internal gills are located on the sides of the gill slits; external gills are feathery extensions of the integument above the gill openings and are limited to the larvae of a few bony fishes and amphibians. Water with its dissolved oxygen is brought in through the mouth and expelled through the gill slits, therefore, there is a constant flow of water over the surface of the vascular internal gills. External gills lay bathed by the surrounding medium.

A fusion of ectoderm from the furrow and endoderm from the pouch lines the gill slits. As in the formation of the oral and cloacal cavities, the precise boundary line between the two germ layers cannot be determined. The mesenchyme caught between the gill slits consists of vertical columns of tissue. This division imparts a seg-

mental appearance to the mesenchyme, but it is not considered true segmentation, since it does not correspond to the segmentation of the myotomes. Instead it is referred to as *branchiomerism*. The mesenchyme of the arches differentiates into cartilage that supports the gills, muscles that move the gills, and blood vessels that help in the exchange of gases.

Although gill construction among the fishes varies, we can describe a basic pattern. The lining of the gill slit is thrown into folds, or *gill filaments*. Each gill filament, in turn, forms extensive outpocketings, or *gill lamellae*. The strip of tissue on which the gills are located may extend to the body wall as the *interbranchial sep-*

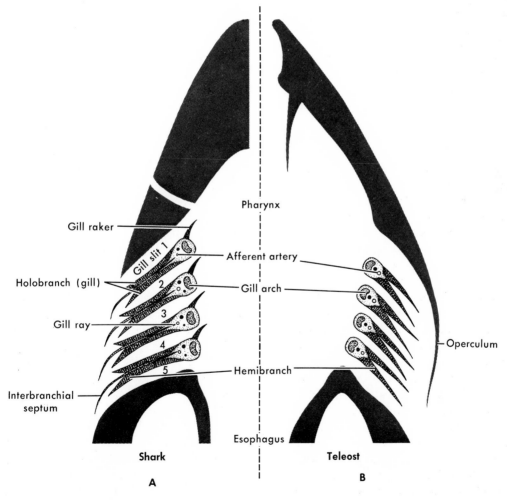

Fig. 13-10
Diagram of gill structure in sharks, **A**, and teleosts, **B**. See text for discussion.

tum (or *gill septum*). Such a septum is present in the elasmobranchs whose name in fact, means "straplike". The gill filaments on one side of the gill slit make up a *hemibranch*, or half gill. Two hemibranches, one on each side of the gill septum, form a *holobranch*, or a *gill*, as shown in Fig. 13-10, *A*.

A dorsoventrally oriented cartilaginous or bony *gill arch* supports the gills. Projections from this arch, called *gill rays*, are embedded in the tissue of the gill filaments, stiffening them, and offering further support. *Gill rakers*, project fingerlike from the inner edge of the skeletal arch and extend into the cavity of the pharynx where they function as a sieve. They prevent large pieces of food or debris from passing into the gill region by diverting them to the esophagus.

The surface of the gill lamellae functions in the exchange of gases, since there is a rich capillary network located immediately under the epithelium. In amphioxus, branches from the ventral aorta pass dorsally through the many visceral arches to the dorsal aorta. These arches are believed to have little respiratory value, since an exchange of gases occurs through the thin integument of this protochordate. When gill filaments form on the sides of the clefts, become vascularized, and function as a respiratory organ, they interrupt the ventrodorsal flow of blood in the aortic arches. Consequently, these aortic arches divide into two segments and differentiate into afferent (to the gills) and efferent (away from the gills) branchial arteries. During the evolutionary process, a system of capillaries develops in each gill lamella connecting the afferent with the efferent blood vessels. We shall delay any further discussion of the evolutionary changes of the aortic arches until the chapter on the circulatory system.

Goblet cells that secrete mucus are distributed among the epithelial cells covering the gill lamellae. In some fish, large acidophils or chloride cells also are present and contain a vesicle presumed filled with excreted salt. In marine animals the salt content of the body constantly increases and the kidneys are unable to handle all salt excretion. The gills act as an accessory excretory structure for salt excretion. In those animals whose external environment contain more salt than their tissues can tolerate, the chloride cells are believed to remove chlorides actively from the blood, against a concentration gradient. Such cells are absent from the gills of animals with blood isotonic to that of seawater, elasmobranchs, for example. The gills, therefore, not only function in respiration, but in certain marine teleosts they are also concerned with osmoregulation.

In the bony fishes another structure is added to the gill system: the *operculum*, or gill cover (Fig. 13-10, *B*). It develops as a bony extension from the hyoid arch on either side of the body. A bony armor is thus placed over the branchial region of the fish. It protects the gill slits and the fragile gill lamellae and forms a *branchial chamber* between the operculum and the gills. In some cases this chamber opens to the outside by way of a semicircular slit; in other forms, this slit is reduced to a single small opening.

External gills. External gills are highly vascular extensions of the integument above the gill region. The larvae of *Polypterus* and lungfishes have external gills, and they are believed to have been present in the crossopterygian ancestors of the tetrapods. They are present in amphibian larvae and function in water-dwelling urodeles.

Amphibians represent a transitional stage between aquatic and terrestrial animals; this is clearly evident in their respiratory system. They use external gills during the larval stage, but the urodeles and tailless amphibians undergo metamorphosis and shift to lungs in adult stages. The aquatic larva (7 mm. frog) has external gills located above the four gill slits. By the 10 mm. stage a fold of tissue covers the gill slits, as well as the forearm limb buds. The fold lacks skeletal support and is referred to as an operculum, although it is not homologous with the operculum of the bony fishes. The opercular cavity surrounding the gills opens to the outside by way of a small opening, the *spiracle*, as shown in Fig. 13-11. The gills that form within the cavity are vascularized filaments and represent modified external and internal gill structures. During metamorphosis (which occurs under the influence of the thyroid hormone) the gills are absorbed. The forearms rupture and push through the opercular cavity, and the frog shifts

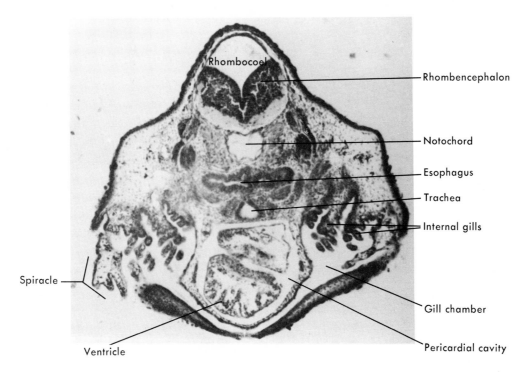

Fig. 13-11

Transverse section through 10 mm. frog tadpole at level of spiracle. Internal gills are protected within an opercular or gill chamber until they are lost at metamorphosis. (× 4.)

to its lungs and integument as respiratory organs.

Air sacs. According to some authorities, a pair of posterior pharyngeal pouches failed to open to the outside in the early vertebrate, and they became an accessory respiratory organ. Such a supplementary supply of air would be a definite advantage to the animal if the water became stagnant and foul and the exchange of oxygen through the gill surface was inadequate. Devonian placoderms possessed paired sac-like structures according to fossil records, and we assume that these extinct, primitive gnathostomes used the sacs as accessory respiratory structures.

Primitive air sacs probably evolved along two different pathways as illustrated in Fig. 13-12. One pathway led to the tetrapod lung. Lungs are present in all primitive, living Dipneusti but are lacking in most Actinopterygii and all Chondrichthyes. The crossopterygian ancestors of the first tetrapod probably had primitive lungs; they were present, therefore, before the first tetra-

pod evolved. The second developmental pathway followed by the primitive pouches gave rise to the ventral diverticulum that produced the swim bladder found in modern fishes. This structure, however, in most forms functions as a hydrostatic organ rather than as a respiratory one. The chronological appearance of lungs and swim bladders remains controversial, although evidence seems to indicate that the lung is the more primitive of the two. However, there is usually agreement that both lungs and swim bladders are homologous structures that had a common origin, a posterior visceral pouch that did not open to the outside.

Swim bladder. The swim bladder of present-day actinopterygian fishes is either connected to the digestive tract by a *pneumatic duct* or is an entirely separate structure. It is usually located as an oval sac beneath the vertebral column and dorsal aorta, outside the coelomic cavity. Its walls contain smooth muscle. In some fish, air is taken in or released through the mouth and

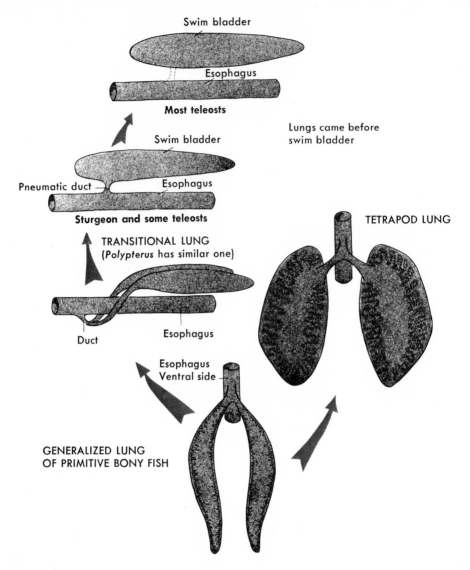

Swim bladder

Esophagus

Most teleosts

Swim bladder

Pneumatic duct

Esophagus

Sturgeon and some teleosts

TRANSITIONAL LUNG
(*Polypterus* has similar one)

Duct

Esophagus

Esophagus
Ventral side

GENERALIZED LUNG
OF PRIMITIVE BONY FISH

Lungs came before
swim bladder

TETRAPOD LUNG

Fig. 13-12

Fossil records indicate that Devonian placoderms possessed sac-like structures believed to be used as accessory respiratory structures. The pouches apparently evolved along two different pathways: one to the tetrapod lung and the other to the swim bladder of modern teleosts. (From Hickman, C. P., Sr., Hickman, C. P., Jr., and Hickman, F. M.: Integrated principles of zoology, ed. 5, St. Louis, 1974, The C. V. Mosby Co.)

passed into the sac by way of the duct, but in most teleosts the pneumatic duct is closed. In these forms, special gas glands are present in the anterior region of the swim bladder, and they secrete oxygen (or other gases) from many capillaries present in this organ (the vascular *rete mirabile,* or *red body*). Another structure, the *oval,* in the rear of the swim bladder is responsible for absorbing gases back into the bloodstream. The secretion of the gland and, therefore, the pressure in the bladder, can be adjusted since the gland appears to be under the control of the nervous system. The specific gravity of a fish's body is greater than that of the surrounding water, but if the bladder is filled with air, the fish can regulate its buoyancy and thus its depth.

The swim bladder is sensitive to pressure

changes and also functions as a hearing aid in some teleosts. The bladder in these fishes expands into sacs that project anteriorly, contact the ear, and act as a kind of tympanic membrane. It transmits sound waves to the Weberian ossicles (modified parts of the anterior vertebrae), which, in turn, convey pressure movement from the air bladder to the perilymph of the inner ear. The swim bladder also functions in sound production in any of several ways. It may act as a resonator, audibly releasing gas through the duct, or function by contracting certain "drumming" muscles associated with its walls.

Lungs. A midventral diverticulum from the gut at the level of the fifth or sixth branchial pouch gives rise to the primordium of the lungs in those vertebrates that use them as respiratory organs. The further development of the lung primordium gives rise to different degrees of lung complexities in different species. The diverticulum (lung bud) grows posteriorly, forming the primordium of the trachea. This single structure soon bifurcates and gives rise to the two primary bronchi, which lead to the two lungs. In some forms (snakes) the left lung remains rudimentary. The glottis opens into the larynx and trachea. The two bronchi, surrounded by mesenchyme and coelomic epithelium (splanchnic mesoderm), grow ventrally to the esophagus and posteriorly. The mesenchyme gives rise to the skeletal structures of the larynx, trachea, and bronchi.

There is evidence that this investing mesenchyme induces the endodermal bud to branch. If the pulmonary mesenchyme is eliminated in tissue culture, the epithelial cells form spherical aggregates or layers and are unable to form the budding bronchial tree. This is one of many examples emphasizing the importance of cellular interaction during normal development.

The lung primordium, common to vertebrate embryos, develops into a variety of adult forms. It ranges from the smooth-walled sac of certain fishes and amphibians to the specialized tubular lungs of birds and the highly developed lobular lungs of mammals. The complexity of the lung is correlated with the metabolic needs of the organism. The poikilothermic animals have simple sac-like structures, but in homoiothermic forms, with higher metabolic rates, a more complex lung develops, providing a greater amount of internal surface for the exchange of carbon dioxide and oxygen.

In amphibians the lung sacs branch off from the pharynx by a short tube (the larynx), thus the trachea is almost nonexistent. Vocal cords, consisting of three lateral ridges, appear for the first time in the frog. The aquatic urodeles have the simplest lungs; their inner surface is almost smooth, and they must depend on their external gills and integument to fulfill most of their respiratory needs. The lungs of frogs and toads are slightly more advanced and reflect their more terrestrial existence. The internal surface of the lungs is thrown into folds, or *septa,* which divide the large sac into smaller chambers. The epithelial lining of these smaller chambers evaginates between the septa and forms projections that further divide the lung into *infundibula,* as illustrated in Fig. 13-13. Small pockets, the *alveoli,* are located in the infundibula.

In some reptiles *(Sphenodon)*, the lung shows little advance over that of amphibians, but in others (crocodiles), it resembles the mammalian lung. In these forms the septa grow inward and further divide several times, giving the lung a spongelike consistency. A distinct neck appears in terrestrial forms when a shift from gill to lung breathing occurs. The trachea of these animals become correspondingly long.

The trachea and bronchi of amniotes are supported by bars and rings of hyaline cartilage, which we shall learn in detail later are derived from the skeletal support of the gill arches. Bronchi extend the air passageway from the trachea to the lungs and are present in reptiles, birds, and mammals. The mammalian lungs consist of three lobes on the right side and two on the left. A branch of the primary bronchus enters each lobe and then further divides many times (Fig. 13-14, *D*). In the human embryo of 2 to 6 weeks, the primary bronchi branch dichotomously as many as 16 to 23 times, finally ending in *respiratory bronchioles* that open into several alveolar ducts.

As shown in Fig. 13-14, *E*, alveolar sacs and alveoli arise from the alveolar ducts and represent the "dead ends" of the conducting system. The air-conducting channels are usually described as consisting of primary bronchi, secondary bronchi, bronchioles, terminal bronchioles, respiratory bronchioles, alveolar ducts, and alveoli. Blood vessels follow the branching of the air-conducting tubes. As the branchial divisions become smaller, their walls become thinner and they lose their cartilaginous support until, at the level of the alveoli, only an extremely thin layer of cells remain. The nature of the epithelial lining of the alveoli has been one of the controversial problems in histology. However, recent electron micrographs reveal that a continuous cellular layer covers the alveoli and separates it from the endothelium of the blood capillaries that loop in its walls. The cytopasm of the epithelial cells is extremely thin where it contacts

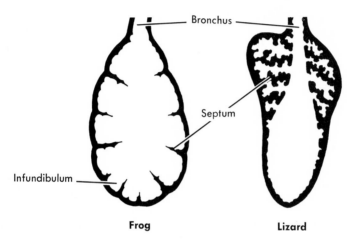

Fig. 13-13
Diagrammatic sections of frog and lizard lungs. The surfaces of the sac-like structures are increased by septa and ridges.

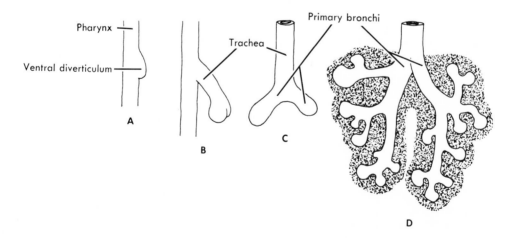

Fig. 13-14
Diverticulum, **A**, from the ventral wall of the pharynx gives rise to the trachea, **B**, which bifurcates to form the primary bronchi, **C**. The primary bronchi divide many times, **D** and **E**, finally terminating in respiratory bronchioles that open into several alveolar sacs, **E**. (**E** from Anthony, C. P., and Kolthof, N. J.: Textbook of anatomy and physiology, ed. 8, St. Louis, 1971, The C. V. Mosby Co.)

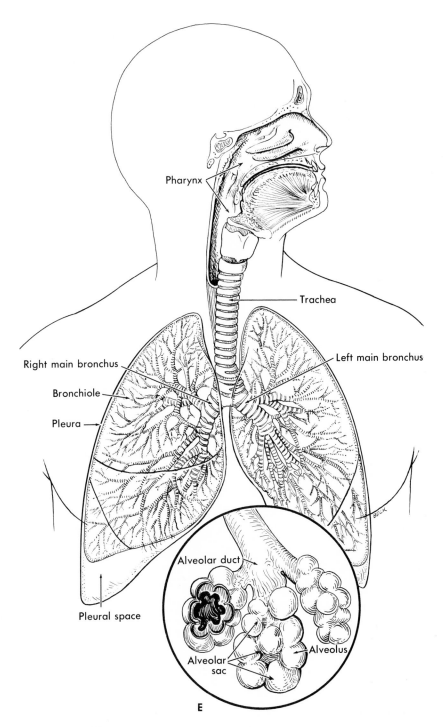

Fig. 13-14, cont'd
For legend see opposite page.

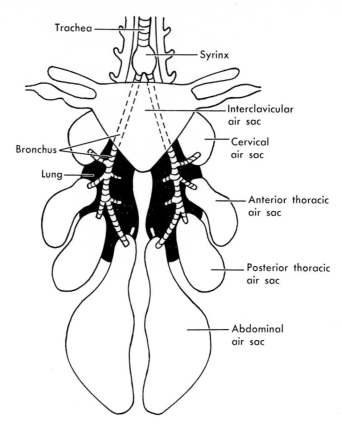

Fig. 13-15

Diagram showing relation of bronchi, lungs, and air sacs of pigeon. (From Hickman, C. P., Sr., Hickman, C. P., Jr., and Hickman, F. M.: Integrated principles of zoology, ed. 4, St. Louis, 1970, The C. V. Mosby Co.)

the walls of the blood vessel; it can barely be seen with the light microscope. It is through these two thin membranes that the exchange of gases occurs.

Since birds have a high metabolic rate and thus a great demand for oxygen, they have a highly specialized tubular lung. Birds lack a larynx, but a sound-producing organ, the *syrinx*, is located at the point where the trachea branches into the bronchi. As each bronchus enters the lung, it becomes known as a *mesobronchus*. From the mesobronchus secondary bronchi extend into nine air sacs (typically) that are located in the major parts of the body (Fig. 13-15). The names of the air sacs indicate their specific location in the bird. They are the angular interclavicular air sac and the paired cervical, anterior thoracic, posterior thoracic, and abdominal air sacs.

The mesobronchi extend caudally through the lungs and open into the most posterior air sacs, the abdominals. The air sacs have smooth, avascular walls and are not involved in respiration. Apparently the avian air sacs function in regulating body temperature by acting as a cooling device. They also help give the animal buoyancy, since they are connected with air spaces in the skeleton, partially replacing the marrow in long bones and in spaces between muscles. These structures act as a bellows, forcing air through the lungs during both inspiration and expiration. When the bird is at rest, the forward movement of the ribs expands the body cavity and draws air in, as by a suction pump. The muscles used in flight produce a similar result when the bird becomes active. Most of the air bypasses the lungs and travels by way of the secondary bronchi into the air sacs. As the air is expired, it is forced out of the air sacs and enters smaller tubes that lead to the parabronchi of the lungs.

The actual exchange of gases occurs in the *air capillaries* of the lung, structures unique to birds. In the lungs a series of tubes, the *parabronchi*, form loops from the bronchi. The air capillaries branch from the parabronchi and form anastomosing tubes. The relationship of the cytoplasm of the air capillaries with the walls of the blood vessels is extremely intimate and resembles the relationship of the alveoli and blood vessels in the mammalian lung. Diffusion occurs across the respiratory epithelium of the air capillaries and the endothelium of the blood vessel.

ORGANS OF DIGESTION. Posterior to the pharynx, the foregut gives rise to the esophagus and the stomach in most vertebrates. The splanchnic mesoderm surrounds the endodermal lining of these structures, as well as the entire digestive tract. The dorsal mesentery suspends them from the dorsal body wall. A pylorus region, containing the pyloric valve separates the original foregut from the embryonic midgut regions.

Histology of gut tube. Although there is much variation, the esophagus, stomach, and the more posterior intestine, are all constructed according to a common histologic pattern. Four concentric layers compose their walls, shown in Fig. 13-16. Each layer is modified and adapted to perform a specific function. For example, the stomach, reflecting its "churning" function, is composed of much more muscle than other segments of the gut and the muscles are more complexly arranged.

The innermost layer is the *mucosa*, consisting of epithelial cells derived from the endoderm. The mucosa acts as a barrier between the outside of the animal (that is, the lumen, or cavity, of the intestine) and the internal environment of the organism. These cells are also responsible for secretion and absorption. The outer three layers of the gut, derived from the closely apposed splanchnic *mesoderm,* are the *submucosa, muscularis,* and *serosa.* The submucosa, consisting of a meshwork of connective tissue, not only ties the mucosa to the muscularis, but also carries the lymphatic and blood vessels that vascularize the mucosa (see Fig. 13-23). Large numbers of lymphocytes accumulate in the submucosa, often

pushing aside and distorting the epithelial cells. These clusters of lymphocytes in the intestinal region of man are known as *Peyer's patches. Meissner's plexus,* also located in the submucosa, contains the postganglionic fibers of the sympathetic system and the cell bodies (ganglia) of the parasympathetic system.

Smooth-muscle fibers arranged in an *inner circular layer* and an *outer longitudinal layer* make up the *muscularis.* They give the gut tone and are responsible for peristaltic movement. *Auerbach's plexus* consists of preganglionic fibers of the parasympathetic system synapsing with the postganglionic cells of this system. The processes of these latter cells terminate on the muscle fibers. Postganglionic fibers of the sympathetic system are also present. As a result, the gut receives a dual (antagonistic) innervation from the autonomic nervous system, as described for the visceral organs in Chapter 12. Simple squamous or cuboidal cells usually compose the outer layer of the gut, the *serosa.*

ESOPHAGUS AND STOMACH. After the food leaves the oral cavity and the pharynx, the esophagus transports it to the stomach. However, the esophagus does not gain prominence until land animals evolve. It is a muscular, distensible structure, the mucosa of which is thrown into branched *papillae.* Unlike the trachea, the esophagus lacks skeletal support. In birds, it is modified to form the *crop,* a sac-like dilation, important in maintaining a constant food supply. In male and female doves and pigeons, it also supplies a secretion of fat, lecithin, and protein (pigeon's "milk") to the young.

Amphioxus and some of the cyclostomes, lungfish, and teleosts lack a true stomach. In these forms, this part of the foregut merely leads into the intestine. The stomach is apparently not essential for food digestion. The act of chewing breaks the food down into smaller particles in the oral cavity. In the stomach, it is further physically reduced in size by the churning action of the thick muscular walls. Glands that secrete pepsin initiate the chemical digestion of proteins. The stomach also secretes the intrinsic factor necessary for the absorption of vitamin B_{12}. The addition of liquid reduces the food material to a pulp, referred to as *chyme.* The stomach can also

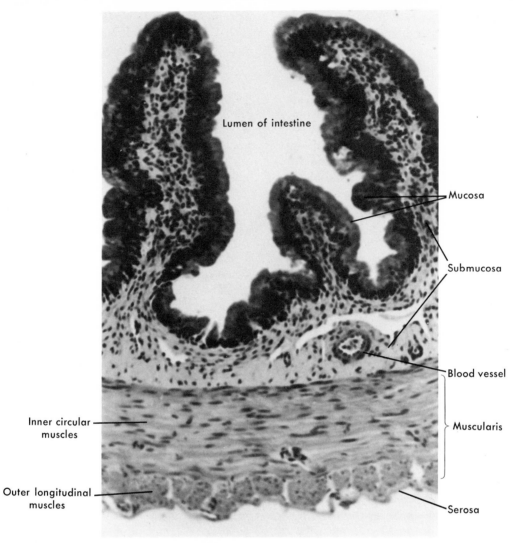

Fig. 13-16
Portion of transverse section through frog duodenum showing the basic four-layer plan of the digestive tract: the mucosa, submucosa, muscularis, and serosa. (× 100.)

act as a storage chamber allowing large meals to be taken infrequently, as demonstrated in snakes. Several large fishes can be stored in the shark's stomach until the intestine is able to digest them, and camels have developed special pockets to hold water. The stomach absorbs some water, alcohol, and certain drugs, but, in general, absorption occurs in the intestine. To carry out these functions, the stomach has muscular walls and mucous and digestive glands.

The stomach is usually a J- or V-shaped structure, but it may be present merely as a straight tube as seen in Fig. 13-17. In mammals, the outer (left) border of the stomach is referred to as the *greater curvature;* the inner, or right, border is designated the *lesser* curvature. The contents of the esophagus enter the *cardiac region* of the stomach and leave by way of the *pyloric region* into the intestine. Although all parts of the stomach have glands, the expanded part, the *fundus,* usually contains most of the tubular glands associated with digestion.

The walls of the stomach are thrown into folds, the *rugae,* the surfaces of which are dotted with

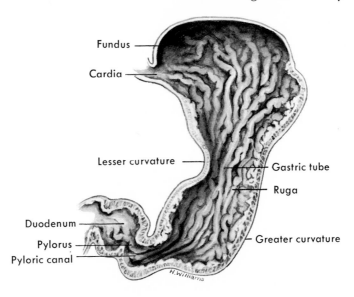

Fundus
Cardia
Lesser curvature
Gastric tube
Ruga
Duodenum
Pylorus
Pyloric canal
Greater curvature

H. Williams

Fig. 13-17
Longitudinal section showing general structure of the stomach. (From Francis, C. C.: Introduction to human anatomy, ed. 6, St. Louis, 1973, The C. V. Mosby Co.)

gastric pits that extend down through the mucosa for a distance of about one fifth its thickness. The glands empty their contents into the pits, as shown in Fig. 13-18, from which their secretions make their way to the surface. Mucus-secreting cells are located at the neck of the gland. In lower animals, one type of cell appears to be capable of secreting both pepsin and hydrochloric acid. In mammals, however, *chief cells* and *parietal cells* located in the deeper portions of the gland secrete, respectively, the digestive enzyme (pepsin) and hydrochloric acid (necessary for the action of the enzyme).

The stomach is capable of great distention and movement within the body cavity. In such animals as the ruminants (cows, deer, sheep), it is divided into as many as four compartments (Fig. 13-19). Food is chewed and then temporarily stored in the first two compartments, where bacteria act upon it. It is then regurgitated as the "cud" and chewed further. When it is returned to the stomach, it bypasses the original two chambers and enters the last two chambers where it is acted upon chemically. Since the abomasum (the most posterior chamber) contains the digestive glands, it is compared to the fundus of most mammalian stomachs.

The stomach is also adapted to the food habits in other animals. In crocodiles and birds, the stomach divides into an anterior, thin-walled *proventriculus*, which functions in food storage, protein digestion, and HCl secretion, and the highly muscular *ventriculus*, the *gizzard*. Birds swallow small pebbles, which lodge in the gizzard and turn it into a grinding organ, which replaces the teeth of other animals.

Liver and pancreas
Development of liver

In all vertebrates the *liver* originates as a ventral diverticulum of endoderm between the foregut and midgut regions. In most forms, it divides into two chambers destined to become the right and left lobes. It grows forward and downward in the ventral mesentery and develops into a massive structure in the anterior part of the body cavity. It is one of the largest organs in the body and may weight as much as 3 pounds in the adult man. The *falciform ligament* anchors the liver to the ventral body wall and the *coronary ligament* attaches it to the transverse septum or diaphragm. It expands laterally until it touches the body wall.

From the original liver diverticulum, fingerlike projections of endodermal cells grow in toward the heart along the pathway of the vitelline veins.

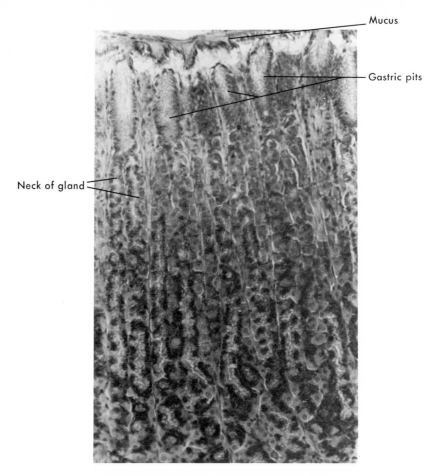

Fig. 13-18

Gastric mucosa of fundic region of stomach. Gastric glands, composed of different types of secretory cells, are oriented perpendicular to surface of mucosa. The cells secrete into the lumen of the gland and the contents enter the stomach cavity by way of gastric pits. A layer of mucus protects the surface of the stomach. (× 60.)

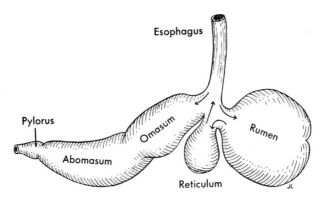

Fig. 13-19

Ruminate stomach may be divided into as many as four compartments. See text for discussion of their function. (From Kent, G. C.: Comparative anatomy of the vertebrates, ed. 3, St. Louis, 1973, The C. V. Mosby Co.)

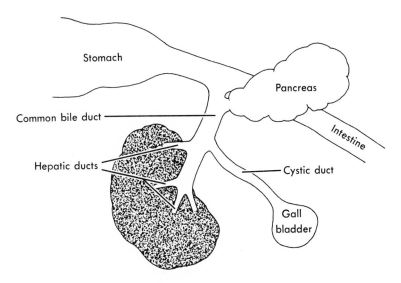

Fig. 13-20
Diagram showing relation of liver and ducts.

These blood vessels are encompassed by the growing liver and, as a result, the veins become divided into *sinusoids,* wide vascular channels separated by cords of epithelial cells. An evagination from the proximal portion of the liver diverticulum gives rise to the *cystic duct* that ends in a blind sac, the *gallbladder.* This becomes a thin-walled sac that stores the bile secreted by the liver. That part of the original duct leading from the hepatic cords is considered the *hepatic duct.* It joins with the cystic duct to form the *common bile duct,* as shown in Fig. 13-20. In some animals, the pancreatic duct also joins the common bile duct as it enters the duodenum.

Structure of liver

The functions of the liver involve the distribution of the food after it has been chemically broken down and absorbed. They concern the metabolism and storage of this material, as well as the secretion of bile. The hepatic portal system transports the food-carrying blood from the stomach and intestine to the liver. A system of tubes (canaliculi) carries the bile away from the liver cells. A hepatic artery brings food and oxygen to the hepatic cells themselves.

In mammals the morphologic unit is the *hepatic lobule,* a polyhedral block of cells that appear to radiate out from a central vein, as one may see in Fig. 13-21. A portal area, located at each angle of the periphery of the lobule, contains a hepatic artery, a hepatic portal vein, lymphatic vessels, and a bile duct. Twigs of the hepatic portal vein or hepatic artery, or both, carry blood to the lobules. The blood "percolates" through the sinusoids, the vascular spaces in the liver, with the materials "filtering out" along the way. The blood then drains into the central canal and is carried away to the heart via the hepatic vein and vena cava.

The liver cells secrete the bile into the bile canaliculi between the cords of parenchyma cells from where it is carried to the bile duct in the portal area. These merge with larger bile ducts, eventually emptying into the large hepatic duct. The cystic duct usually transports the bile to the gallbladder where it is temporarily stored.

The presence of fat, fatty acids, dilute acids, and peptones in the intestine stimulates the mucosal cells to secrete a hormone, *cholecystokinin.* This hormone causes the gallbladder to contract periodically, releasing its products into the duodenum by way of the cystic and common bile ducts. The breakdown products of degenerating red blood cells (the bile pigments derived from the hemoglobin), lecithin, and cholesterol pri-

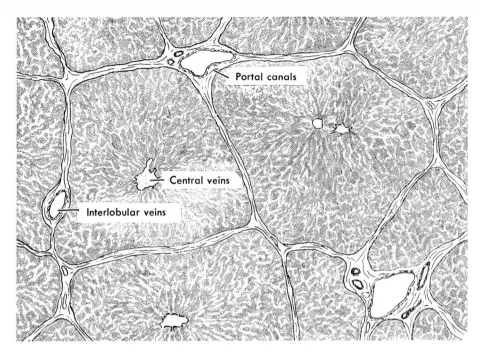

Fig. 13-21

Low magnification drawing of pig liver showing several liver lobules. The hepatic cells are arranged in cords that radiate out from central veins. Blood from the hepatic portal vein and hepatic artery flow by way of sinusoids to the central vein. (With permission of Bevelander, G.: Essentials of histology, ed. 7, St. Louis, 1974, The C. V. Mosby Co.)

marily make up the bile. The liver cells also secrete bile salts that act as emulsifying agents in the intestine, aiding in the chemical digestion and absorption of fats.

Pancreas

Except in cyclostomes, which lack a discrete pancreas, the gland arises as dorsal and ventral diverticula from the gut near the origin of the liver outgrowth. In some animals, the ventral diverticulum arises from the proximal end of the hepatic evagination. These endodermal pockets grow rapidly, branching many times. The dorsal pancreas usually constitutes the bulk of the gland. The two lobes may remain as separate glands in the adult or, as in most vertebrates, merge to form a single gland. Each may retain its original connection to the gut as a duct for *exocrine* secretion, or only one functional duct may remain, with the other atrophying. The *acini,* spherical units of the secretory portion of the pancreas, arise at the ends of the many ducts

and release their secretory products into the ducts. Other cells bud off from the ducts and tubules of the exocrine pancreas and migrate out into the gland, losing their connection with the duct system. These cells function as the *endocrine* (ductless) portion of the pancreas and were first described by Langerhans (1869). They are considered specializations of the duodenal mucosa because of their origin and are usually referred to as the *islets of Langerhans* (Fig. 13-22).

The islets differentiate histologically into four different kinds of cells, designated as alpha (A), beta (B), clear (C), and delta (D) cells. Electron micrographs show three, if not four, of the cell types present in all vertebrates, with the possible exception of the cyclostomes. The A cells are responsible for glucagon secretion and the B cells for insulin. The roles of C cells (when present) and D cells have not been definitely established. The cyclostomes have no pancreas, but "follicles of Langerhans," embedded in the

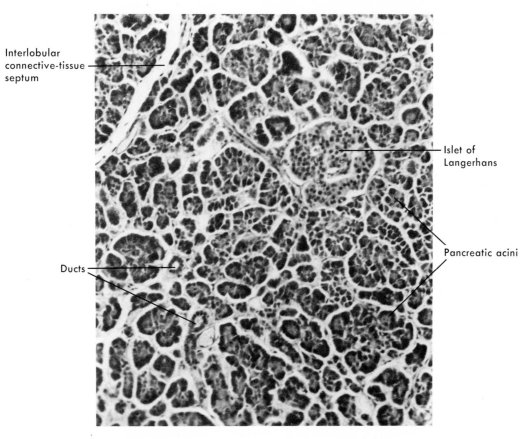

Interlobular connective-tissue septum

Islet of Langerhans

Pancreatic acini

Ducts

Fig. 13-22
Islet of Langerhans surrounded by acinar cells. (× 100.)

submucosal wall of the anterior end of the intestine, help regulate carbohydrate metabolism. They are probably homologous to the islet cells of higher vertebrates.

Insulin and glucagon are the two hormones secreted by the endocrine portion of the pancreas. Insulin facilitates the utilization of glucose by the body cells and inhibits excessive breakdown of stored glycogen in the liver and muscle. It also regulates fat metabolism and promotes the synthesis of protein. The action of glucagon is usually antagonistic to insulin. It brings about a decrease in glucose oxidation and an increase in blood sugar (hyperglycemia) by stimulating the liver to release its glycogen stores and the body cells to convert protein to sugar. Endocrine glands release their secretions into the vascular system where they are then carried to various parts of the body.

The exocrine function of the gland involves the secretion of pancreatic juices, containing digestive enzymes, into the intestine by way of the pancreatic duct. The exocrine secretion consists of enzymes that digest all the major categories of food, that is proteins, carbohydrates, and fats. *Pancreatic amylase* hydrolyzes starches, glycogen, and most carbohydrates (except cellulose) into disaccharides. *Pancreatic lipase* breaks down neutral fats into glycerol and fatty acids. There are several proteolytic enzymes (proenzymes). *Trypsin* and *chymotrypsin* digest whole or partially broken proteins. The pancreatic cells release the proteolytic enzymes in an inactive form. They pass by way of the pancreatic duct into the intestine where they come in contact with the chyme and the secretion of the intestional tract. When the inactive proenzymes reach the lumen of the duodenum, an intestinal enzyme (enterokinase) converts trypsinogen to the active form, trypsin, and this enzyme, in turn activates the proenzyme, chymotrypsinogen to active chymotrypsin.

Midgut

As we stated earlier in the chapter, the midgut contributes the greatest proportion of the *intestine*. Most of the chemical processes related to digestion occur in the lumen of the intestine. The final materials are absorbed into the bloodstream or lymph from this region of the digestive tract, and those unabsorbed products are eliminated by way of the cloaca or anus.

The walls of the intestine contain many glands that add their secretions to the food. Mucus mixes with the food and helps it move smoothly down the tubes; digestive enzymes reduce the complex sugars to simple ones, split fats, and break down the peptides into amino acids. The chemical action of both the pancreatic and intestinal enzymes complete the digestion of the food materials, leaving them in a simple absorbable state. The muscular walls, capable of "mixing" movements, make certain the enzymatic contents are mixed with the chyme from the stomach. The intestine also secretes hormones that control the secretion of pancreatic enzymes, bile, and intestinal juice.

A large inner surface must be present if absorption is to occur, the second important function of the intestine. Vertebrates use a variety of means to increase this absorptive area. In some teleosts outpocketings (ceca) form from the gut; sharks have a longitudinal fold, called the *spiral valve,* that twists down the lumen of the intestine like a spiraling staircase. The intestine may greatly increase in length, as in amphibian larvae, or it may contain branched mucosal folds. Among mammals it may be four or five times the length of the body in carnivores; but in herbivores, it is often as much as 20 times the body length.

In man, three regions of the small intestine are usually distinguished; the *duodenum,* the *jejunum,* and the *ileum.* It is difficult to tell externally where one region begins and the other ends. However, histologically the areas are distinguished on the bases of their glands, thickness of walls, and presence of lymphoid tissue. Leaf-like projections (the *villi*) and folds (plicae circulares) are present in both avian and mammalian intestine and increase the absorptive capacity of the surface. The epithelial surface of villi is richly supplied with vascular and lymphatic vessels as shown in Fig. 13-23.

Not all animals have a large intestine, or colon, but when it is present, a small outpocket, the *cecum,* is usually located at the proximal end. In man, the blind pouch ends in the *vermiform appendix.* In sharks a *rectal gland,* a finger-shaped structure, lies in the dorsal mesentery and opens by a duct into the intestine. Although it resembles the cecum of land animals, the rectal gland secretes a solution of sodium chloride that is about twice as concentrated as plasma or seawater. It apparently has no digestive function. It is considered a "salt gland," functioning in the removal of sodium chloride from the blood.

An *ileocecal valve* may divide the small intestine from the large intestine of some mammals. In these vertebrates the colon assumes a characteristic shape of an inverted U and the terms *ascending, transverse,* and *descending* colon, adequately describe the various sections. The primary function of the colon is the absorption of water, any remaining food materials, and certain other substances produced by the bacteria present in this region of the gut. The residue remaining is condensed and collected together as *feces* and expelled from the body.

Hindgut

The hindgut gives rise to the *tailgut,* the *cloaca,* and certain diverticula, the *allantois* and the *bursa of Fabricius.* The tailgut is an embryonic transitory structure that forms to various degrees in different embryos. It is present at the end of neurulation but is lost in the adult. The cloaca becomes an important collecting chamber; the term "cloaca" literally means 'sewer.' The intestines and urinary and genital ducts open into the cloaca of most vertebrates. It becomes partitioned in adult mammals. Since its evolution is related to that of the urogenital tract, we shall discuss its modifications in more detail in Chapter 18, which deals with the urogenital system.

The proctodeum forms in much the same manner as the stomodeum discussed early in this

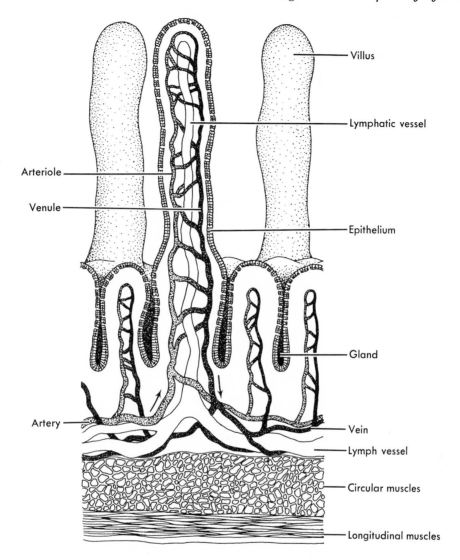

Arteriole

Venule

Artery

Villus

Lymphatic vessel

Epithelium

Gland

Vein

Lymph vessel

Circular muscles

Longitudinal muscles

Fig. 13-23
Microscopic structure of three villi. Each contains an arteriole, a venule, and a lacteal (a lymphatic vessel).

chapter. A ventral evagination of the hindgut endoderm meets the invaginating ectoderm resulting in the double *proctodeal anal membrane,* which eventually ruptures, forming the *anus.*

The allantois forms as an outpocketing of the midventral region of the hindgut and was discussed in Chapter 9. It is important as a respiratory organ in the embryo but is lost in the adult, with the exception of those animals that retain a portion of it as the urinary bladder.

The *bursa of Fabricius* is a dorsal projection from the hindgut in the cloacal proctodeal region of the chick. In the past, most anatomy and embryology texts devoted a sentence or two to this structure. During the past decade, however, it has received a great deal more attention, because of its suggested relationship with the immune system of the bird. It is a thymuslike organ found in no other vertebrate and is important in the development of the cells that form antibodies in the chick. Since some of the lymphocytes appear to originate from the endodermal lining of the bursa, they are of endodermal origin. The bursa mimics the growth of the thymus in that it is large in small chicks and involuted in older ones.

Removal of the bursa produces a deficiency in gamma globulin, but there is little or no effect on the cell-mediated immunity. It is possible to take the immune system apart selectively in the chick; that is, remove the thymus and note the effects and then remove the bursa and note the different effects. The corroboration of these results by patients with immune deficiency diseases leads to the central dogma of immunology: the immune system consists of two types of cells, the B cells and T cells, discussed earlier in this chapter.

SUGGESTED READINGS

1. Biology of immunity in amphibians. A symposium, Am. Zool. **11**:169-237, 1971.
2. Brown, M. (editor): Physiology of fishes, Vol. I and II, New York, 1957, Academic Press Inc.
3. Burnet, F. M.: The mechanism of immunity, Sci. Am. **206**:58, 1961.
4. Burnet, F. M.: The thymus gland, Sci. Am. **207**: 50-57, 1962.
5. Comparative aspects of parathyroid function. A symposium, Am. Zool. **7**:823-897, 1967.
6. Comrol, J. H., Jr.: The lung, Sci. Am. **214**:57-66, 1966.
7. Culliton, B. J.: Immunology: Two immune systems capture attention, Science **180**:45-47, 1973.
8. Etkin, W.: How a tadpole becomes a frog, Sci. Am. **214**:76-88, 1936.
9. Fange, R., and Wittenberg, J. B.: The swimbladder of the toadfish (*Opsanus tau* L.), Biol. Bull. **115**: 172, 1958.
10. Keys, A., and Willmer, E. N.: Chloride secreting cells in the gills of fishes, with special reference to the common eel, J. Physiol. **76**:368, 1932.
11. Miller, J. F. A. P.: The thymus and the development of immunologic responsiveness, Science **144**: 1544, 1964.
12. Sorokin, S.: Recent work on developing lungs. In DeHaan, R. L., and Upsprung, H. (editors): Organogenesis, New York, 1965, Holt, Rinehart & Winston, Inc.

CHAPTER 14

BODY CAVITIES AND MESENTERIES

In the embryo, the largest body cavity is known as the *coelom,* a generalized term referring to a cavity lined with mesoderm. Although it can refer to any mesoderm-lined space, it is usually used synonymously with the term "body cavity." In adult vertebrates, the coelomic cavity becomes partitioned, with each new chamber fulfilling a specific function.

The coelom is a fluid-filled space that in primitive forms was probably used as a temporary reservoir for wastes and reproductive cells (Smith, 1960). In a hypothetical prechordate stage, the coelom may have communicated directly to the outside by pores through which the metabolic wastes and reproductive products passed. Later in evolution, the waste-containing fluids of the coelom entered the kidney tubules by way of ciliated funnels, and, in some ancestral forms, may have emptied to the outside by way of dorsally arranged pores present in each segment. No such arrangement is found in any living vertebrate; the pores are lost and the ciliated funnels have disappeared in most adult vertebrates. However, two *abdominal pores* remain in the ventral, cloacal region of some fishes, turtles, and crocodiles. No one has determined whether these ventral pores are remnants of the dorsal pores. They seem to allow the coelomic fluid to leave the body cavity and, possibly, water to enter it. In the cyclostomes they function for the exit of sperm and eggs, but the elasmobranchs and other vertebrates have developed ducts for this purpose.

Although we speak of the "body cavity," there is actually little free space available. Only a potential cavity exists, since the viscera fills it. The gut and its various diverticula (lungs, pancreas, and liver) primarily occupy the cavity, but the heart also is located there.

The various organs of the body do not embed in solid tissue but are usually located immediately outside the coelom or are suspended in it. Many of the surrounding organs actually bulge into the cavity although they always remain covered by one wall of the coelom. We say their location is *retroperitoneal,* in back of the coelomic lining. The kidneys, ureters, urinary bladder, inferior vena cava, and abdominal dorsal aorta are examples of such organs. Other organs

315

are suspended in the body cavity by double-layered *mesenteries* that allow them to move about with relative freedom as they carry out their functions. For example, the stomach moves downward or upward with each inspiration or expiration, although it is anchored to the dorsal wall by the mesogaster.

PRIMITIVE COELOM

A coelom is present in all modern vertebrates although the introduction of new major organs, such as the lungs, modifies it. We have already learned about the embryonic formation of the coelom in Chapter 8, but we might review this knowledge by referring to the primitive body form shown in Fig. 8-10.

The bilateral mesodermal tubes, along with the gut tube and neural tube, arrange themselves about the solid notochord. The mesoderm divides into the segmented epimere and mesomere and the nonsegmented hypomere. The hypomere pushes toward the midline on either side enclosing the gut. Unlike the epimere, the hypomere retains its cavity as the *primitive coelom*. In vertebrates with a rounded gastrula, the hypomere develops into two longitudinally arranged tubes that extend posteriorly from the pharyngeal region to the anus. In amniotes, on the other hand, the development of extraembryonic membranes complicates the picture, and the coelom in the body extends outward past the lateral folds into the extraembryonic regions. In fact, since these membranes are used for nutritional purposes in the mammalian embryo, the splitting of the mesoderm (hypomere) occurs first in the extraembryonic regions and then proceeds into the body proper. The *intraembryonic coelom* is the cavity within the developing embryo; the *extraembryonic coelom* is the space associated with the developing membranes. During development, the completion of the floor of the gut produces two coeloms separated from one another in the midline. In this chapter, we shall confine our discussion to the intraembryonic coelom of amniotes, since its differentiation is almost identical to that found in the anamniotes.

The mesoderm that forms the walls of the coelom further differentiates into *somatic mesoderm* lining the body wall (the *parietal peritoneum*

of the adult) and the *splanchnic mesoderm* covering the viscera (*visceral peritoneum*, or *serosa*, of the adult). The splanchnic mesoderm from each side fuses dorsally above the gut to establish a complete, longitudinal, double sheet of tissue, the *dorsal mesentery*, and below the gut to form the *ventral mesentery*, thereby separating the right coelomic space from the left. Although these paired cavities are present early in the embryo, they are not retained in any living adult vertebrate.

FATE OF EMBRYONIC MESENTERIES

Adult vertebrates lose part of the embryonic dorsal mesentery and most of the ventral mesentery. For example, in adult sharks the intestine lacks a dorsal mesentery, and in skates and *Necturus* only a portion remains, suspending the stomach. Most reptiles and mammals retain the dorsal mesentery intact although it may also be incomplete in the intestinal region in these forms.

In the adult, the dorsal mesentery differentiates regionally and is referred to by specific names that reflect the organs suspended. For example, there is the *mediastinum*, the mesentery surrounding the esophagus; the *mesogaster*, the mesentery suspending the stomach; the *mesorectum*, which suspends the rectal gland or large intestine; the *mesocolon* (mesentery of transverse colon); the *mesoappendix*; etc. Through common usage, the general term "mesentery" has come to refer to the mesentery of the small intestine. Some of the mesenteries adhere to one another or to the body wall. Adhesions are especially prominent in the mesenteries suspending the intestine. As the intestine coils around in the body cavity, the mesenteries overlap, fuse, and grow together. These mesenteries are very important, since they not only suspend the organs but also serve as passageways to the organs for arteries, veins, nerves, and lymphatics.

In some vertebrates the mesogaster changes from a simple dorsal mesentery to a complicated structure, as shown in Fig. 14-1. As the parts of the gut differentiate, that area destined to form the stomach grows larger and twists to the left. As a result, the original dorsal region of the gut becomes oriented laterally. As the stomach undergoes bending, it pulls the dorsal mesentery

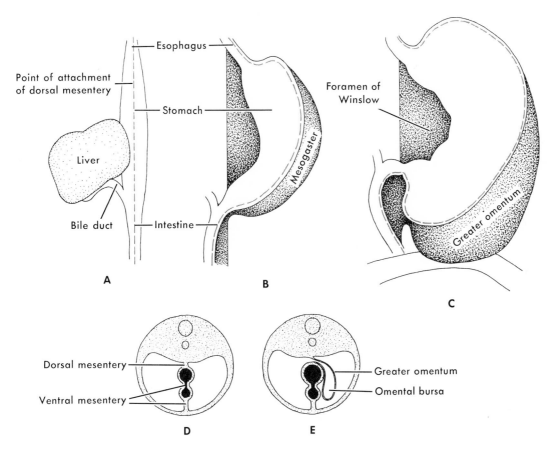

Fig. 14-1
Formation of greater omentum from dorsal mesentery. The primitive tubelike gut, **A,** undergoes growth and bending, **B,** pulling the dorsal mesentery (mesogaster) with it. The mesentery, attached to gut *along dotted line,* continues to grow **B, C,** and **E,** forming a large double-walled pouch, the omental bursa.

with it, and there is a tendency in all gnathostome embryos for the mesogaster to form a pocketlike structure. In some mammals this dorsal mesentery continues to grow, forming a large double-walled pouch, the *omental bursa.* The walls of this pouch, the *greater omentum,* attach to the greater curvature of the stomach. They become fat-laden and fall apron-fashion over the front of the intestine. In the dissection of the cat, this "lacy" membrane is one of the first structures you meet once the abdominal wall is pulled open to reveal the body cavity. The entrance into this double-walled pouch, the *foramen of Winslow,* is located in the region of the smaller curvature of the stomach between the caudate lobe of the liver and the mesoduodenum.

The spleen and pancreas also are associated with the dorsal mesentery of this region. The spleen is not a derivative of the gut, but arises as a condensation of mesenchyme cells along the left edge of the mesogaster. The spleen serves important functions in both the embryo and the adult. It plays a role in the formation, storage, and destruction of blood cells. It also participates in the body's defense mechanisms. During development the spleen increases in size and projects from the surface of the mesogaster. Sometimes folds of the mesentery are referred to as ligaments because they tie organs to one another or to the body wall. That part of the mesogaster between the spleen and stomach is known as the *gastrosplenic ligament.*

The pancreas, described in the previous chapter, arises as one or several diverticula of the duodenum. These grow into the dorsal mesentery where fusion occurs among the various rudiments. The original diverticula branch and re-branch many times in the mesentery, forming an elaborate duct system and producing a compound, alveolar gland. The adult pancreas along with its main excretory duct or ducts rests in the mesoduodenum and mesogaster near the spleen.

The ventral mesentery is a transitory structure and is soon lost, except in the regions of the heart and liver. As a result, the intestines coil and move about freely as they carry out their peristaltic movement. Since the heart forms ventrally to the gut, it is surrounded by the ventral mesentery, referred to in this region as the *mesocardium.* We should take a few minutes at this point to consider the formation of the heart since it is related to the partitioning of the coelom. The details of its development will follow when the morphogenesis of the circulatory system is considered in Chapter 17.

An inner layer of endocardium, derived from the fusion of blood capillaries (vitelline veins) in the region of the pharynx, and a surrounding epimyocardium, constituted from splanchnic mesoderm, compose the heart. When the hypomeric mesoderm on each side of the embryo pushes medially in the area of the heart, it fuses in the midline as described above, enclosing the gut and the endocardial tube beneath it. This fused membrane beneath the gut is the ventral mesentery. Part of the walls of this ventral mesentery (splanchnic mesoderm) thickens and gives rise to the epimyocardium (shown in Figs. 14-2, A and 17-1). In lower vertebrates the heart forms as a single primordium. However, in higher animals, the embryo forms flat on the surface of the yolk and the yolk prevents the hypomeric mesoderm from fusing in the midline. So the heart forms two rudiments (Fig. 17-4). In these animals two endocardial tubes form, each surrounded by splanchnic mesoderm. When the body folds undercut the embryo at the anterior ends, the pharynx develops a floor and the epimyocardial rudiments are brought to the midline. Here they fuse and form a single tube enclosing the endocardial vessels (which also fuse). The ventral mesentery is then completed above and below the heart primordia, as in the lower vertebrates.

The splanchic mesoderm gives rise to the epimyocardium of the heart. That part of the original ventral mesentery dorsal to the heart, that is between the gut and the heart, is called the *dorsal mesocardium;* the mesentery between the heart and ventral body wall becomes the transitory *ventral mesocardium.* These mesenteries are illustrated in Fig. 14-2, A. They are soon lost in the older embryo as the heart tube takes on its typical vertebrate form. The specific fate of the

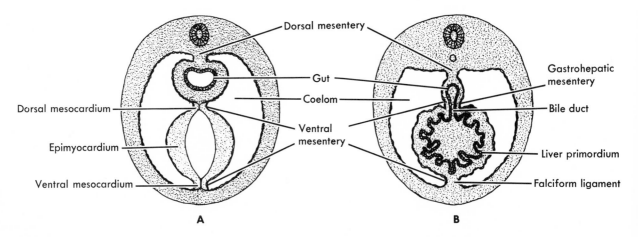

Fig. 14-2

Transverse sections of body at level of heart, **A**, and liver, **B**, showing relation of mesenteries. Dorsal mesentery suspends the gut. Ventral mesentery becomes involved in the formation of heart and liver but is lost in other parts of the body. See text for discussion.

mesocardia is described in greater detail when the morphogenesis of the heart is discussed in Chapter 17.

The liver is the second embryonic organ involved with the ventral mesentery. It forms slightly posterior to the heart (as a diverticulum from the gut) and expands ventrally, laterally, and posteriorly in the ventral mesentery. Its position and growth are important factors in forming the septum that divides the body cavity into anterior and posterior chambers. That part of the ventral mesentery between the liver and gut remains as the *gastrohepatic mesentery*, or *lesser omentum*. The bile duct, the connection between the liver and gut, is located in the lesser omentum. The hepatic portal vein and hepatic artery also pass through this mesentery on their way to the liver. That part of the ventral mesentery between the liver and the ventral body wall remains as the *falciform ligament* (Fig. 14-2, *B*).

The falciform ligament anchors the anterior ends of the shark oviducts. As described in Chapter 3, the oviducts of the adult shark pass forward along the dorsal coelomic wall, curve forward anterior to the liver, and enter the falciform ligament. They are, of course, always covered by the coelomic wall. In the ligament the two oviducts fuse to form the ostium, a wide funnel-shaped structure oriented toward the body cavity and into which the eggs pass when released by the ovaries. Although the falciform ligament does not support the oviduct of all vertebrates, ostial openings, of course, are present in all vertebrates above the cyclostomes. Since the ostium receives the eggs released into the coelomic cavity, it must, of course, perforate the wall of the coelom; it is one of only two openings into the coelom found in vertebrates. The other example is represented by those few primitive vertebrates with peritoneal funnels associated with their kidney tubules. Except for the two examples cited above, the lining of the coelom is a continuous membrane.

A portion of the ventral mesentery that supported the allantois remains to support the urinary bladder. It becomes the *median ligament* and attaches the medial ventral surface of the urinary bladder to the ventral body wall.

PARTITIONING OF COELOM
Formation of pericardial cavity

Amphioxus, the primitive chordate, lacks a definite heart but contains a blood vessel in the midventral region under the pharynx. As the pharynx changed its function from a food-gathering device (such as found in amphioxus) to a respiratory organ (present in fish), the ventral blood vessel in this region evolved into a muscular pump with sufficient power to send the blood through the gill capillaries. This enlargement occurred below the pharynx in the posterior region and pumped blood through the aortic arches located in the visceral arches of the pharynx. The heart had four chambers by the time the cyclostomes evolved.

It is postulated that early in the evolution of vertebrates the coelom extended anteriorly and ventrally under the pharynx, incorporating the newly evolved heart into the coelomic cavity. In all present-day vertebrate embryos, the heart forms in the anterior portion of the large coelomic cavity. Although this part of the coelom is continuous with the rest of the body cavity, it is called the pericardial cavity in the embryo. The splanchnic mesoderm gives rise to the mesocardium and the somatic mesoderm to the outer wall of the pericardial cavity (coelom). In the adult of the earliest known fish, however, a separate pericardial cavity exists. A transversely placed membrane (septum) partitions the coelom into a separate anterior *pericardial cavity* (lodging the heart) and a more posterior *peritoneal cavity* (containing the viscera). This *septum transversum* forms in all vertebrate embryos and is composed of two parts: the lateral mesocardium and the ventral mesentery associated with the growth of the liver.

The sinus venosus, the most posterior chamber of the embryonic heart, receives the veins returning blood from the anterior and posterior regions of the body. The right and left common cardinal veins are two important venous trunks located dorsally on each side of the body wall at the posterior level of the developing heart. They enter the ventrally located sinus venosus by passing diagonally across the coelomic cavity. As we learned previously, nerves, arteries, and veins do not freely cross cavities but are embedded in tissues or protected by mesenteries. In this instance, on each side of the body an infolding of the somatic wall forms a bridge to the heart, the *lateral mesocardium*. The common cardinal veins leave the dorsal, lateral walls and grow ventrally into the sinus venosus along this bridge. As a result, the lateral mesocardium anchors the posterior regions of the heart in place and partially divides the body cavity into an anterior and a posterior chamber. However, these two cavities communicate with one another over the top of the lateral mesocardium (dorsal canals) and beneath the lateral mesocardium (ventral canals), as shown in Fig. 14-3, A.

The gut diverticulum destined to give rise to the liver is located at the level of the lateral mesocardium. In most embryos the liver grows in the ventral mesentery between the two splanchnic mesoderm layers until it contacts the lateral mesocardium. The liver substance then continues to grow laterally and ventrally until it touches the body wall. It also expands anteriorly where its anterior surface flattens in the region of the lateral mesocardium and blocks the area identified as the ventral canals.

That part of the ventral mesentery covering the surface of the liver fuses with the somatic mesodermal bridge, as illustrated in Fig. 14-3, *B*, giving rise to the *septum transversum*. As a re-

sult, the septum divides the general coelom into a *pericardial cavity* and a *peritoneal cavity*. The anterior surface of the septum forms the posterior wall of the pericardial cavity, and the posterior surface forms the anterior wall of the peritoneal cavity. This relationship can be seen in the sagittal section of the 10 mm. pig (Fig. 14-4). In man, the partition is completed in a slightly different manner, but the results are the same. Projections from both sides of the body wall under the lateral mesocardium grow medially and form a membrane; the liver then grows into this membrane and incorporates it into its anterior surface.

As the liver grows posteriorly, it eventually pulls away from the septum but remains attached to it by the *coronary ligament*. The vitelline veins that carry blood from the liver to the heart enter the sinus venosus by way of the coronary ligament. In the adult shark, these veins are identified as the hepatic sinuses. Most of the ventral mesentery degenerates except in an area near the septum transversum. The remnant of this membrane was previously identified as the falciform ligament. The coronary ligament anchors the liver anteriorly to the septum transversum and the falciform ligament ties it to the ventral body wall.

In a few adult fish (some cyclostomes and elasmobranchs) the septum transversum remains

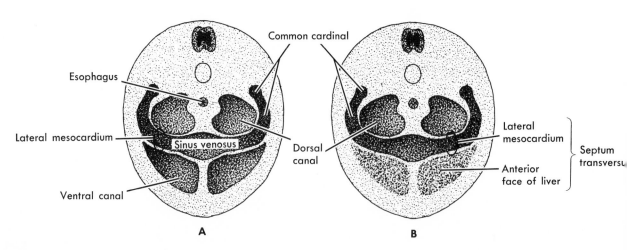

Fig. 14-3

Horizontal section at region of sinus venosus showing formation of septum transversum. Paired common cardinal veins enter sinus venosus by way of somatic mesodermal bridges, lateral mesocardia, **A.** Liver grows anterior in ventral mesentery until it contacts lateral mesocardia and blocks ventral canals, **B.**

as it was in the embryo, an incomplete membrane across the coelom. Dorsal canals above the septum connect the pericardial cavity with the peritoneal cavity. In most adult fish, however, the formation of *dorsal closing folds* blocks these dorsal canals. These dorsal folds of splanchnic mesoderm arise on both sides of the embryonic foregut and grow laterally and ventrally, eventually fusing with the dorsal part of the lateral mesocardium. This fusion produces in the adult fish a septum transversum that completely separates the pericardial cavity from the peritoneal cavity.

Formation of pleural cavity

Both lungs and gills are present in the Crossopterygii and Dipneusti and in some amphibians (salamanders). In these animals, the lungs

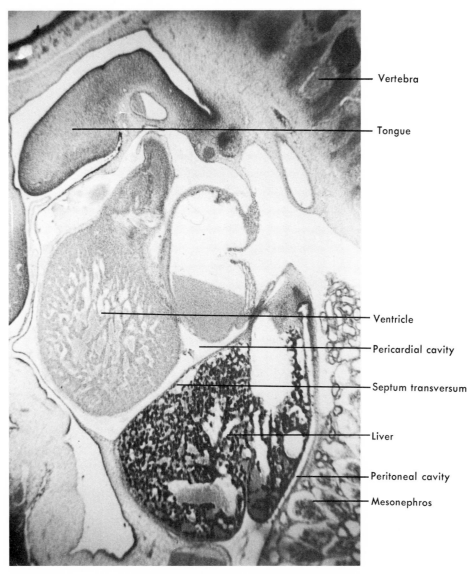

Fig. 14-4

Sagittal section of 10 mm. pig showing midventral region. The anterior surface of the septum transversum forms the posterior wall of the pericardial cavity and the posterior surface, the anterior wall of the peritoneal cavity. The liver is pushed against the septum. (× 4.)

have little function and protrude from the pharynx into the coelomic cavity (Fig. 14-5, *B*). A neck region develops in the area of the pharynx when functional gills are lost in amphibians such as frogs and in reptiles, birds, and mammals. When the long esophagus forms, the heart, transverse septum, and liver push posteriorly and the transverse septum and the dorsal folds become obliquely arranged. This membrane is now referred to as the *oblique septum*. It develops in the tetrapod embryo as seen in Fig. 14-5, *C*. The old transverse septum now not only forms the posterior limits of the pericardial cavity, but because of its oblique position also contributes to the membrane that separates the lungs from the heart.

As a result of the posterior migration of the structures mentioned above and the formation of the oblique septum, the peritoneal cavity pushes anteriorly and dorsally on both sides of the dorsal mesentery and occupies most of the space formerly held by the large pharynx. As shown in Fig. 14-5, *C* and *D*, and Fig. 14-6, two pleural cavities are established dorsally to the heart. The lung buds appear as outgrowths of the gut anterior to the liver diverticulum and project into the anterior extension of the cavity on both sides of the gut. The body cavity is now considered a *pleuroperitoneal cavity*. The lungs are much larger than those of the salamander, for example, and are capable of expansion and contraction. The relationship of the pericardial

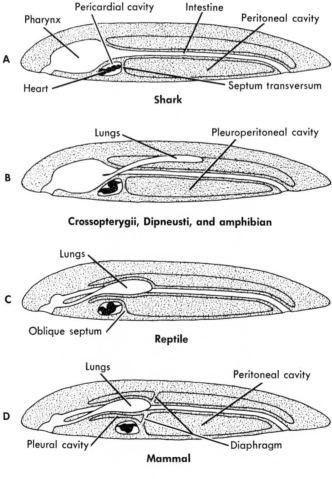

Fig. 14-5
Relation of vertebrate body cavities. See text for description.

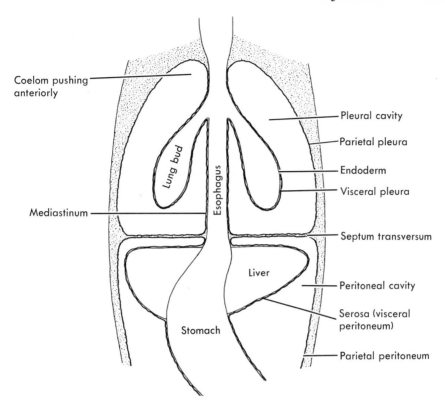

Fig. 14-6
Longitudinal section of Fig. 14-5, **D**, at level of lung buds showing anterior extension of coelom and lung buds covered with visceral pleura.

cavity to the pleuroperitoneal cavity changes from a cavity anterior to the peritoneal cavity as found in the shark (Fig. 14-5, *A*) to one that is ventral to its anterior regions (Fig. 14-5, *C* and *D*) in the typical amphibian and reptilian condition.

As the growing lung buds push out into the cavity, their surfaces are covered with a serous membrane derived from the splanchnic mesoderm as illustrated in Fig. 14-6. Like the gut, the lungs do not lie freely exposed in the cavity, but the visceral pleura (splanchic mesoderm) covers the root of the lung, the bronchi, and blood vessels, as well as the surface of the lung proper. It dips into the interlobular fissures of the adult lungs and at the root of the lung is reflected back and becomes continuous with the *parietal pleura,* which lines the pleural cavities. These anterior extensions of the coelom in which the lungs rest are referred to as the *pleural cavities.* The gut and dorsal mesenteries, known spe-

cifically as the *mediastinal septum,* separate the two pleural cavities. At this stage of development, the mediastinal cavity contains the esophagus and dorsal aorta.

The pleural cavities of amphibians and some reptiles never develop past this embryonic stage but remain continuous posteriorly with the rest of the body cavity. In higher reptiles (crocodiles, snakes, and some lizards) and birds these pleural cavities are partitioned off from the peritoneal cavities by one of several methods and separate pleural cavities form. In some cases a partial membrane appears or, for example, the lungs may be tied to the dorsal body wall in such a fashion that they are separated from the peritoneal regions. In birds, three pairs of longitudinal septa wall off the coelom and form chambers for the air sacs. The presence of air sacs in birds complicates the division of their coelom as compared with other vertebrates. In mammals, the muscular diaphragm, a uniquely mammalian structure, completely separates the two pleural cavities from the abdominal coelom.

The lungs of the mammalian embryo are at first small and dorsally located above the heart in the two pleural cavities, one located on each side of the gut and the dorsal mesentery. This relationship can be seen in a cross section through a 10 mm. pig embryo (Fig. 14-7). The cavities are separated from the pericardial cavity. During early development the pericardial cavity stretches laterally and caudally.

As the lungs continue to grow within their pleural cavities and reach the body wall, they push the parietal pericardium (somatic mesoderm) before them, separating it from the lateral body wall and eventually from the ventral body wall (Fig. 14-8). In this way, the pleural cavities grow at the expense of the pericardial cavity. As the lung cavities approach one another ventral to the heart (Fig. 14-8, *C*), the medial walls of the pleural cavities contact one another, fuse, and form a delicate median strand of tissue connecting the pericardium to the ventral body wall. This tissue is the *ventral mediastinum* and is one of the two mammalian innovations in the division of the embryonic coelom. The formation of the diaphragm is the other. At the level of the heart, the two walls of the pleural sacs separate and a larger space, enclosing the heart and its pericardial sac, is formed.

When the growth of the pleural cavities is completed, the pericardium is also separated

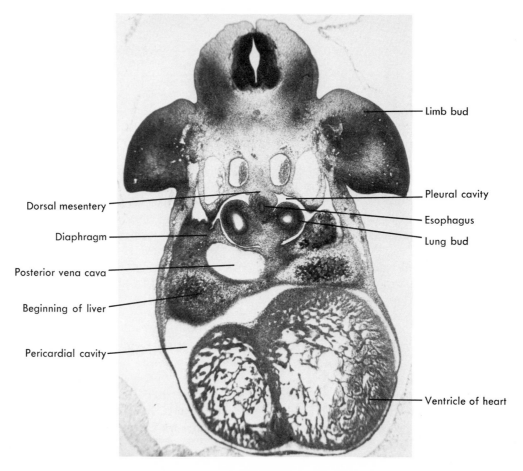

Fig. 14-7
Transverse section of 10 mm. pig embryo through lung buds. (× 4.)

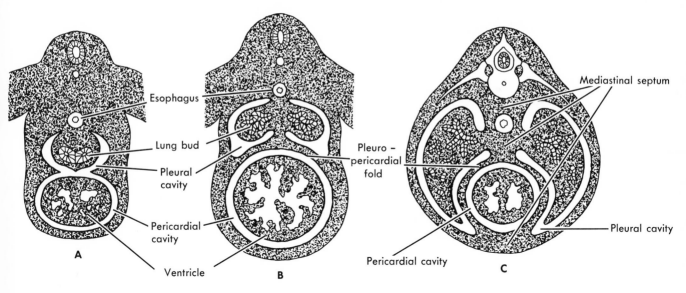

Fig. 14-8
Formation of pleural cavities and mediastinum of mammal.

from the anterior surface of the diaphragm and the heart now occupies a ventral position in the mediastinum between the two pleural sacs. The parietal pericardium, which has been pushed completely away from the body wall and ventrally from the diaphragm, continues to cover the heart and in the adult becomes the *pericardial sac*. This is a thin tissue enclosing the heart, attached to it only where the large blood vessels enter the heart.

The series of steps involved in the formation of the expanded pleural cavity is illustrated in Fig. 14-8. The lungs of the adult mammal are dorsal, lateral, and somewhat ventral to the heart. The parietal pleura (somatic mesoderm) not only lines the pleural cavities but also covers the anterior surface of the diaphragm and forms the ventral mediastinum. The adult mediastinum now not only holds the esophagus, dorsal aorta, and postcaval vein (as in the lower animals) but it also contains the heart and its pericardial sac, the trachea and part of the bronchi, certain nerves such as the vagus and phrenic nerves, thymus gland, lymph nodes, and lymph vessels. The formation of the ventral mediastinum not only allows for a larger pleural cavity and

growth of the mammalian lungs, it also cushions the heart against shocks as the mammal raises its body on its limbs, exposing its ventral surface.

Formation of diaphragm

In mammals, the embryonic coelom is completely divided into four main compartments: two pleural cavities, a pericardial cavity, and a peritoneal cavity. The *diaphragm,* the primary alteration made by mammals in the partitioning of the coelom, replaces the septum transversum of lower animals and separates the thoracic cavity with its two pleural and one pericardial cavities from the abdominal parts of the coelom. The diaphragm is a composite structure formed from four main embryonic sources.

In the mammalian embryo, as in other vertebrates, the septum transversum initiates the division of the embryonic coelom. It is present in a 14-somite human embryo and a 9 to 12 mm. pig embryo and will contribute to the formation of only the ventral part of the adult diaphragm. At this early stage, the septum is incomplete dorsally on each side of the gut above the lateral mesocardium. Two dorsolateral folds of tissue project medially from the body wall where the common

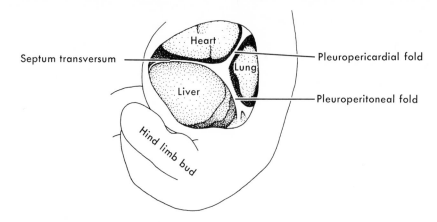

Fig. 14-9

Division of mammalian embryonic coelom. See text for discussion.

cardinal veins swing into the coelom on their way to the sinus venosus. These folds, known as the *pleuropericardial* and *pleuroperitoneal folds,* form a triangular structure, the base of which faces the dorsal body wall, with the apex joining the dorsal part of the transverse septum. This can best be visualized by referring to a sagittal view through the left side of a young mammalian embryo, as shown in Fig. 14-9.

The pleuropericardial fold is added to the septum transversum and completely separates the pericardial from the pleural cavities. The two pleuroperitoneal membranes grow medially and block the dorsal canal. The dorsal mesentery, containing the gut, is caught between the pleuroperitoneal folds and the septum transversum and represents the third embryonic contribution to the diaphragm. A fusion of all these membranes forms a complete partition that transversely separates the body cavity into anterior and posterior regions. The muscles from the body wall represent the fourth contribution to the diaphragm. They invade the septum and convert it into a muscular structure. This muscular sheet is now referred to as the diaphragm.

The adult diaphragm is a curved structure consisting mostly of striated muscles but containing a *central tendon* of connective tissue. It is located anterior to the liver and stomach and below the ribs and pleural cavities. The esophagus, dorsal aorta, and postcaval vein penetrate the diaphragm in the dorsal region. The diaphragm is under voluntary control and is involved in respiration in mammals; when it is lowered, the size of the pleural cavity enlarges and air rushes into the lungs.

SUGGESTED READINGS

1. Goodrich, E. S.: Studies on the structure and development of vertebrates, London, 1930, Macmillan & Co.
2. Patten, B. M.: Foundations of embryology, New York, 1958, McGraw-Hill Book Co., Inc.
3. Nelsen, O. E.: Comparative embryology of the vertebrates, New York, 1953, McGraw-Hill Book Co., Inc.
4. Smith, H. M.: Evolution of chordate structure, New York, 1960, Holt, Rinehart & Winston, Inc.

CHAPTER 15

SKELETAL SYSTEM

EMBRYONIC MESENCHYME CELLS

Cells that leave the mesoderm layers of the embryo and migrate singly or in groups into the spaces of the body are called *mesenchyme cells*. They are predominantly mesodermal in origin, although neural crest, ectoderm, and even, to a limited extent, endoderm also contribute to them. These loosely aggregated cells are usually star shaped (stellate) with extending processes that contact one another. Unlike other cells of the body (muscle, nervous, etc.), mesenchyme cells secrete a semifluid *intercellular substance* that becomes caught in the meshes of the network formed by their processes. Especially in the early stages of development, mesenchyme cells undergo ameboid movement and wander over the body, inserting themselves between developing organs. They are the *packing tissue* of the early embryo and fill in the spaces between the various body tubes (neural, notochordal, gut, etc.) in the primitive embryonic form.

The mesenchyme cells not only act as packing tissue, but they also undergo differentiation and develop into various types of specialized cells. They give rise to a number of other cells that in the adult function in a variety of ways, as shown in Table 15-1. In some cases, they are referred to as wandering cells and in others as fixed cells. They differentiate into *myoblasts*, which form muscle; *hemocytoblasts*, which give rise to the blood cells; *macrophages*, which participate in the body's defense; *mast cells*, which synthesize and store heparin; *lipoblasts*, which store fat; *melanoblasts*, which synthesize melanin; *endothelium, myocardium*, and other important parts of the circulatory system; *fibroblasts*, which contribute to the connective tissue proper; *chondroblasts*, which mature to form cartilage; and *osteoblasts*, which become the bone-secreting cells. Some investigators suggest that a few mesenchyme cells remain in reserve in the undifferentiated state in the adult body. When needed, they develop into specialized cells. For example, they are considered important in tissue repair.

Most of the cells that differentiate from mesenchyme have names that end in "blast" (which means *germ* in Greek), indicating a formative stage of a specific cell type. For example,

TABLE 15-1. Contribution of mesenchyme to the body's structure

Embryonic source of mesenchyme cells	Adult tissue		
	Type of cells derived from mesenchyme	Type of tissue formed	Examples
Myotome	Myoblast	Muscle	Cardiac, smooth, skeletal
Dermatome	Hemocytoblasts	Stem blood cells	Erythrocytes, leukocytes, blood platelets
Sclerotome	Mesenchyme	May remain in adult body	Important in body repair
Splanchic mesoderm	Mast cell	Connective tissue	Synthesizes and stores heparin
Somatic mesoderm	Lipoblast (fat cell)		Adipose
	Macrophages (histiocytes)		Phagocytic cells important in the body's defense
Neural crest cells	Fibroblasts	Connective tissue proper	
		Loose	Areolar packing tissue, serous membrane, endo-thelium, fascia
		Dense irregular	Dermis, capsules of organs, sheaths of tendons, peri-osteum, perichondrium
		Dense regular	Ligaments, tendons, apo-neuroses
	Chondroblasts	Cartilage	Embryonic skeleton, hyalin, elastic, fibrous
	Osteoblasts	Bone	Skeletal support of verte-brates
	Osteoclasts		Remodeling of bone

the word "osteoblast" refers to a mesenchyme cell that has started down the pathway leading toward bone formation. An osteoblast, in turn, will mature and become a specialized osteocyte, surrounded by the intercellular substance of bone.

CONNECTIVE TISSUE

Some of the mesenchyme cells become fibro-blasts and secrete fibers that are deposited in the intercellular substance to give it additional strength. The appearance of large amounts of intercellular material and fibers in association with the fibroblasts is the basis for classifying the tissue as *connective tissue.* Since it is one of the four fundamental tissues of the body, it plays a very important role in its construction. The other three tissues are muscle, nerve, and epithelium. Connective tissue exists in varying degrees of compactness. In the adult it acts as packing tis-sue; it binds tissues and organs together; it gives the body form, allows it to maintain posture,

and provides a substrate for fluid to pass from one organ to another. In this chapter we shall consider the formation of connective tissue from mesenchyme. The other functions of mesenchyme cells listed in Table 15-1 are taken up in ap-propriate chapters.

In connective tissue the number of cells varies in proportion to the intercellular matrix (ground substance). There may be many cells, as in the loose type, or relatively few cells, as in cartilage or bone. The fibers present in the ground sub-stance are usually considered either *collagenous,* *reticular,* or *elastic,* but there is some evidence that these fibers may be different expressions of the same fibrous protein. Further classification of connective tissue is based on the chemical nature of the matrix, the types of cells present, and the kind and compactness of fibers. There are three main groups of connective tissues: *con-nective tissue proper* (loose and dense), *carti-lage,* and *bone.* The intercellular matrix is soft and fluid in loose connective tissue; is firm and flexible and can be cut in cartilage; and is hard and rigid in bone because of the deposition of salts in the ground substance.

Connective tissue proper

When all the tissues of the embryo have formed, the remaining mesenchyme becomes the *loose connective tissue* of the adult. The three types of intercellular fibers are loosely arranged in a somewhat gelatinous matrix, containing mucopolysaccharides, proteins, and water. When exposed, as in a dissection, spaces in the tissue trap air, giving it a bubbly or frothy appearance. Loose connective tissue is spongelike and surrounds ducts, blood vessels, and nerves. It forms the membranes of the pleural, peritoneal, and pericardial cavities. It composes the mesenteries and some of the fasciae. In Chapter 10 we discussed its contribution to the subcutaneous layers of the skin. Adipose (fat) and pigmented connective tissue are usually classified as special types of loose connective tissue.

In other places in the body, the fibers are more compactly arranged and form what is known as *dense connective tissue*. The fibers are principally collagen, and there are fewer cells and less ground substance present. When the fibers are randomly oriented, they are found in the dermis of the skin, in capsules (testis, for example), sheaths of tendons, periosteum (surrounding the bones), and perichondrium (surrounding cartilage).

If the fibers are arranged more compactly, in closely packed bundles, they give rise to *ligaments*, *tendons*, and *aponeuroses*. The tough cordlike tendons attach muscles to bones and offer resistance to a pulling force. They are usually shiny white in appearance and consist primarily of longitudinally arranged collagenous bundles. Fish lack most tendons, and therefore their flesh is more tender than that of the tetrapods whose tendons are highly developed. Ligaments are similar to tendons but contain more elastic fibers. As an illustration, they tie together the neural arches of tetrapods. Aponeuroses and fasciae are broad flat sheets of tissues composed of layers of fibers, often running in different directions. These interwoven layers cannot be dissected. For example, the connective tissue wrapping on one muscle may extend as a flat sheath (aponeurosis) and attach to another muscle.

Notochord

The notochord is a special kind of connective tissue that does not exactly fit into the general classification. It resembles cartilage in that it functions as a skeletal support and is considered embryonic tissue but differs from it in one important aspect. The rigidity of cartilage is attributable to extracellular matrix, but in the notochord it is the intracellular component that allows it to function as a supportive rod. The cells composing the notochord appear as large vacuolated cells, with the cytoplasm pushed to one side. There is little or no extracellular matrix present. The pressure of the water in the swollen cells keep the structure turgid much as in a plant stem. Dense connective tissue sheaths of varying widths, believed to be produced by the notochordal cells, usually envelop the notochord (Fig. 15-1). The sheaths consist of an inner layer of dense connective tissue and an outer one of elastic tissue.

The notochord, one of the three distinguishing characteristics of chordates, is present in the embryos of all members of the phylum and is retained in the adult stages of some. It appears first in the Urochordata. It is present in the tail of tunicate larvae where it supports the extended body (fish form) as it swims by side-to-side movements. In the cephalochordates (amphioxus), the notochord extends forward beyond the end of the neural tube. In the vertebrate embryo, it arises from the cells of the dorsal lip (rounded gastrulas) or anterior region of the primitive streak (flattened forms). During gastrulation, it separates from the other germ layers and takes up a position beneath the dorsal neural plate as the rod-shaped axial skeleton of the primitive embryonic form. It is one of the first organs to appear in the embryo. In developing fish, it is relatively large, but in embryos of birds and mammals, it is small. It is unsegmented but flexible. From cyclostomes to mammals, the notochord projects anteriorly in the embryo only as far as the hypophysis and infundibulum.

When the notochord is retained as an adult structure, as in amphioxus, electron micrographs

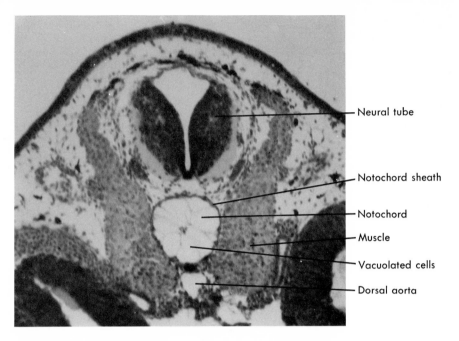

Fig. 15-1
Section through the notochord of 10 mm. frog embryo showing large vacuolated cells and notochordal sheath. (× 4.)

reveal that it undergoes certain changes, becoming more highly organized than in its embryonic state. In those lower vertebrates that keep the notochord in the adult stage, the connective tissue sheaths usually become very thick and strong, imparting to the structure greater rigidity. In some cyclostomes, small paired segmentally arranged cartilages reinforce the cord. In higher vertebrates, a vertebral column surrounds and replaces the notochord. In these animals, as the vertebral column forms, it squeezes the notochord out of existence.

Cartilage

In vertebrate embryos, most of the axial and appendicular skeleton first forms in cartilage. In most adults, bone replaces the cartilage, with the exception of the members of the classes Petromyzontes, Myxini, and Chondrichthyes. In these animals, bone never forms. Cartilage also plays a role as a supporting tissue in the adult body. Its pliable but firm support prevents the collapse of certain tubes (respiratory, for example).

Wherever cartilage occurs, it is basically the same material, differing mainly in the type and amount of fibers secreted into the ground substance. It consists of cells, the *chondrocytes,* an *amorphous gel* of chondroitin sulfate, and *collagenous* and *elastic fibers.* There is more intercellular material present than cells. Cartilage contains no nerves or blood vessels. This lack of vascular and lymphatic vessels definitely limits the size of the tissue since the chondrocytes must obtain their nutrition by diffusion. A compact connective tissue covering, the *perichondrium,* encloses cartilage. Based on the amount of matrix and kind of fibers present, cartilage is divided into three types: *hyaline, elastic,* or *fibrocartilage.* Hyaline cartilage is somewhat elastic, smooth, and glasslike. It is the most common and characteristic cartilage and some histologists regard the other types as modifications of it.

Hyaline cartilage is present in long bones during their period of growth and, in the adult, continues to cover their articulating surfaces. It provides a hard, even surface, allowing the bones to move smoothly against one another. It forms the only support for the larynx, trachea, and bronchi. Elastic cartilage is present in the external ear, epiglottis, walls of the external auditory canal, and the eustachian tubes. Fibrocartilage composes the intervertebral disks, pubic symphysis, ligamentum teres femoris, and certain sites of attachment of tendons to bones.

Development and growth of cartilage

In the embryo, migrating mesenchyme cells concentrate at the site of cartilage formation. Here they undergo mitosis and differentiate into chondroblasts. They withdraw their stellate "arms," round up, and form large spherical cells with centrally placed nuclei. These dense clusters of cells are referred to as *centers of chondrification.* The mesenchyme (fibroblasts) surrounding the centers forms layers of dense connective tissue that give rise to the *perichondrium* as shown in Fig. 15-2. This membrane is composed of two components: an outer layer, adjacent to the surrounding connective tissue (packing tissue), and an inner one, in contact with the chondroblasts. The inner layer is able to add cells (chondroblasts) to the centers and, therefore, is said to be *chondrogenic.*

In the centers of chondrification, the chondroblasts mature and become chondrocytes, capable of secreting a metachromatic hyaline matrix around themselves. As identified in Fig. 15-2, the space in the intercellular matrix surrounding each cell is the *lacuna;* the clear matrix immediately around the lacuna becomes the *capsule.* In the embryo, the continuing growth of cartilage occurs in two ways: (1) The mass of cartilage expands from within. Each cartilage cell undergoes mitosis and divides into two; a second di-

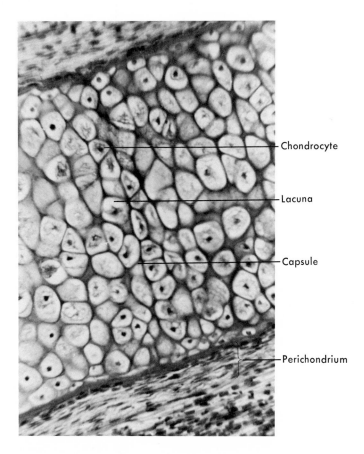

Fig. 15-2
Section showing a center of chondrification. Each chondrocyte rests in a lacuna surrounded by a capsule. The mass of cartilage cells is covered by a connective tissue sheath, the perichondrium. (×40.)

vision may also occur, forming a cluster of four cells. Each daughter cell secretes intercellular matrix and, as a result, becomes surrounded by its own lacuna and capsule. The newly deposited matrix separates the daughter cell from the other cells. The whole process is repeated. Growth that occurs by expansion of the internal mass of cartilage because of the division of chondrocytes is referred to as *interstitial growth*. It occurs in young cartilage before the matrix becomes too rigid. (2) *Appositional growth* takes place as described above except that it goes on at the surface of the cartilage. The inner layer of the perichondrium gives rise to chondroblasts that secrete matrix and fibers and add to the surface of the mass. As a result of this type of surface growth, the inner layer of the perichondrium enlarges and pushes outward. However, it always remains in contact with the cartilaginous mass. In the adult, the perichondrium retains its ability to form cartilage but normally is not actively chondrogenic unless specifically stimulated.

Bone

Bone, the connective tissue with the most rigidity and support, is present in the oldest vertebrate skeleton. It is a unique vertebrate characteristic since it is found in no invertebrate group. Like other connective tissues, it consists of cells, fibers, and an intercellular matrix. However, it also has inorganic matter, composing about two thirds of its weight, in the form of calcium phosphate (85%), calcium carbonate (10%), and small amounts of calcium and magnesium fluoride. It has great tensile strength, which makes it ideal for carrying out its particular supportive and protective functions. Bone is the main internal support of the body, providing attachment for the muscles and tendons. It encases the brain, lungs, and heart, protecting them from injury. Its marrow is the center of blood-forming activities, and it represents a storehouse for calcium in the body.

Unlike cartilage, bone is vascular. A series of small canals carry nutrients to the bone cells (osteocytes) deep in the center of bone. Metabolic wastes are removed in a similar manner. Bone is a dynamic tissue that is constantly eroded away and re-formed throughout the life of the individual. In fact, some of the long bones of man are not completely ossified until the individual reaches his early twenties. Bone is affected by dietary and hormonal conditions.

Macroscopic structure

Depending on its gross organization, two types of bone can be distinguished: *cancellous* (or *spongy*) and *compact (dense)* bone. Their names indicate something of their structure. When a long bone in its formative stage is cut lengthwise, most of it will be found to be filled with cancellous bone. Hard, compact bone composes only the outside rim. Cancellous bone is made up of spicules or trabeculae that anastomose with one another forming a three-dimensional latticework. The growing spicules of apatite crystals (primarily calcium phosphate) are oriented in such a way that maximum strength is obtained. Many irregular spaces are formed, giving bone a spongy appearance.

Although compact bone is composed of the same cells, matrix, and fibers as cancellous bone, it is more dense. Most bones consist of both cancellous and compact bone but in varying amounts. In the adult, cancellous bone is present in the *epiphyses* (ends of the shaft) and *diaphysis* (shaft) of the long bones. It also is found in the center of some of the flat bones of the skull and ribs. Wherever present, compact bone always covers the surface of cancellous bone. Compact bone, in turn, is sheathed with dense connective tissue, the *periosteum*.

Adult bones are not solid but have spaces in the center filled with either yellow or red marrow. Yellow marrow, consisting chiefly of fat and a network of blood vessels, fills the cavity of most vertebrate long bones. In reptiles and birds, hemopoietic tissue is also located in the yellow marrow. In birds, diverticula from all the air sacs (except thoracic) extend into the spaces of long bones, thereby lightening them even further. In the tetrapod's epiphyses, skull, ribs, vertebrae, and girdles (flat irregular bones), the spaces between the trabeculae of cancellous bone contain red marrow. In adult birds and in mammals, myeloid tissue primarily concerned with the production of erythrocytes and granulocytes make up the red marrow. We shall refer again to the red marrow when we discuss blood formation in Chapter 17.

Microscopic anatomy

Bone is too hard and rigid a tissue to be sectioned in the normal manner unless demineralized, but thinly ground sections are available for microscopic examination. (Fig. 15-3). These sections show bone to consist primarily of interstitial substance and to contain only a few cells. Each osteocyte (bone cell) is located in a small almond-shaped space, the *lacuna*. Radiating out into the intercellular matrix from each lacuna are slender tubular structures, the *canaliculi*. They make contact with the canaliculi of other lacunae, thereby establishing in the intercellular matrix an anastomosing network of canals that communicate with one another as may be seen in Fig. 15-3. The osteocytes extend their cytoplasmic processes into the canaliculi, but there is no evidence that they actually contact one another.

Electron micrographs show the osteocytes resting in an amorphous nonfibrillar material that fills not only the lacuna but also the canaliculi. It probably acts as a medium for the exchange of materials between the blood vessels in the Haversian canal and the bone cells. The deposition of calcium salts in the matrix of bone appears to inhibit diffusion and, unlike cartilage cells, the osteocytes cannot depend on this mechanism for their nutrients.

Microscopic studies further reveal the *lamellar* or *layered* structure of bone, one of its most char-

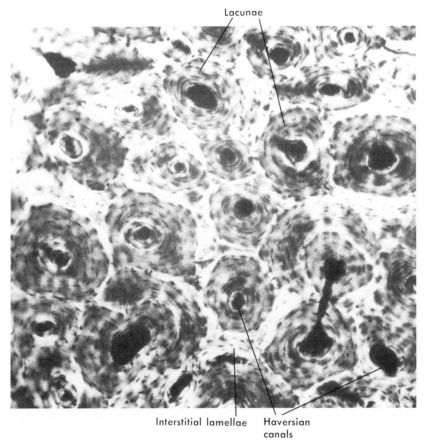

Lacunae

Interstitial lamellae   Haversian canals

Fig. 15-3
Ground section of compact bone showing Haversian systems composed of Haversian canals (a central vascular channel) surrounded by concentric rings of lacunae. Interstitial lamellae are wedged between the Haversian systems. (× 10.)

acteristic features. Although present in both cancellous and compact bone, the layers are more obvious in the compact type. They are arranged in various ways, three of which may be mentioned. At the outer and inner surfaces of compact bone the layers run parallel with the periosteum and endosteum (the lining of the marrow cavity). These relatively thin continuous layers around the shaft are known as the *outer* and *inner circumferential lamellae*. However, most of compact bone is penetrated by branching, longitudinal vascular channels that anastomose with one another. Osteoblasts follow these channels and arrange themselves in rings around the blood vessels. Here they deposit their bony matrix forming lacunae and radiating canaliculi. As many as 8 to 15 concentric rings of lacunae may surround these circular openings. The central vascular channel, the *Haversian canal*, together with its layers of intercellular matrix and osteocytes make up structural units known as *Haversian systems* or *osteons*. These structural units may be seen in Fig. 15-3. The third type of bony layer, the *interstitial lamellae*, is represented by irregular-shaped layers wedged in between the Haversian systems. These lamellae represent the remnants of old Haversian systems.

Since bone consists of a rigid matrix, it is obvious that, unlike cartilage, interstitial growth cannot occur. All growth must be appositional. In a newborn child, as the bones grow in width and length, a remodeling of the skeleton must also occur. Otherwise, almost solid bones would result as layer after layer is deposited. However, anyone who has examined a longitudinal section of a long bone knows that bones are not solid. A cavity, which contains marrow and gives lightness to the bone, is present.

The remodeling does not occur as one would remodel a bone in clay but involves the removal of bone and the deposition of new bone. Remodeling is a continuous process that goes on not only in young organisms but in adults, and not only on the surface of the bone but internally as well. Absorption begins in the center of the bone and contributes to new and larger cavities. Bone is constantly deposited by the periosteum at one area and absorbed at another. Both pro-

cesses occur simultaneously. In this way, bone is able to maintain a constant shape.

The *osteoclasts* are a second type of cell derived from the primitive mesenchyme and present in microscopic preparations of bone. These are giant cells containing as many as 15 to 20 nuclei. Although their function is not clearly understood, most investigators view the osteoclasts as cells that play a major role in the remodeling of bone. They have been seen enveloping the ends of the spicules in a region of bone absorption and therefore are usually assumed to be the cells responsible for bone removal.

Histophysiology

Calcium and phosphate in the form of ions and elements are extremely important and necessary in the proper functioning of the body. Calcium ions play a vital role in membrane permeability, enzymatic activity, neuromuscular response, clotting of blood, acid-base balance, and hormonal effects. Inorganic phosphate is necessary for many enzyme-controlled activities, for example, the metabolism of glycogen. Aided by vitamin D, most calcium is absorbed from the duodenum. According to radioactive calcium (^{45}Ca) studies, about 99% of the body's calcium is rapidly deposited in the skeleton. Bone, therefore, is an important storehouse of mobilizable calcium. Under normal conditions there is a constant interchange between the calcium of the plasma and the calcium of the bone. Calcium levels depend on a balance between the amount absorbed from the intestine and the amount resorbed from bone and the amount lost in feces and urine and the amount deposited in bone. Despite these variables, the calcium levels in the plasma remain remarkably constant. If the ionized calcium level falls in the circulating plasma, the body draws upon the bone to maintain its circulating levels.

The formation and resorption of bone is controlled by the action of several hormones. Parathyroid hormone (PTH) and thyrocalcitonin (TCT) are the principle hormones involved. The parathyroid hormone increases serum calcium and decreases serum phosphate levels by directly affecting bone and kidney. It appears to act on the bone collagen and apatite crystals to cause the release of calcium and phosphate into the circulation. The parathyroid is sensitive to the fluctuating levels of calcium and is regulated by a negative-feedback mechanism. Thyrocalcitonin, produced by the thyroid gland (or probably the ultimobranchial bodies embedded in the gland), is believed to act as an antagonist to PTH. It affects bone by suppressing calcium resorption or by increasing its deposition in bone. As a result, plasma calcium is lowered.

The pituitary growth hormone, somatotrophin (STH), also affects the rate of bone formation. It is especially important in young growing animals. It usually complements the action of the thyroid hormone, encouraging maturation. Both hormones (somatotrophin and thyroxine) are important for normal growth to occur. Gonadal hormones also modify the rate of bone maturation. When there is precocious sexual development, the skeleton matures early and growth is stunted.

Obviously a diet lacking certain minerals or vitamins will affect bone. If a deficiency in dietary calcium occurs, the parathyroid gland is stimulated (negative feedback) and, in turn, induces the osteoclasts to increase their activity. As a result the bone salts are broken down and calcium is released into the circulation. Vitamin D increases the rate of calcium absorption from the gastrointestinal tract. When there is a lack of vitamin D, calcium cannot be absorbed from the intestine, even though it may be present in adequate amounts, and rickets may result. A deficiency in vitamin C interferes with the production and maintenance of the intercellular matrix of bone. Vitamin A regulates the action of the osteoblasts and osteoclasts during development. If a deficiency in this vitamin occurs, the remodeling of the skull is impaired, compressing the growing brain and causing serious damage to the developing nervous system.

Osteogenesis

In the embryo, bone forms in two different ways (osteogenesis), but always develops by transforming preexisting connective tissue. Embryologists refer to these two types as *intramem-* *branous*, or *dermal*, and *intracartilaginous*, or *endochondral*, *ossification*.

In the first type, the bone forms *directly* from primitive mesenchyme and is called *membranous bone*. Bone is deposited on a membrane secreted by mesenchyme cells. In the primitive animal, this membrane was formed in the dermis of the skin. For this reason it is also referred to as dermal bone. In the second type of bone formation, the replica of the bone is first laid down in hyaline cartilage. The cartilage is then removed and replaced by bone. It is, therefore, indirectly produced and is referred to as *"cartilage" bone*, or *replacement bone*. Despite the different names, the chemical, macroscopic, and microscopic composition of the two types of bone are the same. Only the specific osteogenic pathway differs. Also, an extra step is inserted in endochondral (cartilage) bone formation, since the cartilage must be eroded away before the bone can be deposited. In general, membranous bone gives rise to certain skull bones; endochondral bone composes the bones at the base of the skull, the vertebral column, the pelvis, and the appendages.

FORMATION OF MEMBRANE BONE. Mesenchyme cells concentrate and proliferate in those regions where membrane bone forms, in the skull region, for example. They arrange themselves in sheets, with their stellate processes touching one another. Blood vessels invade the area, forming loose networks. The mesenchyme cells differentiate into fibroblasts and osteoblasts. They secrete a clear gel-like ground substance between the cells and deposit randomly oriented reticular and collagen fibers in the intercellular matrix. The mesenchyme can now be compared to a loosely woven membrane. For this reason bone formed in this manner is referred to as membranous bone. However, at this stage only the organic part of the matrix is present; it is soft and can be cut, since there are no minerals deposited in it.

Once the organic matrix forms, bone salts are next deposited in it by the osteoblasts. They are able to remove the inorganic material from the contents of the surrounding blood vessels and deposit the salts on the collagen fibers. Bone first appears as anastomosing spicules equidistant between the meshlike blood vessels. Since the spicules follow the blood vessels, they also appear in a branching and anastomosing pattern as shown in Fig. 15-4. Bone forms as a result of an intimate union of collagen fibers (of the intercellular matrix) with minerals in the form of very minute crystals. These crystals, containing primarily calcium phosphate, are responsible for the calcification of the matrix. As the matrix continues to be laid down, some of the osteoblasts are trapped in the bone, leaving small spaces around the cell body and processes. These spaces become the *lacunae* and *canaliculi,* respectively. Once entrapped by bone matrix, the osteoblasts cease their synthetic activities and differentiate into *osteocytes,* cells responsible for maintaining the bone.

Since the matrix is secreted in the concentrated area of mesenchyme cells, certain osteoblasts remain on the surface of the matrix. As

bone grows, these surface cells are added to the bony mass and new cells take their place. Their numbers are maintained by mitosis and by surrounding mesenchyme contributing more osteoblasts. During embryonic and postnatal growth, these surface osteoblasts, in direct contact with the bone, arrange themselves as an *osteogenic layer* and contribute to the inner layer of the periosteum, the connective tissue covering over all bone. The outer layer of the periosteum is composed of blood vessels and dense connective tissue, formed from the surrounding mesenchyme cells. In actively growing bone, when the osteoblasts on the inner surface of the periosteum are added to the growing bony mass, the periosteum, must of course, move outward. The bone laid down on the surface by the periosteum is the same as that in the interior except that it is more compactly arranged. There are fewer spaces present and the bone is in the form of sheets or

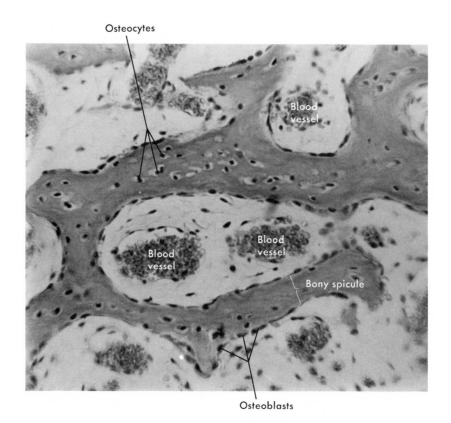

Osteocytes

Blood vessel

Blood vessel

Blood vessel

Bony spicule

Osteoblasts

Fig. 15-4
Section showing deposition of membrane bone as anastomosing spicules equidistant between blood vessels. (× 40.)

compact bone. Cancellous bone composes the more central areas, where spicules are present. The spaces between the spicules are filled with marrow.

In the adult, the inner layer of osteoblasts composing the periosteum is usually in a resting state and cannot be distinguished from the surrounding connective tissue. Should a bone be broken, however, they are stimulated to differentiate into functional osteoblasts and lay down new bone.

FORMATION OF ENDOCHONDRAL BONE. In endochondral ossification, a number of sequential steps must occur for normal development to take place. The first step begins when the replica of the bone is laid down in cartilage. In the area of bone formation, the mesenchyme differentiates into chondrocytes that undergo hypertrophy and assemble in three main areas. They first collect in the middle of the future shaft or *diaphysis* of the bone and later in the middle of the two adjacent areas at the top and bottom of the shaft designated as the *epiphyses*. The epiphyses and the diaphysis join together to form the adult bone. The femur of the leg and the humerus of the forearm are two examples of long bones formed in this manner. They are represented in the human embryo of about the seventh week as a cartilaginous model covered by a perichondrium.

Primary centers of ossification are established in man in the center of the future shaft as early as the eighth week of fetal life. Here, the lacunae of the hypertrophied cartilage cells grow at the expense of the surrounding matrix until only thin partitions or spicules remain between them. An enzyme, secreted by the chondrocytes, diffuses out of the cell into the surrounding matrix and splits off the phosphates of the phosphorylated sugars present in the ground substance. As a result, the free calcium ions combine with the phosphate to form apatite crystals (calcium phosphate) and are deposited in the matrix. As a result of the deposition of insoluble salts, the hyaline cartilage becomes calcified. As stated earlier, cartilage is avascular, and when calcification occurs, oxygen and nutrients can no longer diffuse from the vascular system at the surface of the cartilage mass through the ground substance to the individual cartilage cells in the interior. Consequently, the hypertrophied cartilage cells undergo degeneration and death and are eventually removed. Degeneration begins in the center of the future shaft and proceeds outward toward the periphery. The formation of calcified cartilage and the death of the cartilage cells at the primary center of ossification represent the second step in endochondral ossification (Fig. 15-5).

Concurrent with the changes in the center of the future shaft of the bone, the cells in the inner layer of the perichondrium develop osteogenic abilities and secrete a *bony collar* or band around the primary center of ossification. The fibrocellular membrane (perichondrium) is now referred to as the *periosteum*. The bony collar is considered membrane bone, since it forms directly by the periosteum and does not first pass through a cartilage stage. This third step, the formation of the collar, strengthens and supports the weakened area of degenerating cartilage.

The periosteum is stimulated to send *periosteal buds* into the degenerating areas of calcified cartilage. These buds, consisting primarily of blood vessels from the outer layer of the periosteum (Fig. 15-6), carry with them connective tissue cells (mesenchyme) as they erode openings through the collar and penetrate the central area of the diaphysis (shaft). Some of the connective tissue cells differentiate into osteoclasts that dissolve some of the narrow islands of cartilage between the hypertrophied cartilage cells and lacunae. As a result larger spaces are formed by the merging lacunae, the *primary marrow spaces*. Other connective tissue cells carried in by the periosteal buds become hemopoietic elements and take up a position in the marrow where they will give rise to blood cells described in more detail in Chapter 17. Finally, some of the connective tissue cells differentiate into osteoblasts and deposit bone matrix on the remaining spicules of calcified cartilage. Eventually all the calcified cartilage is eliminated, leaving only bone in its place. As a result of these activities the center of the growing bone has a spongy appearance and is composed of cancellous or spongy bone; compact bone covers the periphery of the bone.

Bones continue to grow in length and width. Starting at the primary center of ossification, an orderly sequence of events takes place that extends the zone of ossification in either direction to the ends of the cartilage model. At the same time, the bony collar is also increased in length and diameter by the additional deposition of bone. At the end of the shaft, in the epiphysis, a *secondary center of ossification* appears. In many long bones there is an epiphyseal center at either end of the bone. However, in some bones, such as the smaller phalanges, only one such center forms. In these smaller bones, the epiphysis may be distally or proximally located. Irregularly shaped bones such as the scapula or pelvic girdle may have more than one primary center of ossification and several secondary centers.

Bone is deposited in the cartilage model of the epiphysis in a manner similar to that in the diaphysis. Eventually only a thin transverse plate of cartilage remains between the epiphysis and diaphysis. This *epiphyseal plate* is a proliferative zone responsible for all future growth of the long bone until sometimes in adulthood. After the ossification of the epiphysis and diaphysis, cartilage cells continue to leave the cartilage

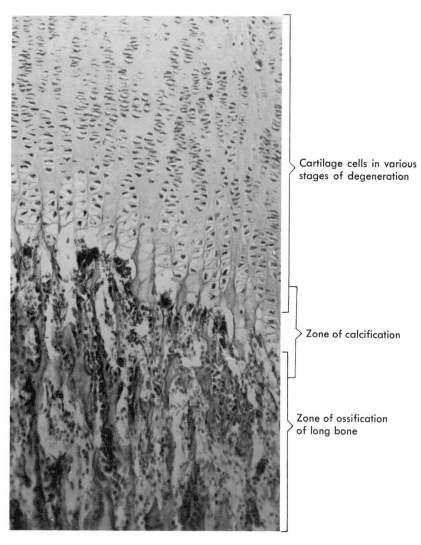

Cartilage cells in various stages of degeneration

Zone of calcification

Zone of ossification of long bone

Fig. 15-5
Section through portion of long bone showing endochondral ossification. (× 10.)

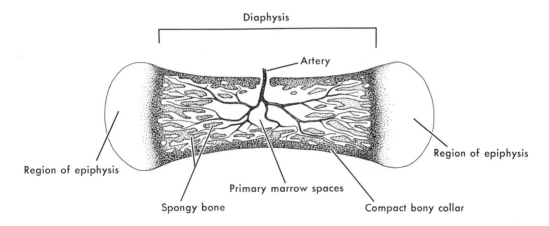

Fig. 15-6

Diagram of primary center of ossification in long bone. Blood vessels perforate the bony collar deposited around cartilaginous model. They penetrate the center of the cartilage carrying osteoclasts and osteoblasts with them. These cells dissolve the calcified cartilage and replace it with bony trabeculae.

plate and pass into the shaft. They are then replaced by bone. As a result, the epiphyseal plate remains the same thickness and the diaphysis continues to grow in length. The epiphyseal plate is especially sensitive to the growth hormone (somatotrophin). In fact, it is so sensitive that the increase in width of the epiphyseal cartilage after injections of the hormone into an experimental animal is the basis for one of the bioassays of STH.

Eventually, the epiphyseal plate ossifies and growth of the long bone ceases. In man, this usually occurs by the time the individual reaches his late teens or early twenties.

VERTEBRATE EXOSKELETON

Bone is exceedingly ancient and is the primary skeletal material of vertebrates. As pointed out in Chapter 2, it was present in the earliest known vertebrates, the ostracoderms. In general, cartilage is considered an embryonic skeletal material, since it is pliable and its size, shape, and form are easily altered. Just why modern lampreys and sharks have lost their bony skeleton and retained their embryonic form is not known. However, since the earliest vertebrates possessed bone and the lampreys and sharks came later, we assume that they, too, originally had a bony skeleton. Perhaps a more flexible skeleton offered certain advantages, possibly lightening it, as the

animal left the bottom of the oceans to pursue a more active life near the surface.

The oldest bones, phylogenetically speaking, are considered to be those formed directly from mesenchyme in the dermal regions of the integument, the membrane or dermal bones. They were responsible for the exoskeleton of bony plates that covered the body of the early ostracoderms and placoderms. The term "dermal bone" has a phylogenetic connotation and refers specifically to the bones derived from the dermal region. All dermal bones are membrane bones, but all membrane bones are not dermal bones. As we mentioned earlier, membrane bone gives rise to compact bone of long bones. Also, certain bones of the vertebral column form directly from mesenchyme and do not first form in cartilage.

The phylogenetic history of dermal bones is an interesting one and is a story of progressive loss. In general, higher vertebrates have lost their exoskeleton and only retain the dermal bones as part of the skull, jaw, and pectoral girdle. In higher animals the term "dermal bone" is used somewhat loosely. For example, the frontal bone of the mammalian skull no longer forms directly in the dermis. However, since it did form in this manner in piscine ancestors, it is considered homologous and therefore a true dermal bone.

According to fossil evidence, the dermal bones of ancestral vertebrates were a part of the integument and formed a continuous armor about the body. Since they were derived from mesenchyme (mesoderm) and not epidermal ectoderm, in Chapter 10 only reference was made to this component of the integument. These plates, present in the integument of the extinct ostracoderms and placoderms had a basic structure: a layer of spongy bone sandwiched between two layers of compact bone (Fig. 15-7). Spiny structures

(denticles), composed of dentine, covered the surface of the plates.

In modern elasmobranchs, the bony regions of the plate regressed and the denticles are retained as *placoid scales.* These scales are conical in shape and contain a pulp cavity. Their surface is covered with a hard enamel-like material with most of their bulk consisting of dentine (refer to Fig. 10-1). They are similar to vertebrate

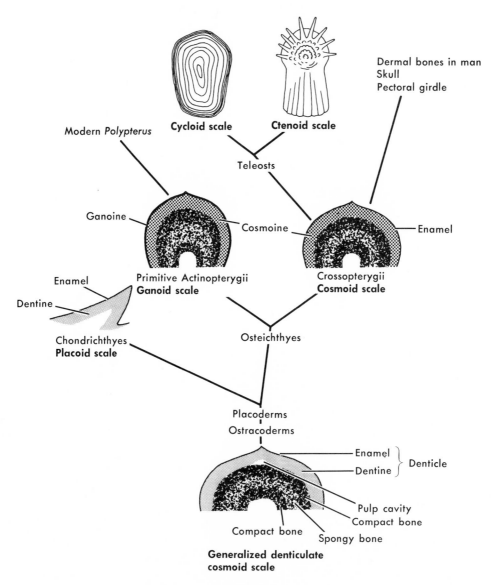

Fig. 15-7
Evolution of dermal armor. See text for details.

teeth, and indeed both scales and teeth are believed to represent the last remnants of the armor that wrapped the body of the early vertebrates. Once jaws evolved, it is not difficult to imagine some of the scales located about the mouth migrating into the oral cavity and their denticles giving rise to teeth. The teeth of the placoderms are homologous to teeth of modern vertebrates and both are considered vestiges of the original ostracoderm plates.

The scales of the early Osteichthyes varied in composition, but as time past, they evolved toward a simpler form. The crossopterygian line of fishes retained the bony composition of the scale but lost the denticles. Cosmine, rather than dentine, composed the main substance of the plates. The resulting cosmoid scale, therefore, did not have the same structure as the placoid scale of the shark. The crossopterygian fish had such scales but no living vertebrate possesses them today. In the head region, they were arranged topographically according to size and shape. Ultimately, it is believed that it is these regularly occurring cosmoid scales of the crossopterygian fish that were incorporated as part of the skull and pectoral girdle of higher animals.

In primitive actinopterygians, the scale evolution followed a different line. There was retention of the bony layer and several layers of hard enamel-like ganoine replaced the outer enamel layer. These scales became the *ganoid scale,* present today only in *Polypterus,* and the garpike. Most modern actinopterygians have a much simpler scale. Both the ganoine and cosmine layers were lost by the time the teleosts evolved. Their scales consist primarily of flat, overlapping sheets of acellular bonelike material (produced by the dermis) resting on a fibrous layer. They are covered by a thin layer of epidermis, except where the spines protrude. Two slightly different scale types can be distinguished in living teleosts. One of these (cycloid) has a smooth margin, whereas the other (ctenoid) is equipped with a comblike series of teeth (cteni) along one edge.

The early amphibians, recently descended from fish, retained some of the bony plates in the ventral regions of the skin. Modern amphibians, however, lack scales except for a few vestiges buried in the skin of Apoda. Gastralia, V-shaped rods located in the abdominal region of modern lizards, crocodilians, and *Sphenodon,* represent remnants of the ancestral bony armor. It is (with a few exceptions) completely lacking in birds and mammals. The armadillo, for example, still retains an exoskeleton.

VERTEBRATE ENDOSKELETON

The skeleton inside the body, the *endoskeleton,* is composed of cartilage and bone. The skeletal system is sufficiently rigid to give support and protection but flexible enough to allow movement. Muscles are anchored to bones. Their contraction causes the bones to change position in relation to one another and to act as levers. In this way, body posture is maintained and motion can take place. The two systems (muscular and skeletal) function in close relationship with one another.

Based on the parts of the body served, the skeletal system of all vertebrates is divided into two main subdivisions: the axial skeleton and the appendicular skeleton. These are illustrated in Fig. 15-8, for man. More specifically, the skeletal elements may be organized as follows:
1. Axial skeleton
   a. Skull
   b. Pharyngeal skeleton
   c. Vertebral column
   d. Ribs
   e. Sternum
2. Appendicular skeleton
   a. Pectoral girdle
   b. Pelvic girdle
   c. Appendages

Articulations

Bones and cartilages join with one another at *articulating surfaces* or *joints.* Depending on their degree of movement, these joints may be of two general structural types: rigid *(synarthroses)* or movable *(diarthroses).* Some anatomists add a third type of joint to their classification by distinguishing between slightly flexible joints (symphyses) and fully movable ones (diarthroses). Connective tissue fibers from the perichondrium or periosteum connect the two cartilages or bones together.

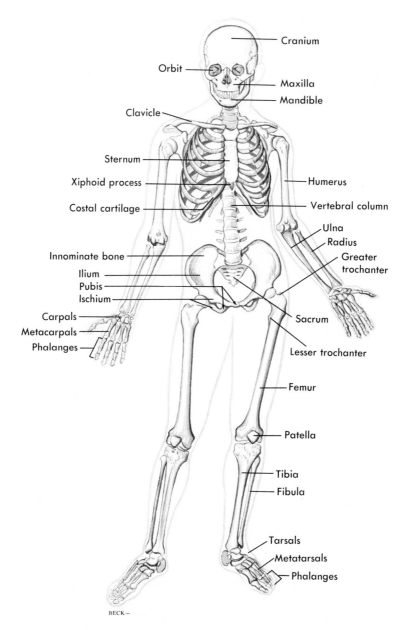

Fig. 15-8
Anterior view of axial and appendicular skeleton of man. (From Anthony, C. P., and Kolthoff, N. J.: Textbook of anatomy and physiology, ed. 8, St. Louis, 1971, The C. V. Mosby Co.)

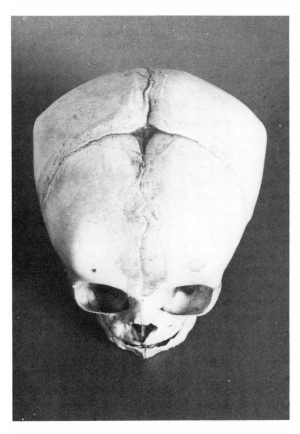

Fig. 15-9
Skull bones abut directly against one another and allow no movement. The connective tissue separating the two bony pieces becomes calcified or ossified and only a thin line or suture remains as shown in this skull of an infant. An example of a synarthrosis joint. (From Hickman, C. P., Sr., Hickman, C. P., Jr., and Hickman, F. M.: Integrated principles of zoology, ed. 4, St. Louis, 1970, The C. V. Mosby Co.)

There is no movement between the membranous bones of the skull. In this example of the simpler type of joint (synarthrosis), mesenchyme cells located between the developing bones differentiate into connective tissue, separating the two bony pieces but holding them tightly together. In some instances, however, the connective tissue becomes calcified or ossified, and only a thin line or *suture* remains, as shown in Fig. 15-9, or the bones may be so closely apposed that the line separating them may not be visible at all. In this type of articulation, a synovial membrane does not develop.

The pubic symphysis in female mammals is an example of a flexible (but in most vertebrates not freely movable) joint. In this type of articulation, the mesenchyme cells between the bones differentiate into cartilage. At the time of parturition a hormone, *relaxin*, secreted by the ovary or placenta, or both, acts upon the plate of fibrocartilage (or in some cases dense fibrous connective tissue) increasing its flexibility. As a result of this hormonal action, the ligaments holding the bones of the pelvis together relax and the birth canal distends, facilitating delivery.

In a diarthroidal joint, a cavity lined with a *synovial membrane* is present (Fig. 15-10). In this type of articulation (for example, that between humerus and ulna), hyaline cartilage covers the articulating surfaces of the bone. At the point of contact between the two bones the periosteum is reflected back, contributing to the membrane of the joint capsule. A liquid, the *synovial fluid*, fills the space formed between the

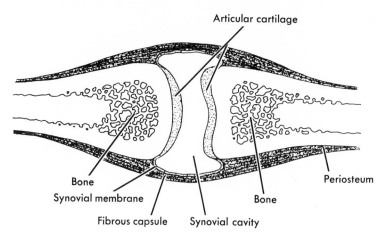

Fig. 15-10
Longitudinal section through typical diarthrodial joint.

two juxtaposed skeletal elements, bathing the articulating surfaces and acting as a lubricant. The capsule about the joint is composed of an outer tough, fibrous layer and an inner ill-defined synovial membrane, believed to secrete the synovial fluid.

Axial skeleton
Skull

The cranial skeleton, or skull, occupies the anterior portion of the axial skeleton of vertebrates. Since the nervous system is one of the earliest to differentiate, the brain and nerve cord are well developed before there is evidence of any skeletal support. Three primary embryonic components give rise to the bony skull: (1) the cartilaginous brain case, *chondrocranium,* (2) contributions from the visceral arches, the *splanchnocranium,* and (3) a dermal roof, or *dermatocranium.*

First evidence of the formation of a cranial skeleton is the appearance in the embryo of a cartilaginous shelf beneath the primitive brain. Later, lateral walls are added and finally a roof. With the exception of adult cyclostomes and Chondrichthyes, bone partly or completely replaces the cartilaginous components. Ossification centers are established, and bone replaces cartilage by one of the two methods previously described, that is, either by membranous or endochondral bone. With few exceptions, these basic parts fuse together to form the bony skull. The skull is a very complex structure. The presence of well-preserved fossil records has allowed paleontologists to study extensively its evolutionary development. We shall attempt to simplify its discussion as much as possible, limiting ourselves primarily to a general consideration of representative modern forms.

EMBRYONIC CRANIUM

Chondrocranium. In the embryo, the notochord extends anteriorly as far as the hypophysis and is immediately ventral to the posterior regions of the brain. The earliest indication of a head skeleton occurs when mesenchyme cells surround the early neural tube and condense, forming a membrane that encapsulates the developing brain. In the human skull, this occurs as early as the fifth or sixth week. Several centers of chondrification give rise to independent rudiments. Later, these fuse and provide the floor of the braincase. The formation of these rudiments is best followed in the shark, since in higher animals the stepwise formation of the floor is less clear.

First, cartilaginous *parachordal plates* appear on both sides of the anterior end of the notochord beneath the posterior regions of the brain, as shown in Fig. 15-11, *A.* They soon expand laterally toward the otic region and posteriorly to the occipital vertebrae. The plates form from mesenchyme derived from the sclerotome of the head somites. Therefore, although they lack segmentation, they resemble the rudiments of the vertebrae not only in their origin but in their location on either side of the notochord.

Paired elongated *prechordal* or *trabecular* cartilages develop in front of the parachordal plates. The mesenchyme that contributes to their anterior region is believed to be produced from neural crest sources. At the same time the prechordal and parachordal plates are forming, cartilaginous or connective tissue capsules surround the special sense organs (nose, ear, and eye). The *nasal capsule* develops anteriorly and the *otic capsule* forms posteriorly. The *orbital (optic) capsule* surrounding the eye is first formed in connective tissue and is known as the *sclera.* In man, it is not cartilaginous. In some animals bony rings form in the sclera and offer greater protection to the eyes. These separate chondrocranial cartilages are shown in Fig. 15-11, *A.*

In lower animals such as the shark, the para- chordal cartilages grow medially, posteriorly, and laterally, fusing with the notochord, occipital vertebrae, and otic capsule to form the basilar plate, as illustrated in Fig. 15-11, *B.* In man, a single plate is present from the beginning. Anterior to the basilar plate, the prechordal cartilages fuse with one another and with the nasal capsule to form the *ethmoid plate.* Further growth of the ethmoid plate gives rise to the rostrum of the shark. The posterior ends of the ethmoid plate fuse with the basilar plate. At the point of union, an open space remains, the pituitary space or *hypophyseal fenestra.*

As a result of the growth and fusion of the various cartilaginous components, a floor forms beneath the forebrain, midbrain, and hindbrain, as illustrated in Fig. 15-11, *C.* This basic plate is flat in the shark but more compressed in higher forms. Contributions from the nasal and otic capsules provide side walls to the structure. The posterior regions of the parachordals grow dorsally, fusing above the hindbrain, encasing this

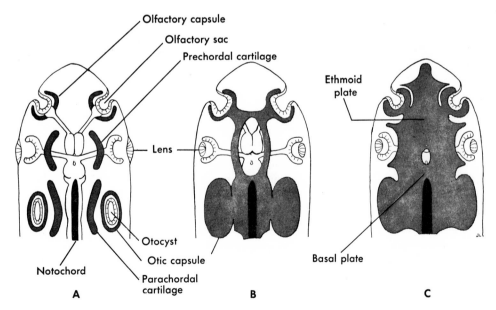

Fig. 15-11

Diagram illustrating major embryonic components of braincase. Parachordal and prechordal plates and nasal and otic capsules first appear, **A.** These fuse, **B,** and form a cartilaginous floor consisting of the basilar and ethmoid plates that incorporate the notochord, **C.** (From Kent, G. C.: Comparative anatomy of the vertebrates, ed. 3, St. Louis, 1973, The C. V. Mosby Co.)

area of the brain and forming the *foramen magnum,* the opening through which the spinal cord leaves the braincase. Only the eyes remain independent, movable orbits, with their capsules being free of the other cartilages. Such a basic structure appears uniformly throughout the embryos of all vertebrate classes. It is comprised of four main areas: an anterior ethmoid region followed by orbital, otic, and occipital components.

The next step in the formation of a cranium is the completion of side walls and a roof. Cartilaginous walls are gradually added, extending dorsally from the nasal and otic capsules. In the shark these lateral walls fuse over the brain, forming a roof. In this animal the brain becomes completely enclosed in a cartilaginous braincase. Such a single structure is known as a *chondrocranium.* Although it grows larger as the animal and its brain increase in size, it never becomes ossified. In other animals, complete sides and roof are limited to the otic and occipital regions. In reptiles, birds, and mammals, the cartilaginous floor is replaced by bone. The rest of the braincase (sides and roof) consists of a connective tissue membrane formed by the condensation of mesenchyme cells. This lack of a rigid support early in development allows for the growth of the brain. Later, dermal bone is deposited in the membrane, contributing to the roof of the skull.

There are several openings, *foramina,* in the braincase, allowing cranial nerves and blood vessels to pass to and from the brain. In general, these openings occur in the spaces between the various components of the chondrocranium. For example, there must be spaces for all the cranial nerves to pass to their respective effector or receptor organs. We have already mentioned the largest opening, the foramen magnum, located at the posterior end of the chondrocranium.

Splanchnocranium. Although the visceral arches arise completely independent of the chondrocranium, during the course of evolution, the first two arches became associated with the skull. They contribute to the upper and lower jaws and their articulating hinge. Neural crest cells, located dorsal to the neural tube at the end of neurulation, soon migrate laterally and ventrally.

They give rise to the visceral arches, the substance between the gill clefts. Although most skeletal material is formed from mesoderm, as mentioned at the beginning of this chapter, neural crest cells can also differentiate into mesenchyme cells capable of forming chondroblasts and osteoblasts. It was originally believed that the splanchnic mesoderm gave rise to the visceral arches, thus the term "splanchnocranium." However, one can trace streams of neural crest cells, labeled with radioactive substances, as they migrate into the spaces between the gill slits. Authorities generally agree that in most cases, at least, it is the neural crest cells that form the cartilaginous or bony bars supporting the gill arches. The arrangement of the clefts and pouches is presented in Fig. 13-5.

In the cyclostomes, as many as 12 to 14 pairs of visceral arches are present. In gnathostomes, there are usually seven pairs. The mass of neural crest cells anterior to the first pouch becomes the first, or *mandibular, arch.* It is divided into dorsal and ventral halves that transform into upper and lower jaws (Fig. 15-12). In the shark, each half of the dorsal arch is a *palatoquadrate cartilage;* together they form the upper jaw. Each side of the ventral part of the first arch is called a *Meckel's cartilage.* They contribute to the lower jaw, the *mandible.* Teeth are born on both the palatoquadrates and Meckel's cartilages.

The accumulation of neural crest cells between the first and second pouches gives rise to the second or *hyoid arch.* In fishes, this second gill arch acts as a hinge in the articulation of the upper and lower jaw. It consists of an upper part, the *hyomandibula,* that is attached to the otic capsule by connective tissue fibers. A slender lateral *ceratohyal* and a lower median *basihyal* complete the hyoid arch. The latter supports the tongue. The remaining pairs of visceral arches are associated with the branchial (gill) apparatus of fishes and some amphibians *(Necturus).* In higher animals, when the gills are lost, the visceral skeleton becomes modified and contributes support to other structures of the body. Later in this chapter we shall follow in greater detail the alterations of the visceral skeleton. At the present, we shall consider only the first two

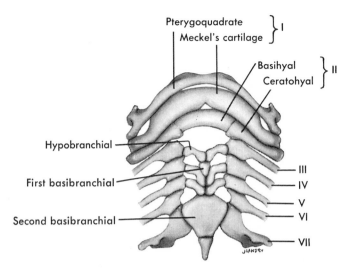

Fig. 15-12
Ventral view of the visceral skeleton of dogfish shark showing upper and lower jaws and ceratobranchial cartilages of visceral arches III to VII. (From Kent, G. C.: Comparative anatomy of the vertebrates, ed. 3, St. Louis, 1973, The C. V. Mosby Co.)

arches. In sharks, these arches form the upper and lower jaw and its articulation; in higher animals, they contribute ossification centers to the formation of the bony auditory ossicles.

Dermatocranium. As indicated earlier, the roof of the cranium is first of a membranous nature. The bones, forming the roof and sides of the skull, develop in this membrane and are collectively referred to as the *dermatocranium.* They are never preformed in cartilage. They represent the remnants of the scales that covered the heads of ancestral ostracoderms and placoderms. Many of these scales fused to form larger skull bones that, in general, are paired. In the early embryo and young postnatal individuals, the dermal bones do not quite meet (Fig. 15-13). Membrane-covered spaces known as *fontanelles* (soft spots) exist between them. In man, the last of the fontanelles usually close about the second year of life. The dermatocranium becomes intimately applied to the chondrocranium and contributes the following components: (1) roof and sides of skull covering the brain, (2) sheath covering certain bones of the upper and lower jaw, (3) roof of oral cavity, the palate, and (4) in bony fish, the bones that strengthen the operculum.

DEVELOPMENT OF ADULT SKULL. The skull re-

mains cartilaginous in adult cyclostomes and elasmobranchs. In the adult of higher forms, bone replaces the three primary embryonic components in part or totally. Each cartilaginous or membranous part establishes an ossification center. More than one center is present in those bones formed by the fusion of several pieces of cartilage, for example, the occipitals.

Ossification of chondrocranium. Ossification centers appear more or less simultaneously in the four regions of the embryonic chondrocranium. The degree of ossification depends on the class of animals considered. For example, ossification is reduced in modern amphibians as compared with reptiles, birds or mammals. Since bone replaces cartilage, it is deposited in the centers by endochondral ossification in much the same way as in the formation of long bones. In man, these centers can be identified as early as the third month. Fig. 15-14 presents a diagram of the endochondral bones that form from these centers.

OCCIPITAL REGION. Varying numbers of occipital arches (resembling the more posterior vertebrae) surround the emerging spinal cord and contribute to the walls of the foramen magnum. Four bones usually form from the cartilaginous arches in the occipital region. Their names indi-

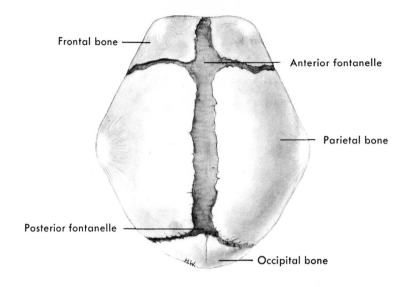

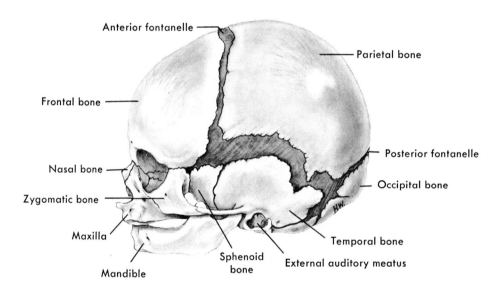

Fig. 15-13
Individual dermal bones of a term fetus do not quite meet and membrane-covered spaces, known as fontanelles, exist between them. (From Francis, C. C.: Introduction to human anatomy, ed. 6, St. Louis, 1968, The C. V. Mosby Co.)

cate their position around the foramen magnum. Ossification centers give rise to the *basioccipital,* which becomes the ventral wall of the foramen magnum and underlying hindbrain. Two bones, the *exoccipitals,* contribute to the sidewalls, and a dorsally located *supraoccipital* completes the roof of the foramen magnum. In mammals, these four bones usually fuse into a single *occipital bone* (Fig. 15-13). It is this bone that articulates

by means of one or two condyles with the first vertebra of the vertebral column. In mammals, a condyle develops on both exoccipitals.

SPHENOID REGION. In the floor of the chondrocranium in front of the basioccipital, ossification centers produce two flat bones, the *basisphenoid* immediately anterior to the basioccipital, and the *presphenoid* in front of the basisphenoid. A bony floor is thus established under the develop-

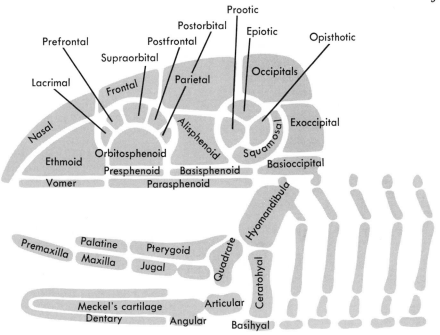

Fig. 15-14
Lateral view of vertebrate skull. Description given in text.

ing brain. The orbit (eye) with its capsule (sclera) lies dorsal to the presphenoid and the *orbitosphenoid* bone forms part of the lateral wall of the orbit. In some reptiles and birds, a *pleurosphenoid* develops in the posterior wall of the orbit above the basisphenoid. In some mammals, the several ossification centers produce bony elements that fuse to give rise to a single *sphenoid bone* (Fig. 15-15).

OTIC REGION. A bony capsule completely surrounds the otic vesicle. In most lower vertebrates a *prootic* forms in the anterior wall of the capsule, an *opisthotic* in the posterior wall, and an *epiotic* in the dorsal wall. In birds and mammals, these bones fuse to form a single *periotic* bone that may unite with surrounding bones. In the cat and man, for example, the periotic bone contributes the endochondral elements to the temporal bone, the *petrous* and *mastoid* portions. The rest *(squamous part)* of the temporal bone is of dermal origin.

ETHMOID REGION. The cartilaginous ethmoid plate, formed when the median prechordal cartilage fused with the lateral nasal capsule, provides the floor of the braincase anteriorly and contributes to the support of the nose. Of all the regions of the chondrocranium, the ethmoid is the most likely to remain cartilaginous.

The *mesethmoid* arises from an ossification center in the middle of the plate and extends to the tip of the nose. In some fishes, the anterior portion of the ethmoid plate is ossified, but in tetrapods, it remains cartilaginous and gives rise to the *nasal septum*. The lateral cartilages form the scroll-like *turbinate bones* composing the nasal passages and supporting the nasal conchae (Fig. 15-15). At first, the central and lateral cartilages of the ethmoid region are not fused and the olfactory nerve passes between them. As development continues, the two are joined by cartilaginous trabeculae, providing a protective sheath to the olfactory nerve. When ossification of these cartilages occurs, many foramina remain, through which the olfactory nerve passes. This region is known as the *cribriform plate*. In mammals, the several centers of ossification may fuse to form a single *ethmoid bone*.

Ossification of splanchnocranium. In sharks, the dorsal palatoquadrate cartilage becomes the

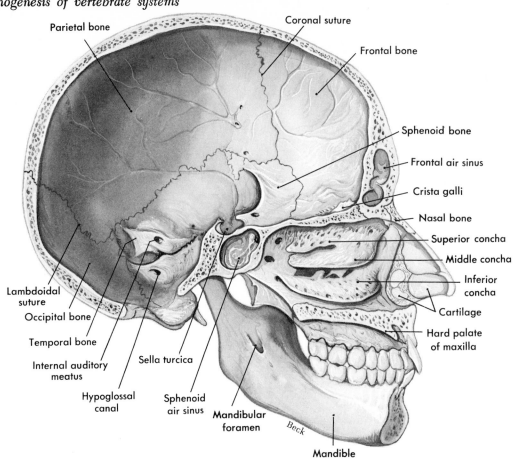

Fig. 15-15
Diagram of left half of skull showing the scroll-like turbinate bones composing the nasal passages and supporting the nasal conchae. (From Anthony, C. P., and Kolthoff, N. J.: Textbook of anatomy and physiology, ed. 8, St. Louis, 1971, The C. V. Mosby Co.)

upper jaw and the ventral Meckel's cartilage becomes the lower jaw. They do not ossify and articulate with the chondrocranium by way of the hyomandibula. In primitive bony fish, several ossification centers may be established along the quadrate part of the arch, but in modern bony fish only the caudal portion ossifies, forming the *quadrate bone*. In tetrapods, the contribution of endochondral bone is greatly reduced or lacking. Instead, dermal bones cover the upper jaw and tie it securely to the skull.

In primitive fishes, Meckel's cartilage has several centers of ossification, but in modern fishes and tetrapods, most of them have disappeared. This part of the arch may remain as a cartilaginous core covered with dermal bone or, as

in the quadrate cartilage, only the proximal or lateral end of Meckel's cartilage may ossify, forming the *articular*. In tetrapods, with the exception of mammals, the quadrate lies in the sidewall of the skull abutted by the articular. This type of jaw suspension is known as *autostylic* since it is suspended directly from the skull. It can be compared with that of the sharks (*hyostylic*) in which the hyomandibula braces the first arch against the chondrocranium.

As a result of the evolution of this new type of jaw suspension in the tetrapods, the hyomandibula no longer functions as a jaw support but rather moves to the middle-ear cavity. It becomes the rodlike *columella* and functions as a transmitting device from the eardrum to the inner ear. In reptiles and birds, it extends from the tympanic membrane to the fenestra ovalis. In mammals, the entire relationship of the jaws is altered and a new type of joint system has evolved. Two bones, the dentary and squamosal (temporal) are involved in the articulation of mammalian jaws with the skull. Consequently, some of the skeletal components of this area are now superfluous. Part of the columella becomes the *stapes,* one of a series of three ossicles that function in the transmission of sound. The articular and quadrate bones present in the sidewalls of the tetrapod skull are freed. They are incorporated into the middle ear and give rise to the *malleus* and *incus,* respectively. Table 15-2 summarizes the fate of the visceral arches in vertebrates.

Ossification of dermatocranium. Dermal bones form the roof and sides of the skull as well as provide substantial contributions to its base (parts that arose primarily as cartilage). In bony vertebrates these dermal bones form in the membrane that invests the brain. An examination of the skull of modern ganoid fishes (sturgeon, garpike, or bowfin) reveals that the brain is protected by typical fish scales located in the head region of the skin. These scales are no different from the rest of the scales covering the body, but they are destined to become the dermal roof of the skulls of higher forms. The roof of the chondrocranium is located beneath this bony covering. It is possible to separate the sheath of dermal scales from the underlying chondrocranium, thus demonstrating the dual origin of the skull. The large scales covering the chondrocranium are given names that correspond to the bones composing the skulls of land animals.

Although the proportion of the various components of the skull has changed during evolution, some bones in the tetrapod skull are believed to be exactly homologous to the head scales and therefore merit identical names. On the other hand, the numerous plates in the roof and snout of the early fish ancestors later fused with other plates or were eliminated. No living tetrapod has retained all bones of the primitive vertebrates, and as a result, homologies of all skull bones are impossible to trace. Mammals, for example, have only a few skull bones because of the fusions and deletions that occurred during their evolutionary development.

ROOF OF TETRAPOD SKULL. Many variations occur in the tetrapod skull, but a generalized pattern exists that can be followed for discussion purposes. In the skull roof of modern tetrapods it is possible to identify a longitudinal series of paired bones along the midline (see Fig. 15-14). The *nasals* are located at the anterior end, posterior to the nares. Behind them lie the *frontals* (between the orbits), the *parietals* (centrally located), and the *occipitals* from the posterior portions of the roof. In man, for example, the frontals develop from paired ossification centers around the ninth week, and the parietal bones make their first appearance in the tenth week (Fig. 15-13).

TABLE 15-2. Evolution of the visceral arches

			Sharks	Amphibians	Reptiles	Aves	Mammals
Visceral arches	1		Pterygoquadrate (upper jaw)	Quadrate	Quadrate	Quadrate	Incus
	1		Meckel's cartilage (lower jaw)	Articular	Articular	Articular	Malleus
	2		Hyomandibular cartilage	Columella	Columella	Columella	Stapes
	2		Remaining hyoid	Hyoid apparatus			
	3		First branchial arch	Portion of hyoid apparatus			
	4		Second branchial arch	Trachea, larynx, and epiglottis			
	5		Third branchial arch	Trachea, larynx, and epiglottis			
	6		Fourth branchial arch	Trachea, larynx, and epiglottis			

BONES OF ORBIT. Ossification centers arise in the orbital capsule and form a series of five bones that surround the orbit, or eye socket. *Prefrontals* and *postfrontals,* located anterior and posterior to the *supraorbital* bone, contribute to the upper wall of the orbit. As indicated in Fig. 15-14, the posterior portion of the upper wall is composed of a *postorbital,* and a rather large (endochondral) *orbitosphenoid* makes up the ventral wall of the orbit. The *lacrimal* completes the orbit and, in amniotes, carries the tear duct on its inner surface.

BONES OF LATERAL SURFACE. In primitive tetrapods, the otic notch, located behind the orbit, probably housed the tympanic membrane. Three bones extend along the dorsal surface in the early tetrapods but tend to be lost in modern animals. The remnants of these membrane bones fuse with endochondral bone to form the *temporal.* The *squamosal* occupies most of the cheek region.

TOOTH-BEARING BONES. Dermal bones in the embryos of lower vertebrates cover the upper jaw. The cartilage core, the remnants of quadrate cartilage, then degenerates in various degrees. In mammals, there is no trace of the cartilaginous ancestry, and the upper and lower jaws form directly from membrane bone derived from mesenchyme. The paired *premaxillas* occupy the anterior portion of the skull, fusing in the mid-

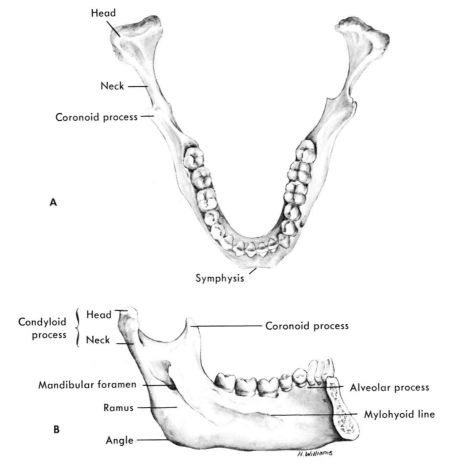

Fig. 15-16
Lower jaw of man viewed from above showing fusion of two dentary bones to form mandible, **A**; medial surface of left dentary bone, **B**. (From Francis, C. C.: Introduction to human anatomy, ed. 6, St. Louis, 1973, The C. V. Mosby Co.)

line. Along with the nasal bones, they surround the external nares. It is premaxillas that bear the anterior incisor teeth. The sides of the upper jaw, composed of the *maxillas,* carry the remaining teeth.

Although strictly speaking the lower jaw (mandible) is not a part of the skull, we shall include it in our discussion. In the embryos of bony fishes and all tetrapods, Meckel's cartilage is present, and in adult Chondrichthyes, it remains as the cartilaginous lower jaw. In adult bony fish and tetrapods, it becomes ossified to various degrees. The posterior portion of Meckel's cartilage, articulating with the upper jaw, becomes the (endochondral) bony *articular.* In lower animals, several dermal bones encase the articular and contribute most of the lower jaw. In mammals, as stated above, the articular moves into the middle ear as the malleus (Table 15-2). A single paired *dentary* bone is retained composing each half of the lower jaw. It articulates with the squamosal and fuses at the anterior midline in a symphysis. The dentary bone has a flat horizontal surface, called the *body,* in which the teeth are embedded, and a more or less vertical *ramus,* articulating with the skull (see Fig. 15-16). Several processes are present, affording ar-

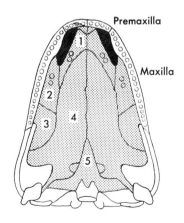

SEYMOURIA

Fig. 15-17
Diagram of primary palate of primitive reptile *Seymouria.* Palatal bones, shown stippled, consist of **1,** vomers; **2,** palatines; **3,** ectopterygoids; **4,** endopterygoids; and **5,** parasphenoid. (From Kent, G. C.: Comparative anatomy of the vertebrates, ed. 3, St. Louis, 1973, The C. V. Mosby Co.)

ticulating surfaces and points of muscle attachment. Foramina allow arteries and nerves to pass within the jawbone and supply the teeth.

PALATE. In sharks, the ventral floor of the chondrocranium is also the roof of the oral cavity. In bony fish and tetrapods, this floor becomes covered by dermal bone, thus providing a new roof for the mouth cavity. Ossification centers are established in the skin lining the oral cavity. They give rise to four bones that are closely applied to the endochondral bones of the braincase floor. In bony fish and lower tetrapods, the paired *vomers* are located laterally beneath the olfactory capsule: the *palatines* are situated more posteriorly, followed by the *endopterygoids* and *ectopterygoids.* The *parasphenoid,* occupying the central region, remains as a single element. The *primary palate,* as formed by these dermal bones in the primitive reptile *Seymouria,* is depicted in Fig. 15-17. By the time the mammalian skull evolved, some of these basic bones were reduced or lost. For example, the parasphenoid is eliminated.

In some reptiles (crocodiles) and in all birds and mammals, a horizontal partition is added below the primary palate, dividing the mouth and pharynx into two chambers. This horizontal shelf of bone is known as the *secondary* or *hard palate* and separates the oral cavity into an upper chamber associated with olfaction and breathing and a lower chamber concerned with the passage of food.

In general, this secondary palate forms when the premaxilla, maxilla, and palatine on each side of the primary palate contribute horizontal shelflike projections of bone that grow medially as shown in Fig. 15-18. In reptiles and birds, these bones do not always meet in the center, but in mammals, the projections of one side fuse with the projections from the other side to give rise to a complete new roof to the oral cavity. Failure of the two sides to fuse in mammals produces a *cleft palate.*

In amphibians, the internal nares open into the anterior region of the oral cavity, the common chamber that functions as a passageway for both food and air. In amniotes, as a result of the formation of the secondary palate, the internal nares are shifted posteriorly. The air is

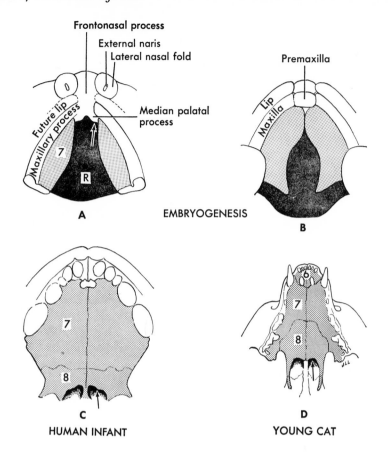

SECONDARY PALATES

Fig. 15-18

Horizontal shelflike projections, the palatine processes of the premaxillas, *6,* and maxillas, *7,* grow below the primary palate *(dark gray)* and toward the midline, in **A** and **B.** They fuse with one another and with the palatine process of the palatine bone, *8,* to form the secondary (false) palate of man, **C.** Rathke's pouch, *R,* the future anterior pituitary gland, marks the primary roof of the skull. A secondary palate of a young cat is included for comparison, **D.** (From Kent, G. C.: Comparative anatomy of the vertebrates, ed. 3, St. Louis, 1973, The C. V. Mosby Co.)

now carried to the back of the throat in a dorsal air passageway before it contacts the mouth cavity proper by way of the internal nares. In mammals, this shelf is extended even further by the *soft palate,* unossified connective tissue that extends the bony roof caudally. The internal nares of mammals, therefore, are brought in closer contact with the glottis, the opening into the trachea leading to the lungs.

Formation of face

The various steps in the formation of the cranial and visceral portions of the skull are easily followed; the modeling of the mammalian face from the mandibular and hyoid arches is more difficult to observe because the embryo's head presses against its thorax. However, in the human embryo, studies show that by the end of the fifth week proliferating mesenchyme cells concentrate on both sides of the midline, forming the primordium of the mandibular arch as illustrated in Fig. 15-19, *A.* This arch furnishes the posterior boundary for the stomodeum, the ectodermal inpocketing described in Chapters 8 and 13 that marks the opening of the mouth. The mandibular arch gives rise to the lips and lower jaw of the fetus.

Also by this stage of development, bilateral convex thickenings of ectodermal cells, the *nasal placodes,* appear as horseshoe-shaped elevations surrounding the *nasal pits.* The pits are located on both sides of the head at the lateral angles of the stomodeal (oral) opening. Laterally these elevations are known as the *nasolateral processes* (or folds) and medially as *nasomedial processes.* The front part of the head housing the forebrain constitutes the *frontal process.*

A swelling develops into a *maxillary process* at the lateral angles of the oral cavity and grows medially toward the stomodeum as shown in Fig. 15-19, *A* and *B.* By the sixth week, the maxillary process has pushed the nasomedial process more medially. It has also contributed a portion of the upper border to the oral opening. The upper lip, upper jaw, and nose will develop from these paired, lateral maxillary processes, paired nasomedial processes, and single median frontal process.

The nasolateral fold separates the developing eyes from the nasal pits. The nasomedial processes continue to grow, pushing away the frontal process and eventually meeting one another in the midline. The developing maxillary processes also move medially. Some embryologists believe that the processes continue medially until they fuse with one another at the midline; others believe that the process first joins the nasomedial fold. According to this last interpretation, the upper arch consists of a fused nasomedial process and a lateral maxillary process on both sides.

The nasal pit deepens to form the *nasal sac* and, in time, develops further into *nasal cavities.* The cavities expand dorsally toward the frontal process and also posteriorly. The two sacs also expand medially but remain separated from one another by a portion of the nasofrontal process, the *nasal septum.* This septum extends as a midline ridge in the roof of the oral cavity. Chondrification and ossification centers produce cartilage and bone (ethmoid) in the mesoderm of the septum, the skeleton of the nose. The superior, middle, and inferior conchae shown in Fig. 15-15 arise as elevations in the lateral wall of the

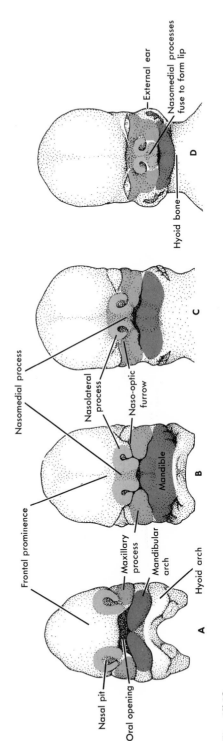

Fig. 15-19
Diagram illustrating the various steps in the formation of the human face from the mandibular and hyoid arches. See text for details.

septum. They become covered with nasal epithelium as described in Chapter 11.

The face is completed when the maxillary process fuses with the frontal process as well as with the nasolateral process (Fig. 15-19, *D*). A solid rod of cells is formed approximately where the maxillary and nasal processes meet. A cavity develops in the rod, converting it into the tubelike *nasolacrimal duct* (tear duct), which connects the eye with the deep olfactory pit. Mesenchyme from the second visceral arch invades the primitive lips and cheeks, supplying the facial muscles.

The nasomedial and maxillary processes also contribute to the formation of the shelflike secondary palate separating the nasal portion from the oral regions of the original stomodeal cavity (Fig. 15-18). The premaxilla region of the upper jaw (nasomedial) gives rise to a median palatine process. The maxillary processes on both sides of the cavity contribute the major portion of the palate. Shelflike projections grow out from these processes toward the midline. They eventually fuse, first with the median palatine process and then with one another, producing the "false" roof of the oral cavity, the secondary palate, previously described.

In humans, the maxillary bones are among the first to calcify. Ossification centers are established in the upper jaw of the human fetus at about 8 weeks. They first form in the nasomedial region of the upper arch (considered to be the area of the premaxilla in lower animals). A second ossification center arises in that portion of the upper jaw formed from the maxillary process (maxillary bone of lower forms). In the human embryo, these two centers fuse to form a single maxillary bone. However, the sutures indicating their dual origin are visible in fetal skulls and emphasize their probable homology with the premaxillae and maxillae of lower vertebrates.

Visceral skeleton

In the jaw-bearing fishes, a series of cartilaginous or bony bars form arches in the walls of the pharynx between the gill slits. These serially arranged bars support the gills and aid in their movement. They compose a set of structures known as the *visceral skeleton*. It

is because the gills are a part of the wall of the pharynx that the term "visceral" is appropriately used. As stated earlier, seven pairs of these arches are present in most gnathostomes. We have already discussed how the first two visceral arches, specifically known as the mandibular and hyoid, are incorporated into the skull to various degrees. The remaining arches have no individual names but are merely numbered, starting at the anterior end. They are referred to as the first branchial or third visceral arch, the second branchial or fourth visceral, etc. (Fig. 15-12).

The arches resemble one another and support the functioning gills. Each one is divided into a number (usually five) of movable, separate parts. In the pharyngeal floor, the paired arches articulate with median basibranchials (copulae), but dorsally they remain separated from the vertebral column. Branchiomeric muscles are responsible for their movement. *Gill rakers* project from their inner margins and act as sieves, preventing large pieces of debris from passing through the gill clefts and injuring the delicate gill structures. Fine cartilaginous *gill rays* are attached to the outer surface of the gill arches and reinforce the septum of the gills.

In sharks, the visceral arches remain cartilaginous, but in bony fish, ossification occurs. Amphibian larvae retain their visceral arches but in adult amphibians (land forms) and in all amniotes, the gills disappear. As the tetrapod adapted to a terrestrial life, the arches underwent profound changes and became available for other uses. In general, they remain cartilaginous although parts of the arches ossify in various animals.

A movable tongue, a characteristic of most land vertebrates, arises in the floor of the oral cavity. The anterior and ventral parts of the second visceral arch (hyoid) are modified to give it support. The *hyoid apparatus* forms at the base of the tongue in the throat region. The more dorsal part of the hyoid arch contributes to the stapes (Table 15-2), but the ventral portion along with arch three and frequently four contribute to the hyoid apparatus. Processes (horns or cornua) may project from the body of the apparatus and extend to the otic region.

The remaining more posterior visceral arches

contribute to the skeletal support of the larynx (vocal organ of amphibians and mammals) and trachea. They are believed to form the C-shaped cartilages in the walls of the trachea and chief bronchi. These regularly spaced cartilaginous segments provide a supporting framework, which keep the respiratory structures from collapsing. The flaplike *epiglottis* covering the glottis (opening into the trachea) of mammals is also reinforced with cartilage derived from the ancestral visceral arches.

Vertebral column

In all vertebrate embryos, the axial supporting system is represented by the notochord. It is retained in adult cyclostomes and modified in adult elasmobranchs. In all other vertebrates, mesenchyme cells derived from the sclerotomes form V-shaped structures that become integrated with the notochord and develop into the neural and hemal arches. The vertebrae composing the vertebral column first form in cartilage. With the exception of the cyclostomes and Chondrichthyes, they are replaced or supplemented with bone in the adult. In fishes, the vertebral column functions primarily in maintaining the body's length when the longitudinal muscles contract. It is especially important in land forms since the trunk muscles are attached to the vertebrae and the column supports the weight of the body.

Embryonic origin of vertebrae. If you recall in Chapter 8 when we discussed the mesoderm, we noted that the segmented epimeres differentiated into dermatome, myotome, and sclerotome. In this chapter, we are particularly interested in the contributions of sclerotomes since they give rise to the distinct segments (vertebrae) that make up the spinal column. Mesenchyme cells proliferate from the ventral medial surface of the epimere, migrate toward the midline, and take up positions as paired masses on both sides of the notochord and neural tube. Since the sclerotomes are derived from the somites, they initially form segmentally arranged blocks that correspond to the number of somites, as shown in Fig. 15-20, *A*.

In some vertebrates (most amniotes) the mesenchyme cells spread out, lose their segmentation, and form a continuous sheath on both sides of the notochord and neural tube. Concentrations of mesenchyme cells in the sheath give rise to nodules of cartilage known as *arcualia*. In other animals, the concentration of sclerotome cells opposite each somite differentiate into anterior and posterior halves. A rearrangement of these cells then takes place. The sclerotomes split and move apart, and the posterior half of one sclerotome segment merges with the anterior half of a second one to form a single vertebral mass or arcualia (Fig. 15-20, *B*).

As a result of the fusion, the position of the arcualia no longer corresponds to the myotome. Instead, a staggering effect is produced and the arcualia develop into vertebrae that alternate with the segments of myotome. When muscle fibers derived from the myotome grow out, they attach to two vertebrae instead of one, thus allowing movement of the vertebral column.

Typically these sclerotomal blocks split vertically and horizontally and give rise to four pairs of cartilages, an anterior and posterior dorsal component and an anterior and posterior ventral group. In some cases, however, the arcualia only form two pairs, one above the notochord and one below (Fig. 15-20, *C*). The dorsal segment (or in the example above the anterior dorsal segment) extends around the neural tube and upward where it fuses with the one on the other side, forming a *neural arch*. The ventral pair grows in a similar fashion ventrally. In the trunk region they give rise to the primordium of the ribs, but in the tail area they form a *hemal arch*. As a result of the fusion of the dorsal segments, the neural tube lies in a protected cavity, the *neural canal*, formed by the series of neural arches. In the tail region the hemal arch protects the caudal artery and vein. Later, in most vertebrates, bone replaces the cartilage; however, the mesenchyme cells are also able to contribute bone directly.

A typical vertebra consists not only of a neural arch but also has a centrum, which replaces the notochord. Apparently the centrum forms in either of two ways. Sclerotomal cells may invade the notochord and deposit cartilage within the notochord and sheath, or the notochordal sheath cells undergo proliferation and add to the cen-

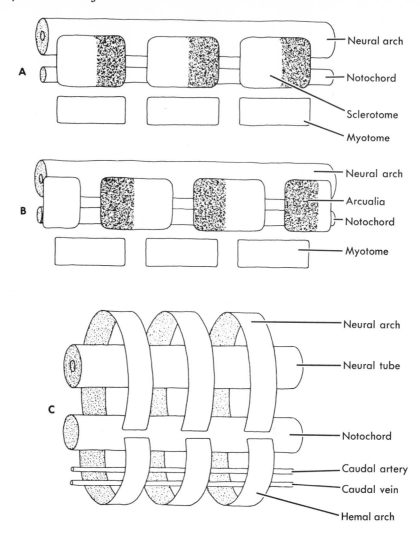

Fig. 15-20

Diagram illustrating the formation of amniote vertebrae. Sclerotome cells are arranged in segments on both sides of the notochord and neural tube. Each segment differentiates into an anterior and posterior half, then splits, and moves apart. Anterior part of one sclerotome joins with the posterior part of a different sclerotome to form arcualia. Arcualia are now staggered in respect to somites. Arcualia grow upward and fuse above the neural tube to form the neural arch and ventral beneath the blood vessels (in the tail region) to form the hemal arch.

trum. In some cases both processes contribute to the formation of the centrum.

The centrum is typically converted to a cartilaginous or bony structure. In the elasmobranchs, the centrum is entirely cartilage and almost squeezes the notochord out of existence as shown in Fig. 15-21. In the shark, the notochord is restricted to only a small central area in each vertebra, but it enlarges to almost embryonic size between successive vertebrae. In amphibians, the centrum consists of some carti-

lage, but bone is also present. In man, the notochord degenerates in the region of the centrum but enlarges to form the pulpy material in the center of the intervertebral disks, the *nucleus pulposus*. The centrum of higher animals is an ossified structure.

The upper surface of the centrum forms the lower surface of the neural canal. The centra articulate at either ends with adjacent centra. Their shape varies among the various groups of animals and forms one of the bases for classifying vertebrates, especially the amphibians. The centrum may be concave at both ends, flat at both ends, or have one articulating surface concave and the other convex. Intervertebral disks, when present, are wedged between two consecutive vertebrae.

The neural arch extends dorsally as the *neural spine* and serves as a point of anchorage for the muscles on the two sides of the body. The spines themselves are tied together by muscles or ligaments. A *transverse process, diapophysis,* located at the base of each arch, serves as a point of rib attachment for the tuberculum, one of the articulating surfaces of the rib. The head of the rib rests on the centrum. These points of articulation on the centrum or transverse processes are small smooth areas referred to as *facets.*

This typical vertebra (Fig. 15-22, *D*), consisting of neural arch and spine, centrum (body), transverse processes, and hemal arches (in the tail), is present in both amniotes and anamniotes. The history of the centrum in fish and amphibia show great variation and is beyond the consideration of this text. However, it is interesting to note some of the general modifications that occur to the vertebral column of vertebrates as they move from the buoyancy of the water to the demands of a terrestrial life.

REGIONALIZATION OF VERTEBRAL COLUMN. In the primitive animal, ribs were present on all vertebrae and remain in modern fish, early amphibians, and some reptiles. Hemal arches are present in the tail region, and the vertebral column of these animals are divided into only two regions: the trunk and the tail. However in higher animals, five regions are usually identified: the (1) cervical, (2) thoracic, (3) lumbar, (4) sacral, and (5) caudal.

Regionalization begins in the amphibians, since they have one cervical and one sacral vertebra. The total number of vertebrae varies not only between the classes but within the classes. For example, among the reptiles, snakes may have several hundred vertebrae and turtles only a few. Modern mammals, in general, show less variation. There are usually 7 cervicals (both giraffe and mouse), about 20 thoracic and lumbar (although the proportion between the two may vary), and 3 to 5 sacrals. Man has 12 thoracic and 5 lumbar, 5 fused sacral, and 4 to 5 fused caudal vertebrae (the *coccyx*).

In reptiles and birds, the cervicals allow greater movement than the more posterior vertebrae and have small, short ribs fused to them. With the exception of monotremes, mammals apparently lack cervical ribs although in the embryo the transverse processes are shown to be actually short, two-headed ribs. Long ribs are usually present on the thoracic vertebrae, and these articulate ventrally with the sternum. In mammals, ribs are absent in the lumbar region.

Most primitive vertebrates possessed long tails

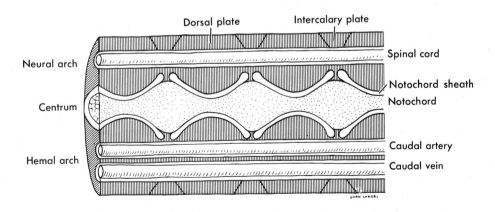

Fig. 15-21
Sagittal section of caudal vertebrae *(Squalus)* shows constriction of notochord within each centrum. Between each successive centrum it enlarges to almost embryonic size. (From Kent, G. C.: Comparative anatomy of the vertebrates, ed. 3, St. Louis, 1973, The C. V. Mosby Co.)

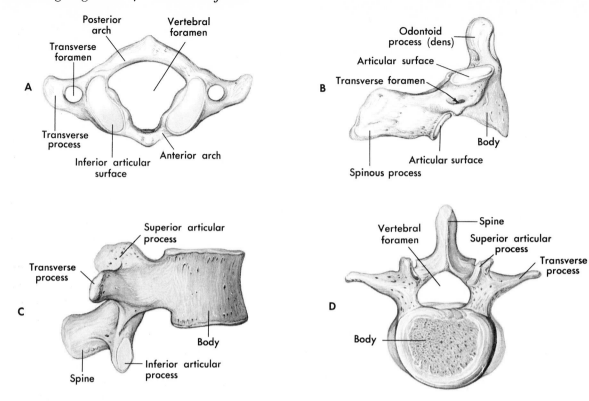

Fig. 15-22
Vertebrae of adult man showing the atlas, which supports the skull, **A**, and the axis with its odontoid process that allows movement of the head from side to side, **B**. Typical vertebra in lumbar region has a body (centrum), neural spine, and transverse processes, **C**. Side view illustrates the superior (anterior) and inferior (posterior) articular processes (zygapophyses), **D**. (From Anthony, C. P., and Kolthoff, N. J.: Textbook of anatomy and physiology, ed. 8, St. Louis, 1971, The C. V. Mosby Co.)

with as many as 50 or more caudal vertebrae. During evolution, no consistent trend can be noted, since both increases and reductions in caudal vertebrae occurred.

CRANIAL MOTILITY. Alterations of the vertebrae allows cranial motility. In fishes, the head and trunk move as a unit, since efficient swimming requires a rigid body. However, motility of the skull, so advantageous to land animals, appears for the first time to a limited degree in amphibians. In fishes, the articulating surface of the skull (condyle) is rounded and fits firmly against the first vertebra. In amphibians, this rounded surface becomes separated into two occipital condyles. Two articulating surfaces also form on the first vertebra, the *atlas*. As a result in frogs, a hinge type of relationship is established, allowing up and down movement of the head. How-

ever, frogs cannot move their head from side to side.

In most amniotes, the second vertebra also becomes modified to form the *axis*, shown in Fig. 15-22, *B*. The first vertebra, the atlas, illustrated in Fig. 15-22, *A*, is a ring-shaped structure that allows further movement in reptiles and birds. In mammals, the centrum of the axis forms a projection, the *odontoid process*, that projects into the ring of the first vertebra and acts as a pivot. The head can now move from side to side by movements of the atlas and axis complex and up and down because of the occipital condyle and atlas articulation.

SUSPENSORY MODIFICATIONS. As vertebrates moved to the land, the weight of the body was supported by the limbs. It was advantageous for these terrestrial animals to have a more solid anchorage of hindlimbs. In amphibians, the articulation of the pelvic girdle with a posterior vertebra, the *sacrum,* provided such a stable support. Fish lack a sacrum. Such a structure would be of little advantage to them since their fins support no weight. In reptiles, the sacrum usually consists of two vertebrae fused with one another. In mammals, the number of fused sacral vertebrae increases to from three to five. In birds, much of the vertebral column (postthoracic, lumbar, and proximal caudals) is fused, adding even greater rigidity and support for the pelvic girdle.

In mammals, the enlarged neural spines slant forward or backward, allowing the attachment of muscles that suspend the body and hold it off the ground. These enlarged neural and hemal spines provide surfaces for the attachment of the powerful tail muscles.

ANTITWIST MECHANISMS. In land animals, each vertebra articulates with the ones anterior and posterior to it by way of interlocking processes on the neural arch known as zygapophyses, or articular processes (Fig. 15-22, *C* and *D*). Each vertebra has an articulating surface that faces upward and inward (prezygapophysis) and one that faces downward and outward (postzygapophysis). The postzygapophysis of one vertebra articulates with the prezygapophysis of the next posterior vertebra. A few vertebrae also have other accessory antitwist processes. These interlocking mechanisms give the vertebral column

more rigidity and prevent torsion of the body, a new problem confronted by the vertebrates as they moved from water to a terrestrial environment.

Ribs

Ribs form from mesenchyme derived either from the sclerotome or from the lateral plate mesoderm. They are first formed in cartilage and later replaced in whole or in part by bone. An exception, of course, are the short ribs of some sharks that remain cartilaginous. Their ossification occurs separately from that of the vertebrae, with distinct centers of ossification appearing in both vertebrae and ribs as depicted in Fig. 15-23. At first, the shaft of the rib ossifies; later, secondary centers are established in the two articulating surfaces of the rib. Epiphyseal plates separate the ends of the rib from the shaft (as described for the long bones) until the adult form is reached.

In most fishes, a horizontal septum divides the lateral muscles into dorsal and ventral groups. These muscles, derived from myotomes, retain their segmented structure and are separated from one another by a myoseptum. With the exception of cyclostomes, which lack ribs, the *dorsal ribs* of fish develop in the myosepta at the intersection with the horizontal septum as shown in Fig. 15-24. A second type of rib, the *ventral* or *pleural ribs,* forms just external to the peritoneal lining where the myoseptum meets

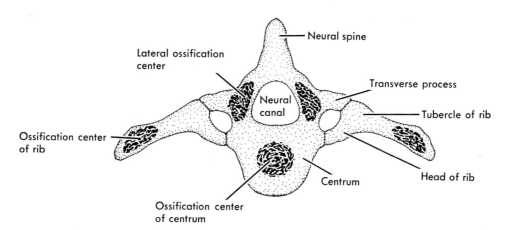

Fig. 15-23

Ossification centers of vertebra and ribs appear separately. See text for details.

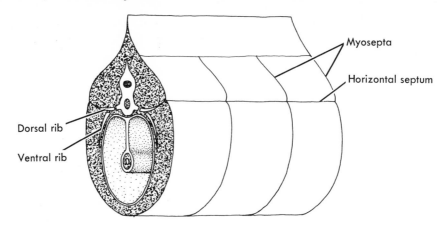

Fig. 15-24
Cross section of typical vertebrate showing location of dorsal ribs developing in the myosepta at the intersection with the horizontal septum. Ventral ribs from externally to the peritoneal lining where myoseptum meets the ventral body wall.

the ventral body wall. Both dorsal and ventral ribs are attached to the centrum of the vertebra by articulating processes. A variety of rib arrangements have developed in fishes. They may have only a pair of dorsal ribs articulating with each vertebra, only ventral, both types, or, in cyclostomes, none. Most teleosts have both dorsal and ventral ribs. The powerful swimming muscles of the fish are attached to them and exert their force on the vertebrae by way of the ribs. Some fish, shad for example, also have intermuscular ribs that add to their swimming efficiency. In the tail region, the ventral ribs bend ventrally around the caudal artery and caudal vein, forming the protective V-shaped hemal arch.

Most investigators agree that the ribs of higher vertebrates are homologs of dorsal ribs. There are no pleural or ventral ribs present. In ancestral tetrapods, each vertebra was attached to a pair of ribs deposited in the myosepta. In general, they were short in the cervical and caudal regions and longest in the thoracic.

Fossil evidence leads us to believe that the ancestral tetrapod rib was *bicipital* (that is, having two heads attached to each vertebra). A *capitulum* (ventral head) articulates with the centrum (or the juncture of two centra), and a *tuberculum* articulates (dorsal head) with the transverse process (diapophysis) of the neural arch. A single head, representing either the tuberculum or capitulum or a fusion of both, may be present in some modern tetrapods (reptiles and some posterior ribs of mammals). In the bicipital rib, a narrow *neck* separates the two articulating surfaces. The remaining part of the rib, the *shaft*, is usually a long slender curved bone. The most curved part of the rib is referred to as the *angle* (Fig. 15-25, *B*).

Modern amphibians lack typical tetrapod ribs. They may be reduced as in urodeles or entirely absent except for the sacrum as in frogs and toads. If present, they are short, attach to the transverse processes, and never encircle the body cavity. Reptiles demonstrate a variety of conditions. Typically, thoracic ribs are composed of two segments: a proximal ossified section and a distal cartilaginous one. A joint between the two allows expansion of the thoracic cavity during respiration. In snakes, ribs are present on all vertebrae except the first two cervical ones. In turtles, the eight trunk vertebrae as well as many neural arches are fused with the underside of the carapace. All five regions in the crocodiles and birds have ribs. Some of the anterior ribs of lizards and eight or nine ribs of the crocodiles encircle the body cavity and at the midventral region articulate with a median ventral structure, the sternum. In birds, all segments of the ribs are ossified.

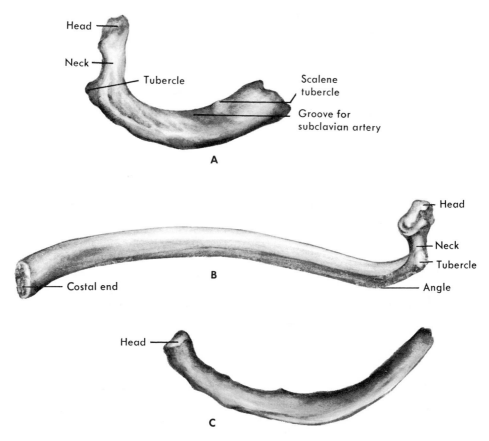

Fig. 15-25
Diagram of three ribs from man. The first rib is short and stocky containing a groove in which the subclavian artery and nerves pass on their way to the arm, **A.** Typical rib has a dorsal and ventral head, a neck, and an angle, **B.** The last two ribs (eleventh and twelfth) are free of the sternum and are called floating ribs, **C.** (From Francis, C. C.: Introduction to human anatomy, ed. 6, St. Louis, 1968, The C. V. Mosby Co.)

In mammals, the remnants of ribs compose the cervical and lumbar processes and only the thoracic region contains well-developed ribs. In man, the first rib is a short, stocky one, containing a groove in which the subclavian artery and nerves pass on their way to the arm (Fig. 15-25, *A*). Each of the first seven ribs are considered *true ribs,* since they curve ventrally and attach to the sternum by costal cartilages. The remaining ribs are referred to as *false ribs.* The ends of the eighth, ninth, and tenth ribs are joined to one another and to the last true ribs. They are, therefore, indirectly attached to the sternum. The last two ribs, the eleventh and twelfth (Fig. 15-25, *C*) are free of the sternum and are called

floating ribs. Ligaments bind them to the anterior longer ribs.

Sternum

The sternum, or "breastbone," is lacking in fish but present in tetrapods where it provides further support for the anterior trunk region. It is associated with land animals where it offers a site of muscle attachment, thereby aiding in locomotion. It forms the ventral portion of the thoracic basket and helps protect the lungs and heart. It arises independently from the ribs and pectoral girdle as bilateral condensations of mesenchyme in the ventral septum. These condensations appear between the midventral edges of the mesenchyme destined to form the costal ends of the ribs and the clavicle. The bilateral condensations merge in the midline and give rise to cartilage. In the birds and mammal, several centers of ossification are established, converting the sternum to a bony structure.

A sternum is absent in some amphibians. In necturus, it consists of a few midventral bars, and in frogs, it forms a part of the pectoral girdle. Some biologists believe that the amphibian sternum is not homologous to that of the amniote and that the reptiles are the first tetrapods to have a true sternum, one that connects with the ribs. Even in the reptiles, however, it is absent in snakes, legless lizards, and turtles. In birds, the ventral portion of the sternum is drawn out to form the *keel,* an important surface for the attachment of the flight muscles.

Although typically the sternum is a cartilaginous plate, in mammals it is composed of a series of ossified elements, *sternabrae:* eight in the cat and six in the rabbit. The sternum articulates with the ribs and with the pectoral girdle supporting the forelimbs. Three regions compose the human sternum (Fig. 15-8). The *manubrium* is the most anterior sternabra and articulates with the clavicle of the pectoral girdle and the costal cartilage of the first pair of ribs. The *mesosternum* or *body* of the sternum consists of the fusion of several sternabrae and supplies articulating surfaces for five ribs. One pair of ribs attaches at the juncture of the manubrium to the mesosternum. The most posterior sternabra, the *xiphisternum,* bears a xiphoid process and is not associated with any ribs.

Appendicular skeleton
Early development

In general, the primordia of vertebrate appendages make their external appearance as a lateral longitudinal ridge of tissue on both sides of the animal. These folds or ridges have a core of mesenchyme cells covered by epidermal ectoderm. The folds may extend from the anterior to posterior regions of the body. Or as in the lungfish (the Dipneusti) and amphibians, rather than folds the future appendages may form as rounded knoblike projections on the side of the body. In amniotes, as development continues,

a reduction in size of the fold occurs in the regions between the future appendages, finally disappearing altogether. Whatever their initial appearance, the future appendages appear as internal concentrations of mesenchyme covered with thickened epithelium. These areas of future limb formation are the *limb buds*.

The mesenchyme that accumulates under the ectoderm arises from two different sources depending on the class of vertebrates. In the fish, dorsal myotomes are believed to contribute the mesenchyme cells. Tongues of mesoderm cells migrate down from the lower surfaces of the myotomes into the limb bud where they give rise to the skeletal and muscular components of the fins (Fig. 16-16). In higher animals, it is the dorsal somatic mesoderm that supplies the mesenchymal elements, although contributions from the myotomes cannot be definitely ruled out. In these animals, mesenchyme cells bud off from the outer surface of the somatic mesoderm. They migrate outward from the lateral plate mesoderm and become attached to the inner ectodermal surface. In amniotes, as the mesenchyme accumulates, the ectoderm also thickens, giving rise to the *apical ridge*.

Interactions between a number of morphogenetic mechanisms produce a normal limb. These interactions have been most extensively studied in the amphibian and chick. The mesoderm apparently is determined earlier than the ectoderm as shown by the following experiment with amphibian embryos. If a piece of lateral plate mesoderm is removed after neurulation and transplanted under the ectoderm of some other area of the body (top of head, for example), the transplanted mesoderm and the ectoderm normal for the head region form a limb heterotopically (in an abnormal position). On the other hand, if instead of presumptive limb mesoderm, the presumptive limb ectoderm is removed from the limb bud region (at the same stage of development as in the first experiment) and transplanted to the head region, no limb forms. Apparently the mesoderm but not the ectoderm has the power to induce limb formation.

The ectoderm, however, plays a definite role in limb bud development. It is possible to demonstrate this role in the chick. In these animals, the presence of an apical ridge is necessary for normal formation of the distal portions of the limb. If the apical ridge is removed, the girdle and at least portions of the proximal skeletal elements (humerus or femur) develop, but the distal portions are suppressed. Experiments in the chick, at least, emphasize the importance of interacting systems in establishing a normal organ of the body. The mesoderm determines the structure of the limb bud (that is, whether it develops into a wing or a leg), but the ectoderm is indispensable for normal growth of the bud and differentiation of the distal parts.

Differential growth contributes to the general form of the future limb. Differential cell death aids in the remodeling of the concentrated blocks of mesenchyme cells into their final form. For example, cellular death is believed to play an important role in the sculpturing of digits from the hand and foot plate (Saunders, 1968). The originally rounded plate becomes pentagonal, with the points indicating the site of the future digits. As the points continue to grow, the cells in between the future digits die and clefts appear. As a result, the digits become free from one another.

As the limb bud continues to grow, the mesenchyme concentrates in the central area of the primordium. Chondroblasts differentiate from the concentrated mass and give rise to skeletal tissue. Muscles, tendons, and connective tissue form from the mesoderm immediately beneath the dorsal and ventral surfaces of the limb bud. Distally, the limb bud develops a paddle-like structure, the *hand* (or *foot*) *plate*. A constriction separates the plate from the rest of the bud. Later, a second constriction divides the forelimb into an *arm* (or *thigh*), *forearm (leg),* and *hand (foot).* Deposition of the separate units of the skeletal system occurs individually. The first skeletal area recognized in the limb bud is that of the humerus (arm) and femur (thigh).

A typical primitive limb bud has both anterior (preaxial) and posterior (postaxial) margins as well as dorsal and ventral surfaces. Although at first, the limb buds point caudad, they soon extend outward at right angles to the body. As the limb elongates, it bends at the elbow and knee. A rotation occurs with further develop-

ment and this primitive embryonic position changes in all vertebrates. At first the future flexor surface is located on the ventral side of the limb bud; that is, the palm and sole face the body and the joints (elbow and knee) extend laterally. Both sets of limbs rotate 90 degrees. The preaxial (anterior) surface of the forelimb rotates ventrally and the postaxial surface is brought into a dorsal position. The opposite occurs in the hind bud. As a result of the torsion, the elbow points posteriorly and the knee anteriorly.

In fish, the appendages make their appearance at different times. In amphibians (*Rana pipiens,* for example) the forelimbs and hindlimbs do not appear at the same stage of development. The anterior limbs form first but remain concealed by the opercular cavity until metamorphosis. The posterior appendages cannot be seen until a little before the initiation of metamorphosis. In the urodele, where no operculum is present, one can see the earlier development of the forelimbs. In amniotes, on the other hand, the rudiments of the appendages and girdles are first identified about the time the primitive body form is established. In man, during the fourth or fifth week, the appendage buds first become visible as paired paddle-shaped structures located relatively posteriorly in the body.

Pectoral girdle

The pectoral girdle, consisting of right and left halves, supports the pectoral fins of fishes and the anterior limbs of tetrapods. In fishes, it is located just posterior to the gills, and in land animals, it is at the junction of the neck and chest region. In tetrapods, it has no connection with the vertebral column; however, ligaments and tendons tie the two together. It is entirely cartilaginous in the Chondrichthyes, but in all vertebrates containing bone, it is composed of both membrane (dermal) and endochondral elements.

The early vertebrates (for example, the placoderms) were covered by an armor of membrane bone, and the supporting chest armor is considered a shoulder girdle. Some of these bony plates, located in the skin of the primitive fish, sank deeper into the body and contributed der-

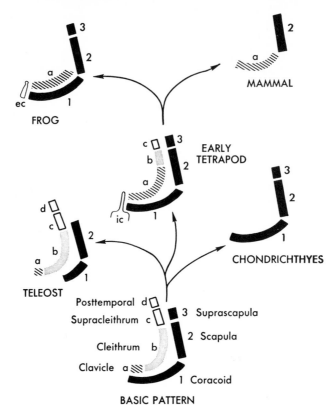

Fig. 15-26
Diagram showing evolution of pectoral girdle from endochondral *(black)* and dermal bones. Girdle of Chondrichthyes remains entirely cartilaginous. **ec,** Epicoracoid. **ic,** Interclavicle. See text for details. (From Kent, G. C.: Comparative anatomy of the vertebrates, ed. 3, St. Louis, 1973, The C. V. Mosby Co.)

mal elements to the endochondral bones present in the endoskeleton.

As illustrated in Fig. 15-26 three main bones are formed from the endoskeleton: the *scapula* and *superscapula* (the shoulder blade) and the *coracoid plate*. Several of the fin elements of fish contact the endoskeleton, but in land animals, only the head of the proximal bone of the forelimb articulates with the pectoral girdle in a ball-and-socket type of joint. The socket is referred to as the *glenoid fossa* and is located at the junction of the scapula and coracoid bones. The endoskeletal portion of the pectoral girdle remains cartilaginous in the Chondrichthyes and in some of the other more degenerate fishes. In higher animals, the cartilage is replaced with endochondral bone.

In fish, at least two membrane bones that ex-

tend dorsoventrally behind the gills are present: a pair of small *clavicles* (collar bones), which meet in the midline, and the larger paired *cleithrums*, which extend vertically and overlie the scapula. In some fish the clavicle is absent, and in others, additional membrane bones that attach to the skull and increase the rigidity of the body during swimming may be present. The loss of this connection with the skull in amphibians is associated with the increased cranial motility of land animals.

An *interclavicle* appears between the clavicles of the amphibians. However, in tetrapods, there is a progressive loss of dermal elements and a progressive increase in importance of the endoskeletal component of the pectoral girdle associated, no doubt, with the increased importance of the limbs. The cleithrum is reduced or absent in amphibians and disappears in reptiles. It is present in no other amniote; only the clavicles and interclavicles of the dermal skeleton remain. The *furcula,* or wishbone, of the bird represents a fusion of these two reptilian bones. Both bones are also retained in the archaic mammals (monotremes) but only the clavicle is present in the higher mammals. It articulates medially with the sternum, but it, too, may be absent or reduced in animals where freedom from the shoulder is advantageous in springing or jumping (cat, for example). The dermal components of the pectoral girdle never articulate with the limb bones; the original endoskeleton elements always assumes this important role.

In higher mammals, the pectoral girdles consist of two components: the scapula and the clavicle. The coracoid is reduced in size and appears as a projection of the scapula, the hook-like *coracoid process.* A ridge, the *scapular spine,* divides the broad scapular plate into the *supraspinous* and *infraspinous fossae.* The spine ends in the *acromion process; a metacromion process* may also be present. The inner surface of the scapula is the *subscapular fossa.* The flat triangular scapula is located external to the front ribs, with the broad part of the blade directed dorsally. Muscles originate in the fossae of the scapula and insert on the humerus, the large bone of the upper arm that fits into the glenoid fossa. Contractions of these muscles extends, rotates, and adducts the humerus.

In man, the clavicle, a membrane bone, is the first bone to ossify in the body. Centers of ossification occur as early as the sixth week of intrauterine life, before chondrification has appeared in any endochondral bone. This is followed by mesenchymatous condensations of the scapula. Since the embryo develops in a cephalocaudad direction, cellular concentrations destined to form the pelvic girdle soon follow.

Pelvic girdle

The pelvic girdle braces the posterior limbs of vertebrates and, when ossified, is constructed entirely of endochondral bone. It is much simpler than the pectoral girdle. In fish, it is free of the axial skeleton. In these vertebrates, it is composed of cartilaginous or osseous plates embedded in muscle and connective tissue and usually located just anterior to the cloaca. However, in some examples (cod), the pelvic girdle shifts far anteriorly. The plates articulate laterally with the fin skeleton at the acetabulum. They usually contact one another along their medial surface, forming a primitive pelvic symphysis. The two plates remain cartilaginous in Chondrichthyes and lungfish, but in most fishes they ossify.

In tetrapods, the pelvic girdle is much more important than in fishes because the femur supports much of the body weight. The girdle increases in size, allowing greater areas for muscle attachment, and is tied to the vertebral column. A fundamental similarity in pelvic structure is demonstrated among all tetrapods.

In the embryo of tetrapods, a pair of cartilaginous plates first form. Although they may remain partly cartilaginous in amphibians, in higher vertebrates two centers of ossification are soon established. As a result, two bones, the anterior *pubic* and posterior *ischium,* compose the pubioischiac plate. An additional dorsal cartilage ossifies and gives rise to the *ilium.* The *acetabulum,* the socket for articulation of the head of the femur, is located at the juncture of these three bones.

Although the pelvic girdle is fundamentally composed of the same three bony elements, variation in size and arrangement occurs. In frogs, the ilium is long and narrow and extends from a sacral rib. When the frog jumps, the ilium partly absorbs the shock of impact. The pubic may remain cartilaginous. The pelvic girdle varies from a reduced structure in certain legless lizards (or entirely absent in snakes) to an enlarged girdle in extinct dinosaurs where it was important as a point of attachment for the huge muscle masses.

In the mammal, the two halves (hipbones) of the girdle are referred to as *innominate bones.* If one examines an innominate bone carefully, it is usually possible to make out the limits of the three embryonic bones despite the fact that they are fused closely together. A large hole is present in each bone, located on each side of the girdle between the two bones of the upper leg. This hole is the *obturator foramen* and al-

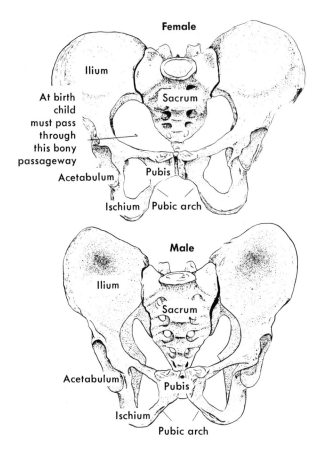

Fig. 15-27

Diagram demonstrating differences between female and male pelvic skeletons. Dorsally the ilium forms a union with the sacrum; ventrally the two halves of the girdle usually unite at the pubic symphysis, thus forming a ring around the posterior regions of the coelom. (From Hickman, C. P., Sr., Hickman, C. P., Jr., and Hickman, F. M.: Integrated principles of zoology, ed. 5, St. Louis, 1974, The C. V. Mosby Co.)

lows the passage of nerves and blood vessels. In life, it is closed by muscles and connective tissue.

Dorsally, the illium forms a union with the sacrum in the posterior region of the vertebral column (Figs. 15-8 and 15-27). In reptiles, two sacral vertebrae articulate with the ilium instead of one (amphibian). In birds, the girdle bones and sacral vertebrae are solidly fused (synsacrum); they are not so firmly attached in mammals. In these animals the innominate bones are firmly tied to the sacrum by tough ligaments and the two pubic bones articulate with one another

at the pubic symphysis, thus forming a ring around the posterior regions of the coelom. All products of the digestive, urinary, and reproductive tracts must pass through this ring before emptying to the outside.

The size and flexibility of the opening leading to the pelvis is of obstretrical importance. In several mammals, during late pregnancy, the pubic symphysis separates and the sacroiliac attachment loosens, thereby enlarging the birth canal in preparation for parturition (delivery of young). These changes are brought about by the interaction of at least two ovarian hormones,

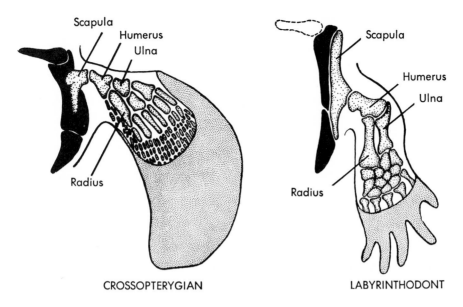

Fig. 15-28

Fin of crossopterygian fish shows many similarities to appendages of labyrinthodont. The radials of the fish are believed to contribute to the ulna and radius of tetrapods. (From Kent, G. C.: Comparative anatomy of the vertebrates, ed. 3, St. Louis, 1973, The C. V. Mosby Co.)

estrogen and *relaxin*. As a result of this expansion of the pelvic outlet, the infant skull can pass through the birth canal in a natural birth.

Appendicular skeleton

There are two pairs of appendages in most modern vertebrates although there are several exceptions. For example, appendages are absent in cyclostomes, in snakes, and in the adult of legless amphibians and lizards. Some have only an anterior pair (certain teleosts and ganoid fish, amphibians, lizards, and mammals), and some have the opposite condition with only a posterior pair.

FINS. It is usually agreed that paired appendages developed from the paired pectoral and

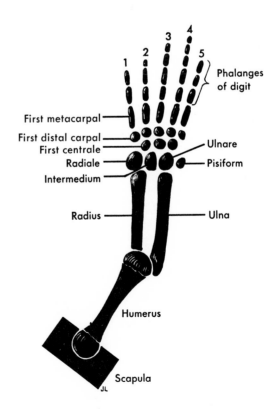

Fig. 15-29

Limbs of tetrapods are divided into three main segments. Proximally, the head of a single bone articulates with the girdles. Two bones compose the second segment and the third segment consists of three divisions, each of which is composed of several bones. The anterior limb follows this plan, as shown in the diagram. (From Kent, G. C.: Comparative anatomy of the vertebrates, ed. 3, St. Louis, 1973, The C. V. Mosby Co.)

pelvic fins of fish, but there is no consensus on how the course of change occurred. Modern jawless vertebrates, in general, lack paired appendages as did the ancient ostracoderms. Apparently, the placoderms experimented with them because some had pectoral but no pelvic fins whereas others developed several fin pairs. In most fish groups, the fins act as steering devices and stabilizing keels, but in land animals, they have evolved into active propulsive organs.

As mentioned in Chapter 2, living and fossil fishes are divided into the ray-finned (Actinopterygii) and lobed-fin (Crossopterygii) fishes. According to fossil evidence a series of parallel bars of cartilage supported the ray fin and a central axial skeleton was absent. In modern ray-finned fish, little support exists for the

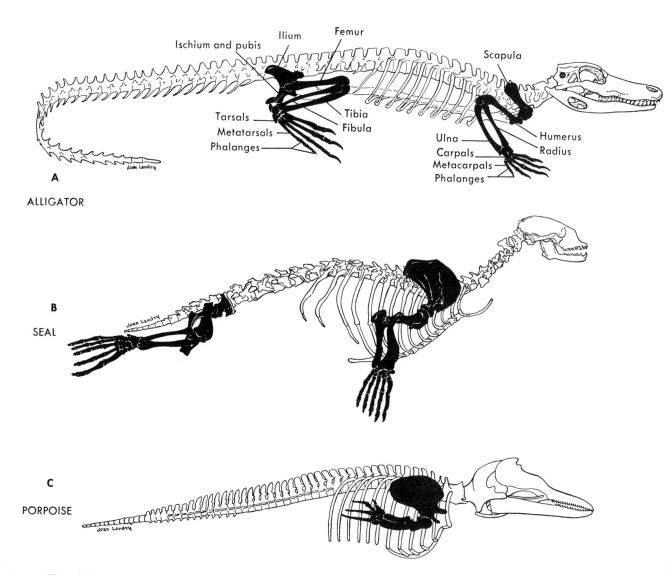

Fig. 15-30
Variations in the typical skeleton of terrestrial animals, **A,** occurred as vertebrates adapted to other environments, **B** and **C.** (From Kent, G. C.: Comparative anatomy of the vertebrates, ed. 3, St. Louis, 1973, The C. V. Mosby Co.)

fins. A few parallel bars that are tied together and support a web of skin remain, but they are incapable of offering much support and are used primarily as keels.

It is from the fleshy-lobed fins that the appendages of higher forms evolved. In this second type of fin, a central pointed axis originally extended to the tip of the fin and a series of radials (side branches) attached to the axial and projected to the margins of the fin. This pattern is modified in most crossopterygian fish. The central axial skeleton is much shortened and the side branches are limited to the anterior margins. The radials contribute to the "ulna" and "radius" of the crossopterygian fin. It is from this type of skeletal arrangement that the limb of the labyrinthodont may have evolved as suggested by Fig. 15-28.

TETRAPOD LIMBS. The limbs of tetrapods, from amphibians to mammals, are remarkably similar and consist of a chain of bones that transmit their support to the body by way of the girdles. They are divided into three main segments as shown in Fig. 15-29. Proximally, the head of a single bone articulates with the girdles, the *humerus* with the shoulder girdle at the glenoid fossa, and a *femur* with the pelvic girdle at the acetabulum. Two bones compose the second segment of a tetrapod limb. The anterior *radius* and posterior *ulna* in the forelimb and the anterior *tibia* and posterior *fibula* in the hind limb. The third segment consists of three divisions, each of which is composed of several bones; that is, some 35 elements may contribute to this distal segment. Many *carpals* form the wrist, and *tarsals* form the ankle; numerous *metacarpals* give rise to the palm, and *metatarsals* give rise to the sole. The *pentadactyl digits*, forming the fingers and toes, are composed of a series of linear bones, the *phalanges*. Although the number of digits may be reduced in some vertebrates, normally they rarely exceed five.

In the early tetrapods and in living urodeles the appendages extend at right angles to the body axis, with elbow and knee pointing dorsally. A great deal of energy is spent in keeping the belly of the animal off the ground. This was changed in the ruling reptiles, many of which were bipedal. The hindlimb was strengthened

and pulled under the animal, and the pelvic girdle articulated with the sacrum of the vertebral column for additional support. Locomotion was further improved when both limbs were pulled under the body. The elbow pointed backwards and the knee forwards, allowing the development of the four-footed gate of therapsids and the later mammals. Variations on this basic limb structure occurred in terrestrial animals as they adapted to other environments, that is, returned to the water (whales and porpoises) or air (bats) or burrowed in the ground (moles). Fig. 15-30 illustrates some of these skeletal adaptations.

SUGGESTED READINGS

1. Amprino, R.: Aspects of limb morphogenesis. In DeHaan, R. L., and Ursprung, H. (editors): Organogenesis, New York, 1965, Holt, Rinehart & Winston, Inc.
2. Bloom, W., and Fawcett, D. W.: A textbook of histology, Phiadelphia, 1968, W. B. Saunders Co.
3. Evans, F. G.: The morphology and functional evolution of the atlas-axis complex from fish to mammals, Ann. N. Y. Acad. Sci. **39**:29, 1939.
4. Hamilton, W. J., Boyd, J. D., and Mossman, H. W.: Human embryology, Baltimore, 1962, The William & Wilkins Co.
5. Holtzer, H.: Aspects of chondrogenesis and myogenesis. In Rudnick, D. (editor): Synthesis of molecular and cellular structure, New York, 1961, The Ronald Press Co.
6. Milaire, J.: Aspects of limb morphogenesis in mammals. In DeHaan, R. L., and Ursprung, H. (editors): Organogenesis, New York, 1965, Holt, Rinehart & Winston, Inc.
7. Nursall, J. R.: Swimming and the origin of paired appendages, Am. Zool. **2**:127, 1962.
8. Patt, D. I., and Patt, G. R.: Comparative vertebrate histology, New York, 1969, Harper & Row Publishers.
9. Romer, A. S.: Cartilage, an embryonic adaptation, Am. Naturalist **76**:394-404, 1942.
10. Romer, A. S.: The vertebrate body, Philadelphia, 1962, W. B. Saunders Co.
11. Saunders, J. W., Jr.: Patterns and principles of animal development, London, 1970, Collier MacMillan Limited.
12. Synder, R. C.: Adaptations for bipedal locomotion of lizards, Am. Zool. **2**:191, 1962.

GENERAL CHARACTERISTICS

Muscles make up one of the four fundamental tissues of the body and are present in almost every organ. They represent one third to one half of the body's bulk. Their primary function is to contract when stimulated and to perform their work repetitively. Specialized contractile protoplasm organized into threadlike units fill the elongated muscle cells. This particular shape allows a greater degree of shortening than if, for example, they were rounded cells. In contrast to the term "fiber" as used in our discussion of the nervous system (which referred to one of the projections from the cell body, in general, the axon), a "muscle fiber" commonly means the whole muscle cell.

Muscles participate in locomotion and are responsible for movement of the various parts of the organism, as in the following examples. The heart muscle pumps the blood (with all its nutrients and wastes) throughout the body. The muscles of the arteries contribute to the maintenance of blood pressure. Contractions of the gut musculature modify the food physically, churn it, mix it with enzymes, and convey it by peristaltic movement down the alimentary canal where absorption or elimination take place. Muscles work against such forces as gravity and give the body tone or tension. Posture and the production of body heat depend on their contraction.

Muscles function specifically in two ways. They are specialized to contract and to conduct electrical impulses. This latter characteristic is especially important in cardiac muscle. Muscles are one of the primary energy converters. Most muscles require stimulation by electrochemical energy (from the nerves) before they are able to convert the chemical energy of nutrients into mechanical energy, heat, or even electrical energy (electric organs).

Classification of muscles

Muscles may be classified histologically as illustrated in Fig. 16-1. Based on their structure as shown by the light microscope, muscles are considered *smooth* or *striated,* each modified to carry out its specific function. The presence or absence of regular, transverse microscopic bands across the fiber is the basis for identifying muscles as striated or nonstriated. Smooth muscles lack these bands. Muscles are also classified on functional grounds according to their innervation. Striated muscles are under voluntary control and are innervated by somatic motor nerves. They are thus referred to as the *somatic,* or *voluntary muscles.* They make up the *axial muscles* of the body (the muscles of the trunk, tail, and eyeball) and the *appendicular,* or limb, muscles. According to standard sources there are 327 paired and two unpaired skeletal muscles in the human body.

Smooth muscles, controlled by the autonomic nervous system, are of the *visceral,* or *involuntary,* type. They usually occur in sheets, forming an integral part of an organ, and cannot be dissected out. Smooth muscles are located under the mucosa of the gut tube as described in Chapter 13. They are also found in the integument, walls of the digestive, urinary, and reproductive ducts, respiratory passages, urinary bladder, uterus, and walls of arteries, veins, and lymphatics. They are also responsible for the elevation of hair (arrector pili muscles). A nerve does not pass to each smooth muscle fiber of the viscera, but rather the muscles react because of their ability to conduct electrical impulses throughout the sheet from a cell that has a nerve supply.

Some histologists further divide striated muscle into skeletal muscle, primarily involved in locomotion, and cardiac muscle. Although nerves regulate the rhythmic contraction of heart muscle, it can undergo contraction even when severed from all nerve supply and completely removed from the body. Cardiac muscle is both striated and involuntary; for this reason, it is often placed in a category of its own.

The branchiomeric muscles present another paradox in the classification of muscles. These muscles operate the gills and, although derived from lateral plate mesoderm of the gut, they are under voluntary control and are striated.

Although muscles vary in gross appearance, they all have common functional and biochemical properties. Studies with the aid of the electron microscope reveal that all muscle cells have contractile elements that consist of aggregates of protein filaments. The variations in gross structure of muscles as shown by the light microscope reflect the different arrangements of these contractile elements. Actin, myosin, troponin, and tropomyosin are the four muscle proteins universally present in all muscle cells (Murray and Weber, 1974).

Muscles, therefore, can also be classified according to their ultrastructure. (1) The first group includes muscles that have their protein filaments arranged in a highly ordered, transverse pattern. The striated and cardiac are examples. (2) The contractile elements of the second group are arranged in longitudinal or oblique patterns. Such a classification includes muscles of the invertebrates, for example, locomotive muscles of annelids and some mollusks. (3) In the third group, the cells contain filaments longitudinally arranged at random. The

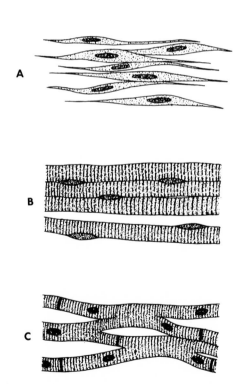

Fig. 16-1
Muscles may be classified as smooth, **A;** striated skeletal, **B;** or striated cardiac, **C.** Transverse lines in **C** represent intercalated disks, which are cell membranes of adjacent cells.

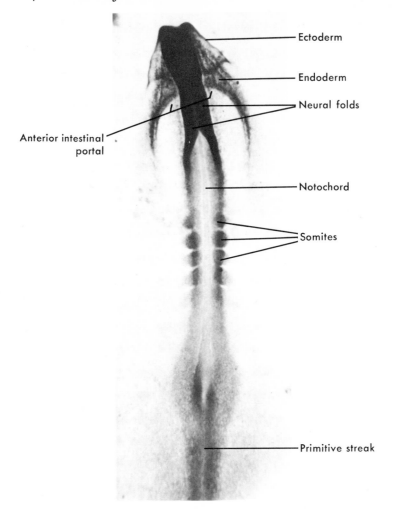

Ectoderm

Endoderm

Neural folds

Anterior intestinal portal

Notochord

Somites

Primitive streak

Fig. 16-2
Dorsal view of chick embryo showing somites.

smooth muscle cells of the gut and reproductive tract of vertebrates are illustrations of this type. It should be emphasized, however, that the mechanisms of contraction in these various cell types are believed to be the same.

Embryonic origin

All muscles are derived from mesoderm, with the exception of the ciliary muscles of the eye and myoepithelial cells of skin glands, which are ectodermal. In general, the skeletal muscles are formed from *myotomes* that originate dorsally from somites in the early embryo, first in the anterior end and then in the posterior regions, laid down one after the other (Fig. 16-2). These myo-

tomes then send buds ventrally in the body as shown in Fig. 16-3. Somatic mesoderm, however, also contributes to the limb muscles of higher animals and trunk muscles of the chick. Each myotome acquires a nerve at its level of origin. The retention of these nerves often helps to reveal the origin of the muscle when it loses its segmental arrangement and changes its position in the adult. For example, the diaphragm divides the pleural and peritoneal cavities. It is located in the lower thoracic region but is innervated by a cervical nerve. Thus the innervation of the diaphragm suggests that its muscles originated from those rectus muscles in the anterior cervical region.

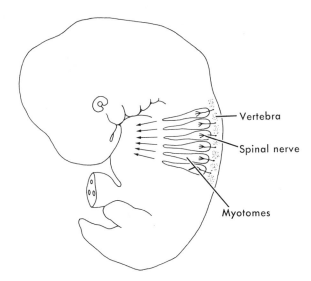

Fig. 16-3
Drawing showing relation of myotomes to vertebrae and spinal nerves. *Arrows* indicate direction of growth of myotomes.

The cells responsible for forming *cardiac muscle* are identified about the time of the onset of gastrulation. By the end of the neurula stage, the splanchnic mesoderm located ventral to the gut in the posterior part of the pharyngeal area gives rise to the contractile cells. In the chick, the cardiac mesoderm contracts as early as 33 hours of incubation, before the cells are differentiated morphologically. The development of the heart will be discussed in the chapter on circulation, but it is interesting to point out here that mesoderm cells destined to form cardiac cells differentiate biochemically at an early stage and demonstrate different nutritional or oxygen needs from other cells. Electron micrographs show that cardiac muscle, once considered to be a syncytium, is actually composed of closely associated cells. The fibers bifurcate and join other fibers to form complex networks, as indicated in Fig. 16-1, *C*. Intercalated disks represent the cell membranes of adjacent cells covered with electron-dense granules.

In general, smooth muscle develops from mesenchyme cells derived from the splanchnic mesoderm of the gut. However, mesenchyme from other sources probably can form smooth muscle, also. Examples of such organs providing mesenchyme include blood vessels, vas deferens, uterus, and ureters. The mesenchyme cells lose their stellate shape and, along with their nuclei, become elongated and spindle-shaped. They line up with their long axes parallel with one another and arrange themselves in layers. Their numbers increase either by mitosis or by transformation of other mesenchyme cells. Smooth muscle cells of the adult appear to retain some mitotic activity, as seen in the pregnant uterus, although the increase that occurs in this structure is also attributable to the growth of individual cells (hypertrophy) and to differentiation of mesenchyme into new smooth muscle cells.

Histogenesis of muscle

By applying the techniques of electron microscopy and cloning to the study of the myoblast, we have accumulated a great deal of information about the morphogenesis and histogenesis of muscle. Although the information is based primarily on chick skeletal muscle, smooth and cardiac myoblasts apparently follow many of the same general developmental patterns.

The precise time of myogenic determination (the formation of myoblasts) is difficult to determine, but for cardiac muscle it probably occurs as early as the gastrula stage and for skeletal muscle it occurs by the time the limb buds fill with condensed mesenchyme. The elongated, spindle-shaped myoblasts develop from mesenchyme cells and enter into a proliferative period. In these early embryonic states, many mitotic figures appear among the myoblasts. Correlated with this augmented mitotic activity is an extensive increase in DNA synthesis. At the cessation of the proliferative period (7 to 11 days in the chick embryo), the mononucleated myoblasts pursue different pathways and differentiate into different muscle types—skeletal, cardiac, or smooth muscle. Chick skeletal muscle differentiates according to the following general procedure:

1. At the end of the proliferative phase the myoblasts aggregate, fuse, and differentiate into thick muscle fibers containing hundreds of nuclei. These multinucleated, ribbonlike fibers are present by the eighteenth day of incubation.

2. At the end of the proliferative phase, the cells no longer produce the enzymes necessary for DNA synthesis and cell division, but start synthesizing the enzymes necessary to carry out the cell's function.

3. Two types of protein appear: those that are involved in the contractile process (actin and myosin) and those that are responsible for supplying the energy for contraction (troponin and tropomyosin).

4. The contractile elements, first present in a disorganized state, organize into myofibrils.

5. The presence of a nerve supply exerts a continuous influence on muscle development as well as on muscle maintenance. (This is also true for muscles of the adult.)

In contrast to skeletal muscle, both smooth and cardiac muscle cells remain microscopically mononucleated.

Muscle contraction

A lipoprotein plasma membrane, the *sarcolemma*, surrounds each skeletal muscle fiber (cell). An axon branch from a motor neuron usually comes in close contact with the sarcolemma at the specialized motor end plates as shown in Fig. 12-8. Many nuclei are located peripherally, beneath the plasma membrane, in adult birds and in mammals. In the embryos of these forms and in all other vertebrates, the nuclei are more centrally situated. Numerous parallel, cross-striated *myofibrils* (representing the smallest unit of contractile material) lie in the *sarcoplasm*, or cytoplasmic matrix. These fibrils impart fine, longitudinal striations to the

fresh muscle fiber. Alternating bands of different refractility compose each myofibril. The parallel arrangement of these closely packed myofibrils results in the cross striations (alternate banding) of the whole muscle fiber. A system of anastomosing tubules, the *sarcoplasmic reticulum*, located in the sarcoplasm, forms a network around each myofibril.

The alternating light and dark bands (best seen under polarized light) of the myofibrils responsible for the cross striations are designated as the I and A bands, respectively. (See Fig. 16-4.) A dark line, the Z *line*, divides each *I band*, and a pale *H band* bisects the dark *A bands*. The distance between two Z lines of a myofibril is regarded as a *sarcomere*, a muscle unit. A myofibril consists of many sarcomeres linked end to end. Sarcomeres measure 2 to 3 microns in relaxed mammalian muscles, but sarcomeres of 14 microns have been described for insect muscle. Invaginations from the sarcolemma penetrate each myofibril at the Z line. The sarcolemma transfers nerve impulses to each sarcomere by way of these invaginations and therefore coordinates the contraction of all the myofibrils of the fiber.

The banding of the myofibrils reflects their fine structure. Four different kinds of protein molecules make up the myofilaments, still smaller submicroscopic units observed in electron micrographs. These aggregated molecules of protein form thick and thin myofilaments. The thick filaments are believed to consist of all the myosin of muscle. The other three proteins concerned in muscle contraction compose the

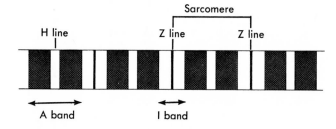

Fig. 16-4

Interdigitation of thick and thin filaments to form a muscle fiber. Thick myosin filaments containing cross bridges (except in a middle area) extend the length of the A band. Thin filaments consisting of actin, troponin, and tropomyosin attach to the Z line (a flat protein structure) and project toward one another in between and overlapping the thick filaments. This alignment of thick and thin filaments gives the muscle a striated appearance.

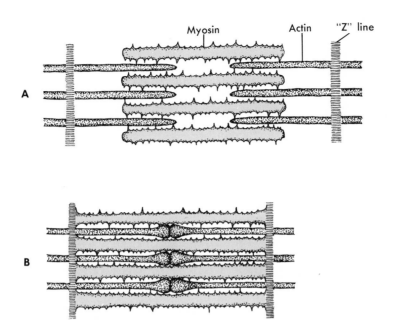

Fig. 16-5

Relation of the filaments (contractile proteins) to one another, **A.** The head of each myosin molecule has projections that extend its length and are identified from electron micrographs as cross bridges. ATP is bound to the surface of each myosin molecule. In the relaxed state thin filaments of troponin and tropomyosin are believed to extend over the twisted filament of actin, preventing it from reacting with myosin. Stimulation of the muscle releases Ca^{++}, which binds with troponin, and myosin is freed to form a myosin-ATP-actin complex. ATP splits, releasing energy that forces the cross bridges to swivel, changing their angle and pulling the actin molecules toward the middle of the myosin filament, **B.** As a result the muscle shortens. (From Turney, T.: Introduction to biology, St. Louis, 1973, The C. V. Mosby Co.)

thin filaments. The small actin particles are arranged like a strand of beads in a thin filament. Troponin and tropomyosin form thin filaments on the surface of the twisted chains of actin molecules (Murray and Weber, 1974).

Fig. 16-5 shows the relationship of the myofilaments to one another. The thinner filaments are attached to the Z line and extend from the midline of one A band to the midline of another A band, that is, to the edge of the H band. The thick myosin filaments line up under the dark band and extend across the length of the A band. According to the *sliding filament hypothesis* of muscle contraction, the thick and thin filaments remain the same length but slide past one another during contraction. As a result, the thin actin filament extends farther into the A band obliterating the H band. In summary, the dark bands consist of both actin and myosin and, therefore, have greater density (Figs. 16-4 and

16-5). Actin only, on the other hand, composes the light I bands.

Physiologists have studied muscle contraction in both living and fixed muscles. In either state contraction produces a shortening and thickening of the fibers. As we stated earlier, all muscle cells appear to have the same physiological and biochemical properties, suggesting that a common mechanism of contractility is present in most, if not all, cells. Authorities agree that the contraction of a muscle is caused by the interaction between the actin and myosin molecules to form actin-myosin complexes. Evidence further suggests that the interaction probably involves *cross bridges*. Each end of a myosin filament contains cross bridges that project outward. In a resting muscle, there is a concentration of calcium in the vesicles of the sarcoplasmic reticulum. Troponin and tropomyosin cover the surface of the actin molecule and prevent it from interacting with myosin (Hoyle, 1970). Stimulation of a muscle causes the sarcolemma to release Ca^{++} into the sarcoplasm. The release of Ca^{++} and its combination with the troponin removes this inhibiting action. As a result, the cross bridges of the myosin attach to the actin molecules and pull them toward the middle of the myosin molecule. The sarcomeres of the many parallel myofilaments shorten and the myofibrils (and ultimately the muscle) are said to be in a state of contraction. When the muscle relaxes, the opposite occurs; the calcium separates from troponin and is recaptured by the sarcoplasmic reticulum. The freed troponin then blocks the actomyosin interaction.

Adenosine triphosphate supplies the energy necessary to bring about the interaction of actin and myosin. There is some evidence that skeletal muscle produces ATP through two routes. Mitochondria produce ATP slowly, but in fast-acting muscle the sarcoplasm generates ATP by anerobic glycolysis. The stimulation of the muscle by a motor nerve impulse in some way triggers the breakdown of ATP by the enzyme myosin ATPase, which is present in the bridges. This results in the formation of ADP (adenosine diphosphate) and the release of energy with the cleavage of each high-energy phosphate bond. The myofibrils utilize this energy in shortening.

Skeletal muscle

We have described muscle as a tissue, a group of similar cells that carry out a single function, and we have stressed the characteristics common to all types of muscles, that is, smooth, cardiac, and skeletal. As tissues, the muscle cells contribute to the formation of most organs and organ systems of the body.

The term "muscle," as generally used, does not apply to these individual muscle fibers but to a muscle mass, an organ consisting of muscle fibers, nerves, and connective tissue elements. It refers to the voluntary muscles of the body, those studied in vertebrate dissections; smooth muscles are identified in the histology of the specific organs. We shall now turn our attention to a study of muscles as organs. We shall limit the rest of this chapter to a consideration of these discrete skeletal muscle masses (biceps or masseter are two illustrations) that combine to form the vertebrate muscular system.

The skeletal muscles compose the body wall and attach to the skeletal components of the body (thus they are responsible for locomotion). They are present as simple segmented myotomes in amphioxus where they stretch in zigzag fashion from the dorsal to the ventral side of the animal. As vertebrates evolved, this segmental condition became obscured by the many splits, fusions, and migrations that took place. These processes have occurred to such a degree that muscle homologies are almost impossible to trace in the higher animals. We only have left as a clue to their origin the specific innervation of some muscles.

Skeletal muscles are of various sizes and shapes. They may be bandlike, long and tapered, short and blunt, or triangular, or they may assume any number of other configurations. The fibers are long, multinucleated cells whose arrangement within an individual muscle mass may also vary.

Two types of skeletal muscle fibers exist in vertebrates: white fibers and red ones. They differ from one another, primarily, in the amount of *myoglobin* they contain. This is a pigment similar in function and structure to hemoglobin. It is present in red fibers but not in white. Myoglobin acts as an oxygen carrier for the red fibers. The white fibers, on the other hand, are able to metabolize their glycogen anaerobically.

Active fishes have many more white fibers than the slower tetrapods. These fibers are fast acting but easily fatigued, as compared to the red fibers. The red fibers associated with land animals are slower acting and tonus maintaining. Although, in general, the evolutionary trend is toward the formation of red fibers, within each class the amount of red and white fibers varies depending on the activity of the animal. Animals of a particular class that dart or sprint about usually have more white fibers than dark.

Histology

Like all other organs of the body, a discrete skeletal muscle is composed of a combination of

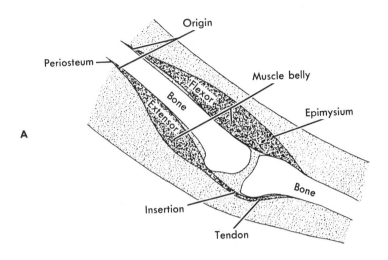

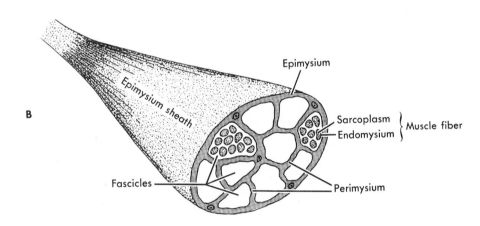

Fig. 16-6
Drawing showing origin and insertion of extensor and flexor muscles, **A.** Transverse section through belly of muscle reveals distribution of connective tissue sheaths, **B.**

other types of tissues; besides the muscle fiber, connective, nervous, and vascular tissues are also present.

A fibrous connective tissue sheath, the *epimysium*, shown in Fig. 16-6, surrounds each mass of skeletal muscle. Muscles never connect to other structures directly. They are attached to bone or cartilage by their epimysium, which is continuous with or merges with either the *tendons* (bands of tough inelastic connective tissue), *aponeuroses* (broad ribbon-shaped bands of connective tissue), or *periosteum* (fibrous connective tissue membrane around the bone). More than one muscle may share the same tendon. The epimysium, and therefore the muscle it surrounds, cannot be separated from this connective tissue (tendon, etc.) without cutting the fibers. Fig. 16-6, *B*, shows the epimysium extending into the muscle mass and dividing it into smaller bundles of parallel muscle fibers, the *fascicles.* It forms a sheath, the *perimysium,* around each of these smaller fascicles. The number of individual fibers within a fasciculus varies depending on the function of the muscle. The perimysium, in turn, surrounds each muscle fiber by a sheath referred to as the *endomysium.* This sheath is in contact with the sarcolemma (plasmalemma) of each muscle cell. Not only does this network of connective tissue sheaths (epimysium, perimysium, and endomysium) bind the various fibers securely together, they also bind the muscle mass firmly to its attachment, ensuring that the muscle will act as a unit.

To function, the muscle must have an adequate oxygen supply as well as a nerve supply. Capillaries ramify in the connective tissue sheaths and form a capillary bed around each muscle fiber. Nerves also run through the muscle in the connective tissue septa.

Muscle terminology

Each end of a skeletal muscle mass is attached to some structure in the body, usually a bone, that acts as a lever. One end, usually the proximal, is attached to a more stationary bone and is referred to as the *origin* of the muscle. The other end, or *insertion,* of the muscle is attached to a movable structure. The *belly* of the muscle makes up the free part of the muscle, the fleshy mass in between the two ends (Fig. 16-6, *A*). Muscles do work by pulling the bone containing the insertion of the muscle toward the one containing its origin. The more stable structure, the origin, is held in place by the contraction of other muscles or as a result of its ligamentous attachment to other skeletal elements. Contractions of the muscle cause the (insertion) bone to move about its joint, which acts as a fulcrum. A thin connective tissue sheath, the *fascia,* binds groups of muscles together; occasionally a muscle originates on the fascia rather than on a bone.

Muscles do not usually work as individual units, but the activity of groups of muscles is coordinated to produce the end results. To do work and produce an action, muscles usually are composed of antagonistic pairs as illustrated by the extensor and flexor muscles in Fig. 16-6, *A*. Controlled movement often results when both muscles of a group contract to different extents. For example, in order for an individual to walk, several muscles must contract to various degrees and several must relax. Other muscles, sometimes referred to as *synergists,* help the main muscles either by contracting or giving stability to some part of the body.

The student should learn to look carefully at the names of the muscles since they often indicate something about the muscles and their actions. There is usually a good rationale for the name, thus making it easier to remember. In some cases a name directs attention to the type of action carried out by the muscle. It may also describe the direction of the fibers, the number of divisions within the muscle, the shape of the muscle, or its attachment. For example, in the cat the *extensor antibrachii* "extends" the forearm. The *thyrohyoid* indicates points of attachment on the thyroid cartilage and hyoid bone, and the *triceps brachii* refers to three divisions (heads) composing the muscle. *Internal oblique* refers to a location and orientation in the body, and the *pectoralis major* indicates location and size. Limb muscles, in particular, are often named according to the type of action they perform.

1. *Flexors* bend a limb (decrease the joint angle); *extensors* open out a joint.
2. *Adductors* draw a part inward toward the median line; *abductors* move the part away from the midline.
3. *Levators* lift a structure; *depressors* do the opposite.
4. *Rotators* rotate or twist the limb (palm) either downward (*pronator*) or upward (*supinator*).
5. *Constrictors* close valves and orifices.

Primitive musculature plan

In the embryos of all vertebrates, the primordia of skeletal muscles first appear as a paired series of blocklike myotomes arranged from the anterior to the posterior end of the

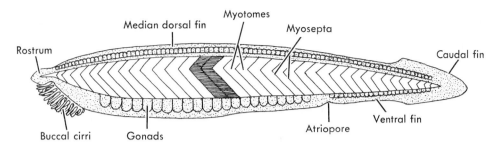

Fig. 16-7
Lateral view of amphioxus showing the v-shaped muscles extending dorsoventrally and separated by connective tissue myosepta. As illustrated, the fibers composing the myotomes run in an anteroposterior direction.

animal. We presume that this simple embryonic plan was retained by the adults of the primitive chordates and is reflected in modern times in the segmented, lateral swimming muscles of amphioxus, as illustrated in Fig. 16-7. In this chordate, the dorsally located myotomes extend ventrally between the somatic mesoderm of the lateral plate and the body wall. About 60 of these myotomes are present from the tip of the snout to the tail. Each is separated from its neighbor by a connective tissue septum, the *myoseptum.* In the adult amphioxus, the myotomes do not run dorsoventrally but bend in the middle to form v-shaped blocks of muscle, with the angles of the v's directed anteriorly. The fibers composing the myotomes, however, run in an anteroposterior direction and a contraction of these fibers tends to bend the body. The contractions pass alternately down the two sides of the body and propel the animal forward. Although gill slits are present in amphioxus, they open into the atrium, a specialized cavity, and do not interfere with the serial arrangement of the myotomes.

In vertebrates, the growth and development of the cephalic region and the appearance of gills in the pharyngeal region interrupt this serial organization of myotomes. The head is no longer involved in swimming movements, and the myotomes become superfluous. Consequently, although some of the myotomes remain in the head region, others appear crowded out by the expansion of the braincase, as shown in Fig. 16-11. Myotomes posterior to the ear (postotic)

become associated with the cervical myotomes. Remnants of the most anterior three myotomes remain in most vertebrates and give rise to the six straplike muscles that rotate the eyes. Slips of the myotomes in the region of the gills provide muscles above and below the gills. However, in general, the muscles that move the gills are not of myotomic origin.

The muscles in the trunk and tail of vertebrates are assembled according to the same fundamental plan. In lower animals, those myotomes posterior to the gills develop into segmentally arranged swimming muscles. In higher animals, this segmentation is lost in the adult, although in the embryo the muscles arise as serially arranged blocks of tissue. In fact, this simple metameric pattern can be seen in the human embryo of 6 weeks. There are 34 pairs of myotomes present at this stage: 4 occipital, 8 cervical, 12 thoracic, 5 lumbar, and 5 sacral pairs. The exact number of myotomes anterior to the ear and in the more poorly defined caudal area is less distinct.

The simple myotomes present in the embryo undergo many changes as they differentiate into the adult muscles of higher animals; it is almost impossible to follow the fate of homologous muscles in the various classes. Some of these changes include the following: (1) The fibers that make up the myotomes shift their direction from anteroposterior to other orientations. (2) A muscle mass may split into two or more muscles or into several layers of muscle. (3) Muscles may fuse with one another to form a larger muscle mass. (4) Some muscles migrate to other parts of the body. (5) Some muscles become vestigial and are lost.

MORPHOGENESIS OF MUSCULAR SYSTEM
Fate of myotomic muscles
Trunk myotomes

Since the trunk musculature is more easily understood, we shall start our discussion with these muscles and work forward. Trunk muscles originate from myotomes that extend on both sides of the animal to the midventral line. They are the swimming muscles used by the aquatic vertebrate and differ from the arrangement found in aerial and terrestrial animals. They are the predominant muscles in forms below tetrapods.

The generalized plan of vertebrates can best be seen in the primitive gnathostomes before the evolutionary changes described above occur. In these animals, a series of massive muscles arranged around the rigid vertebrae compose the trunk and tail regions. The number of muscle segments, or *myomeres*, corresponds to the number of vertebrae. In the tail area the myotomes extend laterally, dorsally, and ventrally between the vertebrae and the skin (Fig. 16-8, cross section through shark); in the trunk region, of course, the body cavity occupies a part of the ventral area, reducing some of the more ventral muscles to sheaths of tissue.

A *horizontal connective-tissue septum*, extending laterally from the vertebral column to the skin, divides the original myotome into a dorsal, or *epaxial*, portion and a ventral, or *hypaxial*, region. The septum appears as a longitudinal, white line running the length of the dogfish in the midlateral region on both sides. This division of the myotomes into dorsal and ventral regions appears for the first time in the Chondrichthyes. It is absent in amphioxus (Fig. 16-8) and in the cyclostomes but is distinguishable in many higher vertebrates. *Dorsal* and *ventral septa* are also present in the middorsal and midventral regions, separating the muscles into right and left sides. The whitish connective tissue in the midventral line is the *linea alba* found in all higher vertebrates, including man.

When viewed laterally the shark myomeres are shaped more like a W than the simple V of amphioxus. Since the myomeres are in close contact with one another, they bend back and forth beneath one another and any cross section reveals a cut through several myomeres, as seen in Fig. 16-8. The myosepta limit the fibers composing the myotomes of the dogfish, as they did in amphioxus, illustrating the basic segmentation characteristic of all vertebrates. The fibers attach to the myosepta, which in turn attach to the vertebrae. As indicated in Chapter 15, the ribs of teleosts develop in these septa where they meet the horizontal septum. This arrangement of epaxial (dorsal) and hypaxial (ventral) musculature makes up the main body of the fish. When tetrapods evolved, body undulation was of little importance, and there was a change in locomotion. There was a corresponding loss in function of the lateral muscles of the body wall. The predominant musculature shifted to the limbs; ribs were inserted, and the musculature, in general, was adapted for terrestrial or aerial living.

EPAXIAL MUSCLES OF TRUNK. In fishes, the dorsal segmented mass above the horizontal septum reaches from the braincase to the tail and remains relatively undifferentiated. It is referred to as the *dorsalis trunci muscle* (Fig. 16-8). It has been modified less than the hypaxial muscles during evolution.

In amphibians, this dorsal musculature is reduced in size but retains its segmented arrangement and remains a relatively simple muscle. It continues to function as a single dorsolateral trunk muscle. The musculature of the urodeles resembles that of the fish more than that of the anurans, since the epaxial muscles are further reduced in these latter jumping animals. The muscles of the tetrapod's back do not project as high above the neural spine as those of the fish. Consequently, the dorsalis trunci in amphibians is restricted to the space between the neural spines and transverse processes (Fig. 16-9). The dorsalis trunci is reduced in the tail and is utilized in bending the vertebral column dorsally and laterally, in side-to-side movements. These muscles also strengthen the column and support the viscera.

In reptiles, birds, and mammals, the epaxial

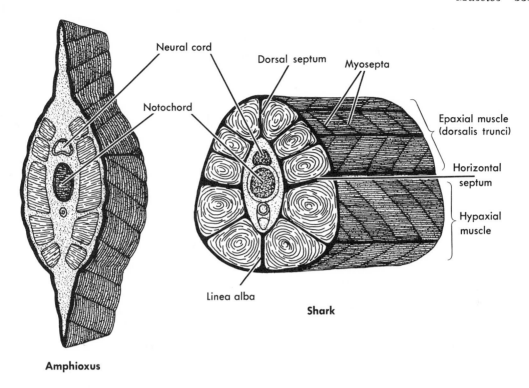

Fig. 16-8

Cross section through the tail of amphioxus and shark. V-shaped myotomes in amphioxus extend from dorsal to ventral region. In shark, a horizontal septum divides the myotomes into epaxial and hypaxial muscles.

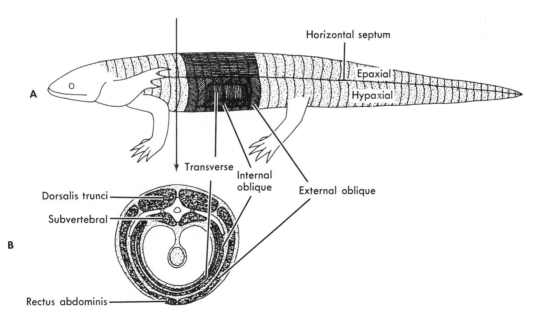

Fig. 16-9

Lateral, **A,** and transverse, **B,** view of segmented trunk muscles of urodele showing horizontal septum and dorsal muscles reduced in size. Hypaxial muscles are divided into three main groups as indicated in dissected area of **A.**

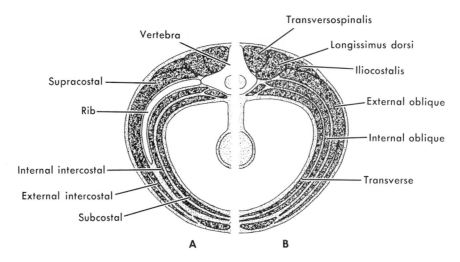

Fig. 16-10
Drawing showing the division of epaxial and hypaxial muscles in higher vertebrates. Presence of ribs, **A**, interrupts the primitive simplicity seen in the lumbar region, **B**.

muscles adapt further to the needs of a terrestrial life. They begin to deviate from the primitive condition found in fish and subdivide into groups to form complex muscles. The fibers are no longer confined to segments but extend beyond the boundaries set by the myosepta. In reptiles and birds, the dorsalis trunci muscle divides into three general groups of muscles. As illustrated in Fig. 16-10, an outer thin sheet, the *iliocostalis*, extends from the pelvic girdle and attaches to the ribs. A *longissimus dorsi*, a major division of the original dorsalis trunci muscle, lies above the transverse processes of the ribs. A crisscrossing series of muscles, the *transversospinalis* system, as the name implies, ties the vertebral spines and transverse processes together.

Segmentation is lost in mammals. They retain the above reptilian divisions and add to them two more lateral muscles, the *sacrospinalis*. These muscles maintain the arch of the back.

HYPAXIAL MUSCLES. The hypaxial muscles show a greater evolutionary change than do the dorsal muscles. In fishes, they are the large muscles in the body wall that extend from the horizontal septum to the midventral line. They are adapted for locomotion (see Fig. 16-8).

When the first fishlike animals migrated to land, they crawled with a side-to-side movement (as if swimming), and as the body bent, the limbs moved backwards and forwards. Friction prevented any kind of rapid locomotion as long as the body remained on the ground. Eventually, as limb muscles grew stronger, the animal lifted its body off the ground in typical tetrapod locomotion. Probably the labyrinthodont amphibians had reached this stage of development.

As a result of the continued growth in importance of tetrapod limb muscles, the hypaxial muscles lost volume. As the myotomes underwent sidewise fusion, the hypaxial muscles decreased to muscular sheets whose fibers ran in different directions. Together, the various layers form a thin but very tough sheath that supports the viscera of the animal. In animals above the amphibians, bony supports (the ribs) insert in the sheath, further dividing it and giving additional support to the body.

The hypaxial muscles of tetrapods act to compress the viscera. We may distinguish three general groups, as illustrated in Fig. 16-9. A subvertebral group runs in a band beneath the rib articulation. A second series of thin flank muscles form the *oblique* system, extending from the transverse processes to the midline. They insert at the linea alba and compress or constrict the abdomen. Their fibers run in diverse directions and provide great strength. The oblique layer is typically subdivided into three parts. The fibers of a broad, flat external sheet, the *external oblique,* slant anteriorly and dorsally from the linea alba. This sheet contributes to the outermost layer of the body wall. Under the external oblique, the fibers of a middle layer, the *internal oblique,* in contrast run posteriorly and dorsally but slant almost at right angles to those of the outer layer. The fibers of the inner layer of muscles run in a transverse direction and therefore are referred to as the *transverse muscles.*

The third general division of the fish's hypaxial muscles consist of a series of midventral longitudinal muscles, the *rectus abdominis,* running from the shoulder region to the pelvis. The fibers of this muscle run on both sides and parallel to the linea alba. The *rectus cervicus* of the neck region and the *geniohyoid* (see Fig. 16-12), covering the hyoid apparatus, are considered anterior extensions of these midventral muscles. Specialized derivatives of the rectus abdominis are believed to contribute to the mammalian diaphragm.

The introduction of ribs in the thoracic region of amniotes interrupts the three generalized divisions of flank muscles, and they become more complicated (Fig. 16-10). In the lower abdominal region (lumbar) the layers retain their primitive simplicity. However, in the rib-bearing regions, the ribs develop in the myosepta and pass laterally between the external oblique and internal oblique layers. The external oblique of amniotes gives rise to two layers: the *superficial*

and the *deep muscles.* The superficial muscles in the thoracic region, located external to the ribs, become the *supracostal muscles.* The deep layer of the external oblique develop into the *external intercostals.* These muscles originate on the posterior margin of one rib and insert on the anterior edge of the next rib; they pull the ribs forward. Beneath the external intercostals is another thin layer, the *internal intercostals,* derived from the internal oblique. They also have their origin and insertion on the ribs and function in lowering the ribs. The intercostals are the chief muscles involved in the respiratory movements of the thorax. The transverse muscles become the *subcostal group* and are confined to the inner wall of the thoracic cavity.

The transverse muscles along with the rectus abdominis make up the most internal layer of muscle in the abdominal body wall. Internal to this muscular layer is the parietal peritoneum, the membrane that lines the peritoneal cavity (coelom).

Pharyngeal myotomes

The presence of gills in fishes disturbs the orderly arrangement of the myotomes in the anterior regions of the axial musculature, as shown in Fig. 16-11. Above the gills, the dorsal myotomes continue anteriorly and attach to the rear of the skull. They make up the epibranchial (*epi,* 'on top of') musculature. In this region they do not differentiate into epaxial and hyp-

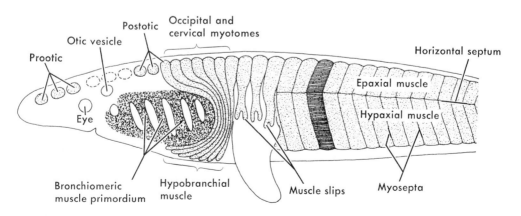

Fig. 16-11
Basic segmented plan of muscles in shark embryo.

axial groups and therefore do not contribute to the formation of the hypobranchial muscles. Myotomes posterior to the gills contribute to these muscles.

The *hypobranchial muscles* are those muscles in the midline of aquatic animals under *(hypo)* the branchial region. We should remember that they are *not* the muscles that move the gills. The muscles that do that job are referred to as the branchial muscles and are derived from the lateral plate mesoderm. They will be discussed in the next few pages. The myotomes of the somites located posterior to the ear and gill regions give rise to the hypobranchial muscles. These myotomes are referred to as postotic because of their position in relation to the ear. They are innervated by branches of nerves that originate in a similar postotic location and follow the migrating myotomic buds.

The hypaxial portion of these postotic myotomes sends buds of mesenchyme ventrally that then turn anteriorly under the gill chamber and grow forward into the jaw. They become the

coracoarcualia, a collective term referring to those hypobranchial muscles that originate on the coracoid region of the pectoral girdle and attach ventrally to the gill bars (Figs. 16-11 and 16-14). In the shark, these muscles strengthen the anterior floor of the body. They also elevate the floor of the oral cavity, aid in opening the mouth, add strength to the walls of the pericardial cavity, and help the branchial pouches expand when water is taken into the pharynx.

In land animals, some of the hypobranchial muscles remain as muscles of the neck region. In tetrapods they attach at the sternum and shoulder area and pass to the thyroid cartilage of the larynx and hyoid and from there to the jaw. These muscles constitute part of the *rectus cervicus,* the forward continuation of the rectus abdominis, and contribute to such muscles as the sternohyoid, sternothyroid, thyrohyoid, and so forth, as shown in Fig. 16-12.

In those lower animals possessing a tongue, the anterior portions of the hypobranchial muscles are carried forward as part of the tongue

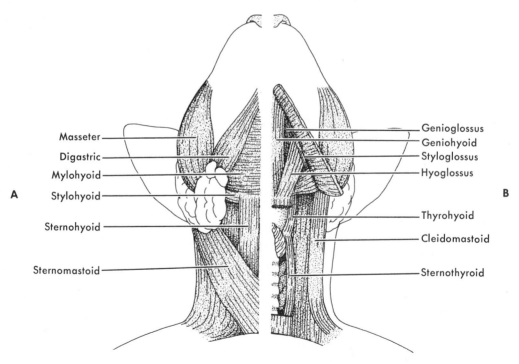

Masseter
Digastric
Mylohyoid
Stylohyoid
Sternohyoid
Sternomastoid

A

B

Genioglossus
Geniohyoid
Styloglossus
Hyoglossus
Thyrohyoid
Cleidomastoid
Sternothyroid

Fig. 16-12
Diagram of superficial throat muscles of the cat, **A.** Left side is cut away to reveal deep muscles of neck.

musculature. In higher animals it is not always possible to follow the migrating buds of postotic myotomes into the tongue. Instead, concentrations of mesenchyme appear, which some investigators believe may arise in situ.

One of the basic rules of muscle organization is that a specific muscle mass is constantly innervated by a specific nerve. In fish, the nerves from the occipital and the anterior cervical regions follow the migratory pathway of the postotic myotomes and enter the throat area. In amniotes, the nerves from this region become the hypoglossal, cranial nerve XII. Despite the fact that migration of myotomes cannot be followed in higher animals, we usually assume that the tongue muscles of man are of myotomic origin. This assumption is based on the innervation of the tongue by nerve XII. Funda-

mentally, the embryonic pathways of tongue formation remain the same but some stages occur so rapidly that they are difficult to identify, a developmental characteristic common to higher animals.

Head myotomes

Although somites are present from the anterior to posterior end of the embryo, only the first few (usually three pairs) remain in the head of the adult. These are present in all vertebrate classes and contribute to the eye muscles. The other prootic somites tend to be crowded out (see Figs. 16-11 and 16-13, *A*).

Following the developmental plan described earlier, a cranial nerve arising at the same segmental level of the body enters each of the first three somites. These are the somatic motor

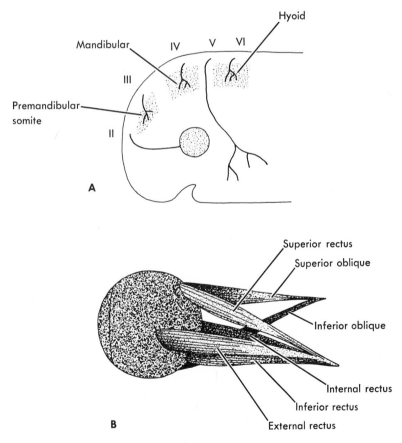

Fig. 16-13
Cranial nerve arising at the same segmental level of the body as the somite enters each of the first three myotomes, **A.** Prootic myotomes give rise to the six straplike eye muscles, shown in the adult from the side, **B.**

nerves III (oculomotor), IV (trochlear), and VI (abducens) (Fig. 16-13, *A*). These anterior myotomes give rise to six straplike muscles, two anterior oblique muscles, and four more posteriorly located rectus muscles (Fig. 16-13, *B*). The condensations of mesenchyme cells in the head region anterior to the ear are referred to as prootic in contrast to the postotic previously described. They are also given more specific names that reflect their locations. The premandibular somite first forms over the mandibular visceral arch and is innervated by the third cranial nerve. The second condensation is the mandibular, and the hyoid makes up the third. The first myotomes (one on each side) each give rise to four of the eye muscles, the *superior rectus, inferior rectus, internal rectus,* and *inferior oblique*. All are innervated by the oculomotor nerves (III). The second myotomes form the *superior oblique muscles* innervated by the trochlear (IV) nerves. The third myotomes develop into the *external rectus muscle* supplied by the abducens nerve (VI).

Fate of branchiomeric muscles

With the exception of the help of hypobranchial muscles, the muscles of the gill region, those that move the gills, are not derived from myotomes; instead, they form from the hypomeric mesoderm caught in the visceral arches when the clefts form. As we mentioned in Chapter 13 when we discussed the pharynx, the visceral clefts impose a type of segmentation on the hypomere in this region. These divisions do not necessarily correspond to the metamerism exhibited by the myotomes. The term "branchiomerism" describes the divisions of the hypomere into *branchiomeric* muscles (see Fig. 16-11).

In the pharyngeal region, the hypomere does not differentiate into splanchnic and somatic mesoderm and therefore the coelom, the cavity formed by the splitting of the hypomere, does not extend into the pharyngeal area. The anterior region of the coelom ends where the pharynx begins. The mesenchyme derived from the pharyngeal hypomere develops into voluntary, striated skeletal muscle. Posterior to the pharynx the splanchnic mesoderm gives rise to the smooth involuntary muscles of the gut. This change in microscopic structure reflects the function assumed and represents only a superficial difference. As pointed out in the beginning of the chapter, all muscles appear to have the same fundamental physiological and biochemical properties.

In the early chordates, the ostracoderms, ciliary movement rather than the pumping action of muscles brought about the flow of water through the branchial basket. As the vertebrates evolved, muscles derived from hypomere became associated with the visceral arches. These branchiomeric muscles functioned primarily to open and close the mouth and to pump water through the gills. When the gills were lost in land animals, the skeletal elements changed in function and the muscles associated with them also changed. For example, during evolution when the modification of the first arch produced an upper and lower jaw, the muscles associated with this first arch became a part of the gnathostome jaw. When gills were lost in land animals, the skeleton along with its muscles were incorporated into the head, neck, and shoulder region.

The gill region of fishes is supplied with cranial nerves V, VII, IX, and X. As indicated in Chapter 12, cranial nerve V supplies the jaw region, VII passes to the second gill arch (hyoid), IX innervates the first typical gill bar, and X sends branches to all the more posterior ones. It is only when we trace these nerves to the muscles of land animals that we can follow the phylogenetic history of these muscles.

Muscles of typical gill bars

In the shark each branchiomere becomes divided into at least four main types of muscles, each responsible for a specific function. These main categories are represented in Fig. 16-14. (1) The largest branchiomeric muscle is the broad, flat *superficial constrictor*. Dorsal constrictors above and ventral constrictors below the gill slits extend outward in the gill septum and surround the pharyngeal region. Contraction of their fibers closes the mouth and compresses the gill pouches, forcing water out. (2) The *levator* series are located dorsal to the constrictors. Their fibers run somewhat diagonally

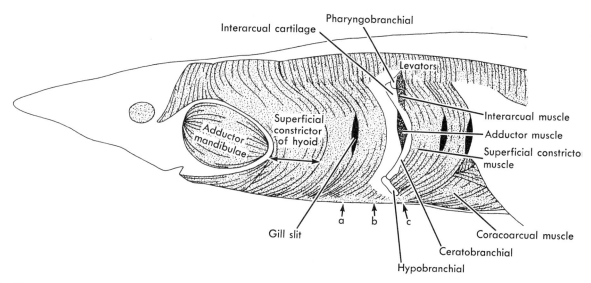

Interarcual cartilage
Pharyngobranchial
Levators
Interarcual muscle
Adductor muscle
Superficial constrictor muscle
Adductor mandibulae
Superficial constrictor of hyoid
Gill slit
a b c
Coracoarcual muscle
Ceratobranchial
Hypobranchial

Fig. 16-14
Lateral view of some of the branchiomeric muscles of the shark. The superficial constrictor, **b,** of one gill septum is dissected away to show a single gill arch with its cartilaginous gill bars and musculature, **c.**

and attach to the gill bars. They raise the gill bars and also help to constrict the pharynx. The more posterior levators are considered the homolog of the tetrapod trapezius muscle. (3) A deep *adductor* series pulls the dorsal and ventral halves of each arch together, and (4) the *interarcual* series bend the dorsal ends of the skeletal arch backwards expanding the gill pouches.

Derivatives of gill bar muscles

MUSCLES OF FIRST PHARYNGEAL ARCH. The basic components of a branchiomeric muscle become further modified, depending on the general function the muscle performs. When the skeletal structure of the first arch becomes modified to form the upper and lower jaws, the branchiomeric muscles of the arch are retained and serve to operate it (Fig. 16-14). An anterior levator (*levator palatoquadrati*) attaches the upper jaw to the chondrocranium and elevates the jaw. The *adductor mandibulae* is the major muscle mass in the shark and incorporates not only the adductor of the first arch but also the dorsal constrictor. The adductor inserts on Meckel's cartilage and acts to close the jaw. It lies outside the angle of the jaw and its action is important in biting or grinding food. The ventral portion of

the constrictor gives rise to the intermandibular, a thin sheet that originates on the midventral raphe (linea alba) and inserts on Meckel's cartilage.

These jaw muscles are always innervated by the trigeminal nerve (cranial nerve V), a fact that allows their homologs to be traced in higher animals. Above the fishes, these muscles associated with the primitive first arch continue to operate the jaws. The ventral intermandibular of primitive forms contributes to the *mylohyoid* muscle and anterior belly of the *digastric* of mammals (Fig. 16-12). The adductor mandibulae gives rise to two main groups of muscles: the *pterygoids,* which originate on the palate and insert on the jaw, and the *temporalis,* the cheek muscle. In mammals, the *masseter* is derived from the temporalis. In higher animals, when the skull fuses with the upper jaw, the levator is lost.

MUSCLES OF SECOND PHARYNGEAL ARCH. The muscles associated with the hyoid (second) arch in sharks represent a modification of a typical gill arch, presumably present in jawless ancestors. In sharks the skeletal elements of the second visceral arch are modified for jaw support and the superficial constrictor associated with it remains, although the deeper muscles are lost. The constrictor gives rise to several divisions. The *epihyoideus* (dorsal constrictor) originates on the otic capsule and inserts on the hyomandibular cartilage; a part of the ventral constrictor may remain to connect the jaws ventrally and contributing to the digastric.

In bony fish, the gill bar of the second arch expands in the gill septum to form a bony operculum that covers and protects the fragile gills. The dorsal constrictor of the hyoid arch controls the movements of the bony operculum.

When the gills are lost in higher animals (and the operculum along with it), the dorsal constrictor of the hyoid expands, forming a thin sheet over the neck and head region. This sheet is referred to as the *sphincter coli*. In the head region of mammals it contributes to the *panniculus carnosus*, a continuous sheath of muscle, of various structural origins, that encircles the trunk and head region (Fig. 16-15). Slips of muscles from the sphincter coli region grow forward over the cheeks and skull and give rise to the muscles of expression. They are innervated by the seventh facial nerve and enable the individual to smile, frown, and kiss.

MUSCLES OF POSTERIOR PHARYNGEAL ARCHES. In fishes, the muscles of arch III are innervated by cranial nerve IX; those of the more posterior arches are served by nerve X. These muscles operate the gills and are responsible for respiratory movements. They run in the gill septa and are more obvious in sharks than in the bony fish because no operculum protects the gills. In bony fish, the operculum that now controls the stream of water through the pharynx covers the septa. The muscles supplying these gill structures are correspondingly more limited in bony fish.

In aquatic tetrapods, the posterior pharyngeal muscles resemble those of the teleosts, but in land forms, they are further modified and reduced. As noted in the preceding chapter, the posterior skeletal arches of aquatic forms become associated with the larynx, hyoid apparatus, and trachea of land forms. Their muscles follow them, become associated with the new structures, and take on new functions. The fate of the levator (trapezius) muscle is one exception to this trend toward reduction of gill arch muscles in higher animals. This muscle survives in land animals as the expanded *trapezius muscle* group and may also divide anteriorly and ventrally into

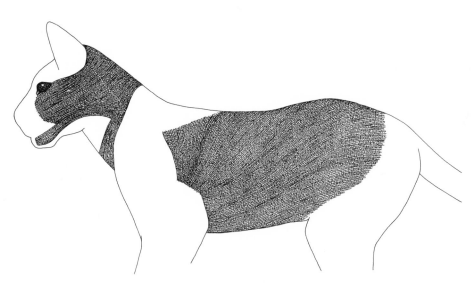

Fig. 16-15
Muscles of skin of cat. A continuous sheath of skin musculature wraps the neck (platysma) and trunk (cutaneus maximus) of most mammals. These muscles, known collectively as the panniculus carnosus, contribute to the facial muscles in head region of man.

the *sternomastoid* (Fig. 16-12) and *cleidomastoid* muscles.

Appendicular muscles

Appendicular muscles attach the limbs and girdles to the axial skeleton. They are derived either from the lower edges of the myotomes or from somatic mesoderm or both. In fishes, paired buds from several myotomes near the base of the paired fins, along with their corresponding spinal nerves, migrate into the developing limb bud and form a common mass of myoblasts, as illustrated in Figs. 16-11 and 16-16, *A*. The original segmentation is lost and the various dorsal and ventral muscles of the fins differentiate from this mass. If the lateral plate mesoderm is removed from a young fish embryo and transplanted near the midline, a fin develops there; but it is devoid of muscles. The inclusion of some myotomic material in this graft causes muscles to appear. Apparently, the somatic mesoderm is unable to form muscle in the fishes.

However, beginning with amphibians it is the somatic mesoderm that is responsible for the formation of muscles (Fig. 16-16, *B*). In these forms, the transplantation of the lateral plate mesoderm to the midline, uncontaminated by myotomic material, produces a complete limb with muscles. The early limb buds are ectodermal sacs of mesenchyme cells. Although myotomic buds do not form in higher animals, it is possible for individual myotomically derived cells to migrate into these sacs; thus myotomic contributions cannot be ruled out absolutely. Both sources may contribute to the myoblasts of higher animals.

Muscles that function in an antagonistic manner to raise and lower the fin are present in all fishes. A dorsal muscle mass extends the length of the pelvic fins and may be regarded as an *abductor, levator,* and *extensor* of the fin. The ventral muscle mass acts as a *depressor, adductor,* and *flexor.* This same pattern remains as the tetrapod limb develops. The two basic divisions of the limb muscle mass are innervated by spinal nerves that also divide into dorsal and

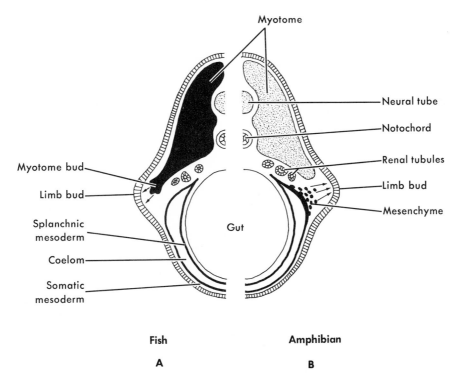

Fig. 16-16
Diagram of origin of limb mesoderm in fish, **A**, and amphibian, **B**, embryos.

ventral branches as described in Chapter 12. The forelimbs and hindlimbs undergo a torsion of 90 degrees as they develop, but in opposite directions, with the result that when their final adult position is reached, the elbow bends posteriorly and the knee points anteriorly. The muscles, therefore, on the inner side of the forelimb are homologous to the ones on the outer side of the hindlimb.

Vertebrates moved out of the water to land as their limb musculature increased in size and importance. Any segmentation was lost and the dorsal and ventral muscle masses gave rise to distinct and separate muscles. The appendicular muscles of the simplest tetrapod (urodele) are much more complex than any present in the fishes.

The musculature of the tetrapod limb is usually categorized as *intrinsic* or *extrinsic*. Intrinsic muscles arise from clusters of mesenchyme cells (blastemas) that condense around the emerging skeleton of the appendage. These blastema cells develop into myoblasts, which give rise to muscles originating and inserting on the limb skeleton. They move parts of the limb rather than the appendage as a whole. Extrinsic muscles of the limbs are defined as those that tie the limb and its girdles to the axial skeleton. These are the muscles that must be cut during dissection if the limbs are to be removed from the body. The extrinsic muscles originate from mesenchyme arising in the limb bud and migrating out toward the axial skeleton or from blastemas in the body wall that grow in toward the limb bud or girdles. Strictly speaking, based on their embryology, some of these muscles that we group together as "limb" muscles should be considered instead as "girdle" muscles.

Integumentary muscles

Two types of "skin" muscles are present in vertebrates: those that are completely embedded in the skin (intrinsic) and those that have only the insertion on the dermis (extrinsic). In general, these muscles are limited to amniotes.

Intrinsic integumentary muscles are derived from the dermatomes and not from myotomes or branchiomeres. Extrinsic muscles, on the other hand, may be derived from either myotomes or branchiomeres. Intrinsic muscles are smooth and involuntary. They are found only in homoiothermic animals and, for example, compose the muscles that move the hairs (arrector pili) or feathers (arrector plumi). When they contract, the hairs or feathers become erect, trapping air and adding to the insulating dead-air space. They are of value, therefore, in controlling the body temperature. It has been suggested that they evolved from those reptilian ancestors possessing muscles that moved epidermal scales during locomotion.

Integumentary muscles are absent in fishes, since the skeletal muscles are closely tied to the skin. They are poorly developed in amphibians and most reptiles, reaching their greatest development in the extrinsic skin muscles of birds and especially mammals. Two major extrinsic muscles have already been mentioned: the sphincter coli, that remnant of the ancient hyoid musculature first to appear in reptiles, and the panniculus carnosus, limited to mammals. The sphincter coli expands into the *platysma* of mammals, a sheet of muscles covering the head and contributing to the facial muscles. In man, this muscle subdivides many times, forming 26 facial muscles that can be identified as originating from the platysma. The fact that it is innervated by cranial nerve VII (facial) reminds us of its branchiomeric origin. The panniculus carnosus wraps the entire mammalian trunk and neck in a continuous sheath. For example, the animals uses these muscles when it twitches its skin to remove insects. It is found only in axillary and inguinal regions of lower primates and is almost absent in the higher apes and man.

Electric organs

Through parallel evolution in seven families of fish, certain embryonic, striated muscle cells were modified to form organs capable of generating electrical shocks. In some cases these "electric fish" can generate an electrical potential great enough to electrocute other fish. In these fishes the muscles become modified to convert food energy into electricity rather than muscle contraction. This ability is of value in paralyzing prey or protecting the fish against predators. Many of these "shocking species" live in murky or turbulent waters, and here the electric organs are believed to act as a kind of guidance or warning system. They seem to operate by establishing a weak electric field around the fish. Disturbances in the field caused by objects entering the field are detected by special sense organs located in the skin. Thus, investigators believe that in these animals electric organs are used as an aid in navigating through waters in which vision is obscured. The lateral line and cerebellum detect and coordinate this electrical field.

Flattened plates, *electroplaxes*, make up the basic structure of the electric organ and may vary in position and appearance among the fish. They are stacked in a series of piles. The positive and negative differences in charge between the two sides of the plate essentially form a battery. In some cases, one muscle fiber composes the electroplax but in other instances, more than one muscle fiber is involved. Typical cross striations are apparent in some species and actin myofilaments are present in all electroplaxes. In a few forms there is also evidence of myosin.

SUGGESTED READINGS

1. Comparative aspects of muscle: A symposium, Am. Zool. **7**(3): 435-669 (entire issue), 1967.
2. Yaffe, D.: Cellular aspects of muscle differentiation in vitro. In Moscona, A. A., and Monroy, A. (editors): Current topics in developmental biology, New York, 1969, Academic Press Inc.
3. DeHaan, R. L.: Morphogenesis of the vertebrate heart. In DeHaan, R. L., and Ursprung, H. (editors): Organogenesis, New York, 1965, Holt, Rinehart & Winston, Inc.
4. Detwiler, S. R.: Experiments on the origin of the ventrolateral trunk musculature in the urodeles, J. Exp. Zool. **129**:45-75, 1955.
5. Hoyle, G.: How is muscle turned on and off? Sci. Am. **222**:84-93, 1970.
6. Huxley, H. E.: The mechanism of muscular contraction, Sci. Am. **213**(6): 18-27, 1965.
7. Huxley, H. E.: The mechanism of muscular contraction, Science **164**:1356-1366, 1969.
8. Konigsberg, I. R.: The embryological origin of muscle, Sci. Am. **211**(2): 61-66, 1964.
9. Konigsberg, I. R.: Aspects of cytodifferentiation of skeletal muscle. In DeHaan, R. L., and Ursprung, H. (editors): Organogenesis, New York, 1965, Holt, Rinehart & Winston, Inc.
10. Murray, J. M., and Weber, A.: The cooperative action of muscle proteins, Sci. Am. **230**:59-71, 1974.
11. Patten, B. M.: Human embryology, Philadelphia, 1946, The Blakiston Co.
12. Porter, K. R., and Franzini-Armstrong, C.: The sarcoplasmic reticulum, Sci. Am. **212**(3):72-80, 1965.

CHAPTER 17

CIRCULATORY SYSTEM

Simple diffusion is an inadequate mechanism to take care of the vital needs of vertebrates since they have a high metabolic rate and a large body volume. Some kind of a transport system is necessary to distribute the food, oxygen, and hormones to the tissues and to carry wastes and carbon dioxide away.

In vertebrates, the blood vascular system carries out these important functions. This system transports food materials stored in the liver, or absorbed from the intestine, to the various cells of the body. It carries oxygen from the skin, gills, or lungs to the metabolizing cells, and waste materials and carbon dioxide to the organs that eliminate them. It transports hormones, secreted by glands in one area of the body to another part of the body where they produce their effect. The blood carries the materials necessary to maintain the proper acid-base balance of the body. Circulating antibodies, lymphocytes, macrophages, and blood-clotting factors preserve the body's defenses. The constant circulation of the fluids maintains stable cellular environments.

In all vertebrates, the organs composing the circulatory system are assembled according to a basic, uniform plan. The system consists of the blood and lymph and the organs that propel and transport these fluids. Included in the system are the hemopoietic (blood- and lymph-forming) organs. A muscular pump, the *heart*, forces the blood through the circuit, and a series of continuous vessels ensure circulation of blood to all parts of the body. *Arteries* carry the blood away from the heart to the anterior and posterior regions of the body. These efferent vessels branch many times, constantly decreasing in caliber as they extend outward. They are continuous with thin-walled *capillaries*, and it is through the walls of these small vessels that diffusion of materials occurs into the microscopic spaces between the cells. Capillaries lead into *veins*, which converge and finally return the blood back to the heart. Such a circulatory plan is referred to as a *closed circulatory system* since the blood never leaves the vessels.

In teleosts and all tetrapods, we find a *lymphatic system*. This system consists of lymphatic capillaries that lead into progressively larger lymphatic vessels. These vessels anastomose (merge) and eventually empty into the vascular system.

In fish, the heart pumps the blood to the gills. After aeration, the blood then passes to the rest of the body. In higher animals, the heart functions as a *double pump* and the circulatory system divides into two circuits. A *pulmonary circuit* carries blood to the lungs and returns it to the heart, and a *systemic circuit* transports fluid to all the cells in the rest of the body and back to the heart again. Embryos of amniotes have additional circuits to the yolk sac (vitelline circulation) and allantois (allantoic or umbilical circulation). Of course, these extraembryonic vessels are modified or eliminated at birth or hatching.

The liquid portion of the blood (plasma), along with the solutes it carries, filters out of the capillaries and surrounds the cells as interstitial (tissue) fluid. These two liquids (plasma of the blood and interstitial fluid of the tissues) are almost identical chemically. However, since the capillary membranes are impermeable to proteins, one would expect to find more proteins in plasma than in the tissue fluids. Also, there is some inequality of electrolytes. There are more sodium ions and fewer chloride ions in the blood. It is the interstitial fluid that provides the internal environment of the body. Although the cell membranes of adjacent cells appear to touch one another, actually a thin layer of fluid surrounds each cell of the body. All nutrients, wastes, and cellular products move by way of the interstitial fluid from the blood capillaries to cells, from cells to cells, or from cells back again into capillaries of the blood or lymphatic systems.

The fluid found in various spaces of the body is similar to interstitial fluid but usually varies somewhat depending on the specific function it serves. Examples are the fluids of the pleural, pericardial, and peritoneal cavities; the cerebrospinal fluid; the aqueous and vitreous humors of the eye; the synovial fluid of the joints; the endolymph of the ear; and tears, secreted by the lacrimal glands. These fluids not only supply nutrients and oxygen to the surrounding tissues and remove wastes, but they also lubricate moving surfaces that come in contact with one another and protect the cells of the various organs from drying as well as from bacterial and mechanical injury.

Because of its importance in the body, the circulatory system forms early in development. In fact, it is the first system to become functional in the embryo. After 118 hours of development at room temperature, the heart is beating in the embryo of the frog *(Rana pipiens)*. In the chick, at the end of 26 hours of incubation, sufficient channels have been completed and the heart pulsations have grown strong enough to start the blood in circulation. In the human embryo, blood starts to circulate by the beginning of the fourth week. In these early stages, the embryo is very small when compared to the size of the yolk of the egg or mass of placental chorion. The vessels that lead to the oxygen and food sources and the heart, which pumps the blood through the channels, are larger proportionately in the embryo than in the adult. By hatching or birth, adjustments must be made in heart size to compensate for the loss of the extra-embryonic circulation.

HEMOPOIESIS

Mesenchyme cells in the embryo known as *angioblasts* give rise to both the blood vessels and to the blood cells. In amphibians, clusters of these mesenchyme cells first appear in the splanchnic mesoderm between the heart and anus. In birds and mammals, they are located in the yolk sac. These originally solid groups of cells, referred to as *blood islands*, rearrange themselves into a flattened outer layer destined to become the *endothelial lining* of the blood vessel and an inner core of cells that develops into hemocytoblasts, the stem cells from which other types of blood cells differentiate (see Table 15-1). The formed elements (cells) float in a fluid, the *blood plasma*, secreted by the cells of the blood islands.

Early in development, one blood island merges with another, until through growth and union they establish a plexus (network) of vessels. For example, they are responsible for the name given to the area vasculosa of the chick. The blood vessels form inside the embryo (intraembryonic vessels) in a similar manner. Mesenchyme cells clump together and then hollow out to form the endothelial lining of the blood vessel. Eventually, all the blood vessels, both inside and outside the embryo, anastomose to form a continuous vascular channel. Once this closed system is established, new vessels form by budding. These buds tap into already established vessels and increase the vascular bed of the tissue.

The process of blood formation is known as *hemopoiesis*. Although the original blood cells first form in the blood islands of the yolk-sac area of very young embryos, the site of origin soon moves to other areas in the prenatal animal. The mesenchyme cells of the body present in liver, spleen, kidney capsule, thymus, lymph glands, and bone marrow successively take over this responsibility. In lower animals, many of these organs continue their hemopoietic function in the adult. However, in birds and mammals as the site of origin shifts, the old sites usually lose their ability to function.

Vertebrate animals produce two general categories of cells: *erythrocytes* (red blood cells) and *leukocytes* (white blood cells). *Blood platelets*, found in mammals, are considered by some to represent a third type of cell. Two kinds of blood-forming tissue have evolved in the birds and mammals. *Myeloid tissue* gives rise to the erythrocytes and the granular leukocytes. As indicated in Chapter 15, the red bone marrow, an example of myeloid tissue, is considered the primary site of red blood cell formation in the higher vertebrates. Red marrow is found in the vertebrae, ribs, sternum, and sometimes epiphysis of the femur and humerus. The hemocytoblasts of bone marrow are often given the more specific term of *myeloblasts*. *Erythropoietin*, a protein that can be extracted from the blood and kidney, appears to be secreted by the kidney and regulates the proliferation and release of red blood cells into the bloodstream.

The second type of hemopoietic tissue is referred to as *lymphoid* and is the source of lymphocytes and monocytes. Examples of this type of tissue include the spleen, tonsil, lymph node, thymus, and patches of lymphoid tissue associated with the gut (Peyer's patches and the bursa of Fabricius).

Plasma

The blood that fills the blood vessels and heart of the circulatory system is a very complex substance. It represents 7% to 8% of the weight of the body and is two to five times more viscous than water. It is considered (by some) a type of connective tissue since it consists of cells, fibers, and a (liquid) matrix. The billions of cellular or formed elements are suspended unattached to one another in a fluid, intercellular substance known as *plasma*.

A little more than half of the blood is plasma and of this, approximately 90% is water. The dissolved organic and inorganic materials make up the remaining 10% of the plasma. All the substances mentioned previously (nutrients, wastes, hormones, gases, etc.), transported from one region of the body to another, are also found in varying amounts in the plasma. A large proportion of the solute is protein, present in one of three forms: albumins, globulins, and fibrinogens. Since proteins are large molecules, they normally remain within the blood vessels where the albumins, especially, help maintain the osmotic pressure of the blood, its viscosity, and volume. The globulins are primarily antibodies or enzymes, and the fibrinogens take part in the clotting of blood. When the endothelium of a blood vessel is injured or the blood is exposed to air, certain constituents of the blood react with the platelets to form a blood clot. As a result, fibrinogen is converted into fibrils of fibrin and the red and white blood cells become enmeshed in the fibers of the clot. *Serum* remains after the blood clots, as a clear fluid.

Formed elements
Erythrocytes

All vertebrate classes have *erythrocytes*, which produce the iron-containing hemoglobin capable of picking up oxygen in the gills, skin, or lungs. In contrast, the blood pigment of invertebrates is usually suspended in the blood plasma and can therefore leak out of the blood vessels. Only a few members of the vertebrates, certain species of fish, lack hemoglobin and have colorless blood.

The size of the erythrocyte varies among the vertebrates from 80 microns in the urodele red blood cell (long axis) to 7.5 microns in man. The cells are usually flattened oval shaped or elliptical. With the exception of the mammals, the erythrocytes of most vertebrates contain a nucleus. It is present in the early developmental stages of the mammalian erythrocyte, but just before they reach maturity, the nucleus is extruded. The enucleated condition is considered more advanced and more efficient than are the nucleated forms, since the amount of hemoglobin per volume of the cell is greater. However, since the cell has lost its nucleus, it is unable to divide; all new erythrocytes must be produced in the mammalian erythropoietic centers in the red marrow.

Blood platelets

Blood platelets appear to be formed in the mammal when large cells, the *megakaryocytes*, derived from the bone marrow undergo fragmentation. These giant cells may be as large as 40 microns in diameter. They are irregular in shape and have a lobulated nucleus. They form pseudopodia that project into the lumen of the marrow sinusoids, break off (forming the platelets), and float away in the circulating fluid. When a blood vessel is cut, platelets aggregate, their membranes rupture, and they release clotting factors. These factors trigger the clotting mechanism.

Leukocytes

The blood of vertebrates also contains *leukocytes* whose exact function is not always completely understood. These white blood cells can be divided into two types depending on the presence or absence of distinct, membrane-bound granules in the cytoplasm: the *granulocytes* and the *agranulocytes*. On the basis of their staining reaction, the granulocytes are further divided into three main types. In general, the granulocytes originate in the bone marrow or in the lymphoid organs, or both.

Eosinophils contain granules in their cytoplasm that stain with acid dyes. They are found in most vertebrate species. In fact, in the fish, they are the most abundant type of leukocyte. We do not understand their exact function, but they are usually associated in man, at least, with allergies; they may have an antihistamine reaction. They are present in great numbers in the tail and gut of the tadpole at the time of metamorphosis. *Basophils* are leukocytes that contain many granules of unequal size that stain with basic dyes. They are much scarcer than other granulocytes. The fact that in humans the granules are water soluble makes them difficult to identify. They appear more numerous in the blood of amniotes than in that of anamniotes. They have been reported lacking in the blood of cyclostomes and elasmobranchs. They may carry heparin and histamine and therefore be similar to mast cells. The blood of all vertebrates contain *heterophils*, leukocytes that have granules that stain best with a mixture of acid and basic dyes (in the human) or with either an acid (rabbit and guinea pigs) or a basic dye. They are easily identified by their lobed nucleus and in man are usually referred to as *polymorphonuclear neutrophils*. They are the scavengers of the bloodstream since they can carry out phagocytic actions. The heterophils invade areas of infection in the body's tissues. They leave the blood vessels in great numbers and make their way to the invasion site where they engulf the microorganism.

The second general type of leukocytes, the *agranulocytes*, are composed of *lymphocytes* and *monocytes;* the lymphocytes are the most numerous. They are found in all vertebrates and are structurally and (supposedly) functionally alike. They have a large nucleus and a small but varying amount of cytoplasm, a characteristic that enables them to be classified as small, medium, or large lymphocytes. The functions of these cells are only now being deciphered. These are the cells described when we discussed the thymus (Chapter 13). They appear to be of two types: the B and T cells and take part in the body's immune reaction. They may also be able to differentiate (transform) into other cell types.

The monocytes are much larger than most lymphocytes, and many have a large indented nucleus. They are almost impossible to differentiate from large lymphocytes in the circulating blood and lymph. They have some phagocytic properties and are usually associated with inflammatory diseases. There is evidence that they can transform into macrophages.

HEART
Development of heart

The heart primordium of all vertebrates develops in the anterior region of the body below the pharynx from splanchnic mesoderm. It represents a specialization of the ventral blood vessel first noted in amphioxus. Early in development, there is formed a longitudinal tube (blood vessel) that bends upon itself and eventually separates into the number of heart chambers characteristic of the species. The main difference in heart formation among vertebrates occurs early in its construction. The heart tube may form in two ways. In animals such as amphibians, an initial single tube of splanchnic mesoderm appears and becomes divided into chambers; in amniotes, man for example, right and left endocardial tubes arise and soon merge to form the single one. This tube becomes the lining of the definitive heart.

The splanchnic mesoderm contributes two layers to the heart of all vertebrates: the inner lining of *endocardium* and an outer *epimyocardial wall*. As described in Chapter 14, the heart lies in the anterior region of the original coelom designated as the *pericardial cavity*. The somatopleure gives rise to the *pericardium*, the membrane enclosing the pericardial cavity and the heart. In the early embryo the septum transversum separates the pericardial cavity from the rest of the peritoneum.

In amphibian embryos, the cardiac mesoderm appears to be determined as early as the neurula or even the gastrula stage. Staining experiments indicate that the mesoderm on both sides of the neural fold at the level of the future hindbrain shifts ventrally into the mesoderm free regions. By the tail bud stage the mesoderm assumes its normal position ventral to the gut. The mesoderm on each side of the embryo, ventral to the gut, gives rise to one half of the heart. When pieces of this mesoderm are excised and cultured during the neurula stage, the cells develop into pulsating tubes of tissue. During its early development, the heart is dependent on induction from the gut. If the endodermal tube is removed,

leaving an ectoderm and mesoderm shell, no heart develops.

In amphibians, at the end of neurulation the lateral plate mesoderm separates into somatic and splanchnic mesoderm. The latter moves toward the midline where it thickens under the gut tube as shown in Fig. 17-1. Loose mesenchyme cells derived from the splanchnic mesoderm congregate in the midline between the converging right and left sides; these mesenchyme cells form a longitudinal tube, the endocardium. At the anterior end, the endocardial tube divides to form the two ventral aortae; the posterior region becomes continuous with the vitelline veins that have grown into the area.

In the embryos of fishes and amphibians, the edges of the lateral plate continue to push ventrally under the gut until they reach the midline. The mesoderm from the two sides of the animal first fuses ventral to the endocardial tube. Later, the splanchnic mesoderm encloses the endocardial tube and fuses in the dorsal region as well. This double-layered membrane (formed from the right and left sides of splanchnic mesoderm) was described when we considered the formation of the mesenteries in Chapter 14. We identified the dorsal portion of the original ventral mesentery as the *dorsal mesocardium*. It remains attached to the anterior and posterior regions of the developing heart but soon ruptures in the middle area leaving the heart tube free to bend on itself. The mesentery ventral to the heart tube is the transitory *ventral mesocardium*. It also soon ruptures, and the right and left pericardial cavities become continuous, except in the region of the remaining dorsal mesocardium. The splanchnic mesoderm adhering to the endocardial tube gives rise to the *epimyocardium*. By the time the frog reaches 5 mm., this layer, in turn, separates into the *myocardium*, which will give rise to the striated, involuntary muscles of the heart, and the *epicardium*, or visceral peritoneum.

The original straight longitudinal tube soon bends upon itself forming an S-shaped structure. It begins to pulsate before the general chambers are established. Starting at the posterior end, one can see four successive dilations of the original tube. Each chamber is separated from

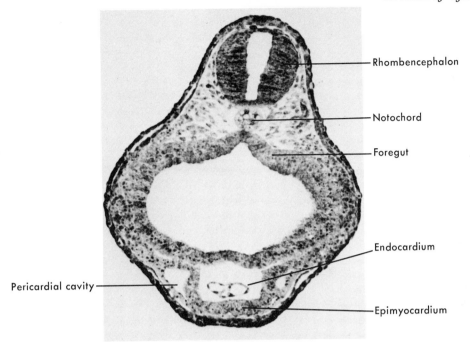

Rhombencephalon

Notochord

Foregut

Endocardium

Pericardial cavity

Epimyocardium

Fig. 17-1
Cross section of frog tadpole showing endocardium, epimyocardium, and pericardial cavity. (× 10.)

the others by constrictions. The vitelline veins penetrate the septum transversum and enter the large collecting chamber, the *sinus venosus.* This chamber also receives the two common cardinal veins (ducts of Cuvier) formed by the union of veins from the head (anterior cardinals) and posterior regions of the body (posterior cardinals). The sinus venosus, the most posterior chamber, is followed by the thin-walled *atrium,* the thick-walled *ventricle,* and the *conus arteriosus* (bulbus cordis of mammals). As shown in Fig. 17-2, the sinus receives the blood and passes it on to the atrium; the ventricle and conus act as the main propulsive chambers. This embryonic S-shaped structure is the generalized basic condition found not only in fishes and amphibians but in all vertebrate animals. The future development of the heart then diverges according to the specific group. The S-shaped structure of the heart appears because of differential growth of the various chambers. It has also been suggested that the hemodynamic force of fluid pressure helps to shape the developing heart, but

such effects on morphogenesis have not been definitely established.

In the flat blastodisk of the amniotes, it is possible to trace the first heart-forming cells to the anterior end of the developing primitive streak. They migrate into the streak and are carried forward with the mesoderm to form a crescent. Their movements are closely associated with those of the endoderm. By the head-fold stage, mapping studies indicate that they take up a position on each side of the animal as "wings" of the lateral plate mesoderm. The formation of the coelom, therefore, is also correlated with the development of the heart. The hypomere splits to form the ventral splanchnic and dorsal somatic mesoderm; the cavity formed, of course, is the coelom. In the region of the heart this coelomic cavity is referred to as the *amniocardiac vesicle,* the future pericardial cavity (see Fig. 17-3).

Loose mesenchyme cells in the region of the amniocardiac vesicles migrate away from the more solid mesodermal layer and form clusters

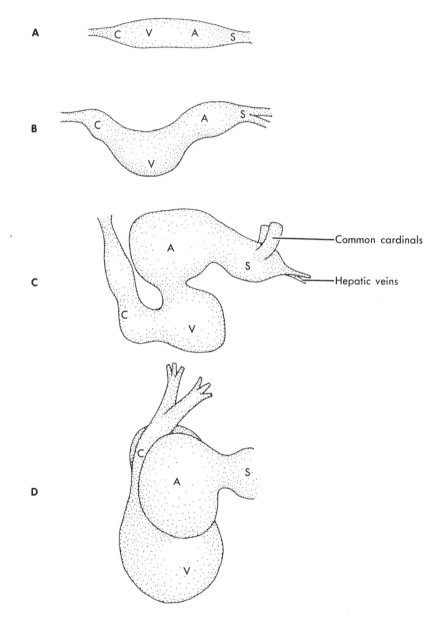

Fig. 17-2

Heart rudiment of frog (and all vertebrates) develops as longitudinal tube that differentiates into four heart chambers. **A,** Starting at the posterior end, they are sinus venosus, S; atrium, A; ventricle, V; and conus arteriosus, C. The heart tube bends on itself, **B,** forming an S-shaped structure, **C.** As a result of the bending, the atrium's final position is dorsal and anterior to the ventricle, **D.**

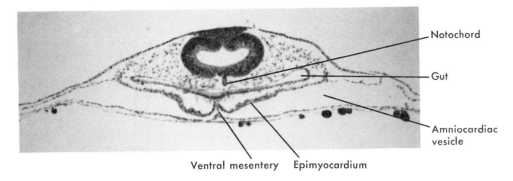

Fig. 17-3
Transverse section of chick embryo showing amniocardiac vesicles and epimyocardium. (× 10.)

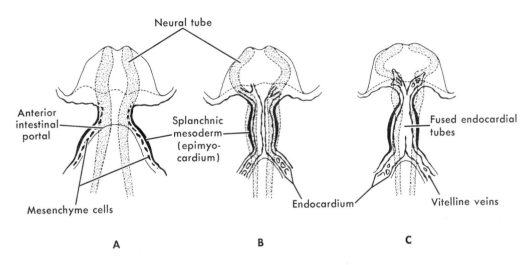

Fig. 17-4
Ventral view of developing chick heart. Mesenchyme cells bud off from splanchnic mesoderm and form tubes. These paired rudiments fuse in the anterior end to form endocardial lining of heart, **A** and **B**. Posteriorly, the tubes are continuous with vitelline vessels, **C**.

or networks of cells between the mesoderm and endoderm. These cells are similar to the cells that formed the blood islands. They soon assemble on each side of the foregut into groups that hollow out to form tubes as shown in Fig. 17-4, *A* and *B*. These tubules are continuous with the vitelline blood vessels and become the endocardium of the primitive heart (Fig. 17-4, *C*). The heart forms in the same manner as the rest of the vascular vessels and can be considered an enlarged, highly muscular blood vessel.

As the developing floor of the foregut moves

posteriorly (see Chapter 8) and the lateral margins of the embryonic disk fold under, lifting the embryo off the yolk, the splanchnic mesoderm pushes ventrally under the gut toward the midline. As a result, on each side of the body below the closing foregut, the splanchnic mesoderm thickens and forms a trough, the epimyocardium. As in the rounded embryonic forms, the epimyocardium swings under the gut where it encloses the presumptive endocardial tube. The heart forms as a progressive fusion of the two troughs of epimyocardium and the paired endo-

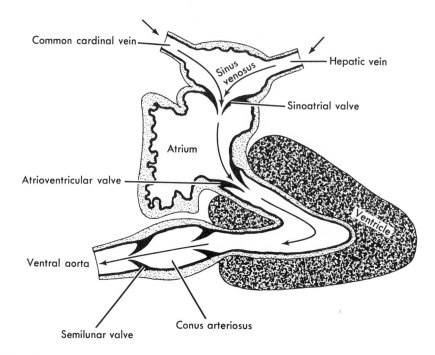

Fig. 17-5
Median longitudinal section of S-shaped fish heart. *Arrows* indicate path of blood flow.

cardial tubes. Fusion occurs first at the anterior region of the heart, the future ventricle, and proceeds posteriorly, with the atrium forming next, followed by the sinus venosus. The result is an almost straight endocardial tube within an epimyocardial tube (Fig. 17-4, *C*). When fusion begins, the cardiac primordium starts to twitch (about the seventh somite stage in the chick), before the cells show the special cytological properties of cardiac muscle and before the anastomosis of all the circulatory channels. In such animals as the rat and the rabbit, pulsations are observed before the completion of fusion.

Adult heart
Piscine heart

The adult of typical fishes retains the simple S-shaped tube. It lies behind the gills, suspended in the pericardial cavity. Because of the bending of the heart during formation, the posterior atrium is situated dorsal and anterior to the ventricle. Blood collects from the body by way of the paired anterior and posterior cardinal veins, which join to form the right and left common cardinals (ducts of Cuvier) (Fig. 17-15). The thin-walled, sac-like sinus venosus acts as a venous collecting chamber and receives the common cardinals laterally and the hepatic vein or veins posteriorly. The chambers of the fish's heart are continuous and all are muscular.

The initiation of the beat occurs in the rear of the heart at the sinus venosus. The venous blood flows forward from this chamber to the thin-walled atrium and then to the thick-walled muscular ventricle. The ventricle provides the main force for sending the blood throughout the body. It pumps the blood to the contractive conus, containing several simple typical heart valves, and into the ventral aorta. Here it is propelled by way of afferent branchial arteries to the gills for oxygenation. Valves present between the heart chambers prevent any backflow. The heart of the fish, as illustrated by the shark heart (Fig. 17-5), is a single pump containing only venous blood. The coronary arteries arise from the efferent branchial arteries (those on the other side of the gills) and supply oxygenated blood to the heart muscles themselves.

Tetrapod heart

The piscine heart pumped blood to the gills where aeration occurred. Efferent branchial vessels carried the blood from the gills to the dorsal aorta, and this vessel then distributed it to the head and to the rest of the body. When tetrapods evolved, the heart chambers were inherited but lungs replaced gills as respiratory organs. Considerable alteration in the development and structure of the heart became necessary because both oxygenated and venous blood now entered the heart. Two pumps were needed: one to pump venous blood to the lungs and one to pump the aerated blood to the body. To be most efficient, the two types of blood should remain separated. Adaptive changes in heart structure necessary to bring about this separation developed slowly and were not completely installed until the evolution of the avian and mammalian heart. Modifications in the piscine heart were introduced in the lungfishes and amphibians, and the atrium became partially or completely divided. As a matter of fact, there appear to have been several different ways in which the division of the atrium occurred. However, apparently no one simple evolutionary pathway was followed.

Associated with the loss of the gills and the development of lungs is the appearance of new blood vessels, the *pulmonary veins,* which carry the blood back to the heart from the lungs. However, in the lungfishes and amphibians, instead of entering the sinus venosus along with the rest of the venous vessels, the pulmonary veins pass directly to the left side of the atrium. The sinus venosus collects the blood from the rest of the body and enters the atrium more from the right. A septum forms in the atrium of the lungfishes and partially divides this chamber into a large right half and a smaller left half. It makes its first appearance in the grass frog at about the 7 mm. stage. By this time, the simple straight heart tube is bent on itself and constricted into the four chambers. An anterior dorsal fold of the wall of the heart grows ventrally and caudally, dividing the atrium into two chambers. The sinus venosus empties into the right chamber and the pulmonary veins into the left. After metamorphosis this septum is more or less complete in most amphibians and there is little mixing of blood

in the atrial chambers. However, only a single opening from the two atria leads into the single ventricle.

When injection of x-ray opaque material is made into one or the other of the atria, the passage of blood can be followed. Aerated and unaerated blood is shown to mix in the ventricle. Modern lungfishes have evolved a partial septum in the ventricle, but such a partition is lacking in amphibians. Since the Dipneusti have a septum, we presume that the crossopterygian fishes, from which tetrapods evolved, also possessed such a structure. This lack of a ventricular septum in amphibians represents a degenerate condition rather than an evolutionary stage halfway between fish and reptiles.

For many amphibians, the mixing of blood in the ventricle may actually be an advantage. It is estimated that more aeration of blood occurs in the amphibian's vascular skin than in the saclike lungs. Blood returning from the integument by way of the pulmocutaneous veins makes its way to the sinus venosus and then into the right atrium. This partially aerated blood from the right atrium then mixes in the ventricle with the blood aerated by the lungs.

The thick-walled ventricle contracts and forces the blood into the contractile conus. An elongated spiral valve, running down the length of the conus, separates it into a dorsal and ventral channel. Blood is projected dorsally into the pulmocutaneous artery, which passes to the lungs and to the skin. Ventrally, blood courses to the head by way of the carotid arteries and caudally to the rest of the body in the systemic arteries, as shown in Fig. 17-12.

Amniote heart

In amniotes there is a tendency for the sinus venosus to merge into the walls of the right atrium. It is smaller in the reptiles than in the amphibians and completely absent in birds and mammals. In fishes and amphibians, the sinus venosus functioned as a pacemaker, regulating and coordinating cardiac contractions. This function can be demonstrated by removing the pulsating embryonic heart and cutting it into three pieces corresponding to the regions of the sinus venosus (and atrium), ventricle, and conus

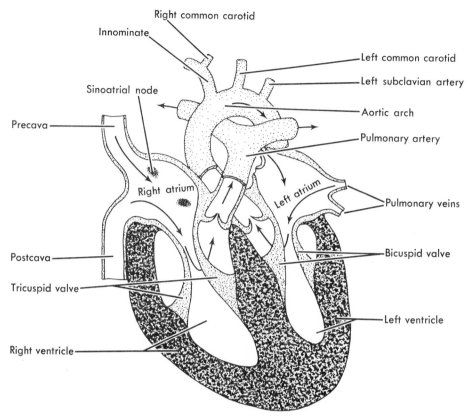

Fig. 17-6
Diagram of chambers of mammalian heart showing sinus venosus incorporated into wall of right atrium as sinoatrial node. Mammals have complete atrial and ventricular septa that divide the heart into a right and left side (double pump). Valves control the flow of blood between atria and ventricles and between ventricles and aorta or pulmonary trunk.

arteriosus. The segments will soon start to pulsate again. Now that the chambers are separated from one another, each portion of heart tissue contracts at a different rate. The contraction is fastest in the sinus, the intake portion of the heart, and slowest in the conus segment. The rate of beat in the intact heart corresponds to that of the sinus segment, indicating that normally its rhythm of beat is superimposed on the other parts.

In the anamniotes, the sinus, functioning as a collecting chamber, fills with blood. A contraction originating at the sinus, efficiently propels the blood through the simple tubular heart and out the other end. In mammals, the sinus is absorbed into the wall of the right atrium but it retains its ability to initiate the heartbeat. The area of excitatory tissue in the right atrial wall, representing the remnants of the sinus venosus,

is referred to as the *sinoatrial node*. In adult mammals, each heartbeat originates from this region of the right atrium, as shown in Fig. 17-6.

The conus is also lost in the amniote heart. Although part of the conus is probably absorbed into the ventricle, most of it splits into channels that form the large arterial trunks leaving the heart. In most reptiles, the conus divides into three large arteries: one carrying blood to the lungs and two systemic arteries. The one leading from the right side of the ventricle passes to the left and is known as the left systemic; the artery originating from the left side of the ventricle passes to the right and becomes the right systemic. Both systemics fuse dorsally and caudally in the reptile to produce a single dorsal aorta. As a result of this division of the conus in reptiles, the three arterial trunks leave directly from the ventricle of the heart. Fig. 17-13 illustrates this rather confusing relationship of arterial trunks to the ventricle. In fishes, semilunar valves in the conus prevented any backflow of blood. In lungfishes and amphibians, these valves fused and gave rise to the spiral valve, separating the single conus into pulmonary and systemic channels. In mammals, when the conus divides, valves are retained at the bases of the pulmonary and systemic trunks as the *semilunar valves.*

The heart of amniotes (as well as amphibians) contains a complete atrial septum; the atrium is thus separated into a left side and a right side, which receive blood from the pulmonary and systemic circulation, respectively. The ventricular septum varies in the reptiles from that of the lizards, in which it is almost absent, to that of the crocodiles, in which it is almost complete. However, according to Romer, even in the crocodiles there is a small gap in the septum where the arterial vessels leave the ventricle and some mixing of the aerated and unaerated blood occurs. The manner in which the ventricular septum arises in the various reptilian orders varies. It is almost horizontal in the Squamata (snakes and lizards) and Chelona (turtles) and vertical in the Crocodilia.

The relationship of the ventricular septum to the atria is such that each atrium now opens separately into one side of the ventricle. The oxygenated blood from the left atrium empties its contents into the left ventricle; the venous blood from the right atrium, in general, passes into the right ventricle. In the reptiles, when the ventricle contracts, the right side pumps blood into the pulmonary trunk and the left side forces blood through the right systemic. In crocodilians, whose heart resembles more closely the mammalian plan, the almost complete ventricular septum forms to the left of the left systemic. As a result, the left systemic also leaves from the right ventricle and carries venous blood (see Fig. 17-13). In those reptiles with incomplete septa, the blood in the left systemic is a mixture of oxygenated and unoxygenated blood.

The higher metabolic rate of the warm-blooded vertebrates demands a highly efficient heart and therefore the separation of oxygenated from unoxygenated blood. In the birds and mammals, this is accomplished by a complete separation of the left side of the heart from the right and the retention of only one of the systemic arteries. Double systemic arches are both inefficient and of little value to the organism. Birds and mammals evolved independently from the primitive reptiles, with mammals diverging earlier from the reptilian stock than did birds. However, through parallel evolution they both developed a four-chambered heart; but different roots from the original conus were used for the systemic artery. Birds retain the right arterial vessel of the original pair; mammals, on the other hand, make use of the left. In either case, the septa forms to the right of the systemic artery and therefore it exists from the left ventricle.

As a result of the interatrial and interventricular septa, the right atrium receives venous blood from the body and sends it to a right ventricle. A left atrium receives the oxygenated blood from the lungs and forces it into a left ventricle. When the ventricles undergo systole (contract), the right ventricle forces the blood into the pulmonary artery, conveying it to the lungs. The blood from the left ventricle passes into the systemic artery, which distributes the blood to the body. With the completion of atrial and ventricular septa the heart becomes a *"double pump."*

Partitioning of mammalian heart. Two problems must be met in the partitioning of the mammalian heart. The heart must not only provide a double circuit (thereby separating oxygenated from unoxygenated blood) but it must also make it possible at birth to convert quickly from the embryonic to the adult condition. This is accomplished by forming temporary partitions in the embryo that at the time of birth fuse to provide a complete division of the heart.

The septa begin to form in the heart of the human embryo by the end of the fifth week of development. At this time, although it lacks partitions, the embryonic tube actively pumps blood. Once the sinus venosus moves to the right of the atrium and the pulmonary veins to the left, the *atrioventricular (A-V) canal,* the opening of the single atrium into the single ventricle, is located near the middle of the heart. Connective tissue outgrowths from the wall of the canal give rise to dorsal and ventral *endocardial cushions.* The two endocardial cushions continue to grow in the walls of the canal, eventually fuse, and divide the original single channel into *right* and *left atrioventricular canals* (see Figs. 17-7 and 17-8).

Valves form between the atrial and ventricular cavities. When the endocardial cushions fuse, dividing the original A-V canal into two canals, folds of endocardium thicken along the margins of the canal. These elevations are invaded by muscle that becomes attached to the walls of the heart by cords of tissue. Three such elevations surround the right A-V canal and two form around the left. These elevations develop into flaps or cusplike structures. Further development converts the flaps into fibrous tissue covered on two sides by endocardium. Their free ends connect with the *chordae tendineae* formed from the muscular cords. These, in turn, remain attached to the *papillary muscles* of the heart and are anchored in place. When the ventricle contracts and the pressure within the chamber increases, these flaps prevent the backflow of blood into the atrium. The three cusps surrounding the right A-V canal become known as the *tricuspid valve*, and the pair on the left side becomes the *bicuspid* (Fig. 17-6).

A fold, the *septum primum,* appears in the roof of the atrium in a manner similar to that noted in amphibians. It grows posteriorly toward the elevations from the wall of the heart. At first, the septum primum and the endocardial cushions do not fuse, leaving an opening, the *foramen primum,* communicating between the two atria. This is a transitory orifice and is obliterated when the septum primum finally fuses with the endocardial cushions. However, this membrane does not remain complete but soon ruptures. A new interatrial opening, the *foramen secundum,* allows the blood once again to pass from the right side of the atrium to the left (Fig. 17-7).

This equilibrium of blood volume in the two atria is necessary since the pulmonary veins carry only a small amount of blood to the left side from the embryonic nonfunctional lungs. The right side, on the other hand, receives the blood from both the body and placenta. The development and growth of the heart apparently depends on the amount of work it does, and this, in turn,

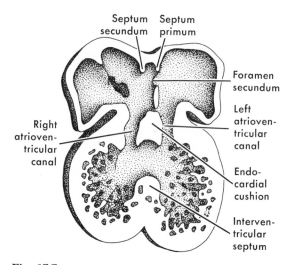

Fig. 17-7

Diagram of heart of mammalian embryo showing septa primum and secundum, endocardial cushions, interventricular septum, and right and left atrioventricular canals.

is related to the volume of blood circulating through its cavities. Therefore, both atria need to do a comparable amount of work to ensure equal growth. The interatrial opening allows the adjustment in blood volumes to occur and each side of the embryonic heart handles similar work loads. Consequently, both atria develop to the same extent.

At a later stage a second partition, the *septum secundum,* appears in the roof of the atrium a little to the right of the primary septum. As it grows downward, it extends over the lower edges of the opening in the original septum. As a result, an oblique slit, the *foramen ovale,* remains between the two atrial cavities. The foramen ovale remains until the lungs function at birth. Until that time the oxygenated blood returns from the placenta to the right atrium. The foramen ovale permits passage of this blood to the left side of the heart where it is eventually carried to the body of the embryo. The fate of the foramen ovale is discussed further when we consider some of the changes in the circulatory system that occur at birth.

In summary, the human right atrium is derived from the primitive atrial chamber, the sinus venosus, which is incorporated into its walls, and the right A-V canal. The left atrium is composed

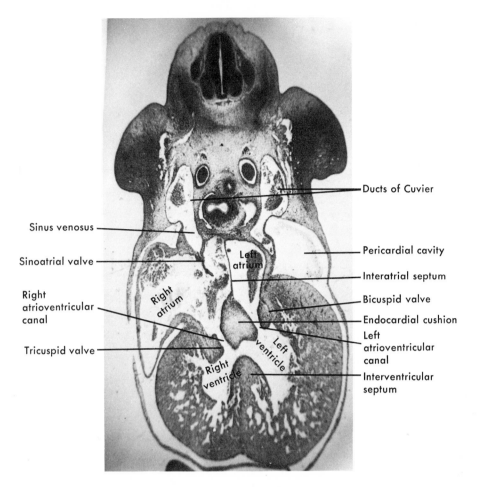

Sinus venosus

Sinoatrial valve

Right atrioventricular canal

Tricuspid valve

Left atrium

Right atrium

Left ventricle

Right ventricle

Ducts of Cuvier

Pericardial cavity

Interatrial septum

Bicuspid valve

Endocardial cushion

Left atrioventricular canal

Interventricular septum

Fig. 17-8
Section through heart of 10 mm. pig embryo at level of sinus venosus and atrioventricular canals. (× 4.)

of the left primitive atria, parts of the roots of the pulmonary veins, and the left A-V canal. The embryonic atria are divided by a septum that allows blood in the right side to pass into the left chamber; at birth, this passageway is obliterated.

The *ventricular septum* begins to form about the time the septum primum is established. A myocardial (muscular) ridge in the floor of the ventricle grows in an oblique direction from the apex of the heart toward the endocardial cushions and partially divides the ventricular cavity into a right and left side (Fig. 17-8). An opening that allows blood to pass from one side of the ventricle to the other remains for a

time. This interventricular foramen is eventually closed when connective tissue proliferated by the cushions fuses with that from the septum and forms the ridges of the conus.

Spirally arranged longitudinal endocardial ridges first appear distally on the sides of the wall of the conus arteriosus and then extend down its length. These ridges continue to grow and push into the lumen of the conus where they finally meet to form a septum. As a result of the fusion of the ridges, the conus arteriosus is divided into two arterial channels: the aortic and pulmonary trunks. The spiral arrangement of the septum is responsible for the slight entwining of the pulmonary and aortic arches as

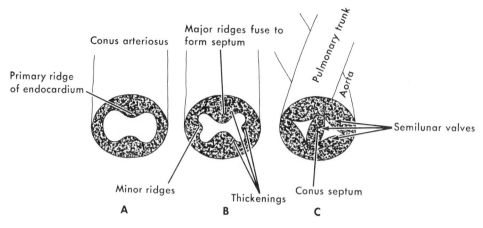

Fig. 17-9
Schematic diagram showing partitioning of conus arteriosus.

they leave the ventricle. The ridges twist in such a manner that the pulmonary side of the septum becomes continuous with the right ventricular half and the aortic side with the left side of the ventricle.

Three semilunar valves are located in the adult mammalian heart at the junction of the pulmonary and aortic trunks with the ventricles. They prevent the blood from flowing back into the heart from these vessels when the ventricles are in the relaxed state. These valves form in the embryo from three local endothelial thickenings (Fig. 17-9, *C*). When the primary ridges fuse to form the septum of the conus, two thickenings occur on each side of the septum and adjacent to it, as shown in Fig. 17-9, *B*. These valves, known as the *semilunar valves*, are able to press against one another in the closed position and thereby prevent any backflow of blood into the heart.

ARTERIAL SYSTEM
Aortic arches

In amphioxus, the ventral aorta, located beneath the pharyngeal region, extends anteriorly and gives off numerous paired blood vessels. These vessels pass laterally upward in the visceral arches between the gill slits to join the dorsal aorta. There may be as many as 50 or more pairs of these blood vessels, usually referred to as *aortic arches*. Amphioxus lacks

a heart, but each arch has a contractile swelling near its base, and pulsations in these bulblike swellings, as well as in some of the major blood vessels, aid in propelling the blood forward. As pointed out in Chapter 10, amphioxus satisfies much of its respiratory needs by the diffusion of gases through its thin skin. Some exchange of gases may occur in the arches, but they are not considered to be primarily involved in respiratory functions.

When ancestral vertebrates evolved, some of the aortic arches were retained and became intimately involved with the respiratory system of the organism. Also, a single pump was added to the circulatory system. As described above, a part of the ventral vessel enlarged and functioned as the heart, propelling the blood forward to the gills. In primitive vertebrates, when gills developed on the sides of the gill clefts, each aortic arch became divided into two parts. *Afferent branchial* vessels carried blood from the ventral aorta to the gills. In the membrane of the gill filaments the afferent vessels broke down into capillaries and aeration of blood occurred. The blood was collected on the other side of the gills by *efferent* branchials and conveyed to the dorsal aorta. This vessel distributed the oxygenated blood to the head and rest of the body.

In the cyclostomes, several aortic arches are retained: eight in lampreys but as many as 15 in hagfishes. By the time modern jawed vertebrates evolved, only six of the aortic arches were included in the general plan. However, the first arch was altered to serve the spiracle and only five functional arches remained, such as in sharks. The "idealized" plan was further modified when gills were eliminated in land animals. The aortic arches of fishes were adapted to fulfill new needs; their evolution in higher animals is one of the interesting stories of comparative anatomy. The fate of these arches is summarized in Table 17-1.

In other chapters in this book it has been easier to discuss common vertebrate characteristics; the processes leading to germ-layer formation as well as the morphogenesis of several organ systems followed generalized patterns of development. On the other hand, the common vertebrate plan of the circulatory system only becomes apparent if we turn to a study of the embryo. It is in the embryo of vertebrates that we find a basic circulatory plan; in the adult it becomes camouflaged by adaptive changes.

The embryos of higher vertebrate forms, including human embryos, follow conservative developmental pathways and, despite the loss of gills, continue to construct the aortic arches according to the blueprint laid down by ancestral forms. As indicated in Chapter 8, it was this similarity of embryonic rather than adult forms that lead to the modification of Haekel's law of recapitulation by more modern embryologists. The development of the aortic arches in higher animals is an excellent example of embryonic structure that can best be explained in the light of the evolutionary past. Their development is quite compatible with De Beer's modification of the old adage to read "Ontogeny repeats fundamental steps in the ontogenies of ancestral forms, especially when these steps are of structural and functional importance to the individual" (De Beer, 1954).

Evolution of aortic arches

The aortic arches of gnathostomes form first in the anterior pharyngeal region of the embryo and are consecutively numbered by Roman numerals in order of their appearance, I to VI (Fig. 17-10). Each blood vessel is located in the center of a visceral arch and is anterior to the gill slit. For example, at first blood can only flow from the ventral aorta to the dorsal aorta by way of arch I. This vessel passes without interruption dorsally between the mouth and spiracle

TABLE 17-1. Fate of aortic arches

Aortic arch	Dogfish	Necturus	Frog	Reptile	Bird	Cat
I	Ventral carotid Hyoidean	Disappears	Disappears	Disappears	Disappears	Disappears
II	Afferent no. 1 (common carotid)	Disappears	Disappears	Disappears	Disappears	Disappears
III	Afferent no. 2 Efferent no. 1	Afferent no. 1 Efferent no. 1	Internal carotid	Internal carotid	Internal carotid	Internal carotid
IV	Afferent no. 3 Efferent no. 2	Afferent no. 2 Efferent no. 2	Systemic arches	Systemic arches	Left lost Right forms aortic arch	Right lost (subclavian) Left forms aortic arch
V	Afferent no. 4	Disappears	Disappears	Disappears	Disappears	Disappears
VI	Afferent no. 5 Efferent no. 4	Afferent no. 3 Efferent no. 3 Pulmonary artery Reduced ductus arteriosus	Pulmocutaneous arch Ligamentum arteriosum	Pulmonary arteries Ligamentum arteriosum	Pulmonary arteries Ligamentum arteriosum	Pulmonary arteries Ligamentum arteriosum (Botalli)

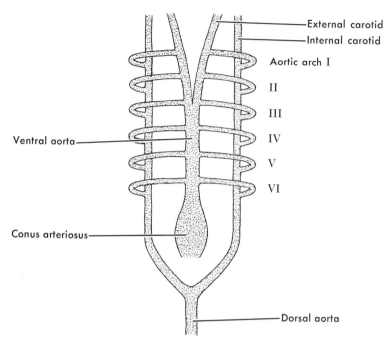

Fig. 17-10
Six embryonic arches form in gnathostomes and are consecutively numbered by roman numerals in order of their appearance. The external carotids are extensions of the ventral aortae that pass to the lower jaw regions. Extensions of the dorsal aortae give rise to the internal carotids, which carry blood to the head area.

(first pharyngeal pouch). The second aortic arch forms between the spiracle and the second pharyngeal pouch.

Although the ventral aorta was probably paired in ancestral forms, in living vertebrates, only one vessel is present posterior to the fourth aortic arch. It is connected to the conus arteriosus of the heart. Anterior to the fourth arch, the ventral aorta is double as seen in Fig. 17-10 and extends into the head region as the *external carotid* carrying blood to the jaws and surface of the body. The blood that passed through the anterior arches (I, II, and III) into the paired dorsal aorta is carried into the head region by extensions of these vessels, the *internal carotids*. They convey blood to the brain and special sense organs. Posterior to the origin of the carotids the blood flows caudally in the dorsal aorta. The paired dorsal aortic roots fuse behind the pharynx to form a single vessel that extends into the tail as the *caudal artery*. The dorsal aorta gives off dorsal, lateral, and ventral arteries along the way. Although all six arches may not be func-

tional at the same time, this basic plan is present in all vertebrate embryos and appears in modified form in adult fishes.

The integument of most living vertebrates is too thick to allow an exchange of gases between the vascular system and the source of aeration. It is necessary to use some other membrane for respiratory purposes. The aortic arches of primitive animals were in proximity to an abundant oxygen supply as they passed dorsally in the gill arches. They were separated from their aquatic environment by only a thin layer of cells lining the pharyngeal gill slits and were admirably suited to carry out a respiratory function. The aortic arches, therefore, became modified to serve the respiratory needs of the primitive ancestor.

In aquatic animals, the nonfunctional gill slits (visceral clefts) of the embryo enlarged to form the gill pouches of the adult. Their membranous lining was elaborated and thrown into folds, the gill filaments and gill lamellae (described in Chapter 13 when we considered the structure

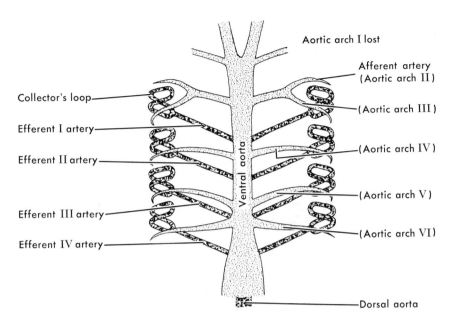

Collector's loop

Efferent I artery

Efferent II artery

Efferent III artery

Efferent IV artery

Ventral aorta

Aortic arch I lost

Afferent artery
(Aortic arch II)

(Aortic arch III)

(Aortic arch IV)

(Aortic arch V)

(Aortic arch VI)

Dorsal aorta

Fig. 17-11
Diagram of aortic arches of shark showing five afferent vessels passing to the gills and four efferent vessels draining the gills. The efferent vessels merge to form the dorsal aorta.

of internal gills). The aortic arch that entered each visceral arch (holobranch) supplied each side of the gill. It broke up into a plexus of blood vessels in the gill lamellae of each hemibranch. As a result, each aortic arch was divided into two parts; an afferent vessel carried blood to the gills and an efferent carried it away.

Six afferent and six efferent vessels were derived from the six primitive aortic arches. In the early stages of their development both afferent and efferent blood vessels leave at a point opposite each gill bar. Although the afferent branchial arteries supplied blood to both sides of the gill, separate efferent vessels drained each hemibranch and then joined one another to give rise to the efferent vessel. The more anterior branch leaving a hemibranch is usually referred to as the *pretrematic branch,* and the posterior branch becomes the *posttrematic branch.*

This arrangement of a circuit around a holobranch does not allow the complete utilization of the membrane surface of a gill pouch. A more efficient arrangement was achieved when the

posttrematic branch of one efferent artery joined the pretrematic branch of the succeeding efferent artery. As a result of this union, a *collector loop* was formed around each *gill pouch,* and the entire inner surface of a gill pouch was then utilized. The collector loops are clearly seen when the dogfish shark's circulatory system is studied (Fig. 17-11). An understanding of their formation explains why the afferent vessels enter each gill arch but the exit of the efferent vessels is shifted and is located opposite the gill slit.

All of the six embryonic aortic arches are not retained in the adult. In adult fishes the afferent portion of aortic arch I is missing and the efferent becomes the spiracular artery that passes from the spiracle (modified first gill slit) to the orbital region. In cartilagenous (and some bony) fishes, the second arch is located anterior to the first regular gill cleft, between the cleft and the spiracle. In most other fishes, both arches I and II are missing as typical aortic arches, and only arches III through VI are fully developed. In

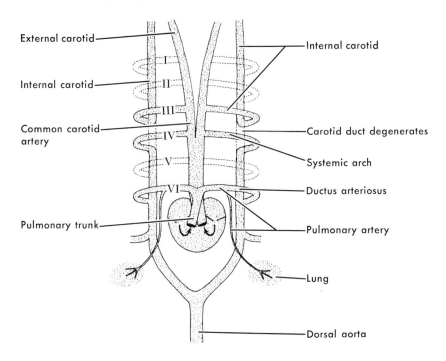

Fig. 17-12
Diagram of aortic arches of frog. Aortic arches I, II, and IV degenerate (although V remains in urodeles). Conus arteriosus divides into a pulmonary and systemic trunk.

those fish with lungs (the lungfish, *Protopterus*) the last four arches remain intact and a new branch from the efferent portion of the sixth grows out into the lungs.

The arches of amphibians represent an intermediate stage between fish and amniotes. In aquatic forms with vascular external gills (urodeles), arches I and II are absent and the other four arches are continuous vessels. The frog larva, on the other hand, since it possesses internal gills, has the typical fish form of afferent and efferent vessels. During metamorphosis the gills are absorbed and the adult frog changes over to lungs. As a result, the adult frog retains aortic arch III, IV, and VI. Arch V present in amphibian embryos and adult aquatic amphibians, is missing in the adult frog and all amniotes.

At first all of the arches empty into the paired dorsal aortae. With the loss of arches I and II, the third arch delivers blood primarily to the head region. In most amphibians, reptiles, birds, and mammals, that portion of the dorsal aorta between the third and fourth arch, known as the

carotid duct, degenerates. With the loss of the duct, the internal carotid is now composed of the third arch and the attached anterodorsal ends of the aorta, as shown in Fig. 17-12. The external carotid forms from the extension of the ventral aorta. That portion of the ventral aorta anterior to the fourth arch that leads into the external and internal carotids becomes the *common carotid artery*.

In adult amphibians, the fourth pair of embryonic arches become the systemic arches and deliver blood to the rest of the body. These right and left fourth arches unite to form the dorsal aorta. The proximal portion of the sixth arch gives rise to a new vessel leading to the lungs, and together they form the pulmonary artery. That part of the sixth arch, distal to the union of the new portion of the pulmonary artery, joins the dorsal aorta and becomes the *ductus arteriosus* (or *duct of Botalli*). The ventral aorta is much shortened in amphibians. As described earlier in the chapter, the spiral valve separates the conus arteriosus into a pulmonary trunk,

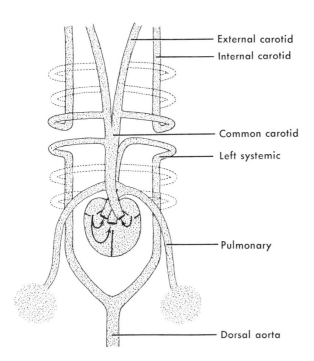

Fig. 17-13
Modification of aortic arches of some reptiles.

External carotid
Internal carotid
Common carotid
Left systemic
Pulmonary
Dorsal aorta

which leaves from the right side of the single ventricle, and the systemic trunk, which leaves from the left side.

When the ventricle contracts, some of the blood passes into the pulmonary side of the conus and, in most amphibian larva (and amniote embryos) with functionless lungs, continues by way of arch VI to the dorsal aorta. Here it joins the contents of the fourth arch and is carried to the rest of the body. At metamorphosis, when the frog shifts to lungs, the ductus arteriosus is lost as a functional vessel, and the heart pumps the blood by way of the proximal portion of the VI and the new pulmonary vessel to the lungs. At ventricular systole some of the blood also enters the systemic side of the conus. This blood then passes by way of the arch IV to the body and to the common carotid (paired ventral aortae anterior to arch IV) where it is shunted either into the internal or external carotid vessels.

The reptilian plan is similar to that of the amphibian. An exception, however, involves the separation of the ventral aorta not only into two divisions, the pulmonary and systemic trunks, but the further division of the systemic trunk into two vessels. As a result, in many living reptiles, a separate vessel connects with the left systemic arch and another one with the right arch. The carotids to the head and subclavian from the forelimbs are attached to the proximal portion of this right systemic arch (Fig. 17-13). Since the right and left sides fuse to form the dorsal aorta, venous blood from the right side of the ventricle mingles with the oxygenated blood from the left side. This inefficiency is eliminated in birds that evolved from reptiles. In birds, only one systemic (the original right one) and a pulmonary trunk remain. As a result of complete partitioning of the heart and the elimination of one systemic vessel, the single systemic trunk leaves the left ventricle and carries blood to the head, forelimbs, and the rest of the body.

Mammalian embryos follow the basic circulatory plan of embryos of other classes of vertebrates. Blood circulates through the heart tube anteriorly by way of the ventral aorta to the pairs of aortic arches partially encircling the pharynx and then into the paired dorsal aortae that distribute blood to the head, body, and extraembryonic membranes. All six pairs of pharyngeal arches are never present at one time in the human embryo. When it reaches the 22-somite stage, the first aortic arch has formed and the second is in the process of appearing. By the time the fifth and sixth arches form, the first two arches disappear; however, the fifth arch is only transitory. In human embryos of about 10 mm. C.R. (crown-rump) length, the third, fourth, and sixth aortic arches are well developed.

The reptilian line that gave rise to the mammals departed from the stem reptiles well before the birds evolved, and probably before the three vessels leaving the heart found in later reptiles had appeared. Instead, mammals apparently evolved from those animals with a pulmonary trunk and a single systemic trunk described for amphibians and presumably existing in ancestral reptiles.

In contrast to birds, mammals utilize the em-

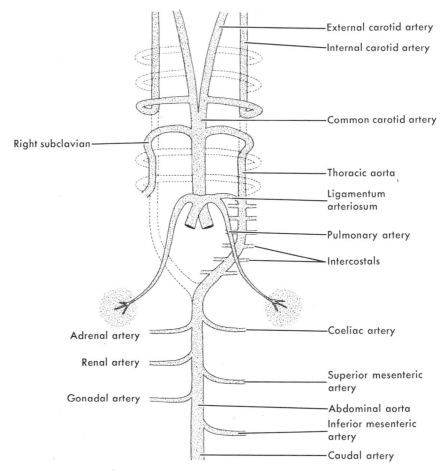

External carotid artery

Internal carotid artery

Common carotid artery

Right subclavian

Thoracic aorta

Ligamentum arteriosum

Pulmonary artery

Intercostals

Adrenal artery

Renal artery

Gonadal artery

Coeliac artery

Superior mesenteric artery

Abdominal aorta

Inferior mesenteric artery

Caudal artery

Fig. 17-14
Basic plan of mammalian arterial system. Only the left systemic arch remains as thoracic aorta. The right becomes the proximal portion of the right subclavian artery.

bryonic left systemic (IV) arch to carry blood to the head, forearm, and rest of the body (Fig. 17-14). The short portion of the right ventral aorta between the fourth and fifth arches becomes the *innominate* or *brachiocephalic* artery. It leads into the right common carotid, and the right systemic arch now becomes the proximal part of the right subclavian. The more distal portion of the right systemic degenerates. The left common carotid and the left subclavian usually enter the left systemic arch. This assymetrical condition can be seen in most dissections of the cat. Although this is the usual plan, it is possible that in the embryonic construction the carotids may leave by a common stem (re-

flecting the old ventral aortic base) or all may enter the systemic circulation separately.

As the dorsal aorta develops in tetrapods, it sends out branches to the three regions of mesoderm: epimere, mesomere, and hypomere.

1. Dorsal branches segmentally arranged and termed *intersegmentals* pass out between the somites and send branches toward the neural tube, epaxial muscles, and hypaxial muscles. They remain in the adult as the *intercostal* and *lumbar arteries*. In the region of the limbs, the intercostals are modified and contribute to the *subclavian* (forelimbs) and *iliac* (hindlimb) *arteries*.

2. Short lateral vessels pass into the mesomere.

In lower adult forms, many renal arteries are present; they usually fuse to form a single *renal artery* in higher vertebrates. Sometimes fusion is incomplete and two renal arteries are present, a condition seen in many cat dissections. These arteries feed the glomerululi of the nephrons. The *genital arteries* of the adult also belong to this lateral series.

3. Ventral branches of the dorsal aorta pass out to the splanchnopleure. The single *coeliac* and *inferior mesenteric arteries* form by the fusion of paired ventral embryonic vessels. In the amniotes, the *vitelline arteries* of the yolk sac and the *allantoic (umbilical) arteries* of the allantois or placenta are examples of ventral embryonic branches. When the yolk sac degenerates, the vitelline arteries unite to form the *superior mesenteric artery* of the adult. When the placental circulation is lost at birth, the original umbilical roots become the *common iliac arteries*.

VENOUS SYSTEM

Veins carry blood from the capillaries of the body to the heart of all vertebrates. These vessels are constructed with thinner walls than arteries and usually contain valves that prevent the backflow of blood. In the dorsal regions of the embryo, paired *anterior cardinal veins* bring blood from the head regions and paired *posterior cardinals* drain the rest of the body. These two vessels join one another on both sides of the body in the midregion to form the paired *common cardinal veins (ducts of Cuvier)*, as illustrated in Fig. 17-15. They cross the body cavity by means of the lateral mesocardium (previously described when we discussed the partitioning of the peritoneal cavity) and enter the ventrally located tubular heart. In the very early embryo of fish and amphibians two sets of blood vessels enter the sinus venosus. Two vitelline veins return blood from the yolk sac or intestine and two common cardinals, from the body proper. In amniotes a third set of veins empty into the sinus venosus. These vessels are the allantoic vessels, which transport blood from the allantois or placenta.

Fishes retain this basic embryonic plan of venous circulation with few modifications in the adult. In higher animals, however, the evolution of the venous system involves a series of pronounced changes involving anastomoses, atro-

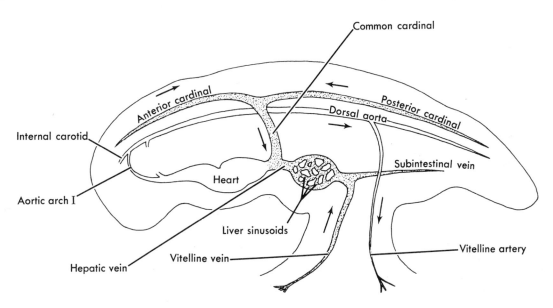

Fig. 17-15
General circulatory plan of early amniote embryo. With the exception of the heart and liver sinusoids, the blood vessels are paired during early developmental stages.

phies, additions, and shifts in blood supply. These changes are summarized in Table 17-2. As a result of these evolutionary changes, the adult mammalian venous system changes from a bilateral plan (seen in adult fish) to one in which only the peripheral regions remain paired (jugulars, subclavians, renals, iliacs, etc.). The main paired venous channels from the head and trunk regions are converted to single vessels: the *anterior vena cava* from the head region and the *posterior vena cava* from the trunk. These vessels converge on the right side of the body where they enter the right atrium of the heart.

The complexity of the venous system is made simpler if veins are classified according to their embryonic development. We should remember that several changes may be going on at one time in the venous system. However, for discussion purposes each one must be described separately. The veins of the early vertebrate embryo may be grouped as follows:

1. Vitelline veins from the intestine or yolk sac
2. Allantoic or umbilical veins found only in amniotes
3. Cardinal veins representing the major intraembryonic veins but later replaced in mammals by the venae cavae
4. Minor group of abdominal veins
5. Pulmonary veins present in lung-bearing vertebrates only

Vitelline circulation

The vitelline circulation is one of the first circuits to develop in vertebrate embryos and consists of two vitelline arteries and two vitelline veins. In the frog, the veins appear as irregular blood channels on both sides of the midgut region, which fuse to form a single subintestinal vein. In such vertebrates as the chick, they are located on both sides of the anterior intestinal portal and extend out over the developing yolk sac. In the anterior pharyngeal regions the vitelline veins become continuous with the endocardial heart primordium as noted earlier in the chapter. It is the embryonic vitelline veins that give rise to the *hepatic portal system* in the adult of all vertebrates.

The vitelline circulation is important in those embryos with large-yolked eggs such as elasmobranchs, reptiles, and birds. Blood from the dorsal aorta travels by way of the vitelline arteries to the meshwork of blood vessels located in the walls of the yolk sac. Endodermal cells secrete digestive enzymes that act upon the yolk granules, breaking them down into smaller units. The

TABLE 17-2. Fate of some of the veins

Shark	Amphibia	Reptile	Bird	Mammal
Anterior cardinal				
Proximal portion	Distal precava ——————————————————→			Right forms part of anterior vena cava
Distal portion	Internal jugulars ——————————————————————————→			
Common cardinal (duct of Cuvier)	Proximal precava ——————————————————→			Right forms proximal portion of anterior vena cava; left forms coronary sinus
Posterior cardinal				
Proximal	Azygous ——————————————————————————→			Part of azygous and hemiazygous
Distal	Renal portal veins ——————————————————————→			Degenerates
Laterals	Fused to form ventral abdominal	Allantoic veins ——————————→		Umbilical in embryo Ligamentum teres in adult
Renal portal	Reduced in some	Reduced	Functionally absent	Degenerates

liquid food diffuses into the blood vessels and is transported to the heart by way of the vitelline veins. These extraembryonic vitelline arteries and veins with their associated capillaries are referred to as the *vitelline arch* and function primarily as a food transport system. Human embryos that have a yolk sac but no yolk continue to form a vitelline circulation. Its presence is considered additional evidence that higher mammals evolved from ancestors with large yolk sacs filled with stored food.

Soon after the vitelline veins begin to form, a *subintestinal vein*, which taps into them, is established. Anterior to the point of this union with the subintestinal vein, fingerlike projections of the developing liver invade the vitelline veins and break them up into sinusoids (vascular channels). In reptiles, birds, and mammals, the two vitelline veins merge in the embryonic liver and establish a large channel, the *ductus venosus*. For a time the blood uses this shunt to pass directly through the liver and enter the heart. At hatching or birth, it degenerates and the blood is forced to "percolate" through the liver sinuses.

As a result of the invasion by the liver primordium, the vitelline veins are divided into three areas, as illustrated in Fig. 17-16, *A*. They form sinusoids within the liver as noted above. Anterior to the liver, the right and left vitelline veins carry blood from the liver to the sinus venosus and become known as the hepatic veins. In adults of lower animals, both these hepatic vessels remain (as in the adult sharks) or merge to form one vessel (most fishes). In higher animals, as we shall see later, the right hepatic vein contributes to the proximal part of the posterior vena cava, a vessel that replaces the cardinals as the main vein from the trunk region. The left hepatic vein degenerates. Posterior to the liver the third division of the vitelline veins gives rise to the *hepatic portal system*, the system that collects blood from the digestive tract and transports it to the liver.

A portal system is usually defined as one that arises as capillaries in one organ of the body, builds up into veins, and breaks down into capillaries in another part of the body. Lower vertebrates have two such portal systems: the hepatic

portal system and the renal portal system. Adult mammals have only a hepatic portal system. As the embryo assumes a shape and the yolk sac disappears, the vitellines associated with the sac also degenerate. The paired vitellines located within the body follow the lengthening gut posteriorly and establish a rich plexus of vessels between them. The hepatic portal system begins with capillaries of the stomach, pancreas, and spleen as well as the intestine and transports the digested food by the most direct route to the liver. Since the stomach and intestine rotate as they develop, the most direct route to the liver does not necessarily involve both right and left vitelline veins. In fact, a part of each side is utilized, with an anastomosis somewhere near the middle area (Fig. 17-16). In general, blood collected from the digestive organs passes into the left vitelline vein. It travels anteriorly in this vessel until it is shunted over by a transverse vessel to the right side where it then continues into the liver. As a result of the abandonment of the cephalic left side and the caudal right, the hepatic portal vein in the adult animal has a curious spiral construction.

Umbilical circulation

The *allantoic* or *umbilical circulation*, as it is usually called in mammals, is also composed of an embryonic arterial and venous system. Since it serves the extraembryonic membranes of amniotes, you would not expect to find these vessels in fishes and amphibians or in the adult of higher vertebrates. However, parts of the embryonic vessels are retained and are incorporated into adult structures of reptiles, birds, and mammals.

As described in Chapter 9, during development the allantoic membrane of the chick pushes out toward the porous shell. The exchange of gases occurs between the outside environment and the plexus of blood vessels located in the membranes immediately beneath the shell. In reptiles and birds, the allantoic circulation is primarily respiratory in function. The situation changes somewhat in those animals with a placenta. In them, the umbilical blood vessels are brought (with various degrees of intimacy) into contact with the circulatory system of the maternal tissues. Not only does an exchange of gases

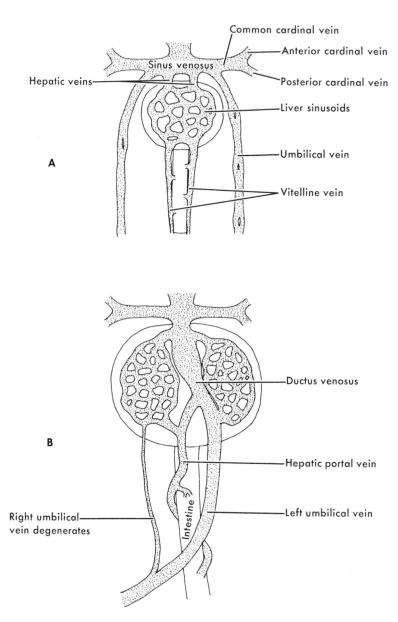

Fig. 17-16

Diagram showing development of hepatic portal system and umbilical veins. **A,** Two vitelline veins establish connections and form a meshwork over gut. **B,** Elimination of parts of each vein results in a hepatic portal vein consisting of a posterior left vitelline vein and anterior right vitelline. At first umbilical veins enter the sinus venosus, **A,** but liver soon grows laterally, incorporating them. The right umbilical joins the hepatic portal vein, forming a large vascular channel within the liver, the ductus venosus.

occur, but also food materials and wastes diffuse between these two sets of vessels. As pointed out earlier, this relationship between maternal and fetal blood vessels can be loose, such as in the pig, or intimate, such as in primates and rodents. Obviously such a transport system must be established early in development in order to supply the vital needs of the fetus. In the human embryo, the umbilical circulation is probably functioning by about 13 days after implantation (20-day-old embryo).

Allantoic arteries carry blood from the embryonic dorsal aorta to the allantois or placenta. Here they break down into capillaries that eventually merge to form the right and left allantoic (umbilical) veins. These vessels pass from the allantoic membrane or placenta to the body of the embryo by way of the allantoic stalk. At first, as illustrated in Fig. 17-16, *A*, the veins pass anteriorly, embedded in the body wall of the embryo, and return directly to the heart, joining the common cardinals and emptying into the sinus venosus. Later, the liver enlarges, expanding until it fuses with the body wall and incorporates the allantoic vessels into its tissue. The allantoic (umbilical) vessels then join the plexus of veins within the liver, contributing to the excavation of the large vascular channel, the ductus venosus. In mammals, the two umbilical veins fuse in the body stalk (umbilical cord). Within the embryo, the right umbilical vein degenerates, leaving the blood to travel to the liver of the embryo by way of the left umbilical vein (Fig. 17-16, *B*). In the liver, the blood from the umbilical vein joins that of the vitellines.

Anterior cardinals and anterior vena cava

Paired *anterior cardinal veins* are present in amphioxus and in the early embryo of all vertebrates. They are located on both sides of the body, dorsal to the coelom. With the exception of mammals, lateral head veins extend the anterior cardinals to the orbital and brain regions where they function as a drainage system for the area. The anterior cardinals, along with the posterior cardinals from the trunk region, join the paired common cardinals in the wall of the embryo. Supported by the lateral mesocardium, these vessels cross the coelomic cavity and enter the ventrally located sinus venosus (Fig. 17-15). During evolution and ontogenetic development, the cardinal system undergoes extensive transformation. However, there are fewer changes in the anterior cardinals than in the posterior ones.

In adult fishes this embryonic system persists relatively unchanged. In general, the anterior cardinals are superficially located in such animals as the dogfish shark. An orbital sinus surrounding the eyeball drains the skull region and connects with the anterior cardinal sinus located near the lateral line, on the dorsal side of the head. The anterior cardinal then turns ventrally, joining the posterior cardinal sinus at the common cardinal vein (Figs. 17-17 and 17-18).

In amphibians that have lost their internal gills and developed lungs, a neck region forms, and the heart is forced more posteriorly. Also in these animals, a new blood vessel, the postcaval vein (rather than the posterior cardinals) carries most of the blood from the posterior areas of the body. As a result of the shift in heart position, the common cardinals are drawn in a more longitudinal direction and become the roots of the anterior cardinals. The anterior cardinal sinuses are superficially located in fishes, but in the amphibians and all animals above them, there develop anterior vessels that become more discrete, are better protected, and accept new tributaries. These anterior vessels are now referred to as the *internal jugular veins*. Superficial vessels on the lateral and ventral surface of the head (probably present as remnants of old anterior cardinals in piscine ancestors) converge into "new" vessels in the tetrapod, the *external jugular veins*. In tetrapods, blood now passes from the brain and orbital region by way of paired internal jugulars (distal part of anterior cardinal) and from the superficial neck region by paired external jugulars ("new" vessels) into the paired common vein (Fig. 17-19). These common veins, usually referred to as the *right* and *left precaval veins*, are formed by the junction of the proximal portion of the anterior cardinals with the common cardinal veins. The *right* and *left subclavian* veins from the forelimbs join the precaval veins near their union with the jugulars.

This pattern remains unchanged in reptiles

and birds, but in many mammals, further modifications are made. As has been indicated several times previously, because of hydrodynamic factors there is a natural tendency for blood to seek the most direct flow to the heart. In mammalian embryos, a new vein develops by diagonally connecting the left side of the head region with the right, representing a more direct route. This new vessel, the *left innominate vein*, joins the anterior part of the left precaval with the posterior part of the right, as illustrated in Fig. 17-20. Blood is now shunted from the left jugulars by way of this new vessel to the right side, and in some mammals (Insectivora, Chiroptera, Ungulates, and Rodential) the embryonic left innominate as well as the left precava remain in the adult. In others (including man and the cat), the left precava between the innominate and heart is lost. In these animals, a Y-shaped structure results, with the left part of the Y formed from the new left innominate. The term *right innominate vein* is now given to the distal part of the right common cardinal and a portion of the old right anterior cardinal that remains between the entrance of the subclavians and jugular and the left innominate. As a result of the anastomosis, a bilaterally symmetrical drainage system from the head, the right and left innominate or brachiocephalic veins form and drain into the vessel now termed the *anterior* or *superior vena cava* (proximal portion of the right anterior cardinal and right common cardinal).

The left precaval vein may remain as a small remnant attached to the left innominate. When the sinus venosus migrates to the right side of the heart and is absorbed into the right atrium, it pulls its left horn (corner) across the dorsal surface of the heart. As the heart muscle grows in bulk, the proximal portion of the left precaval becomes the *coronary sinus* into which the *coronary veins* of the heart drain.

Posterior cardinals and posterior vena cava

The adult fish retains the posterior cardinal veins of the vertebrate embryo. They return the blood from the caudal region of the body to the heart by way of the paired common cardinals. In cyclostomes, blood from the tail, kidney, gonads, and back musculature empty into these

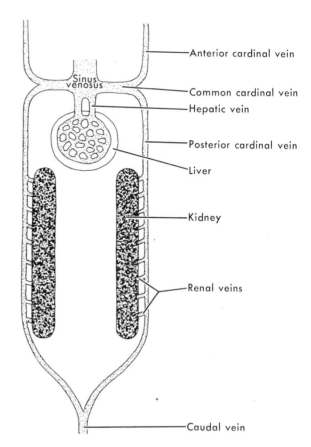

Fig. 17-17
Basic plan of venous system of cyclostome.

veins (Fig. 17-17), but in the elasmobranchs, the circulation of the kidney is inserted into the path of the posterior cardinal vein, dividing it into two parts (Fig. 17-18). Associated with this division is the formation of the *subcardinal sinus* and the development of the opisthonephric kidney. The subcardinals play a major role in the formation of the *renal portal system*. By the time the mammals evolved, the posterior cardinals were reduced in the early embryo, and by birth a new composite vein, the *posterior vena cava*, functions to transport blood from the posterior regions. Its formation in the embryo reflects the various evolutionary stages of mammalian development.

A plexus of blood vessels in the midregion of

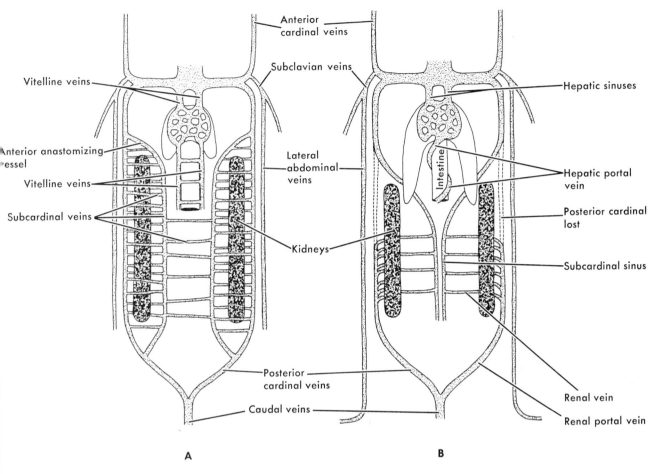

Fig. 17-18
Development of hepatic portal system and renal portal system in embryo, **A**, and adult elasmobranch, **B**.

the body of gnathostome embryos gives rise to the *subcardinal veins*. These longitudinally oriented veins are located ventral and medial to the kidney and parallel to the posterior cardinal vein. Paired segmental veins from the body wall, the parietals, drain into them. The subcardinals make connections with the capillaries encircling the renal tubules (but not those passing to the glomeruli). This plexus of blood vessels then establishes connections between the kidney capillaries and the posterior cardinals. Therefore, from the beginning the subcardinals are closely associated with the posterior cardinal veins at various points of anastomoses along their route. The subcardinals also anastomose with one another, and blood that

collects in them takes the most direct route to the heart. It travels by way of anterior vessels that link the subcardinals to the proximal portion of the posterior cardinal veins. For a time, blood returning from the caudal regions of the body either passes directly to the heart via the posterior cardinals, or it takes an alternate route and travels via anastomosing vessels from the posterior cardinals to the subcardinals, eventually joining the proximal portion of the posterior cardinal veins (Fig. 17-18, *A*).

As the kidney increases in size during development, it bulges toward the midline, pushing the subcardinals together. Although they remain separate in some vertebrates, the two vessels usually fuse, forming the large *subcardinal sinus* in the

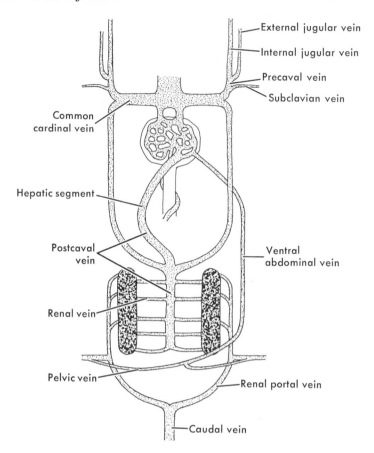

Fig. 17-19
Basic plan of venous system of amphibians. The addition of a hepatic segment offers a more direct route to the heart and contributes to a new vein, the postcaval.

midregions of the body. The renal veins that ramify in the kidney join the subcardinals.

As the kidneys assume more of a filtering function, blood is directed from posterior cardinals into the capillaries that loop around the nephric tubules. In the kidney, the filtered blood collects in the renal vein and empties into the subcardinal sinus. Consequently, in the region of the subcardinal sinus the posterior cardinals degenerate. As a result of the loss of this "middle" portion of the vessel, the old posterior cardinal vein is divided into two parts. The proximal segment connects to the subcardinals by the anterior anastomosing vessels. The isolated distal portion of the paired posterior cardinal veins (that breaks down into capillaries in the kidney) becomes the *renal portal vein* (see Fig. 17-18).

The adult kidney of the elasmobranch does

not develop further. As a result of these changes in the basic structure of the cardinal veins, the blood flows to the kidney from the caudal region by way of the renal portal system. Here it filters through the kidney tissue. Then by way of renal veins it passes into the fused subcardinals and on into the proximal portion of the original posterior cardinals. In the shark, these proximal portions expand to form the large posterior cardinal sinuses. Despite its dual origin (subcardinal sinus and proximal posterior cardinal veins), this pathway in the shark is referred to merely as the posterior cardinal vein and is present in most gnathostome fishes with the exception of the Crossopterygii.

In the Crossopterygii and all tetrapods, a new vessel referred to as the *hepatic segment* appears. This vessel becomes a shunt

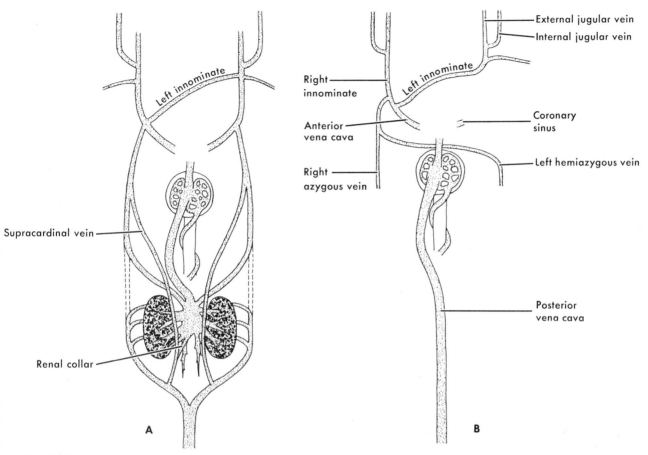

Fig. 17-20

Formation of adult mammalian vena cava. **A,** New embryonic vessel, the supracardinal, contributes to the adult posterior vena cava, **B.** See text for details.

in the adult, providing a single direct route to the heart, the postcaval vein, as shown in Fig. 17-19. The blood now has a tendency to travel forward from the kidneys by way of the fused subcardinals and this right hepatic segment. As a result, the proximal parts of the posterior cardinals begin to lose their prominence as routes of venous return to the heart. Their remnants are present, for example, in *Necturus,* but they disappear in reptiles and higher vertebrates. The cardinals are associated primarily with the mesonephros; when it degenerates and is replaced by the metanephric kidney, the primitive systemic drainage channels degenerate with it. In some reptiles, and to a greater extent in birds that evolved from them, direct channels between renal portal veins and fused subcardinals appear. Venous circulation around the kidney tubules retro-

gresses and disappears entirely in the mammal, leaving only the arterial blood supply to the glomeruli.

In mammals, blood returns to the heart from the posterior regions by way of the *posterior vena cava.* This composite vessel reflects the reptilian plan, since it utilizes parts of the existing reptilian postcaval vein and adds a new segment from the *supracardinal veins* (thoracolumbar veins) (Fig. 17-20, A). The posterior vena cava forms at the time the posterior cardinals degenerate. The changes that bring about its formation are much more radical than those responsible for development of the anterior vena cava.

The development of the mammalian posterior vena cava is another striking example of an embryo following ancient blueprints to form a modern structure (vena cava). Its development repeats the evolutionary stages biologists believe preceded it. The evolution of the system, therefore, can be studied either by comparing its form in representative adults of classes ancestral to the mammals or by studying the various stages of development in the embryo. For clarity, Table 17-3 summarizes the steps taken by the mammalian embryo in establishing the adult vena cava. The adult of various classes that have reached a particular stage and proceeded no further are contrasted.

In the human embryo, the posterior cardinals are present by the 14-somite stage. By the time the embryo reaches 7 to 8 mm. C.R. length, the right subcardinal (which has formed by now) is connected to the liver sinuses by a hepatic segment. By 10 mm. C.R. length, the subcardinals fuse. Soon after the hepatic segment forms, the supracardinals appear between the anterior region of the posterior cardinals and the renal portal veins. Anteriorly they make connections with the proximal part of the old posterior cardinals; distally they tap into the renal portal vein (Fig. 17-20, A). Blood from the posterior regions now returns to the heart more directly, bypassing the renal portal system, entering the supracardinals, and continuing into the old (proximal portion) posterior cardinals and common cardinals.

Since these vessels form in the mammalian embryo, they are presumed to have been present in the mammalian line of reptilian ancestors. A *renal collar* appears, connecting the right supracardinal with the renal vein. Posterior to the renal collar, the supracardinal now becomes the main venous route from the pelvis and legs, since it offers an even more direct route to the heart as may be seen in Fig. 17-20, A. On the other hand, the anterior portions of the supracardinals lose their significance. They remain attached to the proximal portions of the old posterior cardinals and become the *left hemiazygous* and *right azygous veins* that, in general, drain into the right common cardinal.

Knowledge of embryonic vessels normally used in composing the vena cava offers insight into some of the numerous variations found in the adult vessel. In general, the embryo uses the right half of the various paired vessels to construct the posterior vena cava. The following list of vessels summarizes the embryonic components involved in forming the adult mammalian vena cava of such animals as the cat:

1. Caudal vein
2. Small portion of right renal portal vein depending on point of attachment of right supracardinal
3. Right supracardinal

TABLE 17-3. Ontogeny and evolution of mammalian venae cavae

Mammalian vessel	Embryonic components	Evolutionary stage
Anterior vena cava	1. Right and left anterior cardinal joins common cardinal	All fish
	2. Formation of neck and longitudinal stretching of common cardinal to form precava veins	Amphibian
	3. Formation of internal and external jugulars	Amphibian
	4. Anastomosis of right and left sides forming left innominate	Mammal
	5. Formation of right innominate	Mammal
	6. Formation of anterior vena cava and coronary sinus	Mammal
Posterior vena cava	1. Formation of posterior cardinals	Cyclostomes
	2. Formation of renal portal	Elasmobranchs
	3. Formation of subcardinals and their fusion with proximal posterior cardinal	Elasmobranchs
	4. Formation of hepatic segment by vitellines tapping into right side of subcardinals	Choanichthyes
	5. Formation of supracardinals and fusion with proximal postcava and renal portal	Probably close reptilian ancestor to mammals
	6. Formation of subcardinal-supracardinal anastomosis	Mammal
	7. Loss of renal portal veins	Mammal
	8. Establishment of posterior vena cava	Mammal
	9. Formation of azygous and hemiazygous veins	Mammal

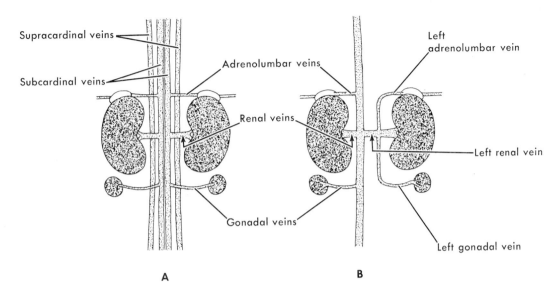

Fig. 17-21
A, In adult mammals, part of the right supracardial and right subcardinal veins contribute to the posterior vena cava. Right adrenolumbar, renal, and gonadal veins empty into this composite vessel. **B,** Left subcardinal becomes the left renal vein, and left adrenolumbar and gonadal veins continue to empty into it. As a result, there is a loss of symmetry in this region of the venous system.

4. Right renal collar
5. Right renal vein
6. Right portion of subcardinals
7. Possibly a small portion of right proximal posterior cardinal depending on point of union with hepatic vein
8. Hepatic vein that passes through the liver (the vena cava does not break up into capillaries in the liver but receives the blood from the liver and from the hepatic portal system)
9. Right hepatic vein (old vitelline) into the sinus venosus (left hepatic degenerates)
10. When the sinus venosus is absorbed into the right atrium of the mammalian heart, the vena cava empties into this chamber directly

The fact that, in general, the right side is used in forming the vena cava explains the asymmetry found in the region of the kidneys (Fig. 17-21). The right renal vein along with the right adrenolumbar and right genital, all of which originally emptied into the right subcardinal, enter the vena cava directly. Since the mammalian renal vein is formed by a fusion of several embryonic veins, the fusion is not always complete and two (instead of one) renal veins may lead from the

kidney into the vena cava. On the left side, portions of the left subcardinal become the left renal vein. The left adrenolumbar and the left genital, which originally entered the left subcardinal, now open into the left renal vein. Approximately 87% of the cat embryos follow this plan in constructing the posterior vena cava, but many other combinations exist. The left side may be used instead of the right or a combination of the two. The subcardinals may remain separated and two venae cavae may be present for a part of the distance. Other embryonic combinations occur. The varieties of form in the posterior vena cava often found when the anatomy student dissects his cat, is a challenge to his embryological knowledge.

Abdominal veins

Paired *abdominal veins* appear in all vertebrate embryos. They are retained in the adult of most lower animals but are lost in the adults of birds and mammals. In fish, the abdominal veins are lateral and ventral in position. Parietal vessels from the body wall drain into them as well as vessels from the pelvic and pectoral fins. They run forward and empty into the common cardinals, as depicted in Fig. 17-18, *B*.

In Crossopterygii and amphibians, the lateral abdominals move ventrally and lose their connection with the common cardinals. They fuse in most amphibians to form a single ventral abdominal vein but remain paired in reptiles. They travel in the body wall, but at the level of the liver move into the falciform ligament. At the posterior regions of the liver they leave their enclosure in the falciform ligament and enter the liver. Here they join the hepatic portal vein. Blood from the hindlimbs may now follow two pathways to the heart (Fig. 17-19). It may pass by way of the renal portals to the postcaval vein or by way of the abdominals into the hepatic portal system. Blood from the forelimbs continues to enter the common cardinals. Since this last vessel is incorporated into the precava, it carries the anterior limb veins with it.

The lateral abdominal veins form in all amniote embryos. However, they assume the names of the allantoic or umbilical veins, since they collect blood from the extraembryonic membranes. At first they join the common cardinals but later enter the liver (Fig. 17-16). The liver of these amniote embryos receives blood from three sources: arterial blood from the dorsal aorta, venous blood from the vitellines (hepatic portal), and venous blood also from the abdomi-nals (allantoic or umbilical). The posterior vena cava passes through the liver; it does not break down into capillaries but collects the blood from the renal veins in the trunk region and from the hepatic veins of the liver. It is the posterior vena cava that transports the blood to the heart. At hatching or birth, the abdominal veins are obliterated as noted in our previous discussions.

Pulmonary veins

When the lungs appear, several new pulmonary veins that drain the branches of the lung buds form. These vessels unite and give rise to one main vessel that enters the left atrium. As the lung grows, the main pulmonary stem is absorbed and several (four) pulmonary branches typically enter the wall of the atrium.

CHANGES THAT OCCUR AT HATCHING OR BIRTH

Two circulatory arcs, intraembryonic and extraembryonic circuits, compose the embryonic circulatory system of amniotes. These are presented schematically in Fig. 17-22. Before birth or hatching, the allantoic or placental circulation assumes the responsibility for respiration. At birth, food and oxygen are no longer supplied to the young animal, and it must receive these

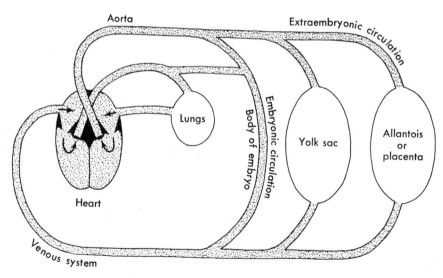

Fig. 17-22
Extraembryonic and intraembryonic circulatory arcs compose the circulatory system of amniotes. See text for a description of the sudden and drastic changes that must occur at birth or hatching.

necessary materials from an external source. Since these are transported to the fetus by way of the circulatory system, it is obvious that the greatest sudden change at birth must occur to this system. The extraembryonic circulation is eliminated, and certain vessels within the body are closed off, first by physical means such as the contraction of muscle fibers in the walls of the vessels that obliterate the lumens and later anatomically by growth of fibrous tissue.

The nonfunctioning lung is a collapsed sac with its air spaces undistended and containing fluid. Although blood flows to the lung by way of the pulmonary artery and away by the pulmonary vein, this circulation is small, merely maintaining the metabolism of the lung tissue. In general, it is bypassed during early developmental stages. Near term, however, lung tissue expands and its circulation increases considerably. As noted when we discussed the growth of the heart, both sides of the heart must do similar amounts of work (that is, pump similar loads) if normal development is to occur. Since little blood returns to the left atrium from the pulmonary veins in comparison to that received by the right atrium, blood from the right atrium pushes through the foramen ovale to the left side, thereby equalizing the pressure on the two sides. The contraction of the two atria forces blood into the right and left ventricles.

Since the atrial output is balanced, the ventricular input as well as its output must also be balanced. The contraction of the left ventricle sends the blood out through the dorsal aorta to be distributed to the body. The contraction of the right sends blood to the sixth arch where some blood passes by way of the pulmonary arteries to the lungs, but the larger portion proceeds into the ductus arteriosus and is carried to the dorsal aorta. The shunt provided by the ductus arteriosus allows the right ventricle to do the same amount of work as the left and thereby develop its capacity to function. At birth it is prepared to pump a large volume of blood to the expanded lungs.

At the time of birth, two events occur. There is a loss of extraembryonic circulation and an expansion of lung area. Both the ductus arteriosus and the valvular structure of the foramen ovale are prepared to adapt to these changes. The ductus arteriosus closes first. The smooth muscles of this vessel contract, shutting off this pathway to the dorsal aorta. In mammals these changes have been studied in detail and found to occur rather suddenly. In chicks, the obliteration of the ductus arteriosus proceeds more slowly since there is evidence that the vessel is still open and carrying blood in newly hatched chicks. Later, fibrous tissue invades the ductus arteriosus converting it to the *ligamentum arteriosum* (duct of Botalli).

As a result of the expansion of lungs and the physiological closure of the ductus arteriosus, the volume of blood sent to the lungs increases greatly. This in turn, necessitates a greater volume returning by way of the veins to the left atrium. The pressure in the two atria now equalize one another as the blood presses on each side of septum primum and septum secundum, forcing the two septa together and obliterating the foramen ovale. Obviously the closure of the foramen ovale must follow that of the ductus arteriosus. Sometime after birth, there is fibrous adhesion of the two components of the septum although it is estimated that in 20% to 25% of adult individuals this is not complete.

At birth when the placental circulation stops because of the ligation of the umbilical cord, circulation in umbilical arteries and veins ceases abruptly. Later, fibrous tissue invades the umbilical vein and converts it to the *ligamentum teres* of the liver. The large vascular channels of the liver, the ductus venosus, develop into the fibrous *ligamentum venosum*. The proximal portions of the umbilical arteries become the *hypogastric* (internal iliac) *arteries,* and the small fetal external iliacs increase in size in the adult and take over the arterial supply to the legs. The original root of the umbilical artery arising from the dorsal aorta becomes the *common iliac.*

LYMPHATIC SYSTEM

The lymphatic system consists of a network of delicate vessels that develop from mesenchyme in much the same way as the blood vessels do. They form later than does the blood vascular system. Once these simple endothelial tubes form, they grow by budding. Because of their diffuse and delicate nature they cannot be followed in an ordinary dissection. In mammals, certain lymphatic organs are also included in this system. The lymphatic organs are collections of lymphatic tissue that are scattered over the body and identified as Peyer's patches, tonsils, thymus, lymph nodes, and spleen. The bursa of Fabricius in the chick may be comparable to Peyer's patches. Solitary lymphatic nodules are often associated with the gastrointestinal, respiratory, or urogenital systems.

Lymphatics are found in most tissues and organs of the body but have not been identified in the central nervous system, bone marrow, liver, fetal placenta, internal ear, and eyeball. Tissue fluid filters through the capillary walls of the blood vessels and surrounds all cells. If it is not constantly removed, the tissue fluid accumulates in the tissue spaces, and the tissues "swell" and become edematous. The veins, along with the lymphatics, collect this fluid and return it to the heart. The lymphatics are, therefore, closely associated with the venous system and may be considered an accessory to it. Unlike the blood vascular system, nothing comparable to arteries are present, and the liquid (lymph) circulates in only one direction, toward the heart. There is no agreement as to the presence of lymphatic vessels in cyclostomes or elasmobranchs, but they are well developed in bony fish and tetrapods.

The blind tips of the lymphatic capillaries, originating in the tissue spaces, anastomose with one another to form sac-like sinuses or vessels. These merge to form larger vessels until they eventually open into the venous system. Since endothelial cells compose the walls of the tiny fine lymph capillaries, the lymphatic system is considered a closed system. There are present in the frog large subcutaneous lymph sinuses that may play a role in maintaining the moist skin needed by these vertebrates in respiration.

In fishes, the lymph enters the veins primarily in the pelvic region. In other vertebrates, the anterior or posterior, or both, cardinals receive lymphatics. In mammals, the lymphatic channels merge to form two main vessels in the embryo, a large *left thoracic duct* and a smaller *right thoracic duct;* both empty into the subclavian veins near their union with the internal jugulars. Some adult mammals retain this plan, but in many the right thoracic vessels join the left, and the lymph enters the subclavian vein. In the heart, the lymph mixes with the blood and recirculates through the body.

Lymph is a colorless liquid similar to tissue fluid except that it is higher in carbon dioxide and lower in oxygen. After a meal the lymph draining the small intestine, referred to as *chyle,* is laden with fat and milky in color. At the end of the digestive process, the carbohydrate and protein products are absorbed into the capillaries of the hepatic portal system, but the fats pass into the *lacteals,* lymphatic vessels of the intestine, bypassing the liver (see Fig. 13-23). They are transported to the thoracic duct and added to the general circulation. Lymph contains few erythrocytes, but the larger vessels, especially of mammals, usually have many small lymphocytes. In mammals, lymph nodes are located in the pathway of the lymphatic vessels and the lymph must filter through the nodes, picking up the lymphocytes along the way.

The lymphatic system is a sluggish system. There is no connection with the arteries and therefore no propelling force. Movement of the lymph is primarily attributable to body movement; the muscles press or massage the liquid forward. Valves occur in pairs along the way with their free edges oriented in the direction of lymph flow and prevent any backflow. In all vertebrates except Chondrichthyes and mammals, two-chambered muscular structures, known as *lymph hearts,* located at the junction of the lymphatics with veins, pump the liquid into the general circulation. They are most numerous in the amphibians where they may vary in number from four in Anura to 200 in Apoda.

SUGGESTED READINGS

1. Angell, C. S., and Hipona, F. A.: Angiographic studies of the anuran double circulation, Am. Zool. **5:** 668, 1965.
2. De Beer, G. R.: Embryonic ancestors, New York, 1951, Oxford University Press.
3. DeHaan, R. L.: Morphogenesis of the vertebrate heart. In DeHaan, R. L., and Ursprung, H.: Organogenesis, New York, 1965, Holt, Rinehart & Winston, Inc.

4. Ebert, J. D.: The first heart beats, Sci. Am. **200**:87-96, 1959.
5. Foxon, G. E. H.: Problems of the double circulation in vertebrates, Biol. Rev. **39**:196-228, 1955.
6. Functional morphology of the heart of vertebrates (symposium), Am. Zool. **8**:179-229, 1968.
7. Mossman, H. W.: Circulatory cycles in the vertebrates, Biol. Rev. **23**:237-255, 1948.
8. Mayerson, H. S.: The lymphatic system, Sci. Am. **208**:80-90, 1963.
9. Patten, B. M.: Foundations of embryology, New York, 1958, McGraw-Hill Book Co.
10. Patten, B. M.: Initiation and early changes in the character of the heart beat in vertebrate embryos, Physiol. Rev. **28**:31-47, 1949.
11. Romer, A. S.: The vertebrate body, Philadelphia, 1962, W. B. Saunders Co.
12. White, F. N.: Circulation in the reptilian heart (*Caiman sclerops*), Anat. Rec. **125**:417-431, 1956.

CHAPTER 18

UROGENITAL SYSTEM

INTERMEDIATE MESODERM
Urogenital system

The intermediate mesoderm *(mesomere)* is a thin plate of cells that connects the dorsal mesoderm *(epimere)* with the lateral plate mesoderm *(hypomere),* as shown in Fig. 18-1. It is destined, along with contributions from the splanchnic mesoderm, to give rise to the excretory and reproductive systems. These systems, usually referred to collectively as the *urogenital system,* function in the elimination of metabolic wastes and the reproduction of the species. Although they are very diverse systems from a physiological standpoint, they share many common embryonic and some adult structures.

Paired kidneys, excretory ducts, urinary bladder, and urethra (in higher forms) make up the excretory system; the paired gonads (ovaries or testes) and their ducts make up the reproductive part of the urogenital system. The primordial germ cells (as described in Chapter 4) originate in a different region of the body and migrate into the embryonic gonads. Since the kidneys and gonads form on each side of the body from the intermediate mesoderm, as explained when we considered the formation of the coelom, they are outside the coelomic cavity (retroperitoneal).

With the exception of adult cyclostomes, a few fishes, and the mammals, both the urinary and reproductive ducts of vertebrates open into a common collecting chamber, the cloaca, an endodermal derivative of the hindgut. In the male embryo, a part of the urinary system becomes incorporated into the reproductive system. The close association of these two systems during development make it impossible to describe one without referring to the other.

Adrenal gland

The intermediate mesoderm also contributes to the *adrenal gland,* one of the endocrine organs present in all vertebrates from cyclostomes to mammals. Adrenal tissue is not considered a part of the urogenital system; however, it can logically be discussed at this time. It is derived from cells located near the embryonic gonad and kidney and usually remains in close spatial relationship with the kidney. Its cortical hormones are ste-

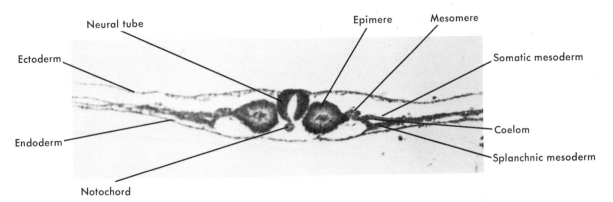

Fig. 18-1
Transverse section of chick embryo showing intermediate mesoderm. (× 100.)

roids, as are those produced by the ovaries and testes. Many biologists do not accept as valid the attempts to relate the histogenesis of the adrenal with that of the interstitial cells of the gonads. There is agreement, however, that a significant functional relationship exists between the two organs.

The adrenal gland is a composite organ, composed of two different cell types, steroid-producing and catecholamine-producing cells. In lower animals these two cell types either coexist or are independently dispersed along the posterior cardinal vein and kidney. In amphibians, the cells form discrete bodies embedded in kidney tissue. In mammals, the cells are arranged in two distinct layers; the steroidogenic cells are restricted to a compact cortex, and the catecholamine-producing cells are found in the medulla of the adrenal gland.

The intermediate mesoderm gives rise to the steroidogenic cells. Along with the ovary, testes, and the placenta, these cells of the adrenal gland are responsible for the steroid secretion of the body. As many as 50 steroids have been isolated from the mammalian adrenal gland. Included among them are progesterone, estrogen, and androgen, hormones usually considered as sex hormones. Because of the similarity in hormones produced, one would expect some overlapping of adrenocortical and gonadal functions.

The catecholamine-containing cells, usually referred to as the chromaffin cells on the basis of their staining reaction, are believed to represent modified postganglionic neurons. They originate from neural crest cells. They are probably under the control of the nervous system and secrete epinephrine or norepinephrine. These hormones function to maintain blood pressure, regulate carbohydrate metabolism, and help the body adjust to stressful situations.

If the adrenal glands are surgically removed, the animal dies within a few weeks. It is the cortex of the gland that is essential for life; its hormones regulate carbohydrate, protein, water, and electrolyte metabolism. Although a variety of functions are attributed to the cortical hormones, recent evidence suggests that the most basic mechanism involves the action of the hormone on the genome in relation to protein synthesis.

EXCRETORY SYSTEM
Function of excretory system

All vertebrate animals must take in nutrient materials. In the digestive tract these materials are broken down into small units that pass through the membranous lining of the gut and enter either capillaries or lymphatics. They eventually find their way to individual cells where they are metabolized and used for growth, maintenance, repair, or some specific activity of the cell, such as secretion. Many of the by-products of metabolism are more or less toxic to the organism and therefore must be eliminated. Carbohydrates and fats are broken down mainly to carbon dioxide and water. The carbon dioxide is removed from the body by the respiratory system. Nitrogenous wastes from protein metabolism compose the largest proportion of wastes, and these are usually excreted in the form of either ammonia (teleosts and crocodiles), urea (sharks, amphibians, aquatic turtles, and mammals) or uric acid (most reptiles and birds).

The regulation of the concentration of the constituents of the blood and body fluids is under the control of the paired *kidneys.* They function primarily to maintain a homeostatic state. As a result of their excretory function, they eliminate nitrogenous wastes, certain nonmetabolites, toxins from bacteria, and surplus water, as well as excessive amounts of certain other substances (such as glucose). These materials leave the body as *urine* and the desirable constituents of the blood and tissue fluids are retained at their optimum levels.

Several other structures of the body can be listed as auxiliary organs of excretion. Salt is excreted by the gills of some bony fishes, rectal glands of elasmobranchs, and the nasal glands of some marine reptiles and birds. The glands of the skin (mucous and sweat glands) also eliminate salt, a small amount of nitrogenous wastes, and water. Salivary glands, liver, intestine, and even the lungs are important organs in regulating the internal environment of the organism. The cells of the body can tolerate only narrow variations in this environment, with respect to ions, oxygen, carbon dioxide, metabolic products, pH, osmotic pressure, and nutrient supplies.

Since vertebrates have adapted to homes in saltwater and freshwater and on land, the problems of secretion and osmoregulation vary greatly from animal to animal. However, the basic morphologic and functional unit of the vertebrate kidney is the tiny *nephron* or *urinary tubule.* Although kidneys of the different classes vary in gross appearance and in location within the organisms, the principle upon which the kidney operates is the same in all vertebrates. It is fundamentally a filtering system. As a result of filtration, selective reabsorption, and secretion, especially in terrestrial animals, the urine that is finally excreted is typically much more concentrated than the blood or the original filtrate.

Because of these processes, the amounts of water and electrolytes leaving the body equal the amounts of these substances entering the body, and the internal environment is maintained in a constant, or homeostatic, state.

The kidney is also a site of enzyme and hormone production. It produces the proteolytic enzyme *renin,* which acts as a catalyst in the conversion of *angiotensinogen* (a blood protein) into *angiotensin.* Angiotensin causes arteriole constriction and thus an elevation in blood pressure. It also stimulates the adrenal to secrete aldosterone, the hormone involved in the regulation of salt balance. The application of fluorescent antibody technique indicates that granules identified as renin are present in the *juxtaglomerular cells,* located in the walls of the afferent arterioles of the glomerulus.

In the embryo, the kidney is a site of red blood cell production and in the adult it is believed to be the source of a hormone, *erythropoietin.* This protein stimulates the bone marrow to proliferate and release red blood cells into the circulatory system. Conflicting information does not allow a satisfactory resolution of the exact site in the kidney for its production at this time.

Embryology of excretory system

The urinary system develops earlier than does the reproductive system. Fig. 18-2 demonstrates this differential growth in a 4 mm. frog tadpole. For example, the genital ridge of the frog, located dorsal to the midgut, does not arise until the time of hatching. On the other hand, by the end of neurulation, the intermediate mesoderm on each side of the embryo, destined to give rise to uriniferous tubules, forms longitudinal ridges down the length of the animal. Present in all vertebrate embryos, this bilateral ridge is called the *nephrotomic plate,* or *cord.* When the epimere divides into segments, the divisions often extend to the mesomere; the nephrotomic plate also separates into serially arranged blocks of tissues, the *nephrotomes.* A nephrotome is capable of forming nephrons (kidney tubules) along its entire length, but local inductors control the specific type of tubule developed. Regardless of the kind of tubules present or their locations

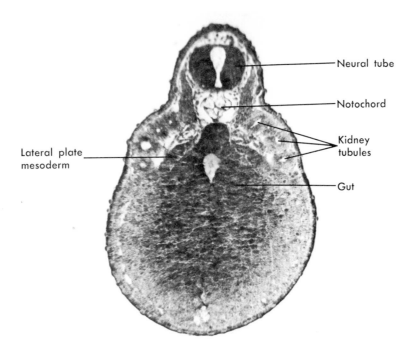

Neural tube

Notochord

Kidney tubules

Gut

Lateral plate mesoderm

Fig. 18-2
Transverse section of 4 mm. frog tadpole showing functional kidney tubules. The gonads do not make their appearance until about the time of hatching (6 mm. stage).

along the nephrotomic plate, the nephrons group together to form the nephros (a Greek word meaning 'kidney'). In some cases the nephrons are held together loosely by connective tissue, as in fishes, but in other animals, mammals, for example, the kidneys are quite compact structures.

Originally each nephrotome probably gave rise to a nephron, whose basic structure is diagrammed in Fig. 18-3. Fossil records of the oldest vertebrates, the ostracoderms, reveal imprints of such structures. In the early vertebrate embryo each anterior nephrotome forms a single nephron containing a cavity, the *nephrocoel,* that remains continuous with the coelom by way of the *peritoneal funnel.* A tube-shaped structure forms as an outgrowth from each nephrotome and extends laterally and dorsally. The cavity of each tubular outgrowth connects to the nephrocoel by way of the *nephrostome.* Lateral branches from the dorsal aorta grow into the medial area of the nephrotome and develop into tufts or coils of capillaries, the *glomeruli.*

Some biologists believe that in the ancestral

vertebrates, each tubule drained the body cavity and opened to the outside of the body as in most invertebrates (Wessells, 1974). In later forms, glomeruli evolved, the connection with the coelom was lost, and the tubules became separated from the surface of the body. A longitudinal duct developed from mesoderm and extended down the length of the embryo. Thereafter, each kidney tubule connected to the duct and emptied its contents into it, instead of directly to the outside by way of an excretory pore.

In some animals this nephric duct (Wolffian duct) forms by the distal ends of the individual tubules turning and growing posteriorly, eventually fusing with the tubule behind it. In other animals (such as elasmobranchs, chicks, and reptiles) the duct develops from the dorsolateral intermediate mesomere and differentiates independently. As a result of the distal growth of the duct, it eventually taps into the cloaca. The factors orienting the backward growth of the nephric duct to the cloaca are not understood, but both chemical attraction and contact guid-

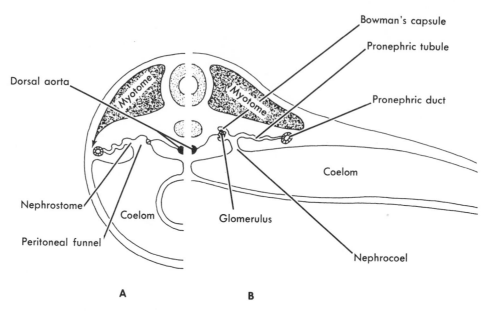

Fig. 18-3
Diagram of cross section through embryo of anamniote, **A,** and amniote, **B. A,** Glomerulus is considered external since branch of aorta pushes into side of coelom. **B,** Glomerulus is surrounded by Bowman's capsule and is referred to as internal. Most amniotes and anamniotes possess internal glomeruli.

ance have been offered as possible explanations. Regardless of the influences involved or its specific origin, an excretory duct forms and collects the urine of the tubules located along its length, transporting it to the cloaca.

Nephron, the basic unit

All nephrons consist of a *renal capsule* and a *convoluted tubule* that varies in length depending on the species (Fig. 18-4). The term "tubule" is used in two different ways. In a general way, it is synonymous with nephron and refers to the excretory unit. More precisely, it refers to the part of a nephron in which reabsorption and secretion occurs.

The proximal end of each nephron is composed of a compact mass of epithelial cells. A cleft within the mass produces a cup-like structure, *Bowman's capsule.* The inner layer of the capsule becomes closely associated with the cells that form the capillaries of the *glomerulus.* Bowman's capsule, together with the glomerulus, make up the *renal corpuscle.* The resistance to the outflow of blood from the glomerulus, pro-

duced by smaller vessels leaving the glomerulus than vessels bringing blood to it, causes the blood pressure in the glomerular capillaries to be higher than in the other capillaries of the body. Most of the liquid, along with the crystalloids and small molecules (under 60,000 mol. wt.), are filtered from the blood into Bowman's capsule. Only two thin layers of cells separate the lumen of the cuplike capsule from that of the capillary.

Large volumes of filtrate are removed from the circulation and collect in the capsule. The filtrate then passes into the lumen of the convoluted tubule, the cavity of which is continuous with the lumen of the capsule. Analysis of samples of this filtrate removed from the frog's kidney show all components of the blood present in the filtrate, with the exception of the blood cells and certain complex macromolecules. Many of the substances that pass into Bowman's capsule are needed by the animal and should not be eliminated. Consequently, as the filtrate moves through the kidney tubules, certain materials (salts and other valuable constituents such as

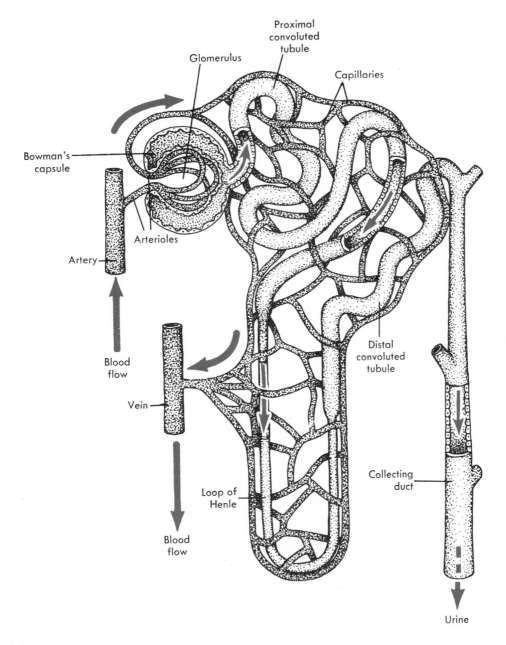

Fig. 18-4
Diagram showing a nephron of human kidney. See text for description. (From Berry, J. W., Osgood, D. W., St. John, P. A.: Chemical villains, St. Louis, 1974, The C. V. Mosby Co.)

glucose) are selectively absorbed back into the circulatory system. More substances are also lost into the lumen of the tubule from the network of capillaries surrounding the convoluted tubule.

The tubular portion of the nephron varies in length, with different segments performing different functions. It is usually possible to distinguish a *proximal* and *distal* portion, each consisting of a *convoluted* and *straight* segment. In mammals, an intermediate thin area, the *loop of Henle,* is located between the two convoluted segments, as illustrated in Fig. 18-4. The kidney tubules actively participate in excretion. The proximal tubules principally reabsorb water and glucose, and the distal tubules reabsorb salts.

Aldosterone, produced by the adrenal cortex controls the absorption of salts by the distal tubules, and the antidiuretic hormone released by the neuronal endings of the posterior gland regulates the water balance. Certain osmoreceptor cells of the hypothalamus react to variations in osmotic pressure of the plasma as the blood flows through the brain. These centers respond to their stimuli by making compensatory adjustments in the amount of vasopressin (antidiuretic hormone, ADH) released into the blood by the posterior pituitary gland. A typical neuroendocrine reflex, therefore, controls the secretion of ADH. When present, the hormone increases the permeability of the walls of the distal tubule and the collecting ducts to water. As a result, an increase in resorption of water occurs as the urine passes through the collecting ducts. If ADH is absent, the filtrate passes down the ducts unaltered and no concentration of urine occurs.

Since kidney function depends on filtration of blood, an adequate blood supply to the glomerulus is a necessity. In those animals that lack a glomerulus (for example, certain teleost fishes), a rich supply of blood vessels enmesh the tubules. In most lower animals, the blood supply to the glomerulus is arterial, but venous blood goes to the tubules; in higher animals, those with a metanephric kidney (see below), the vessels are, in general, arterial, with the renal portal system in reptiles and birds being only slightly functional. Cyclostomes and mammals are exceptions to the above since the blood supply to

the entire kidney is arterial. The kidney of certain teleosts, on the other hand, receive only a venous supply.

Although the nephrons are similar in all vertebrates, the different environments have obviously influenced the evolution of this filtering system. For example, animals that live in freshwater have blood and tissue fluids with a much higher osmotic pressure than their surrounding environment. Thus, the water will pass the semipermeable surfaces of the body by osmosis. The animal must have some means of controlling this excess water and preventing the dilution of its tissue fluids. As noted in Chapter 10, the bony armor of the primitive vertebrates has been considered by some to serve as a bony seal against this influx of water. The problems of marine animals, in which the osmotic pressure may be as high or higher than that of the tissues, and of terrestrial animals, where water must be conserved, are obviously different.

The system of simple kidney tubules by which large volumes of liquid can be collected is particularly efficient for freshwater animals. Such a kidney is found in all vertebrates, including the modern cyclostomes (Agnatha) as well as modern jawed animals (gnathostomes), and presumably indicates that such a kidney evolved before the jawed animals became distinct from the round-mouthed forms. If this is true, then the early ostracoderms also must have possessed this type of kidney. Many consider the large renal corpuscle the best indication that vertebrates evolved from animals that lived in freshwater. There are others, however, who argue that since the same type of kidney is present in some marine animals, then the ancestral vertebrate also possessed such a kidney and that this kidney became adapted to a freshwater environment.

Types of kidneys
Primitive kidney

The primitive plan described above of a series of segmentally arranged, similar tubules connected to a duct that opens into the cloaca, is referred to as the *holonephros* (holo-, 'whole') (Fig. 18-5). It is a hypothetical, idealized, ancestral kidney present in no known vertebrate.

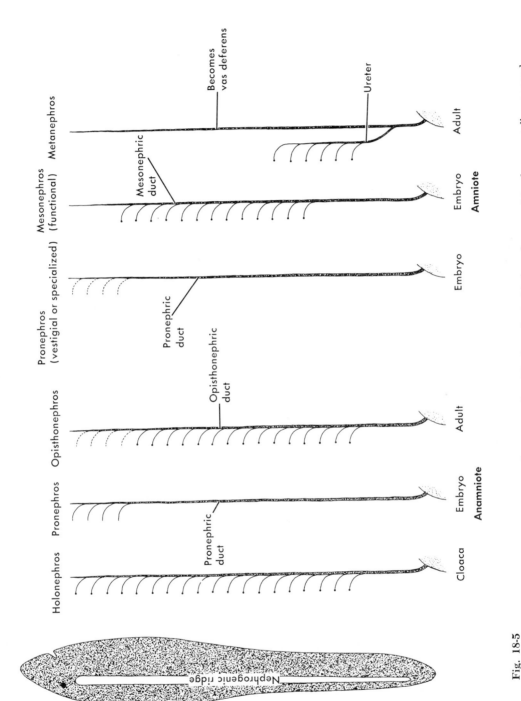

Fig. 18-5
Embryonic origin of kidney types from nephrogenic ridge. The hypothetical holonephros consists of segmentally arranged tubules along the entire ridge. The pronephros is functional in anamniote embryos but vestigial in most higher animals. In amniotes the metanephric kidney develops in the posterior region and the mesonephric duct becomes the sperm duct.

However, its existence is suggested in the kidneys of the larva of the myxinoid cyclostomes. In these embryos, the tubules are segmentally arranged, extending over about 70 segments. They open into a duct that runs the length of the kidney and empties into the cloaca. The anterior tubules lack glomeruli but open into the coelom. On the other hand, the posterior tubules possess glomeruli but lack peritoneal funnels.

Kidneys of anamniotes

This basic plan of the holonephros is modified in most vertebrates. The most consistent changes involve the loss of segmentation and the elimination of peritoneal funnels opening into the coelom. In most vertebrates, the tubules become grouped together into areas. The more anterior tubules function first and are the most primitive in structure. In lower animals the difference among the tubules along the length of the ridge is minimal, but there is a general evolutionary trend toward the utilization of more posterior tubules.

PRONEPHROS. The first tubules to form in the embryo of the fish and amphibian are collectively known as the pronephros, or "head kidney." This kidney consists of only a few nephrons, usually no more than five. Each one grows laterally and then turns posteriorly to fuse with the one behind it (as described above). The duct formed then continues to grow posteriorly until it reaches the cloaca. Since the tubules of the pronephric kidney empty their contents into the duct, it is known as the *pronephric duct.*

The nephrons of the pronephros function for various lengths of time in the embryos of most lower animals. In the hagfish and certain teleosts, the pronephros persists throughout the life of the animal. In the Chondrichthyes, they remain present but nonfunctional.

OPISTHONEPHROS. As the larva develops into an adult, tubules form from the remaining portion of the nephrogenic ridge and take over the excretory function. This type of kidney is referred to as the "back kidney," or *opisthonephros.* The nephrons that give rise to the pronephros, together with those from the opisthonephros, occupy the area of intermediate mesoderm orig-

inally associated with the hypothetical holonephros, as illustrated in Fig. 18-5.

The nephrons that compose the opisthonephros are slightly more complex than those of the pronephros. They arise in the same manner, but each segment may contain more than one nephron, and they usually lack peritoneal funnels. With the loss of access to the coelom, all waste materials must now enter the nephrons from the blood by way of the glomerulus. Fluids can no longer simply drain from the coelomic cavity into the nephrocoel and pass to the cloaca by way of the pronephric duct.

As the embryo develops into an adult, the pronephric tubules eventually degenerate, but their duct remains. The opisthonephric tubules do not form their own duct, but tap into this already present structure. Since it now drains the nephrons that compose the opisthonephric kidney (opisthonephros), the old pronephric duct usually becomes known as the *opisthonephric duct.*

The kidney shows a variety of shapes, ranging from the ribbonlike structure that extends the length of the body in elasmobranchs to the flat compact kidneys of the anurans. The kidney shape of fishes is extremely variable. In male sharks, the anterior portion is more narrow and has lost its excretory function. This portion of the opisthonephros degenerates in the female, but in the male some of the tubules make connection with the testis and take on a sexual function. In amphibians, a similar change in function occurs in the anterior portion of the male opisthonephros. We shall discuss in greater detail the appropriation of the excretory tubules for reproductive purposes when we consider the reproductive system later in the chapter.

Kidneys of amniotes

Despite their structural uniformity in birds, reptiles, and mammals, the succession of tubules are usually grouped for descriptive purposes into three types of kidneys: the *pronephros, mesonephros,* and *metanephros.* The designations of these kidneys depend on their locations along the nephrogenic ridge. The mesonephros and metanephros form from the area designated in

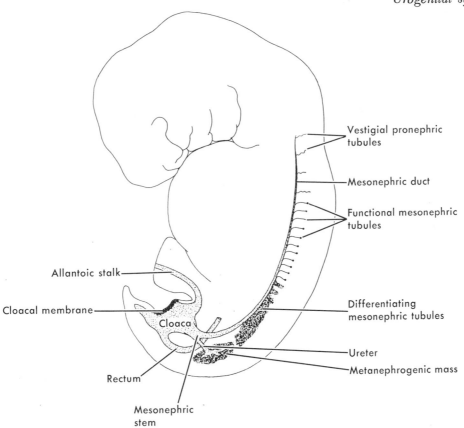

Vestigial pronephric tubules

Mesonephric duct

Functional mesonephric tubules

Allantoic stalk

Differentiating mesonephric tubules

Cloacal membrane

Cloaca

Ureter

Metanephrogenic mass

Rectum

Mesonephric stem

Fig. 18-6
Diagrammatic sagittal section through mammalian embryo showing location of three types of kidneys.

the lower forms as the opisthonephros: the mesonephros (midkidney) derives from the anterior part, and the metanephros develops from the posterior regions, as illustrated in Fig. 18-6. The pronephros and mesonephros function only in the embryo; the metanephros becomes the permanent kidney of adult amniotes. A solid rod splits off from the nephrogenic cord, hollows out, and becomes the nephric duct, usually referred to as the Wolffian duct. Pronephric tubules (if functional) empty into this duct and later, mesonephric tubules also connect to it. In the mammalian adult, the Wolffian duct becomes the ductus deferens.

PRONEPHROS. Actually the pronephros in many amniotes, including man, is a vestigial nonfunctional organ. Several transient condensations of intermediate mesodermal cells form in the cervical region of the human. These clusters of cells

never develop glomeruli or make contact with a nephric duct. In fact, the most cranial of the condensations degenerates before the more caudal vesicles form. However, the presence of even this abortive pronephros in these forms is significant because it represents the remnants of ancestral developmental patterns and demonstrates once again, the conservative nature of the developmental processes.

MESONEPHROS. The mesonephros is considered the functional excretory organ of the embryos of reptiles, birds, and mammals. It has no opening into the coelomic cavity. In general, it is larger than the pronephros but ranges from an almost rudimentary organ in the rat to a huge structure that projects from the coelom wall in the fetal pig, as shown in Figs. 18-7 and 18-10. Its tubules empty into the mesonephric duct.

There may be a correlation between the type

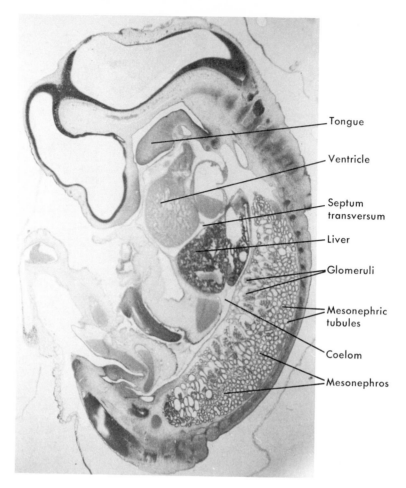

Tongue

Ventricle

Septum transversum

Liver

Glomeruli

Mesonephric tubules

Coelom

Mesonephros

Fig. 18-7
Sagittal section of a 20 mm. pig embryo showing the large mesonephros extending about half the length of the body. Note glomeruli and tubules. (× 4.)

of placentation and the degree of mesonephric development. The pig has a loose, epitheliochorial type of placenta (see Chapter 9) and a well-developed mesonephros. Both the rodents and primates (including man) have the more intimate hemochorial type of placenta and a poorly developed mesonephros. Such a relationship suggests that the intimately structured placenta is able to assume much of the excretory function for the embryo. Whether this is actually true remains to be established.

METANEPHROS. The mesonephros is actively excreting at the time the metanephros forms. The *metanephros* resembles the mesonephros in that it consists of a group of excretory tubules that empty into a collecting duct. Unlike the other types of kidneys, it has a dual origin. A secretory unit and a collecting unit develop separately and then are assembled to form the definitive uriniferous tubules of the metanephros, as illustrated in Fig. 18-8. A new duct, the *ureter*, carries urine from the kidney to the bladder. The old mesonephric duct becomes the sperm duct.

A ureteric bud arises as a diverticulum of the mesonephric duct near its entrance into the cloaca. This bud pushes dorsally into the posterior region of the nephrogenic cord and gives rise to the *ureter*; then the cranial end of the bud enlarges and forms a funnel-shaped struc-

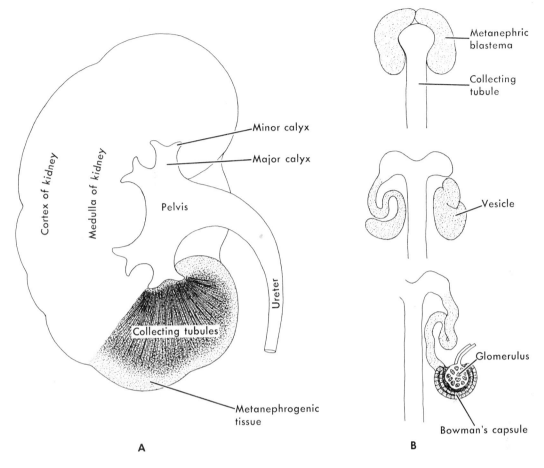

Fig. 18-8

Diagram showing contributions of ureteric bud, **A,** and metanephric blastema, **B,** to amniote kidney. The vesicles unite with the collecting tubules to form the convoluted nephrons.

ture, the *primitive pelvis.* The pelvis is the collecting chamber of the kidney and contains the *renal sinus,* a cavity that is continuous with the lumen of the ureter.

The expanded end of the ureteric bud becomes divided to form several outpocketings, the *major calyces.* These chambers, in turn, give rise to several smaller evaginations, the *minor calyces,* which project into the kidney substance. *Straight collecting tubules,* also derived from the ureteric bud, grow out from the minor calyces. These collecting tubules are grouped together to form 8 to 18 fan-shaped *renal pyramids.* As shown in Fig. 18-9, the bases of the pyramids are toward the outer surface of the kidney and their apices

face the renal pelvis. Several of the collecting tubules composing the pyramids merge at the apex to form *papillary ducts.* Urine collected in these ducts empties into the minor calyces and then into the major calyces and on to the pelvis of the kidney.

The expanded end of the ureteric bud grows into the condensed mass of nephrogenic tissue. The cells in this area of the nephrogenic ridge separate from the more anterior regions and cluster around the end of the ureteric bud as the *metanephric blastema.* The blastema forms a cap about the pelvic dilatation and differentiates into the excretory parts of the kidney, the nephrons. There must be interaction between blas-

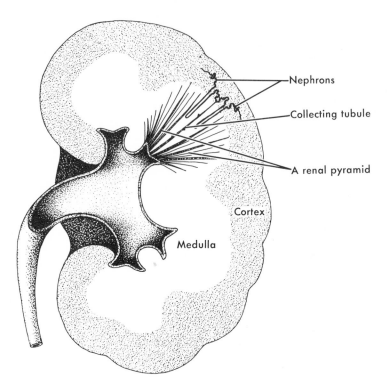

Fig. 18-9
Hemisected adult human kidney showing location of one pyramid and two nephrons in cortex emptying into one collecting tubule.

tema and ureteric bud before normal development can follow. Only when in contact with one another do the collecting tubules and the excretory part of the kidney develop properly. If separated and grown in tissue culture, neither component differentiates. If, for some reason, the ureteric bud fails to reach the metanephric ridge on one side of the animal, metanephric tubules do not develop on that side.

Under normal conditions, the concentration of mesodermal cells associated with the terminal ends of each collecting tubule arrange themselves into a hollow pear-shaped vesicle (Fig. 18-8, *B*). The vesicle develops an S-shaped tubule, makes contact with the collecting tubule, and fuses with it. Blood vessels invade the ends of the S-shaped structure, forming a glomerulus. Growth occurs by an increase in the length of the tubule between two fixed points: the glomerulus and the entrance of the nephron into

the collecting tubule. As a result of this growth, the nephron differentiates into a proximal, distal, and middle portion described above.

The metanephric kidney is usually more compact than are the other types. However, it may range from the extended kidney of snakes to the elongated and lobulated organ of birds and certain cattle. The human kidney is a bean-shaped structure. As shown in Fig. 18-9, the ureter, the large excretory duct that carries urine to the bladder, leaves the kidney at a deep concavity, the *hilus*. It is here also that the renal artery enters and the renal vein leaves the kidney. If a kidney is hemisected, it can be divided grossly into a darker outer *cortex* and a lighter, more centrally located *medulla*. The medulla is made up of the renal pyramids, the fan-shaped regions with papillae opening into the minor calyces. The loops of Henle present in the mammals and some birds are also located in the medulla. The

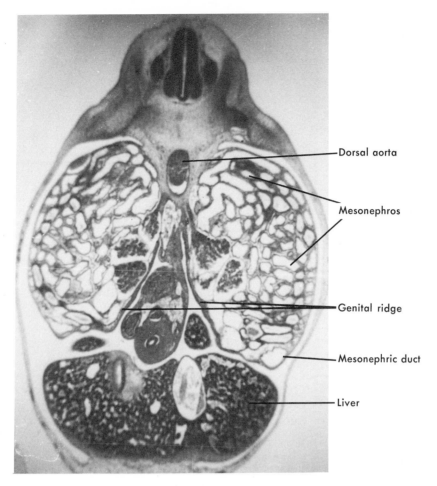

Dorsal aorta

Mesonephros

Genital ridge

Mesonephric duct

Liver

Fig. 18-10
Cross section of 10 mm. pig embryo showing genital ridge.

excretory part of the kidney is located in the cortex and, according to *Gray's Anatomy,* is composed of over a million nephrons.

Urinary bladder

With the exception of fishes, birds, and some reptiles, urinary bladders collect the urine before it is voided. This chamber is typically a sac-like structure with thin muscular walls. In some animals (humans excepted) further processing of the urine may take place in these reservoirs. For example, in reptiles and amphibians, not only is water stored but also urinary sodium is absorbed back into the blood.

In some teleosts and ganoid fish, diverticula from the caudal ends of the mesonephric ducts form these reservoirs. Such bladders, therefore, are of mesodermal origin. However, in most tetrapods the urinary bladder is a ventral diverticulum of the cloaca and is lined with endoderm. It forms at metamorphosis in the frog and has no direct connection to the urogenital ducts. Urine released into the cloaca from the opisthonephric ducts "backs up" into the urinary bladder for temporary storage. It is then released from the body by way of the cloacal opening.

The allantois of amniotes serves as a respiratory organ in the embryo, but in the adult a portion of it remains as the urinary bladder. Although bird embryos have a large allantois, there is no urinary bladder in the adult stage. Snakes and crocodiles also lack urinary bladders. In these animals the urine flows into the cloaca from the metanephric ducts and is then voided by way of the cloacal orifice.

In adult mammals, urorectal folds divide the cloacal chamber into a dorsorectal region and a ventral region containing the allantoic diverticulum. The common mesonephric stem, with its metanephric duct, becomes incorporated into the walls of the bladder. As the bladder enlarges, it engulfs the mesonephric stem; the two mesonephric and two metanephric ducts now enter the bladder at different points. The metanephric duct (ureter) shifts its position and enters the proximal part of the allantois. The mesonephric duct degenerates in adult females. In males, it becomes the ductus deferens and enters the urethra just below the neck of the bladder (see Fig. 18-13, *C*). The bladder releases the urine by way of the *urethra,* a modification of the cloaca.

REPRODUCTIVE SYSTEM

The reproductive system of adult vertebrates was discussed in Chapter 3. Before beginning our study of the individual's development, we needed to know something of the male and female parents. The organs capable of producing the egg and sperm were described as well as the ducts that transported the generative cells to the outside. We noted that hormones not only control the reproductive cycles, ensuring the growth, maturation, and release of the gametes, but they also control the behavior of the animals as well, making sexual reproduction possible. The fusion of the egg and sperm sets in motion a series of orderly, sequential events that ultimately lead to the establishment of a new individual.

Morphogenesis is the story of the specific unfolding of these events; it relates how the basic conditions of the organ systems present in the embryonic body form are rearranged and transformed into adult structures. We discussed a remarkable number of common features that are displayed in the developmental processes and in the organs established. Many of the systems show little variation among the members of the different classes. Basic units adapted for the specific needs of the animal compose many of the organs.

In the present chapter we shall see how the reproductive system originates in the embryo and thereby conclude our survey of the vertebrate systems. We have carried our story to a logical conclusion. The egg has developed into an individual capable of reproducing itself. As we study the reproductive system, here also, we shall find a basic plan unfolding that gives rise to similar structures among the various adult vertebrate animals.

Embryonic origin of genital system
Indifferent stage

There is a period in vertebrate development when all embryos pass through a sexually undifferentiated stage, although the sex of the individual was determined genetically at the time the zygote formed. All the morphological structures (gonads, ducts, and external genitalia) necessary for the development of either sex are present. This stage of vertebrate sexual development in which male and female embryos cannot be distinguished from one another is described as the *indifferent stage.* Cyclostomes and teleosts may remain in the indifferent stage until sexual maturity, at which time they differentiate into males or females. This bisexual stage of development lasts through the larval stage in frogs (a year or more), through the sixth day of incubation in chickens, and as long as the sixth or seventh week in human embryos. In some vertebrates, the indifferent stage continues to adulthood. For example, certain teleosts develop into hermaphrodites with functional ovotestes; such gonads have functional follicles and seminiferous tubules in the same organ. As one might expect, opportunities for sex reversals are greatest among those animals in which the indifferent stage is of longest duration.

The rudimentary gonad consists of structural units, the cortex and the medulla, and the germ cells, which arise independently of the presumptive gonadal tissue. The lateral plate mesoderm and the intermediate mesoderm give rise to the cortex and medulla. The germ cells, which are also bipotential at this stage of development, are believed to form outside the region and migrate into it, as discussed in Chapter 4. As the embryo leaves the indifferent stage and develops in the male or female direction, a competition ensues between the medulla and cortex, resulting in one of these regions of the rudimentary gonad predominating over the other. The cortex will dominate the gonad if it is to become an ovary; the medulla gives rise to a testis. In a few cases, to be discussed later, and in some teleosts mentioned above, both cortex and medulla continue to develop, producing a functioning ovotestis.

The embryo in the indifferent stage of sexual development not only has gonads that are sexless and bipotential primordial germ cells, but it also possesses both female and male gamete-transport systems. The primordia of both the oviduct and the Wolffian duct develop. As the embryo passes into the definitive stage, one of the ducts differentiates and the other remains rudimentary or regresses. For example, the oviduct may be seen as a vestigial structure in some adult male sharks and amphibians. The external genitalia also reflect the bisexual stage, and structures develop that can differentiate into either the male or female sex organs. The young vertebrate embryo has the potentiality of becoming either sex.

Sex determination and differentiation

SEX DETERMINATION. Each individual inherits both autosomes (somatic chromosomes) and sex chromosomes: sex is controlled by the total genome. Genetic dissymmetry is responsible for sex determination, in that one parent is homogametic (forming one type of gamete) and the other heterogametic (with two types of gametes). The types of gametes that get together at fertilization determine the genetic sex of the individual.

In many species, including man, it is the female that is homogametic. The single chromosome that is either paired with its same type or with a different morphological type is designated as the X chromosome, and the different type is the Y chromosome. The females of these species are usually said to be XX. The males are XY, with Y chromosomes varying in size from much larger than the X chromosome to much smaller, or even absent. At meiosis when the gametes are formed, each egg receives an X chromosome and one member of each pair of autosomal chromosomes. However, in the male, half of the sperm will receive an X chromosome and half will receive a Y chromosome. At fertilization the chance combination of XX will produce a genetic female, but an XY yields a male. In other vertebrates (such as certain fish, amphibians, and birds), the females are heterogametic and it is the males that are homogametic. In these cases, instead of assigning an X to the accessory chromosome of the male, some investigators for clarity use Z as their symbol and W instead of Y; others continue to use X and Y. Males, therefore, are ZZ and females, ZW.

All vertebrate animals possess both masculinizing and feminizing genes. However, each animal contains more of one than of the other, thereby dictating the direction it will take in sexual differentiation. The present concept of sex determination involves more than a single chromosome difference; it includes the balance among all the chromosomes in the haploid set. No one gene determines sex by itself. Goldschmidt (1955) suggested that all animals contained both male and female sex determiners and that one of the sex determiners was located on the X chromosome and one on an autosome. Sex was determined by a balance between the two kinds of sex determiners and could result in maleness, femaleness, or intersexuality. According to some investigators, the function of the double X or Z genes is to counteract the opposite influence of the autosomal genes, something that apparently the single X or Z is unable to accomplish.

SEX DIFFERENTIATION. Although the individual's sex is determined at the time of fertilization, all vertebrate embryos first form the bisexual stage. The two competing or antagonistic fields, the cortical and the medullary, are formed in the gonads of most vertebrates, and one becomes dominant over the other. Sex differentiation is a competitive process in which the establishment of this dominance occurs during and after the indifferent stage. It is responsible for the animal's developing in one direction. Intersexes occur when one of the fields establishes only partial dominance. The male toad is an example of medullary dominance. At the anterior end of the toad's testis is a structure, Bidder's organ, composed of suppressed cortical material. If the toad's testes, and presumably the medullary influence, are removed, the animal reverses its sex, and Bidder's organ develops into an ovary capable of producing fertile eggs.

Under normal circumstances, the left ovary of the hen becomes functional and the right remains vestigial. However, the right ovary consists of a great deal of medullary material. Surgical removal of the left ovary causes the right gonad to develop into a *testis*. There are records of chickens who for the first part of their lives laid eggs and demonstrated all the female characteristics. Later they developed into males, complete with combs and wattles of the male and were able to fertilize eggs.

In nature, such factors as environment, hormones, and nutritional levels affect the sexual balance, and individuals that start out as one sex can be influenced in the direction of the opposite sex. Among lower animals sex reversals are common. Low temperature encourages amphibian larvae to differentiate in the female direction, but higher temperatures result in the production of more males. The fact that in amphibians the indifferent stage is a lengthy one offers greater opportunity for the medulla and cortex to continue to develop with neither regressing, or for the cortex to develop for part of the time and then regress, with the medulla taking over. Witchi (1956) describes experiments with two frogs with ovotestes in which the medulla was composed of seminiferous tubules with sperm and the cortex contained ova. According to him, fertile eggs and sperm were obtained from the same individual and by means of artificial insemination they produced normal offspring.

Hormones affect the differentiation of sex in mammalian embryos as illustrated by the famous *freemartin*. The freemartin is an intersexed female calf whose twin is a normal male, but never another female. The female twin has the female type of external genitalia; she may have both oviducts and sperm ducts, and ovaries lacking in cortical development, but with some medullary tubules present. She is always sterile. Lillie (1916) attempted to relate her condition to the fact that male gonads develop earlier than do female ones. The testes produce androgenic hormones, which pass by way of fused placentas (and therefore bloodstreams) from the male to the female twin and affect her sexual development. This epoch-making research focused attention on the relationship between fetal sex hormones and sex differentiation.

Since the primordial germ cells contain the same chromosomes as other cells, it is logical to assume that they would be genetically oriented toward male or female as are other cells of the body. However, they appear to be bisexual and develop into ova or sperm depending on their location in the cortex or medulla of the gonad. Primordial germ cells that wander about and get lost in the embryo are unable to develop further, and thus they degenerate. They must reach either the cortex or the medulla where, regardless of their genotype (ZZ, ZW, WW, XX, XY, or YY) they are induced to develop further in a specific direction. The genetic nature of the gonadal primordium ensures its differentiation into either a testis or an ovary and sets up inductive territories in which one will predominate over the other. The specific inductive field, that is, masculinizing or feminizing, in which the primordial germ cells come to rest, will control their differentiation.

An example of the influence of the field on primordial cell differentiation has been demonstrated by Burns (1961), who induced gonadal reversal in a mammalian embryo. The young of the opossum are born at the bisexual stage, around 13 days, and then crawl into the marsupial pouch where they complete their development. Burns administered estradiol to the young while they were attached to the nipples of the mammary gland, and it induced cortical development in the male gonads. As a result of the cortical proliferation, the testes became ovotestes or, in some cases, normal ovaries. The primordial germ cells located in the cortex differentiated into oocytes instead of spermatocytes, the normal gamete that would have developed had the steroid hormone not been administered.

Individuals that have both male and female generative organs present in the same individual are considered *hermaphrodites.* The hermaphroditic condition may be caused by an abnormal genic balance between the sex and somatic chromosomes that control the functional state of the cortical or medullary components. Although many invertebrates are hermaphrodites, and some fishes can produce both sperm and eggs, the majority of vertebrates are either male or female. The condition occurs rarely in man. Only about 100 cases of true hermaphroditism have been reported in which individuals possessed both an ovary and a testis, two ovotestes, or a normal gonad and an ovotestis. These individuals were sterile. The external genitalia and secondary sex characteristics are usually intermediate between male and female. A condition known as *false hermaphroditism* is more common. In this case an individual has the gonads of one sex, but the secondary sex characteristics and external genitalia resemble the opposite sex, or are indeterminate.

Gonadal development

INDIFFERENT STAGE. The gonads of most vertebrates are paired; those with only one gonad represent a fusion of the paired structure or the degeneration of one side. The development of the gonads is intimately related to the nephric system and the male actually incorporates some of the anterior nephric tubules as the efferent ductules. The gonadal primordia of vertebrate animals first appear as thickenings or ridges of the epithelium on the dorsal surface of the body cavity. These ridges are located on both sides of the dorsal mesentery, medial to the developing kidney, and can be seen in the 10 mm. fetal pig (Fig. 18-10). This epithelial thickening, known as the *genital* or *germinal ridge,* runs longitudinally the length of the embryo and initially is much longer than the actual organ will be. The ridge consists of an epithelial layer derived from the lateral plate mesoderm, covering a mesenchyme core. This epithelial layer is continuous with the peritoneum that lines the coelomic cavity. In the region of the ridge the cells are taller than the neighboring ones and are known by the more specific name of *germinal epithelium.* There is general agreement that this

layer gives rise to the sex cords of the gonads, but whether it contributes to the primordial germ cells remains controversial (see Chapter 4).

The cells composing the ridge proliferate and migrate into the mesenchymal stroma (framework) of the area. These compact strands of cells are referred to as "sex cords" in most vertebrates and make up the medulla of the developing gonad, as illustrated in Fig. 18-11, *A* and *B.* As the *primary sex cords* move inward, they are joined by the primordial germ cells. The genital ridge bulges into the coelomic cavity as the cells proliferate. A peritoneal support that becomes the mesorchium of the testis or the mesovarium of the ovary suspends the bulging gonadal primordium in the coelomic cavity. The structure formed, consisting of germinal epithelium, sex cords, mesenchyme, and primordial germ cells, composes the *gonad of the indifferent stage.*

TESTICULAR DEVELOPMENT. If the gonad is destined to become a testis, the medulla of the indifferent gonad becomes the predominant structure, and the cortex involutes. This relationship is depicted in Fig. 18-11, *C.* The germinal epithelium flattens and loses its ability to undergo mitosis. As the primary sex cords continue to grow, they form elongated masses that twist upon themselves and anastomose with adjoining cords. They eventually differentiate into tubular structures, forming seminal tubules, rete testis, and efferent ductules. Mesenchyme condenses to form the fibrous *tunica albuginea,* which inserts itself between the outer flattened germinal epithelium and the inner mass of cords. It develops into a tough, capsule-like structure. Some of the mesenchyme cells condense and form septa that radiate inward from the capsule, partitioning the testis into lobules. In the human embryo this occurs around the eighth week of gestation.

Blood vessels follow the tunica albuginea and form a network over the gonad. As the tubules develop from the sex cords, the mesenchyme that originally formed the framework of the testis also wraps around each tubule, giving rise to a basement membrane. The primordial germ cells take up a location near this membrane and become the *spermatogonia. Interstitial cells* ap-

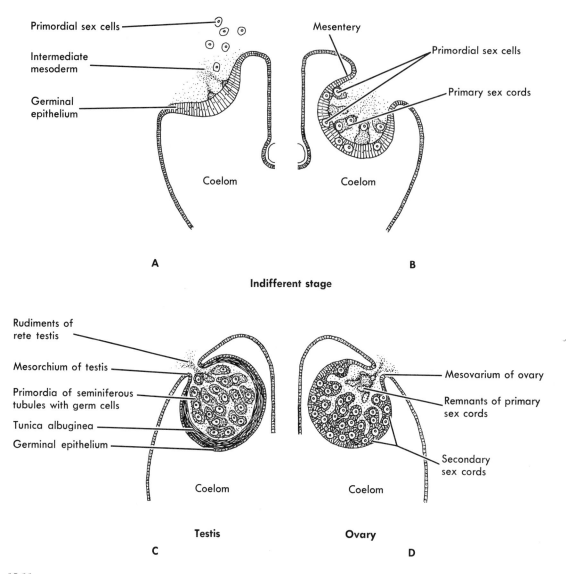

Fig. 18-11

Diagrams showing development of the gonads. In the indifferent stage, germinal epithelium gives rise to primary sex cords, **A.** Later, the sex cells migrate into the sex cords, **B.** Primary sex cords give rise to seminiferous tubules of testis, **C,** but regress in the ovary. Secondary sex cords form and contribute to the primary follicles, **D.**

pear between the tubules and, in the human embryo, proliferate to such a degree that at the time of birth their bulk equals that of the tubules.

The anterior nephrons of the kidney lose their urinary function, as more posterior tubules develop. The anterior ones are incorporated into the male reproductive system as shown in Fig. 18-12. Mesenchyme tissue condenses at the proximal

end of the seminiferous tubules forming the channels of the *rete testis.* The seminiferous tubules converge and join the rete testis, which, in turn, fuses with the anterior tubules of the kidney. These tubules, formerly a part of the urinary system, now become the *efferent ductules.* They connect the *rete testis* with the anterior part of the nephric duct (Wolffian) that becomes the *epididymis* (Fig. 18-12, *B*).

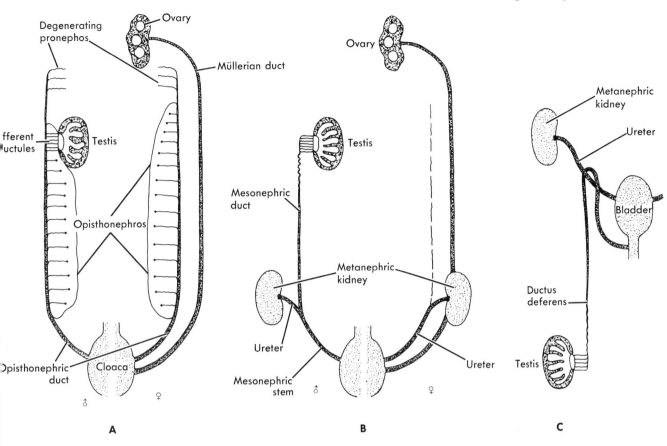

Fig. 18-12
Diagram of male and female urogenital ducts in adult anamniote, **A,** adult amniote with exception of male mammal, **B,** and adult male mammal, **C.**

The remaining part of the opisthonephric duct becomes the sperm duct, as well as the urinary duct in those animals below the amniotes. In higher animals (reptiles, birds, and mammals) the mesonephric duct carries only sperm and is referred to as the *ductus deferens*. The sex cords remain more or less solid until about the time of puberty when cavities appear and coalesce, forming hollow tubules that lead from the seminiferous tubules to the ductus deferens. A continuous system is thus formed in which the processes of spermiogenesis, spermiation, and sperm transport are carried out as described for the adult male in Chapter 3.

OVARIAN DEVELOPMENT. The ovaries of female vertebrates form later in the embryo than do the male testes. They originate, however, from the same primordia. If the gonad is to become an ovary, the medulla does not grow further but remains rudimentary. Instead, the primary sex cords and germ cells located in this region degenerate and are absorbed. Loose mesenchyme fills the area and forms a framework for blood vessels, lymphatics, and nerves. In frogs, for example, cavities form in the medulla and the ovary is converted to a sac-like structure.

The germinal epithelium becomes active again and the cortex dominates the structure as indicated in Fig. 18-11, *D.* A second wave of cells are proliferated, but these *secondary sex cords* break up into isolated masses in the cortex. Some of the cells cluster around the primordial germ cells, forming primary follicles. These small follicles are located in the cortex of the ovary and appear as early as the third month of gestation in the gonad of the human female. They will not differentiate further until the individual reaches puberty. At birth, connective-tissue septa divide the cortex into areas. The germinal epithelium is reduced to a single layer of cells.

Development of ducts

Both oviducts and sperm ducts develop in the vertebrate embryo (with the exception of some fish), although only one of the transport systems remain functional in the adult. The male appropriates part of the nephric tubules and the urinary duct as a sperm-conducting system, and no new structures develop. To transport ova, on the other hand, a second pair of ducts, the *müllerian ducts,* form usually as new structures in both sexes of vertebrates. These later develop into the *oviducts.* In a few animals (sharks for example) the müllerian ducts apparently split off from the opisthonephric ducts. However, they typically develop as bilaterally located grooves in the thickened epithelium of the genital ridge, after the urinary duct appears. When formed in this manner, the müllerian ducts are completely independent of the nephric ducts. The grooves continue caudally as bilateral tubes; the anterior ends of each tube (duct) remain open to the coelom by a funnel-shaped ostium. The two ostia, along with those few anterior pronephric tubules that open into the coelom of some vertebrates, are the only perforations of the coelomic wall. All other structures are covered by a continuous coat of peritoneum.

In lower animals the müllerian ducts grow in a caudal direction, retroperitoneally, along the side of the nephric duct until they reach and join the cloaca (see Fig. 18-12, *A*). The cloaca is modified in mammals and the paired ducts move to the midline where they fuse. This fusion forms the primordia of the uterus and vagina. The cranial parts remain separated as the uterine tubes.

The development of the accessory ducts and glands of the male apparently depends on the presence of a testis. If the testes are removed from a male rabbit fetus in utero at the indifferent stage (19 days), when both oviducts and sperm ducts are present, the sperm duct degenerates, but the oviduct continues its development. Also, if the fetus is castrated, no male accessory structures develop and the external genitalia are of the female type. On the other hand, the oviducts and genitalia appear to be independent of the ovary, since if the ovaries are removed at this time, they continue to develop in the female direction. In the mammal, therefore, it appears that the presence of the testis stimulates the establishment of male structures (sperm duct, accessory glands, and external genitalia) and suppresses female structures (oviduct and genitalia). The opposite appears to be true for birds, in that anything that does not stimulate the cortex allows the medulla to become predominant, resulting in a male.

Modification of cloaca and external genitalia
Differentiation of cloaca

All vertebrate embryos have a ventral chamber or pocket, the *cloaca,* into which the intestine and the urogenital ducts open, and which, in turn, communicates with the outside. This chamber remains in the adults of most vertebrates, with the exception of certain teleosts and ganoid fishes and the higher mammals. A movement toward a separation of urogenital functions occurred during premammalian evolution. Although the prototheria retain a cloaca, it is partitioned in most adult theria. The intestine, gonadal ducts, and urinary ducts open separately to the outside in the female mammal, but in the male, the urethra functions for both urinary and genital systems. Development of the external genitalia is associated with the structural changes in the cloaca.

In the indifferent stage of mammalian development, the intestine, the oviducts, and the allantois open into the cloaca, which at this time is nothing more than an expansion of the hindgut. It is, therefore, of endodermal origin. The mesonephric duct, with its ureteric (metanephric) bud, enters the base of the allantois. As described in Chapter 13, in this region there is an inpocketing of the skin ectoderm that gives rise to the *proctodeum.* A membrane forms, the *cloacal,* or *proctodeal, membrane,* that separates the endodermal chamber of the cloaca from the outside. This is illustrated in Fig. 18-13, *A*.

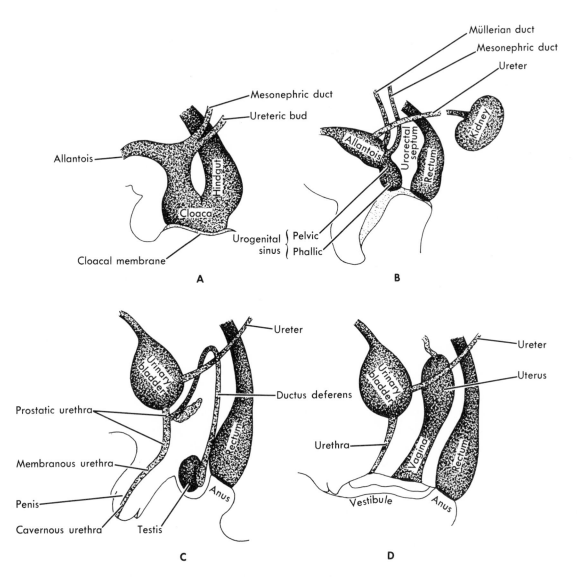

Fig. 18-13
Partitioning of mammalian cloaca. In the early embryo, **A,** the urorectal septum divides the cloaca into a rectum and urogenital sinus, **B.** Structures of the indifferent stage differentiate into adult male, **C,** or adult female, **D.**

Later in the indifferent stage of a human embryo, a urorectal septum develops (Fig. 18-13, *B*) and extends to the proctodeal membrane and divides the cloaca into two parts: a dorsal *rectum* associated with the intestine and a ventral *urogenital sinus* into which open the urinary and genital ducts and the allantoic stalk. The allantoic stalk further differentiates into the *urinary bladder* and a long narrow portion, the

future adult *urethra.* The urethra connects the urinary bladder with the outside. The common stem of the paired ureters (metanephric ducts) and the Wolffian (mesonephric) ducts also become incorporated into the allantoic stalk. As described earlier in this chapter, the growth of the bladder occurs in such a way that it absorbs the urogenital "stems." The ureter and Wolffian ducts thus eventually become separated from one another and enter the bladder through different openings, the ureters into the side of the bladder and the Wolffian duct at the neck of the bladder. The Wolffian duct is usually referred to as the *ductus deferens* in the adult mammal.

By the end of the indifferent stage, the alimentary tract is completely separated from the urogenital system; the oviducts and the urethra empty into the urogenital sinus; and the ureters and ductus deferens have become associated with the base of the allantois.

Once the urorectal fold contacts the ectoderm, the cloacal membrane (ectodermal-endodermal plate) ruptures, forming an anal opening to the outside from the rectum and one from the urogenital sinus. The urogenital sinus differentiates into two regions, the pelvic region, the upper end of which is delineated by the common urogenital stems, and a more distal phallic portion (Fig. 18-13, *B*).

As the female mammalian embryo develops past the indifferent stage, the portion between the allantois and the urogenital sinus elongates and forms the urethra of the adult animal (Fig. 18-13, *D*). The pelvic and phallic areas of the urogenital sinus become the shallow *vestibule* into which the urinary and genital products pass.

The urethra of the adult male forms in the same manner but is a longer canal than that in the female. It differentiates into a prostatic, membranous, and cavernous urethra (Fig. 18-13, *C*). The prostatic urethra is a counterpart of the entire female urethra, the original short tube between the bladder and the urogenital sinus. The pelvic part of the urogenital sinus in the male contributes to the rest of the prostatic urethra and all of the membranous urethra. The phallic portion of the urogenital sinus gives rise to the cavernous urethra, which extends into the male genital tubercle, the forerunner of the penis. Since the male and female urethras receive different embryonic contributions in the construction of the adult organ, they are not considered to be entirely homologous structures. Only the male prostatic urethra is homologous with the female urethra. The prostate and bulbourethral glands arise from endodermal outgrowths of urethral epithelium. The seminal vesicles, on the other hand, are outpocketings from the ductus deferens, and are of mesodermal origin.

Differentiation of external genitalia

External genitalia differentiate in those vertebrates in which fertilization is internal. In the mammalian embryo the appearance of certain structures parallel the modification of the cloaca. An elevation known as the *genital eminence* develops in the midline of very young embryos and ultimately gives rise to either the male or female genitals. Since these structures have the same embryonic origin, they are considered to be homologous with one another. The genital eminence differentiates into structures shown in Fig. 18-14: a phallus, or *genital tubercle*, located just anterior to the opening into the urogenital sinus; a pair of *genital folds* flanking the sinus; and the *genital swellings* lateral to the folds. At this stage, the urogenital sinus is anterior to the anus and separated from it by the urorectal folds. These structures are present during the indifferent stage of development and the young appear sexless. The hormones produced by the differentiating gonads are responsible for bringing about further changes (in either the male or female direction). At the end of the indifferent stage, the external genitalia of the mammalian male develop into the copulatory organs; few profound changes occur in the female.

MALE EXTERNAL GENITALIA. If the embryo is to become a male, several changes are initiated, as outlined in Fig. 18-14, *B*. The genital tubercle becomes the *penis*, the genital folds surround the penis to form the *prepuce*, and the genital swellings increase in size and give rise to the scrotal sacs. As the penis elongates, a groove that extends its length is formed on the caudal surface and is continuous with the more proximal slitlike urogenital sinus, as may be noted in the diagram. The margins of the groove, as well as the edges of the urogenital sinus, fold together and eventually fuse, forming a *raphe*, a ridgelike thickening down the length of the penis. As a result, a small tubular cavity is formed, the *penile urethra*, which extends the length of the penis. The penile urethra is con-

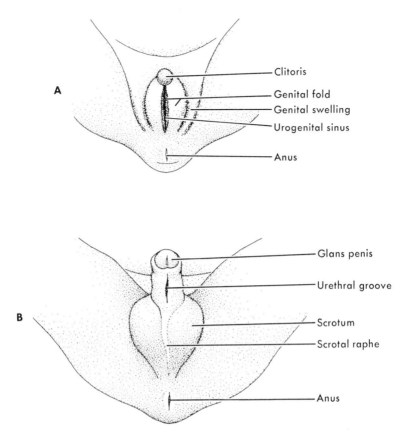

Fig. 18-14
Development of external genitalia in human fetus diverges from common indifferent stage and differentiates in either the female, **A,** or male, **B,** direction. The genital tubercle becomes either the clitoris or the glans penis, the genital folds become either the labia minora or the prepuce of penis, and the genital swellings give rise to the labia majora of the adult female or scrotal sacs of the adult male.

tinuous with that portion of the urethra that develops from the urogenital sinus between the neck of the bladder and the original opening of the urogenital sinus, now considered to be the prostatic urethra. As a result of these developments in the adult male mammal, sperm and urine are discharged through a continuous channel and expelled through the urogenital orifice at the tip of the penis. This channel consists of the prostatic urethra, which is homologous with the female urethra, a middle portion comparable to the female vestibule, plus the additional penile urethra formed by the fusion of the urethral groove and for which there is no counterpart in the female.

FEMALE EXTERNAL GENITALIA. If the animal develops into a female, the genital tubercle differentiates into the *clitoris,* the genital folds become the *labia minora,* and the genital swellings, the *labia majora.* The clitoris and its homolog, the penis, end in sensitive areas, the *glans clitoris* and *glans penis,* respectively, and contain cavernous bodies that become distended with blood during sexual excitement. In the female, the anterior part of the urogenital sinus remains as the urethra. The more posterior areas become flattened and widened and give rise to the *vestibule.* In the adult, the vagina opens into the vestibule, and the urethra also opens into the vestibule rather than into the clitoris as might be expected in comparison with the penis of the male.

SUGGESTED READINGS

1. Arey, L. B.: Developmental anatomy, Philadelphia, 1954, W. B. Saunders Co.
2. Bentley, P. J.: Adaptations of amphibians to arid environment, Science **152:**619-623.
3. Bentley, P. J.: Endocrines and osmoregulation, New York, 1971, Springer-Verlag.
4. Burns, R. K.: Urogenital system. In Willier, B., Weiss, P. A., and Hamburger, V. (editors): Analysis of development, Philadelphia, 1955, W. B. Saunders Co.
5. Burns, R. K.: Role of hormones in the differentiation of sex. In Young, W. C. (editor): Sex and internal secretions, Baltimore, 1961, The Williams & Wilkins Co.
6. Fox, H.: The amphibian pronephros, Q. Rev. Biol. **38:**1-25, 1963.
7. Fraser, E. A.: The development of the vertebrate excretory system, Biol. Rev. **25:**159-187, 1950.
8. Lillie, F. R.: The theory of the free-martin, Science **43:**611, 1916. Reprinted in Willier, B. H., and Oppenheimer, J. M. (editors): Foundations of experimental embryology, Englewood Cliffs, N. J., 1964, Prentice Hall.
9. The reproductive system, Section VI. In DeHaan, R. L., and Ursprung, H. (editors): Organogenesis, New York, 1965, Holt, Rinehart & Winston, Inc.
10. Schmidt-Nielson, K.: Salt glands. In Vertebrate structure and functions. Readings from Scientific American, San Francisco, 1974, W. H. Freeman & Co.
11. Smith, H. W.: The kidney, Sci. Am. **188**(1):40-48, 1953.
12. Smith, H. W.: From fish to philospher, Boston, 1954, Little, Brown & Co.
13. Torrey, T.: Morphogenesis of the vertebrate kidney. In DeHaan, R. L., and Ursprung, H. (editors): Organogenesis, New York, 1965, Holt, Rinehart & Winston, Inc.
14. Wessells, N. K.: Introduction. Section IV. Water balance and its control. In Vertebrate structures and functions. Readings from Scientific American, pp. 206-211, San Francisco, 1974, W. H. Freeman & Co.

INDEX

A

Abdominal veins, 425-426
Abducens nerve, 279
Abductors, function of, 380
Accommodation, 238
Acetabulum, 367
Acetylcholine, release of, by somatic neurons, 277
Acini, 310
Acorn worm, 16-17
Acoustic nerve, 279
Acousticolateralis placodes, 227-234
Acromion process, 367
Acrosomal reaction, 98, 99-102
Acrosome, function of, 83
Actin in myofilaments, 376-377
Actinopterygii in vertebrate evolution, 31
Activation
  of egg in fertilization process, 89
  of genes in embryonic differentiation, 158-166
Adaptation in evolutionary process, 14
Adaptive radiation in vertebrate evolution, 27-28
Adductor mandibulae, 389
Adductor muscles of gill, 389
Adductors, function of, 380
Adenine as nucleotide base in DNA molecule, 75
Adenosine triphosphate (ATP) in muscle contraction, 378
Adrenal gland, derivation of, 430-431
Adrenergic system, 278
Afferent branchial vessels, function of, 408, 411
Afferent neurons, function of, 250
Age of reptiles, 181, 182
Agranulocytes, 397-398
Air capillaries, 305
Air sacs as organs of respiration, 299
Alar plate, dorsal, of neural tube, 244, 245
Albumen, function of, in cleidoic egg, 183
Albumins in plasma, function of, 396
Allantoic arteries, formation of, 415

Allantoic circulation, 417-419
Allantois, 149, 312, 313
  formation of
    in mammals, 187
    in reptiles and birds, 184, 185-186
  function of, in cleidoic egg, 183
Alleles, 10
Alveolar glands, 211, 212
Alveoli, 301-302, 304
Ameloblasts in development of teeth, 287, 289
Amino acid, coding of, codon for, 160
Amniocardiac vesicle, 399, 401
Amnion, formation of
  in mammals, 186
  in reptiles and birds, 184, 185
Amniote egg
  developmental changes associated with, 182-183
  in vertebrate evolution, 32
Amniote heart, 403-408
Amniotes, 24
  definition, 178-179
  extraembryonic membranes of, 179-195
  kidneys of, 438-443
Amniotic cavity, formation of, 146
  in reptiles and birds, 185
Ammocoetes, 25, 27
Amphibia, 23-24
Amphibian(s)
  blastula of, 125, 126
  gastrulation in, 134-141
  modern, in vertebrate evolution, 31-32
  and reptiles, developmental differences and similarities, 182-183
  stem, in vertebrate evolution, 31-32
Amphioxus, 18, 20, 21
  development of, significance of, 132-134
  gastrulation in, 130-134

Amphioxus—cont'd
  in phylogenetic origin of vertebrates, 25-27
Ampulla, 47, 230
Anal plate, formation of, 176
Anamniotes, 24
  definition, 179
  extraembryonic membranes of, 179
  kidneys of, 438
Anatomy, comparative, in study of vertebrate structure, 3, 5
Ancestral pond, amniotic fluid as, 185
Anchored villi, 193
Androgens
  in feedback regulation of, pituitary gland, 58-60
  gonadal synthesis of, 41, 42
  physiological effects of, 42-43
Andromerogons, formation of, influence of male genes on, 159
Androstenedione
  gonadal synthesis of, 41, 42
  physiological effects of, 42-43
Angioblasts, 395
Angiotensin, function of, 432
Angiotensinogen, 432
Angle of bicipital rib, 362
Animal pole, 109
  in egg organization, 85-86
Animalculists, 6
Animals, meroblastic, formation of gut in, 284
Anlagen, 9
Anterior cardinals and anterior vena cava, 419-420
Anterior chamber, 234, 239
Anterior intestinal portal, 284
Anterior semicircular canal, 229
Antidiuretic hormone, secretion and function of, 436
Antifertilizin
  in Lillie's fertilizin theory, 95
  in Tyler's fertilization theory, 95-97
Antitwist mechanisms, 361
Antrum, 49

455